Documentation for Medical Records

Barbara Odom-Wesley, PhD, RHIA, FAHIMA,
and Diann Brown, MS, RHIA, CHP
Editors

Chris L. Meyers, RHIA
Technical Editor

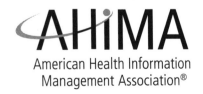

AHIMA

American Health Information
Management Association®

The Web sites listed in this book were current and valid as of the date of publication. However, Web page addresses and the information on them may change or disappear at any time and for any number of reasons. The user is encouraged to perform his or her own general Web searches to locate any site addresses listed here that are no longer valid.

ISBN 1-58426-183-8
ISBN-13 978-1-58426-183-4
AHIMA Product Number AB100708

AHIMA Staff:
Claire Blondeau, MBA, Senior Editor
Cynthia Douglas, Project Editor
Katherine Greenock, Assistant Editor
Beth Hjort, RHIA, CHPS, Reviewer
Melissa Ulbricht, Editorial/Production Coordinator
Ann Wiedemann, MS, RHIA, Reviewer
Ken Zielske, Director of Publications

AHIMA strives to recognize the value of people from every racial and ethnic background as well as all genders, age groups, and sexual orientations by building its membership and leadership resources to reflect the rich diversity of the American population. AHIMA encourages the celebration and promotion of human diversity through education, mentoring, recognition, leadership, and other programs.

American Health Information Management Association
233 North Michigan Avenue, 21st Floor
Chicago, Illinois 60601-5800
ahima.org

Contents

Chapter 12

Part III   Organization and Management of the Health Record   277

Appendices and Resources on CD-ROM

Appendix A   The Complete Medical Record in a Hybrid EHR Environment
(Parts I, II, and III)

Appendix B   Surveying the RHIO Landscape: A Description of Current RHIO Models,
with a Focus on Patient Identification

Appendix C   Guidelines for Defining the Legal Health Record for Disclosure Purposes

Appendix D   Maintaining a Legally Sound Health Record—Paper and Electronic

Appendix E   Building an Enterprise Master Person Index

Appendix F   Standards for the Content of the Electronic Health Record

Appendix G   Principles of Form and Screen Design

Appendix H   Electronic Document Management as a Component of the Electronic
Health Record

Appendix I   Guidelines for Developing a Data Dictionary

Check Your Understanding

About the Editors and Authors

Barbara Odom-Wesley, PhD, RHIA, FAHIMA, is chair of the HIT Program at DeVry University in Dallas, Texas, and HIT curriculum manager for DeVry University, Inc. She is also president of the ambulatory healthcare consulting firm, Medpro Services, in Arlington, Texas. Dr. Odom-Wesley has worked in various healthcare facilities and as a HIM program director for University of the Incarnate Word and Texas Woman's University. Active in HIM since 1968, she is the past president of the Texas HIMA and AHIMA, and currently serves as a MyPHR coordinator for Texas. She was awarded the TxHIMA Distinguished Member Award twice (1991 and 2002). She also serves as vice-chair of the FORE Board of Directors and Chair of the Triumph Awards committee. Because of her long history of distinguished service, she earned the recognition of AHIMA Fellow in 2004. Odom-Wesley is a published author including four editions of the *Medical Record Handbook for the Physician's Office* published by the Texas Medical Association. She is a frequently requested speaker specializing in personal health records and HIM education. Her community volunteer service includes serving as co-chair of the Health Impact Council for United Way of Tarrant County and member of the Ethics Commission for the City of Arlington.

Diann Brown, MS, RHIA, CHP, is the director of health information services at Harris Methodist Fort Worth Hospital (a 710-bed acute care facility) located in Fort Worth, Texas. Brown serves as a liaison for Texas Health Resources Corporate on various task forces and committees. She supports the education of other HIM professionals and has served as an Advisory Committee Member of Tarrant County College Health Information Technology Program in Hurst, Texas, for more than 25 years and is currently the chair of the Health Information Technology Advisory Committee at DeVry University in Dallas, Texas. She serves as Clinical Site Director for several colleges and universities located in North Carolina, Oklahoma, Tennessee, and Texas. In 2000 she served as president of the Texas Health Information Management Association, and she is currently serving a four-year term as a commissioner on the board of Commission on Accreditation for Health Informatics and Information Management Education (CAHIIM). Brown is a published author and speaker on diverse HIM topics. Recently, she was honoree of the 2007 YWCA Tribute to Women in Business in Fort Worth and Tarrant County, Texas. In May 2007, she received the President's Award for Harris Methodist Fort Worth Hospital.

Chris L. Meyers, RHIA, is the President of eCatalyst Consulting, a healthcare consulting firm located in Phoenix, Arizona. eCatalyst Consulting specializes in the design and implementation of electronic health record systems, HIM process redesign, healthcare software development, enterprise content management, eDiscovery and legal holds, legal health records, and personal health records. Chris has more than 18 years of experience in healthcare administration. Before founding eCatalyst Consulting, Meyers was the administrative director of health information management and patient financial services for Banner Estrella Medical Center in Phoenix, where she implemented IT systems and created processes to support a paperless clinical environment at the patient's bedside. Meyers' previous experience includes regional HIM positions for large hospital systems, standalone hospitals, and military facilities. Positions in these facilities included admitting, central scheduling, case management, quality, Joint Commission, and Social Services. She has extensive knowledge in implementing electronic health record systems and is recognized nationally as a leader in health information management transformation. Meyers frequently speaks at national events and is an active participant in Arizona's eHealth Connection. In June 2005, she was awarded the Distinguished Member Award from the Arizona Health Information Management Association. Meyers is the Co-Director of AHIMA's Electronic Health Record Practice Council and Director of AzHIMA's Board of Directors.

Ella L. James, MS, RHIT, CPHQ, is director of corporate health information management and health information security and the privacy officer at Hospital for Special Care in New Britain, Connecticut. James is past president of and twice sat on the board of directors for the Connecticut HIMA and is an AHIMA Community of Practice (CoP) facilitator for long-term care. She chairs the coding committee for the National Association of Long Term Hospitals (NALTH). James has presented programs on HIPAA at the state, regional, and national levels, and has presented educational programs for coders and physicians on long-term acute-care coding for NALTH. She consults on coding and documentation issues for many long-term acute-care hospitals through NALTH. She is the author of *Documentation and Reimbursement for Long-Term Care* and contributing author of the AHIMA publication *Health Information Management Compliance*.

Kathy Munn, RHIA, is the Privacy Officer and Director of Client Records for Mental Health Mental Retardation of Tarrant County in Fort Worth, Texas. She has spent her career in home health, public health, and behavioral health care and continues to consult for long-term care and other community-based services. Munn has spoken on HIM topics for local, regional, and national organizations. She has supported her profession by mentoring many HIM students as an internship instructor and serves as Chair of the HIT Advisory Committee for Tarrant County College.

Susan Rossiter, RHIA, is the operation manager of the HIM Department for 35 university clinics at University of Texas Southwestern Medical Center in Dallas, Texas. Prior to that, she was the Hospital Compliance Officer for Terrell State Hospital and has several years experience in management of HIM departments for acute care, behavioral health and ambulatory care organizations. Susan graduated with honors from Texas Woman's University, where she received the Outstanding Senior Student in the State award from the Texas Medical Record Association and the Dallas Outstanding Senior Student award from Texas Woman's University. As chair for the Executive Women in Texas Government, Dallas Affiliate, she supports and promotes women in leadership service to the state of Texas.

Margaret J. White, MS, NHA, RHIA, CPHQ, has 30 years experience in the healthcare industry with the last 15 years in long-term care. She is a co-chair of AHIMA's Long-Term Care Practice Council and is co-chair of the Special Interest Council of the Ohio Health Information Management Association. She is on the Ohio Health Information Partnership Advisory Board representing OHIMA and post-acute care and is participating on the adoption and exchange of health information subcommittees. Margie also serves on the HISPC project steering committee for Ohio as well as being involved in the various working groups representing health information management and post-acute care. Additionally, Margie is an adjunct faculty member for several HIT programs. Margie is the assistant licensed nursing home administrator for Columbus Colony Elderly Care of Westerville, Ohio, the only facility in the country "for the deaf, by the deaf."

Preface

Clinical documentation and health records play a vital role in every aspect of healthcare delivery and decision making, whether the setting is acute care, ambulatory, long-term, home care, hospice, or behavioral healthcare. Documentation is also a central focus in current efforts to improve healthcare quality and patient safety as well as the efficiency of the U.S. healthcare system. The development and implementation of electronic health record (EHR) systems promise to revolutionize the collection, use, and management of healthcare data over the next decade. Quality healthcare records will be critical to the establishment of accurate databases and will still serve as the primary source of information to promote quality healthcare.

Ensuring the accessibility, accuracy, and integrity of health records has been the primary mission of health information managers since the profession emerged almost eighty years ago. Just as important, health information management professionals continue to champion the protection of patient privacy and the confidentiality of health information. As experts in the documentation requirements of external governmental agencies and accreditation organizations, they also play an invaluable role in managing their facilities' regulatory compliance and accreditation performance.

The goal of this publication is to help health information management students understand the role of health records and clinical documentation in the delivery of direct patient care and the operation of individual healthcare organizations. The book also explains the external environment in which health records function and the documentation requirements of local, state, and federal governments. The process of voluntary accreditation and the development of external practice standards are also explored.

This publication will also be informative for practicing health information management professionals, especially in the preparation for EHR systems. It provides an integrated overview of all of the external standards relevant to clinical documentation and health records. Included are AHIMA practice guidelines, acute care accreditation standards, Medicare Conditions of Participation for Hospitals, national health informatics standards, and state and federal statutory and regulatory requirements.

Specifically, chapter 1 explains the importance of clinical documentation in the context of the U.S. healthcare delivery system. Further, it addresses the role of documentation as we evolve toward the electronic health record. Chapter 2 describes the various uses of health record information in patient care, healthcare operations, healthcare reimbursement, public health, clinical education, and biomedical research. It focuses on distinguishing the legal health record, identifies emerging issues including the personal health record, and looks at the future of clinical documentation. Chapter 3 explores the multiple functions of health records, focusing on ancillary applications. Record access and disclosure are also discussed in this chapter. Chapter 4 reviews the uses of health records for research, statistical reporting, and public health. Vital statistics and specialty registries are included. The content of acute care records is explored in detail in chapter 5, which includes dozens of sample health record forms and reports. Chapter 6 explains the organization of acute care health records, including health record formats and identification/storage systems in both paper-based and computer-based systems. The chapter also provides basic information on the technological infrastructure for EHRs and clinical support technology. The hybrid health record and various storage systems are presented. Chapter 7 explores documentation improvement programs including quantitative and qualitative analyses. The data dictionary is explained, as are guidelines for EHR documentation. The function of managing data in the electronic world is also discussed. Chapter 8 focuses on accreditation and regulatory guides for healthcare documentation in a variety of specialty settings. Chapter 9 concentrates on ambulatory care documentation, accreditation, liability, and standards. Long-term care is the primary topic for chapter 10, which includes documentation for skilled nursing facilities. Chapter 11 covers home care and hospice documentation. Accreditation, liability, and various standards are included. Chapter 12 focuses on documentation in the behavioral healthcare environment. Documentation issues, content, and external forces are discussed.

This publication also includes a glossary of all key terms and nine appendixes containing relevant AHIMA practice briefs in print format. These practice briefs, as well as additional resources including "Check Your Understanding" learning tools for each chapter, are available on the accompanying CD-ROM.

AHIMA hopes that the publication of this up-to-the-minute book on documentation for acute care services will help new professionals, as well as those already in practice, to meet the current demands and future challenges of health information management.

Barbara Odom-Wesley, PhD, RHIA, FAHIMA

Acknowledgments

The authors and the AHIMA publications staff extend our heartfelt thanks to the dedicated professionals acknowledged below, whose time and efforts made this publication a reality. It's a huge accomplishment to provide a comprehensive resource that can be used to educate other health information management professionals, and we are grateful for their contributions.

Ella James, MS, RHIT, CPHQ, who provided her expertise in writing the chapter on long-term acute care and long-term care.

Chris L. Meyers, RHIA, who served as technical editor and reviewed the content for its technical accuracy.

Kathy Munn, RHIA, whose knowledge and expertise in behavioral health provided the content for chapter 12.

Susan Rossiter, RHIA, who contributed the content and her expertise in the area of ambulatory care.

Margaret White, MS, NHA, RHIA, CHPQ, who wrote the chapter on home care and hospice.

In addition, we are grateful to Mona Calhoun, MS, RHIA, and Fran Gray, RHIA, who reviewed several chapters early in their development and offered suggestions for improvement.

A special thanks from Barbara and Diann to their families for their support and encouragement during the writing of this book.

PART I

Clinical Documentation and the Healthcare Delivery System

Chapter 1

Healthcare Delivery

Diann Brown, MS, RHIA, CHP

Learning Objectives

- Outline the basic structure of the U.S. healthcare delivery system
- Explain the significance of recent trends in healthcare delivery
- Describe the distinction between inpatients and outpatients
- Explain the concept of continuum of care
- Describe healthcare's migration to the electronic health record
- Explain current challenges of the hybrid health record
- Describe the use of personal health records
- Explain the role that health information exchange collaborations play in improving healthcare

Key Terms

Acute care

Ambulatory care

Behavioral healthcare

Continuum of care

Diagnosis-related groups (DRG)

Electronic health record (EHR)

Emergency and trauma care

Health information exchange (HIE)

Home healthcare

Hospice care

Hybrid health record

Inpatient

Integrated healthcare network

Long-term acute care

Long-term care

Medicaid

Medical specialties

Medicare

National Health Information Network (NHIN)

Outpatient

Personal health record (PHR)

Primary care

Regional health information organizations (RHIOs)

Rehabilitation care

Secondary care

Skilled-nursing care

Subacute care

Surgical specialties

Tertiary care

Tethered record

Untethered record

Introduction

In colonial America, many communities opened public hospitals for the purpose of caring for the poor and isolating the sick. Until the twentieth century, physicians with little formal training performed most medical care in the homes of patients. In remote areas of the new settlements, there often was little or no help available for the injured and sick, and the mortality rate among early settlers was very high.

Reform movements that began during the late nineteenth century improved the overall quality of medical care in the United States. Specific quality improvement efforts directed at medical school training and hospital care helped improve overall quality. The new, more scientific approach to medicine set the stage for unprecedented advances in biomedicine that were under way at the turn of the 20th century.

The number of hospitals and hospital admissions increased dramatically during the first decades of the twentieth century. Organized efforts among healthcare reformers and private foundations led to the standardization of hospital care, and many private hospitals were established. Care in the new, privately funded hospitals, however, was available only to those who could pay for the services, and underfunded public and charity hospitals continued to serve the poor and indigent.

The development of modern surgical techniques and new pharmaceuticals as well as the more widespread use of antibiotics after World War II created an even greater demand for hospital care. As a result, the late 1940s and 1950s saw a hospital-building boom.

Until the late 1980s, hospitals continued to provide most of the diagnostic and therapeutic healthcare services in the United States. Long hospital stays were the norm rather than the exception. Patients usually stayed in the same hospital facility from the time they were admitted for diagnostic testing, through their treatment, until they were well enough to care for themselves at home. Prior to the development of endoscopic and laser surgery, many routine surgical procedures involved long periods of recovery with weeks or even months of professional nursing and follow-up care. Hospitals provided most of that care, and hospitals became places where terminally ill patients went to spend the last days of their lives.

After World War II, employers began offering health insurance coverage to employees and their dependents. This benefited workers and their families because it provided more access to healthcare services and hospital care. However, due to rising costs, many Americans were still unable to pay for healthcare services. As a result, an amendment in 1965 to the Social Security Act established two federal programs, **Medicare** and **Medicaid,** to provide health insurance coverage to the aged and poor populations. With the implementation of Medicare and Medicaid, these federal programs played a pivotal role in the U.S. government becoming the largest payer for healthcare services.

The last decades of the twentieth century brought another wave of revolutionary advances in the biomedical sciences. The development of new pharmaceutical treatments has made it possible for patients with chronic illnesses to stay healthy longer and to postpone or avoid debilitating complications. Developments in surgical technology and anesthesia have shortened surgical recovery times dramatically. Today, many routine surgeries that once meant lengthy hospitalizations now require patients to spend only a few hours or days in the hospital. Organ transplantations that were innovative just a few years ago have become almost commonplace. Many transplant patients now go home in a matter of days rather than weeks or months after surgery.

Since colonial times, physicians and other healthcare providers have documented the customer services they provide, but increasing costs and the complexity of healthcare delivery requires progressively more sophisticated documentation and data collection processes. Documentation of healthcare services and computerization of health record systems have become critical components of healthcare services and affect the quality and efficiency of the national healthcare delivery system.

Modern Healthcare Delivery

The U.S. healthcare delivery system is made up of thousands of independent providers and facilities that offer a bewildering array of health-related services. Provider reimbursement for healthcare services is accomplished through a complex system of private insurance plans and government-funded programs. The cost of medical–surgical care and pharmaceuticals has grown so much over recent years that many Americans who do not qualify for private or government-sponsored health insurance are unable to find affordable healthcare.

According to the U.S. Census Bureau (2006), the number of Americans with health insurance dropped between 1987 and 2005. (See table 1.1.) In 2005, 46.6 million Americans were without health insurance coverage. The percentage of Americans who qualified for employer-based health coverage decreased from 59.8 percent in 2004 to 59.5 percent in 2005. At the same time, the number of people covered by government-sponsored health insurance programs continued to rise, and in 2005, was 27.3 percent. Today, healthcare is more expensive than ever, and economists continue to worry about its impact on the nation's future economic health.

Table 1.1 Health insurance coverage in the United States, 1987–2005

Year	Percentage Covered
2005	84.1
2004	84.3
2003	84.4
2002	84.8
2001	85.4
2000	86.0
1999	84.5
1998	83.7
1997	83.9
1996	84.4
1995	84.6
1994	84.8
1993	84.7
1992	85.0
1991	85.9
1990	86.1
1989	86.4
1988	86.6
1987	87.1

Source: U.S. Census Bureau 2006.

Healthcare Providers and Facilities

Professional healthcare providers include the following, among others:

- Physicians
- Midlevel practitioners such as physician's assistants and nurse practitioners
- Nurses
- Psychologists and clinical social workers
- Physical, respiratory, speech, and occupational therapists
- Dentists, dental assistants, and dental hygienists
- Medical technologists and cytotechnologists
- Clinical nutritionists
- Patient-care technicians and paramedics
- Podiatrists and chiropractors

Healthcare services, provided in innumerable public and private facilities, include the following:

- Public and community hospitals operated by local governments
- Teaching hospitals affiliated with university medical schools

- Specialty hospitals dedicated to providing specialized services (for example, behavioral health, and rehabilitation care)
- Private hospitals affiliated with religious organizations
- Private hospitals affiliated with for-profit corporations
- Private hospitals operated by nonprofit organizations
- Integrated healthcare networks (made up of hospitals, postacute-care facilities, and ambulatory-care facilities operated by the same corporate entity)
- Physicians' offices, group practices, and private medical clinics
- Community-based clinics and public health departments
- Urgent care clinics
- Hospital-based and freestanding ambulatory, diagnostic, and surgical centers
- Hospital-based and freestanding ambulatory rehabilitation centers
- Skilled-nursing facilities
- Long-term care and assisted-care residential facilities
- Home healthcare and hospice-care agencies
- Facilities providing immediate care for the developmentally disabled

Healthcare Services

Generally, healthcare services are categorized according to the setting in which the services are provided and/or the illness toward which services are directed. For example, **acute care** can be defined as the short-term medical and nursing care provided in an inpatient hospital setting to treat the acute phase of a patient's injury or illness. Following are descriptions of other broad categories of healthcare services.

- **Ambulatory care**: The preventive, diagnostic, and therapeutic medical services provided on a nonresidential basis in healthcare practitioners' offices, group practices, private clinics, community-based clinics, and hospital-based outpatient departments
- **Behavioral healthcare**: The psychiatric and/or psychological care provided to address mental disorders, developmental disorders, and substance-abuse disorders; provided in a variety of settings, including dedicated units in acute-care hospitals, psychiatric hospitals, community-based clinics, and physicians' offices
- **Emergency and trauma care**: The medical–surgical care provided to individuals whose injuries or illnesses require urgent care to address conditions that could be life threatening or disabling if not treated immediately; provided through a network of designated hospitals and emergency transportation systems
- **Home healthcare**: The medical and/or personal care provided to individuals and families in their place of residence with the goal of promoting, maintaining, or restoring health or minimizing the effects of disabilities and illnesses, including terminal illnesses
- **Hospice care**: The medical and/or personal care provided to individuals with life expectancies of six months or less who elect to receive palliative care in place of

standard medical treatment for their illnesses; provided in patients' homes and in residential treatment facilities

- **Long-term acute care**: The medical care provided to individuals who are clinically complex with multiple acute and chronic conditions requiring an average length of stay greater than 25 days in long-term care hospitals certified as acute-care hospitals

- **Long-term care**: The medical- and/or personal-care services provided to chronically ill, aged, disabled, or mentally handicapped individuals who reside in dedicated nursing facilities on a permanent basis

- **Rehabilitation care**: The therapeutic medical services (speech, physical, and occupational therapy) provided to patients who have been disabled by injuries or illnesses; provided in dedicated rehabilitation hospitals, community-based facilities, patients' homes, and hospital-based outpatient departments with the goal of helping patients recover as much function as possible

- **Skilled-nursing care**: The professional nursing care and related medical, therapeutic, psychosocial, and personal services provided in a residential setting to individuals recovering from injuries or illnesses or the residual effects of injuries or illnesses after the acute phase of the condition has resolved; sometimes called **subacute care**

Trends in Healthcare Delivery

Often, medical services provided in the United States are described as being the best in the world. Nonetheless, many critics of the healthcare delivery system consider it too costly and inefficient. The current system is a complex amalgam of payers, providers, and facilities that function more or less independently. There are ongoing concerns related to uneven accessibility, quality, over- and underutilization of services, and cost inflation.

In 2005, more than 15.9 percent of Americans had no health insurance coverage according to the U.S. Census Bureau (2006). Families who do not receive insurance coverage through their employers and do not qualify for Medicaid assistance are finding it difficult or impossible to obtain and pay for medical care. Public healthcare facilities are overcrowded and underfunded and are unable to fully address the needs of their communities. Some economists fear that the high cost of pharmaceuticals will threaten the future stability of the Medicare and Medicaid programs. The federal government passed a drug benefit plan so that everyone with Medicare, regardless of income, health status, or prescription drug usage would have access to prescription drug coverage starting January 2006. The new Medicare drug benefit addresses access for only the elderly and disabled older than age 65, while many low-income and uninsured people younger than age 65 must still rely on community resources to get needed medications. Low-income and uninsured people face many barriers because community resources are limited and do not adequately meet growing prescription drug needs according to findings from a study by the Center for Studying Health System Change (2003), a nonpartisan policy research organization.

Since the 1960s, the cost of healthcare services has grown at a rate much faster than overall inflation. For example, in 2000, the cost of inpatient hospital services increased by about 6 percent, while the overall consumer price index increased by less than 4 percent. In 2002, the cost of inpatient hospital services increased almost 9 percent over the previous year, and the overall cost of medical care rose almost 5 percent. In contrast, overall cost inflation for that period was less than 2 percent (Agency for Healthcare Research and Quality 2002).

Concerns over the growing cost of healthcare services have brought significant changes in the healthcare system over the past two decades. The most significant change has been the movement of most diagnostic services and noncritical therapeutic services away from the acute-care hospital setting. The **diagnosis-related groups (DRG)** prospective payment system, implemented in the 1980s, started the movement to outpatient services.

In response to competition from ambulatory-care facilities, many hospitals have enhanced their service offerings in the areas of ambulatory, diagnostic, and surgical services and subacute nursing care. In addition, many hospitals have merged with other general and specialty hospitals and subacute and ambulatory-care providers to form integrated healthcare networks. An **integrated healthcare network** is a group of healthcare organizations that collectively provides a full range of coordinated health-related services. These services range from simple, preventive care to complex surgical care.

Hospital-based Services

Acute-care hospitals reserve inpatient services for the sickest patients and the most invasive medical procedures. It is routine to perform noninvasive diagnostic procedures, same-day surgery, chemotherapy, and radiation therapy in separate ambulatory-care facilities or in the outpatient departments of acute-care hospitals. Most convalescent care is provided in dedicated skilled-nursing facilities or through home health agencies, but some hospitals have opened dedicated nursing units to care for patients who no longer require acute-care services but are too ill to return home. Similarly, most rehabilitation care has transitioned to dedicated rehabilitation hospitals, skilled-nursing facilities, freestanding community-based facilities, or hospital-based outpatient departments.

Patients who receive healthcare services in a hospital are categorized as either inpatients or outpatients. An **inpatient** is an individual who receives healthcare services as well as room, board, and continuous nursing care in a hospital unit dedicated to providing around-the-clock patient care.

An **outpatient** is an individual who receives healthcare services in a hospital-based clinic or department but who is not admitted to a dedicated acute-care unit. For example, a patient treated exclusively in the emergency department of a hospital is considered an outpatient rather than an inpatient. However, if that same patient is admitted to an acute-care unit of the hospital after receiving emergency services, the patient is then considered an inpatient for the rest of his or her hospital stay.

Continuum of Care

Hospital-based services make up only one component in the broad spectrum of healthcare services available to Americans today. The current healthcare delivery system is extremely complex, and until recently, little effort was made to coordinate services offered by the hundreds or thousands of independent healthcare practitioners and providers working in any one community. Since the early 1990s, healthcare organizations, accreditation and standards organizations, healthcare-related trade and professional associations, and federal agencies have been attempting to integrate the components of the delivery system. The goals are to improve the quality of medical care provided to Americans and at the same time make healthcare services more affordable and accessible.

The concept of a continuum of care was initially developed during the mid-1990s in response to increasing healthcare costs. According to the 1995 hospital accreditation manual from the Joint Commission on Accreditation of Healthcare Organizations, an integrated continuum of healthcare services would match "an individual's ongoing needs with the appropriate level and type of medical, psychological, or social care . . ." (Joint Commission 1995). Ideally, every customer would receive the appropriate service at the appropriate time from the appropriate practitioner or facility.

The **continuum of care** can be defined as the sum of all the healthcare services provided in all settings, from the least intensive and specialized (the least expensive) to the most intensive and specialized (the most expensive). The services that make up the continuum can be further categorized into three levels of care: primary, secondary, and tertiary. The levels of care reflect the cost of the services as well as the intensity of the services provided. For example, the basic services provided in physicians' offices are generally the least expensive, and the intensive medical services provided in acute-care hospitals are generally the most expensive.

Primary Care

The most appropriate setting for routine healthcare services falls at the **primary-care** level. Physicians working in private offices, group practices, private clinics, or community-based clinics generally provide primary-care services. Primary-care physicians usually receive their training in the more general fields of medicine: family practice, pediatrics, and general internal medicine. In addition, many women of reproductive age receive primary-care services from physicians specializing in gynecology. Nurse practitioners (nurses who hold advanced clinical degrees) and physician's assistants also provide primary-care services under the supervision of physicians.

Primary-care services include the following:

- Preventive care (such as immunizations)

- Early detection of neoplastic diseases and other serious illnesses through routine screening and laboratory tests (such as mammograms and blood tests)

- Periodic physical examinations (such as well-baby checkups, well-child checkups, and annual checkups for adults)

- Diagnosis and treatment of minor infectious illnesses (such as influenza and other viral infections) and common bacterial and fungal infections (such as strep throat and athlete's foot), which may be diagnosed with a combination of examination and laboratory testing and treated with prescription drugs

- Diagnosis and management services for chronic illnesses (such as asthma, hypertension, and diabetes), which are monitored through periodic examinations and laboratory testing and treated with prescription drugs

- Diagnosis and treatment of minor injuries (such as lacerations, sprains, and uncomplicated orthopedic injuries)

Primary-care physicians also coordinate their patients' hospital care and diagnostic services, specialty-care consultations, and psychosocial services.

Secondary Care

Secondary care encompasses the diagnostic and therapeutic services provided by medical specialists working in private offices, specialty group practices, private clinics, community-based clinics, and general and community hospitals. Patients may arrange to consult specialists directly. However, it is more common for primary-care physicians to refer patients to specialists for the diagnosis and treatment of complex conditions that require more intensive services than the primary-care physician can provide.

Specialty care can be divided into two groups of services: medical and surgical. The **medical specialties** include the following:

- Internal medicine
- Pediatrics
- Cardiology
- Endocrinology
- Psychiatry
- Oncology
- Nephrology
- Neurology
- Pulmonology
- Gastroenterology
- Dermatology
- Radiology and nuclear medicine

The **surgical specialties** include:

- Obstetrics/gynecology
- Ophthalmology
- Orthopedics
- Cardiovascular surgery
- Otorhinolaryngology
- Trauma surgery
- Neurosurgery
- Thoracic surgery
- Urology
- Plastic and reconstructive surgery
- Anesthesiology
- Pathology

Most medical and surgical specialists provide both office-based and hospital-based care. However, because of the nature of their specialties, some specialists, such as pathologists, radiologists, and anesthesiologists, work predominantly in hospitals and ambulatory-surgery settings.

Tertiary Care

Tertiary care is centered on the provision of highly specialized and technologically advanced diagnostic and therapeutic services in inpatient and outpatient hospital settings. Medical specialists working in large, urban hospitals and specialty clinics affiliated with nearby medical schools and universities provide most tertiary care.

Tertiary-care services include medical–surgical services such as trauma care; burn care; organ transplantation; and medical–surgical intensive care for neonatal, pediatric, and adult patients. In addition, tertiary-care hospitals perform medical research and conduct resident-training programs for physicians and other healthcare practitioners.

Clinical Documentation in Healthcare: Moving Toward the Electronic Health Record

Hospitals, like other American businesses, began applying computer processing to operations and management in the 1960s. Until then, clinical documentation consisted of paper-based documentation methodologies. The first hospital applications of computer technology were implemented in the areas of financial management, admissions, and billing. By the year 2000, virtually every clinical laboratory in the United States had implemented computer-based diagnostic systems with automatic reporting capabilities. Many of today's sophisticated diagnostic, medical, and surgical procedures would not be possible without the support of accurate and reliable software systems.

In contrast, the application of electronic information management to health record systems has progressed slowly. Many acute-care organizations now depend on mixed-media health record systems made up of computer-generated laboratory reports, digital images, transcribed medical–surgical reports, and handwritten orders and progress notes. The cost of electronic clinical documentation systems certainly has been one reason why progress has not accelerated as quickly as expected. However, the biggest factors delaying the universal implementation of **electronic health records (EHRs)** have likely been the lack of shared vision and an absence of functional standards. Healthcare organizations have been reluctant to undertake complex and expensive technology projects without national guidelines that define EHR systems, including parameters (what the records should include), format (how the records are included), and function (how the records should and can be used).

President Bush's Information Plan

The quality of routine, acute, and chronic care coordination among various healthcare providers and settings is contingent on the communication between the consumer, the primary healthcare provider, and the healthcare specialist. The Institute of Medicine estimates that between 44,000 and 98,000 Americans die each year from medical errors (Kohn, Corrigan, and Donaldson 2000). Many more die or have permanent disability because of inappropriate treatments, mistreatments, or missed treatments in ambulatory settings. In his Health Information Technology Plan (The White House Office of the President, April 2004) President George W. Bush expressed his concerns regarding current healthcare services in the United States:

> Despite spending over $1.6 trillion on health care as a Nation, there are still serious concerns about preventable errors, uneven health care quality, and poor communication among doctors, hospitals, and many other healthcare providers involved in the care of any one person (The White House Office of the President, 2004).

President Bush cited the following challenges to the current healthcare system:

- A patient's vital medical information is scattered across medical records kept by many different caregivers in many different locations—and all of the patient's medical information is often unavailable at the time of care. For example, patients with medical emergencies too often are seen by doctors with no access to their critical medical information, such as allergies, current treatments or medications, prior diagnoses, and medical history.

- Physicians keep information about drugs, drug interactions, managed care formularies, clinical guidelines, and recent research in memory—a difficult task given the high volume of information.

- Medical orders and prescriptions are handwritten and are too often illegible, misunderstood, or not followed in accordance with the physician's instructions.

- Consumers lack access to useful, credible health information about treatment alternatives, which hospitals and physicians are best for their needs, or their own health status.

- Physicians do not always have the best information to select the best treatments for their patients, resulting in an unacceptable lag time before new scientific advances are used in patient care. They also do not have ready access to complete information about their patients; do not know how other doctors are treating their same patients, or how other healthcare providers around the country treat patients with the same condition. These conditions set the stage for preventable medical errors.

The above challenges are closely connected to our failure to use information technology as an integral part of healthcare coordination. President Bush's vision for the U.S. healthcare system involves putting the needs of patients first and is more efficient and cost effective. The President's goal is that, within the next ten years, most Americans will have their complete healthcare information available to them at the time and place of care. This initiative raises the bar for all healthcare providers to have accurate, complete, and timely information and documentation as soon as possible after the patient-care visit or encounter, no matter the ambulatory-care setting.

President Bush believes that innovations in health information technology, such as electronic health records, and the secure exchange of medical information will help transform healthcare in America by reducing paperwork, preventing medical errors, improving administrative efficiencies, improving healthcare quality, reducing healthcare costs, and increasing access to affordable healthcare. Steps we need to take across the nation are already underway in some places. Health information technologies—such as electronic health records, computerized ordering of prescriptions and medical tests, clinical decision support tools, and secure exchange of authorized information—improve quality, reduce medical errors, and prevent deaths. During the past three years, some communities, hospitals, clinicians, patient groups, and information technology companies have acted to improve their health information systems. These pioneering communities are taking the initiative and showing that healthcare can and must be modernized.

Most healthcare facilities, while busy with implementing the many components of the electronic health record, operate with patient data and information in paper and electronic formats. The American Health Information Management Association (AHIMA) practice brief titled "The Complete Medical Record in a Hybrid EHR Environment" (2003) defines a **hybrid health record** as "a system with functional components that

- include both paper and electronic documents, and
- use both manual and electronic processes."

AHIMA's practice brief (2003) notes that managing health information in the hybrid environment is challenging and may risk the quality of care provided to patients. (See appendix A on the accompanying CD.)

Personal Health Records

Personal health records are new and have varying formats, but all are designed to achieve the same goals of having more information at the point of care, better communication between patient and physician, and greater consumer engagement in healthcare. The personal health record is growing in recognition and can play a major role in helping consumers and their caregivers make better health decisions.

AHIMA defines the **personal health record (PHR)** as an electronic, universally available, lifelong resource of health information needed by individuals to make health decisions. Individuals own and manage the information in the PHR, which comes from healthcare providers and the individual. The PHR is maintained in a secure and private environment, with the individual determining rights of access. The PHR is separate from and does not replace the legal record of any provider.

It is important to emphasize that the consumer, not the provider, maintains the PHR and that it does not replace any provider's legal health record. Simply put, the PHR is the consumer's compilation of his or her health information from all providers. This "**untethered**" model differs from a "**tethered**" record (sometimes also called a PHR), which is a subset of information compiled by the provider and offered to the consumer, often through the provider's Web site. A tethered record functions as a patient view into the provider's electronic record. Some providers offer consumers the opportunity to build and maintain their PHRs through the providers' Web sites. Tethered and untethered models can thus offer similar benefits—the two-way sharing of health information between consumer and provider—but the untethered definition stresses patient control and the inclusion of information from multiple providers.

PHRs are gaining in popularity with more than consumers and physicians. The Office of the National Coordinator for Health Information Technology includes PHRs as part of its strategy for implementing electronic health records and the **National Health Information Network (NHIN)**. Vendors have introduced a proliferation of PHR products in recent years. For consumers to embrace PHRs, the healthcare industry must provide education on the proper use of PHRs—including security and confidentiality—and the technical standards that facilitate the exchange of PHR information.

The future of the PHR is electronic. At this point, however, with the various PHR formats in use, neither the provider community nor the consumer is ready to rely exclusively on electronic health records. Today, people create and maintain their PHRs using four common media: paper, a personal computer, the Internet, and portable digital assistant (PDA) devices.

Health Information Exchange

Public and private sector stakeholders are focusing efforts on **health information exchange (HIE)** because there is increasing evidence that health information technology can improve healthcare quality and customer safety by reducing errors and unnecessary expenditures. Health information exchange projects have brought a diverse group of stakeholders together to plan, finance, and implement systems to share electronic health information. Stakeholders include hospitals, clinicians, laboratories, pharmacies, payers, employers, public health departments, quality-improvement organizations, and consumers.

Health information exchange collaborations are known by many names, but the most common is **regional health information organizations (RHIOs)**. Although the term *RHIO* has become standard language in healthcare, there is no legal definition in federal or state law. The main purpose for forming a RHIO as facilitating information sharing among enrolled members of the RHIO using common, nonproprietary standards for data content and exchange over existing networks and the Internet. The main goals in sharing patient-specific data are to (AHIMA 2006):

- Improve healthcare delivery by providing immediate, secure, confidential exchange of health information between authorized users

- Enable providers and patients to make decisions based on near real-time access to health information

- Provide warnings and reminders at the point of care

- Reduce medical errors

- Prevent adverse drug reactions

- Encourage participation of patients in their own healthcare and chronic disease management

- Allow patients, payers, and providers to evaluate quality of healthcare and to make informed choices in where and from whom they obtain care

AHIMA describes existing RHIO models in its 2006 practice brief, "Surveying the RHIO Landscape: A Description of Current RHIO Models, with a Focus on Patient Identification." See appendix B on the accompanying CD for the complete text of this practice brief.

Purpose and Funding of RHIOs

The main purpose for forming a RHIO is to facilitate information sharing among enrolled members of the RHIO using common, nonproprietary standards for data content and exchange over existing networks and the Internet. The main goals in sharing patient-specific information include the following:

- improve healthcare delivery by providing immediate, secure, confidential exchange of health information between authorized users;

- enable providers and customers to make decisions based on near real-time access to health information;

- provide warnings and reminders at the point of care;

- reduce medical errors;

- prevent adverse drug reactions;

- encourage participation of customers in their own healthcare and chronic disease management; and

- allow customers, payers, and providers to evaluate quality of healthcare and to make informed choices in where and from whom they obtain care.

This emerging area in healthcare supports the NHIN; however, RHIOs are not an integral part of the healthcare delivery system today.

Summary

Healthcare services in the United States are distributed via a complex delivery system made up of numerous clinical professionals, allied health professionals, healthcare administrators, and healthcare provider organizations. Many more organizations and governmental agencies manage healthcare reimbursement processes, institute healthcare standards and policies, and conduct healthcare-related research. Although the U.S. healthcare system is considered one of the best in the world, the cost of providing services and the challenge of meeting the needs of every American remain a concern in the twenty-first century.

Clinical documentation in today's healthcare environment is migrating from a paper-based health record to an electronic health record. President Bush developed an information plan that puts the needs of the patient first, is more efficient, and is cost effective. Most healthcare facilities are in the throes of implementing electronic health records—a daunting and costly undertaking. Those healthcare entities implementing electronic health record systems are managing hybrid health records that contain paper-based and electronic health information.

The personal health record is an electronic, universally available, lifelong resource of health information for a particular individual. Personal health records are gaining in popularity and are a strategic focus of the National Coordinator for Health Information Technology. The future of the PHR is electronic. However, neither the provider community nor the consumer has completely migrated to a standardized personal health record.

Access to patient information has proven to be critical in improving the care of patients. Stakeholders involved in RHIO projects today are pioneers navigating new terrain as they develop regional networks to improve the health of their communities. As this trend continues to evolve and improve, RHIOs may prove to be a valuable stepping stone on the road to a national system in which a customer's medical information is available anywhere, at anytime, to authorized users.

References

Agency for Healthcare Research and Quality. 2002. *Health Care Costs*. Rockville, MD: U.S. Department of Health and Human Services.

AHIMA e-HIM Work Group on Health Information Management in a Hybrid Environment. 2003. Practice brief: The complete medical record in a hybrid EHR environment. *Journal of American Health Information Management Association* 73(6).

AHIMA e-HIM Work Group on Patient Identification in RHIOs. 2006. Surveying the RHIO landscape: A description of current RHIO models, with a focus on patient identification. *Journal of American Health Information Management Association* 77(1):64A–D.

American Hospital Association. 2006. Health Information Exchange Projects: What Hospitals and Health Systems Need to Know. Prepared by Manatt Health Solutions. Chicago: AHA.

Center for Studying Health System Change. 2003. Tracking health care costs. *Data Bulletin* 25: 1–2.

Joint Commission on Accreditation of Healthcare Organizations. 1995. *Accreditation Manual for Hospitals*. Oakbrook Terrace, IL: Joint Commission.

Kohn, L. T., J. M. Corrigan, and M. S. Donaldson, eds. 2000. *To Err Is Human: Building a Safer Health System.* Washington, DC: National Academies Press. Available online from www.nap.edu/catalog/9728.html.

U.S. Census Bureau. 2006. *Current Population Survey, 1988 to 2006 Annual Social and Economic Supplements.* Washington, D.C.: U.S. Census Bureau.

The White House Office of the President. 2004 (April). Transforming Health Care: The President's Health Information Technology Plan. Washington, DC: The White House.

Chapter 2

Clinical Documentation and the Health Record

Diann Brown, MS, RHIA, CHP

Learning Objectives

- Discuss the purposes of health records
- Describe the functions of clinical documentation and health records
- List users of health records
- Explain the importance of defining the legal health record
- Review documentation requirements in the health record
- Discuss factors driving healthcare organizations toward the electronic health record

Key Terms

Administrative information

Allied health professional

Certification Commission for Healthcare Information Technology (CCHIT)

Computer-based record (CPR)

Derived data

Destruction

EHR Collaborative

Electronic health record (EHR)

Health Insurance Portability and Accountability Act (HIPAA)

Health Level Seven (HL7)

Health record

Hybrid health record

Legal health record

Longitudinal health record

National Committee on Vital and Health Statistics (NCVHS)

National Council for Prescription Drug Programs (NCPDP) Script

National Health Information Network (NHIN)

Personal health record (PHR)

Picture archiving and communications systems (PACS)

Protected health information

Release and disclosure

Release of information (ROI)

Retention

Systematized Nomenclature of Medicine–Clinical Terms® (SNOMED CT®)

Source-system data

Working documents

Introduction

Regardless of the healthcare setting, accreditation and regulatory standards require a separate healthcare record for each individual patient. Healthcare organizations must meet regulatory and accreditation standards when collecting and storing health information. These standards address minimum documentation requirements to ensure health records provide continuity of patient care among providers. The health record serves many purposes such as providing documentation of services for reimbursement, outcomes management, and quality care; protecting legal interests; and supplying clinical data for research. It supports the operational management of the healthcare organization as it is used for training and education as well as planning of services that support community health needs.

Each organization must define the parameters of its legal health record, taking into account the practice setting and state laws. Using a paper-based record as the legal health record seems simplistic when compared to the considerations of an electronic record. An electronic health record (EHR) can have multiple versions, different views of displaying the same information, and features that are not present in paper-based records.

The healthcare industry lags behind other industries in the application of information technology in communications and operations usage. Factors influencing the development of information technology in healthcare have advanced the development of standards for EHR conformity and interoperability.

Clinical Documentation and the Health Record

Every healthcare provider is required to document the clinical services performed on behalf of individual patients. Providers include healthcare organizations such as hospitals, physician offices, clinics, home care, hospice, and ambulatory or long-term care settings. Healthcare providers include licensed practitioners such as physicians, nurses, psychologists, **allied health professionals**, clinical social workers, and licensed independent practitioners (for example, physician's assistants).

Accreditation and regulatory standards require healthcare providers to create and maintain a separate record for each individual patient that is treated, regardless of the healthcare setting.

Clinical documentation may be stored in a paper-based format, in a mixed-media format, or in a computer-based electronic format. Regardless of the format, specific data elements are required.

Accreditation standards, licensing requirements, and federal and state statutes determine the specific health-related information that must be collected for each patient. Standards and regulations specify when the information must be collected and by whom. The content and style of clinical documentation depend on a combination of other factors, including the following:

- the profession and specialty training of the healthcare provider (for example, a physician, surgeon, registered nurse, or respiratory therapist);

- the healthcare setting (for example, a physician's office, ambulatory surgery center, or acute-care hospital); and

- the type of healthcare service provided (for example, routine screening, cataract surgery, or pulmonary intensive care).

Purpose and Value of Documentation

Federal and state statutes, licensing requirements, and accreditation standards provide minimum guidelines to ensure accurate and complete documentation. The purpose and value of documenting in the patient's health record is effective communication to other caregivers for continuity of patient care.

The **health record** is the means that healthcare providers use to collect and store the clinical documentation they create for individual patients. In the context of the overall healthcare delivery system, health records serve several important purposes, including the following:

- ensuring the continuity of patient care among providers and along the continuum of care;

- providing a means for evaluating outcomes, quality, and peer review;

- providing documentation to substantiate reimbursement claims and medical necessity of care;

- protecting the legal interests of customers, caregivers, and healthcare organizations;

- providing clinical data for biomedical research;

- supporting professional education and training for physicians, nurses, and allied health professionals;

- supporting operational management of healthcare organizations; and

- providing health-services data for public health planning and governmental policy making.

Owners of the Health Record

Health records and other documentation related to patient care are the property of the hospital or healthcare provider that created them; however, the information in each record belongs to the individual patient. To ensure their validity and confidentiality, health records must remain under the facility's physical control except in certain legal situations.

Consumers have a right to control how information in their health records is used. Patients can review, copy, and amend their records when necessary. Outside healthcare providers, third-party payers, clinical researchers, and others who have a legitimate interest in the contents of health records need access. To meet the growing demand for healthcare information, hospitals and other healthcare providers must develop processes for fulfilling legitimate requests for health information while protecting the confidentiality of health records and the privacy of patients. Hospitals and providers in other healthcare settings must ensure records remain accessible for legitimate purposes for a reasonable period after the original healthcare episode is complete.

Until 2002, few federal regulations protected the confidentiality of health information. Federal laws did protect a few specialized records in settings, such as chemical dependency treatment and human immunodeficiency virus (HIV) status. Many states had laws in place to govern the use and disclosure of health information, but the protection of patient privacy and health record security generally was the responsibility of individual healthcare providers. In the hospital setting, health information management (HIM) professionals primarily managed the privacy of confidential health information and the security of health records.

The implementation of the **Health Insurance Portability and Accountability Act (HIPAA)** Privacy Rule in 2003 established a consistent set of privacy and security rules for the first time. The rules, designed to protect the privacy of patients, also attempted to simplify the sharing of health information for legitimate purposes. For example, before implementation of HIPAA, a healthcare provider who needed access to a health record maintained by another provider usually could not directly request the information. The former provider required the patient's written authorization to release information to the current provider. In many cases, the patient or the patient's legal representative had to facilitate the transfer of medical information to a current healthcare provider. Under federal privacy regulations, the healthcare provider can directly request protected medical information, and a written authorization from the patient is not required when the information is used for treatment purposes. The privacy rule states that **protected health information** used for the purposes of treatment, payment, or healthcare operations does not require patient authorization to allow providers access, use, or disclosure. However, only the minimum necessary information needed to satisfy the specified purpose can be used or disclosed. The release of information for purposes unrelated to treatment, payment, or healthcare operations still requires the patient's written authorization.

Health information regulations under HIPAA established the rights of consumers to access and amend their own health records. Before the Internet and widespread applications of information technology, most patients had little awareness of the contents of their health records. In fact, state regulations and provider policies allowed patients limited access to their records. Today, patients are more aware of the huge wealth of personal information stored in their health records, and they are more concerned about the information's accuracy and the record's security.

Users of the Health Record

The number of organizations and individuals who have a legitimate need for access to confidential patient information has grown along with the complexity of the healthcare delivery system. Physicians, nurses, allied health professionals, and other healthcare providers administer clinical services directly to patients. Staff working in administrative and nonclinical roles support healthcare providers and have a legitimate need to use the health record. During a short hospital stay, dozens of clinicians, ancillary staff, administrative staff, and support staff will access the information in the patient's health record.

The processes that make health record information available to legitimate users are known collectively as **release and disclosure.** *Release of information* **(ROI)** is another term used when disclosing patient information. The processes entailed in storing health information and destroying it when it is no longer needed are called **retention** and **destruction.** These processes are subject to specific regulations in many states. Federal regulations and accreditation standards also include specific guidelines on the release and retention of patient-identified health information.

The Institute of Medicine broadly defines the users of health records as "those individuals who enter, verify, correct, analyze, or obtain information from the record, either directly or indirectly through an intermediary" (Dick et al. 1997, 75). All users of health records influence customer care in some way, but they use the information for various reasons and in different ways. Some users (nurses, physicians, allied health professionals) refer to the health records of specific patients as an integral part of their daily work responsibilities. In contrast, researchers, statisticians, and others never have direct access to the records of individual patients. Instead, they use aggregate (summarized and deidentified) clinical and demographic data derived from health record documentation.

The main users of health records are the clinicians responsible for direct patient care. They are authorized to record and access clinical documentation for the patients to whom they provide services. It should be noted that most clinicians are only authorized to access the records for their own patients. Accessing or disclosing health record information without a valid reason is considered a violation of the ethical principles of every healthcare profession and the federal privacy rule (HIPAA 2003). Either of these practices would also violate institutional policies protecting the confidentiality of patient information.

Interns and students supervised by hospital, clinical, or medical staff access patient-identifiable information for the purpose of training and learning. Coding and billing staff consult patient-identifiable information as the basis for clinical coding and reimbursement. Figure 2.1 provides a list of representative users of health record information.

Patients (along with their next of kin and/or legal representatives) have the right to access their health records. However, HIM professionals must validate the appropriateness of access. Whenever a patient's next of kin or legal representative requests information belonging to the patient, HIM professionals should be familiar with their state and federal laws regarding the right to access and who can authorize the use or disclosure of the information at issue.

A number of healthcare-related organizations use information derived from health records. Healthcare providers such as HMOs and physicians' practices use patient-identifiable information, as do third-party payers. Quality improvement organizations and other entities working under contracts with hospitals or with third-party payers such as Medicare often review copies of health record documentation. Many other organizations use aggregate health information in activities related to accreditation, research, and policymaking. (See figure 2.2 for a more comprehensive list of the institutions that rely on information from health records.)

Definition of the Health Record for Legal Purposes

Until the widespread use of computer technology in the last part of the twentieth century, the definition of what constituted a legal health record seemed relatively straightforward. The contents of the paper-based health record became the provider's legal business record of the services it provided to specific patients.

Figure 2.1. Representative users of the health record: individuals.[a]

Patient Care Delivery—Providers	Patient Care Management and Support
• Physicians	• Health information management professionals
• Residents	• Administrators
• Nurses and nurse practitioners	• Financial managers and accountants
• Dental hygienists	• Quality managers
• Dentists	• Allied health professionals
• Dietitians	• Risk managers
• Laboratory technologists	• Unit clerks
• Chaplains	• Utilization review managers
• Nurses	
• Pharmacists	**Patient Care Reimbursement**
• Physical therapists	• Benefit managers
• Behavioral health providers	• Insurers (federal, state, and private)
• Social workers	
	Other
Patient Care Delivery—Consumers	• Accreditors
• Patients	• Government policy makers and legislators
• Families	• Lawyers
• Patients' legal representatives	• Healthcare researchers and clinical investigators

Source: Dick et al. 1997, 76.
[a]This is a representative (not exhaustive) list of users.

Defining the "legal record" becomes complex as organizations transition to electronic health records and the inherent capabilities that do not exist with paper-based records. For example, the EHR can have multiple versions, offer multiple ways of displaying information, and contain features, such as alerts and reminders, that provide clinical decision support. These functions and features are not available in a paper-based health record; therefore, it is necessary for a healthcare organization to determine which parts of the EHR are included in the legal record and which parts are not.

In a 2005 practice brief, the American Health Information Management Association (AHIMA) recognizeda the need to reassess the definition of the legal health record regardless of the technologies employed or users involved (AHIMA e-HIM Work Group 2005b). This practice brief is included as appendix C on the accompanying CD. The need to define the legal health record for disclosure purposes is paramount.

There is no one-size-fits-all definition of the legal health record. Laws and regulations governing the content vary by practice setting and state. However, following common principles when creating a definition ensures that a health record serves the legal needs of the provider or facility, whether in a paper-based, hybrid (a combination of paper and electronic), or electronic state. Each organization must consider individual state laws and federal regulations that permit the health record to serve and represent the legal business record. Regardless of the physical state of the health record, it must represent and fulfill the legal and business needs of the organization.

Legal Health Record

The **legal health record** can be defined as the official business record created by or for the healthcare organization (AHIMA e-HIM Work Group 2005b). The legal health record is the portion of the health record that will be disclosed upon request to parties outside the organization. It does not affect the discoverability of other information held by the organization.

Figure 2.2.   Representative users of the health record: institutions.[a]

Healthcare Delivery (Inpatient and Outpatient)
- Alliances, associations, networks, and systems of providers
- Ambulatory surgery centers
- Donor banks (blood, tissue, organs)
- Health maintenance organizations
- Home care agencies
- Hospices
- Hospitals (general and specialty)
- Nursing homes
- Preferred provider organizations
- Physician offices (large and small group practices, individual practitioners)
- Psychiatric facilities
- Public health departments
- Substance abuse programs

Management and Review of Care
- Medicare peer review organizations
- Quality management companies
- Risk management companies
- Utilization review and utilization management companies

Reimbursement of Care
- Business healthcare coalitions
- Employers
- Insurers (federal, state, and private)

Research
- Disease registries
- Health data organizations
- Healthcare technology developers and manufacturers (equipment and device firms, pharmaceutical firms, and computer hardware and software vendors for patient record systems)
- Research centers

Education
- Allied health professional schools and programs
- Schools of medicine
- Schools of nursing
- Schools of public health

Accreditation
- Accreditation organizations
- Institutional licensure agencies
- Professional licensure agencies

Policy Making
- Federal government agencies
- Local government agencies
- State government agencies

Source: Dick et al. 1997, 77.
[a]This is a representative (not exhaustive) list of users.

The legal health record includes documentation of healthcare services provided to an individual during any aspect of healthcare delivery in any type of healthcare organization. The legal health record contains individually identifiable information, stored on any medium, and collected and directly used in documenting healthcare or health status. AHIMA states:

> . . . legal health records must meet accepted standards as defined by [the] Centers for Medicare and Medicaid Services (CMS) *Conditions of Participation*, federal regulations, state laws, and accrediting agencies, such as the Joint Commission, as well as the policies of the healthcare provider. (AHIMA e-HIM Work Group 2005b)

Legal health records are records of care in any health-related setting used by healthcare professionals while providing patient-care services or for administrative, business, or payment purposes. Some types of documentation that compose the legal health record may physically exist in separate and multiple paper-based, electronic, or computer-based databases. The result is a **hybrid health record** that is defined as one that consists of information created with both paper documents and electronic media.

Organizational policies should document and identify the source (paper or electronic) of all information contained in the legal health record. A transition plan and policy should define the "legal source of truth," reflecting whether the legal health record is paper, hybrid, or fully electronic. This should include a specific schedule that provides both retrospective and prospective dates wherein the user can identify sources of all information in the record. There must be a clear indication of the locations where portions of a patient's legal health record are located.

An **electronic health record (EHR)** system is the portal through which clinicians' access patients' health records, order treatments or therapy, and document care delivered to patients. Although healthcare providers may eliminate the paper record when documenting in an electronic system, hard copies (typically paper) are still released for disclosure purposes. This may change with acceptance of technical standards for interoperability that enable health information exchange between providers and other users of health records.

Portions of the EHR are usually located in various electronic systems such as laboratory databases, pharmacy information systems, **picture archiving and communications systems (PACS)**, cardiology information systems, results reporting systems, computerized provider order entry systems, nurse care-planning systems, word-processing systems, and fetal trace monitoring systems. Depending on their size and structure, healthcare providers may store structured clinical and administrative data in a database or clinical data repository. In addition, healthcare providers may store unstructured patient clinical data in separate databases or repositories (such as PACS and fetal trace archives) and provide pointers from the clinical portal to these various repositories.

Defining the Subset of Information That Constitutes the Legal Health Record

The challenge for HIM professionals in defining a legal health record in an EHR system is to determine which data elements, electronic-structured documents, images, and video and/or audio files become part of the legal electronic health record.

- **Step 1**: Determine which legal entities enforce regulations, guidelines, standards, or laws to the healthcare organization defining its legal health record. Although various entities may have defined a legal health record in paper terms, their definition is still the basis for defining the legal health record in the electronic environment.

- **Step 2**: Determine whether the records are created in the regular course of business of the healthcare provider or entity.

- **Step 3**: Create a matrix (or other document/tool) that defines each element in the legal health record and determines the medium in which each element will appear. (See figure 2.3.) Such a matrix could include a column indicating whether a particular element will be released on first request or following a subpoena. Guidelines for release of information vary by state.

Figure 2.3. Elements of the legal health record.

Document/data element	Medium	Released on first request or subpoena (Y/N)
Patient name	Electronic	
History and physical	Electronic	
Lab findings	Electronic	
Progress notes	Scanned images	
Patient consent forms	Paper documents	

Source: Adapted from Servais 2008.

As stated previously, there is no one-size-fits-all definition of the legal health record because laws and regulations governing the content vary by practice setting and by state. Final definition of the legal health record rests with individual healthcare organizations and their legal counsels. When defining the content of the legal health record, organizations should consider the items listed in figure 2.4.

Patient-identifiable Source Data

Various types of patient-identifiable source data are collected and stored in source systems. Source-system data must be evaluated for inclusion in the legal health record.

Source-system data are the data from which interpretations, summaries, and notes are derived. Examples of source-system data are radiological film or scans, laboratory values, pathology slides, video and/or audio recordings, and EKG tracings. They may be designated part of the legal health record, whether or not they are integrated into a single system or maintained as part of the source system.

Historically, reports or findings upon which clinical decision making is based are part of the legal health record. For example, the written result of a test such as an x-ray, ECG, or other similar procedures are always part of the record, whether these reports are integrated into a single system or part of a source system.

Working notes used by a provider in completing a final report are not considered part of the legal health record unless they are made available to others providing care to a patient. However, documents that are kept in a separate record system, such as notes from a particular area of specialty that are kept separately but are final products, are always considered part of the record.

The determining factor in whether data are considered part of the legal health record is not the format or location but, rather, how the data are used and whether it is reasonable to expect the data to be routinely released when a request for a complete health record is received.

Legal health records exclude health records that are not official business records of a healthcare organization, such as personal health records (PHRs).

Figure 2.4. Items to consider when defining legal health record content.

- Advance directives
- Allergy records
- Alerts, reminders, and pop ups
- Anesthesia records
- Care plans
- Continuing care records
- Consent forms for care, treatment, and research
- Consultation reports
- Diagnostic images
- Discharge instructions
- Discharge summaries
- E-mail messages containing patient-provider or provider-provider communications regarding care or treatment of specific patients
- Emergency department records
- Fetal monitoring strips from which interpretations are derived
- Functional status assessments
- Graphic records
- History and physical examination records
- Immunization records
- Instant messages containing patient-provider or provider-provider communications regarding care or treatment of specific patients
- Intake and output records
- Medication administration records
- Medication orders
- Medication profiles
- Minimum data sets (MDS, OASIS, IRF-PAI)
- Nursing assessments
- Operative and procedure reports
- Orders for treatment including diagnostic tests for laboratory and radiology
- Pathology reports
- Patient-submitted documentation
- Patient education or teaching documents
- Patient identifiers (such as a health record number)
- Photographs (digital and analog) for identification purposes only
- Post-it® notes and annotations containing patient-provider or provider-provider communications regarding care or treatment of specific patients
- Practice guidelines or protocols and clinical pathways that imbed patient data
- Problem lists
- Progress notes and documentation (multidisciplinary, excluding psychotherapy notes)
- Psychology and psychiatric assessments and summaries (excluding psychotherapy notes)
- Records received from another healthcare provider if they were relied on to provide healthcare to the patient (see "Continuing care records," above)
- Research records of tests and treatments
- Respiratory, physical, speech, and/or occupational therapy records
- Results of tests and studies from laboratory and radiology
- Standing orders
- Telephone messages containing patient-provider or provider-provider communications regarding care or treatment of specific patients
- Telephone orders
- Trauma tapes
- Verbal orders
- Wave forms such as ECGs and EMGs from which interpretations are derived
- Any other information required by the Medicare *Conditions of Participation* (2006), state provider licensure statutes or rules, or by any third-party payer as a condition of reimbursement

Administrative Information

Administrative information includes patient-identifiable documentation used for administrative, regulatory, healthcare operations, and payment (financial) purposes. Administrative information should have the same level of confidentiality as the legal health record. Two types of administrative information are created and maintained by healthcare organizations. The first type consists of documentation that is typically part of the health record such as consents for treatment, surgery, and research forms that would be produced in response to a subpoena. The second type of administrative information should not be considered part of the legal health record and would not be produced in response to a subpoena for the health record. Examples of administrative information not considered part of the health record are included in figure 2.5. Healthcare organizations might more appropriately consider such administrative information as **working documents**.

Figure 2.5.   Administrative information (working documents) not considered part of the health record.

• Abbreviation and do-not-use abbreviation lists • Audit trails related to the EHR • Authorization forms for release of information • Birth and death certificate worksheets • Correspondence concerning requests for records • Databases containing patient data • Event history and audit trails • Financial and insurance forms • Incident or patient safety reports • Indexes (disease, operation, death) • Institutional review board lists • Logs	• Notice of privacy practices acknowledgments (unless the organization chooses to classify them as part of the health record) • Patient-identifiable claims • Patient-identifiable data reviewed for quality assurance or utilization management • Protocols and clinical pathways, practice guidelines, and other knowledge sources that do not imbed patient data • Psychotherapy notes • Registries • Staff roles and access rights • Work lists and works in progress

Derived data

Derived data consist of factual details aggregated or summarized from a group of health records that provide no means to identify specific patients. These data should have the same level of confidentiality as the legal health record. However, derived data should not be considered part of the legal health record and would not be produced in response to a subpoena for the health record.

The following are examples of derived data:

- Accreditation reports

- Anonymous patient data for research purposes

- Best-practice guidelines created from aggregate patient data

- OASIS reports

- ORYX, Quality Indicator, Quality Measure, or other reports

- Public health reports that do not contain patient-identifiable data

- Statistical reports

- Transmission reports for MDS, OASIS, and IRF-PAI

Emerging Issues

As EHR technology evolves, a number of challenges to the definition of the legal health record are emerging. Organizations must resolve these challenges with their legal counsel and information technology departments. Many of these items have not historically been included in the legal health record and will entail new storage and retrieval costs if they are defined as part of the record. Following are some examples of documents and data that should be evaluated for inclusion or exclusion in the legal health record:

- Audio files of dictation

- Alerts and reminders (including resolutions/responses)

- Audio files of patient telephone calls

- Audit trails
- Nursing shift-to-shift reports (handwritten or audio)
- Patient-physician e-mail
- Telephone consultation audio files
- Videos of office visits
- Videos of procedures
- Videos of telemedicine consultations

Personal Health Records

Organizational policy should address how personal health information provided by the patient will or will not be incorporated into the patient's health record. Copies of **personal health records (PHRs)**, created, owned, and managed by the patient, are considered part of the legal health record when used by the organization to provide treatment. Organizations must address how and when to incorporate PHRs into their legal health records: They must determine when information is used to provide patient-care services; review patient data; or document observations, actions, or instructions. This includes patient-owned, managed, and populated tracking records, such as medication records and glucose and insulin records.

Documentation Guidelines

Health records may be called by different names in different healthcare settings, for example, as follows:

- Resident records (in long-term care facilities)
- Client records (in behavioral health hospitals and clinics)
- Patient records (in physicians' offices)
- Medical records (in hospitals)

The style and content of health records depend on the setting in which the healthcare services are provided. Regulatory and accreditation requirements for the various healthcare settings are quite different, as are the reimbursement requirements, patient demographics, and services mix.

Documentation requirements for acute-care facilities are unique to the setting, and different types of acute-care hospitals must comply with different specialty documentation requirements. For example, the documentation for diagnostic and therapeutic services and care of developmental disabilities and behavioral conditions is somewhat different from the documentation for acute-care medical-surgical services. Other specialty hospitals, such as children's hospitals and women's hospitals, provide services similar to general acute-care facilities and follow the same general guidelines, although there are also specific and unique types of documentation for pediatric care and obstetrics and gynecology specialties. The same is true of critical-access hospitals, very small and geographically isolated hospitals that provide a limited range of services.

Long-term acute-care hospitals treat patients who require intensive medical services for acute and chronic conditions. Rehabilitation hospitals provide nursing, medical, and rehabilitative services to individuals (such as stroke patients) who require physical, speech, and/or occupational therapy—in addition to medical and nursing services—but are no longer in the acute phase of their illness.

Almost all healthcare settings must comply with federal documentation guidelines established by the CMS (2006) for Medicare participants. In addition, most hospitals choose to participate in voluntary accreditation programs, which also publish health record documentation standards.

Regardless of setting, good documentation contains sufficient data and information to identify and support the diagnosis/condition and treatment of the patient. Documentation justifies the care, treatment, and services, and promotes the continuity of care among providers. Although differences exist depending on the setting, high-quality documentation practices are required regardless of the setting.

Organizations face a transition when migrating from paper to hybrid to fully electronic health records (AHIMA e-HIM Work Group 2005a). (See appendix D on the accompanying CD.) An attorney should review policies related to legal documentation issues to ensure adherence to the most current standards and case law. HIM professionals should fully understand the principles of maintaining a legally sound health record and the potential ramifications when the record's legal integrity is questioned. Documentation guidelines that originally applied to paper can translate to electronic documentation; however, additional guidelines will need exploring to maintain a legally sound health record. The ultimate goal for managing EHR information is that it is kept in a manner that supports a facility's business and legal processes and eliminates the need for maintaining a duplicate paper process.

Figure 2.6 lists guidelines that organizations should consider to establish sound documentation principles for health records.

Future of Clinical Documentation

Healthcare has lagged far behind other fields in the application of information technology to operations and communications. However, the development and implementation of computer-based systems, including electronic health record systems, is inevitable for all types of healthcare organizations.

The evolution of computer-based systems in acute-care facilities began with the development of automated systems for administrative operations (admissions, billing, and claims processing). In the 1980s and 1990s, automated systems for laboratory and pharmacy services were implemented in most hospitals. Today, hospitals use a wide variety of computer-based technologies to provide clinical services and support administrative functions. Yet, the application of advanced computer technology to health record documentation has been slow to evolve. The term *electronic health record* is now preferred over **computer-based record (CPR)**, a term that was in use during the 1990s.

HIPAA is driving the movement toward the universal adoption of EHR systems (1996). Standardized transactions and code sets, when electronically transmitting healthcare information, must comply with HIPAA format and content. Standardized transactions include items such as claims information, encounter information, payment, remittance advice, claim status inquiry and response, and eligibility inquiry and response. Code sets identify specific diagnoses and clinical procedures on claims and encounter forms. The International Classification of Diseases, Ninth Revision, Clinical Modification (ICD-9-CM), Current Procedural Terminology, Fourth Edition (CPT®-4), and Healthcare Common Procedure Coding System (HCPCS) are examples of code sets for procedures and diagnoses (Medicare 2003).

Figure 2.6. Health record documentation guidelines.

- Policies should be based on all applicable standards, including accreditation standards, state and local licensure requirements, federal and state regulations, reimbursement requirements, and professional practice standards.
- Content and format of health records should be uniform.
- Health record entries should be legible and complete.
- Individuals documenting the health record should have the authority and right to document as defined by the organization's policies and procedures. The authorship of health record entries should be clearly identified in the documentation.
- The definition of a legally authenticated entry should be established, and rules should be set for prompt authentication of every entry in the health record by the author responsible for ordering, providing, or evaluating the service furnished.
- Entries should be made as soon as possible after an event or observation is made at the point of care. An entry should never be made in advance.
- All entries in the health record should include the complete date and time. Time must be included in all types of narrative notes, even if it may not seem important to the type of entry. Narrative documentation should reflect the actual time the entry was made. Effective January 2007, CMS added a new requirement: hospitals must now "time" all entries in health records (CMS 2006).
- The record should always reflect factual information and be written using specific language and factual statements. Avoid using vague or generalized language.
- For patient safety reasons, organizational policies must address the use of approved abbreviations in the health record. Hospitals may publish a list of abbreviations and symbols that are prohibited when documenting in the health record (Joint Commission 2006).
- Policies should specify the parties responsible for receiving and transcribing verbal or telephone orders of physicians.
- All entries in the health record, regardless of form or format, must be permanent (manual or computerized records). The Rules of Evidence require that policies and procedures be in place to prevent alteration, tampering, or loss.
- Documentation errors should never be obliterated or changed. Instead, documentation errors should be corrected according to the procedure established in the organization's documentation policy and/or medical staff rules.
- Organizational policies should address how the patient or patient's representative can request corrections and amendments to the record. The amendment should refer back to the information questioned and include date and time. At no time should the documentation in question be removed from the chart or obliterated in any way. The patient cannot require that information in the record be removed or deleted.
- The qualitative and quantitative analysis of health record documentation should be conducted according to procedures developed and implemented by the hospital's health information management department.
- Organizational policies should differentiate whether research records are part of the legal health record or if the research center maintains its own records. This should be verified with the institutional review board, since this may influence whether research records are part of the legal health record.

The **National Committee on Vital and Health Statistics (NCVHS)**, a public policy advisory board made up of representatives from numerous healthcare, trade, and professional organizations, recommended to the U.S. Department of Health and Human Services (2003) that standard-developing organizations be encouraged to adopt standards that promote interoperability of electronic health records and PHRs. The NCVHS recognizes that the interoperability of EHRs provides an opportunity to improve the safety and quality of customer care. Providers will need to use specific terminology, data structure, and transport and security standards to connect healthcare entities. In a 2006 report to the Department of Health and Human Services, NCVHS recommended the minimal functional requirements needed for the initial definition of the National Health Information Network (NHIN) to exchange data (NCVHS 2006).

National Health Information Network (NHIN) efforts play a major role in the future of health information exchange. The primary objectives of the NHIN are to interconnect networks of clinicians, make information portable, and move consumers from one healthcare provider to another. This requires an interoperable infrastructure that allows clinicians access to critical healthcare information to make clinical or treatment decisions. The NCVHS has developed and released prototype architecture that contains functional requirements, security, and business models for information exchange. State and regional health information networks will compose the NHIN (Cohn 2006).

The **Health Level Seven (HL7)**, an organization that develops standards related to healthcare delivery, released the draft version of a new EHR functional model in late 2003. The **EHR Collaborative**, which consists of organizations representing key stakeholders in healthcare, worked with HL7 to publicize and refine the draft model. The model was revised several times before industry representatives voted to adopt it in April 2004. The adoption of the universal EHR guidelines has stimulated momentum in the development of new technology that supports the interoperability of EHRs and establishes a messaging standard for the consistent transmission of information between senders and receivers. In February 2007, HL7 announced it had passed the first American National Standards Institute (ANSI)-approved standard specifying the functional requirements for an EHR system. This standard advances key developments in EHR systems and contains functions that support the maintenance of a legal EHR for business, regulatory, and accreditation purposes. Key healthcare stakeholders are encouraged to participate in the development of profiles that support specific uses. The profiles represent functions needed by clinicians using EHR systems for special purposes or care environments. For example, the functional model standard paves the way for additional development of EHR system standards, and these efforts will serve as a framework for the legal EHR (HL7 2007). EHRs and EHR networks are certified by the **Certification Commission for Healthcare Information Technology (CCHIT)**.

The **Systematized Nomenclature of Medicine–Clinical Terms (SNOMED CT)** provides a common language for indexing, storing, retrieving, and aggregating clinical data across specialties and healthcare providers. The NCVHS recommended SNOMED CT as the standard for nonlaboratory interventions and procedures, laboratory test results, anatomical locations, diagnoses, problem lists, and nursing care. The National Library of Medicine purchased a license for SNOMED CT that allows its free use in the United States. This purchase is intended to accelerate the adoption and interoperability of EHR systems (Foley and Garrett 2006).

The **National Council for Prescription Drug Programs (NCPDP)** specifies **SCRIPT** standards (2007) for the electronic transmission of prescription drug information between providers and pharmacies. Medicare has mandated e-prescribing for Medicare plans to reduce prescription errors due to illegible handwriting. The NCPDP is the official standard for HIPAA pharmacy claims.

The implementation of EHR systems may also support the development of longitudinal health records. A **longitudinal health record** is a health record that includes all of the health-related information generated for an individual during his or her lifetime. A longitudinal health record has many benefits for consumers. However, the maintenance of such records for every American will be impossible until every healthcare provider in the country has implemented an EHR system.

Under the current system of mixed-media records, providers keep a separate health record for every patient they treat. As a result, an individual's medical history is documented in hundreds of separate records created over the span of a lifetime. The NHIN would provide the necessary connectivity to link one or more of the customer's EHRs to a single, longitudinal health record, regardless of where the information resides. The NHIN is a critical component to reaching the longitudinal record.

It is possible for individuals and their families to create and maintain their own longitudinal records. Health records maintained by consumers are called personal health records or PHRs. Several tools for creating and maintaining PHRs are available via the Internet, including one from the AHIMA. Personal health records, however, are not considered legal documents; so they cannot be included in the official records of healthcare providers at this time.

Summary

The quality of the clinical documentation in patients' health records is vital to virtually every aspect of healthcare, including delivery, reimbursement, education, and research. Health information management (HIM) professionals play a vital role by ensuring the availability, completeness, and accuracy of health record documentation. HIM professionals protect the consumers' right to confidentiality and privacy. To be effective, HIM professionals must understand every aspect of the healthcare environment, including state and federal laws and regulations, accreditation standards and processes, quality improvement practices, and information system technology.

References

AHIMA e-HIM Work Group on Maintaining the Legal EHR. 2005a. Update: Maintaining a legally sound health record—paper and electronic. *Journal of American Health Information Management Association* 76(10): 64A–L.

AHIMA e-HIM Work Group on the Legal Health Record. 2005b. Update: Guidelines for defining the legal health record for disclosure purposes. *Journal of American Health Information Management Association* 76(8): 64A–G.

Centers for Medicare and Medicaid Services. 2006 (Nov. 27). Conditions of participation for hospitals; Final rule. 42 CFR Part 482. *Federal Register* 71(227): 68672–68695. Available online from http://a257.g.akamaitech. net/7/257/2422/01jan20061800/edocket.access.gpo.gov/2006/pdf/E6-19957.pdf.

Cohn, S. 2006. Functional Requirements Needed for the Initial Definition of a Nationwide Health Information Network. Report to the Secretary of the U.S. Department of Health and Human Services.

Department of Health and Human Services. 2003 (Feb. 20). Health insurance reform: Modifications to electronic data transaction standards and code sets; Final rule. 45 CFR Part 162. *Federal Register* 68(34): 8381–8399.

Dick, R., et al., eds. 1997. *The Computer-Based Patient Record: An Essential Technology for Health Care,* revised edition. Washington, D.C.: National Academy Press.

Foley, M. M., and G. S. Garrett. 2006. Code ahead: Key issues shaping clinical terminology and classification. *Journal of American Health Information Management Association* 77(7): 24–30.

Health Insurance Portability and Accountability Act (HIPAA) of 1996. Public Law 104-191. Available online from www.gpoaccess.gov/cfr/index.html.

Health Level Seven. 2007 (February). HL7 Announces Industry's First Electronic Health Record System (EHR-S) Functional Requirements Standard. Available online from www.hl7.org/documentcenter/public/ pressreleases/20070221.pdf.

Joint Commission on Accreditation of Healthcare Organizations. 2006. *2006 Comprehensive Accreditation Manual for Hospitals; The Official Handbook.* Oakbrook Terrace, IL: Joint Commission.

National Committee on Vital and Health Statistics. 2006. Press Release: Personal health records and personal health record systems. February 2006. Available online from www.ncvhs.hhs.gov/0602nhiirpt.pdf.

National Council for Prescription Drug Programs. 2007. Press Release: NCPDP releases new versions for the Telecommunication Standard, Medicaid Subrogation and SCRIPT Standard implementation guides. July 15, 2007. Available online from www.ncpdp.org/press/PR07_07-17-2007_New_version_telecom.pdf.

Servais, Cheryl. 2008. *The Legal Health Record.* Edited by Neil Olderman and Kelly Trahan. Chicago: AHIMA.

PART II

Utilization of the Healthcare Record

Chapter 3

Principal and Ancillary Functions of the Healthcare Record

Diann Brown, MS, RHIA, CHP

Learning Objectives

- Identify and explain the principal functions of a health record

- Define the terms *information* and *data* and distinguish their differences

- Identify the ancillary functions of the health record; explain the special roles health records play in accreditation, licensure, and certification, biomedical research and education, credentialing and privileging, legal proceedings, and reporting morbidity and mortality rates

- Discuss right to access, release and disclosure, and retention and destruction of health records; list the most common secondary indexes, registries, and databases maintained by hospitals and explain the content and purpose of each

Key Terms

Accreditation

Accreditation organizations

Advanced decision support

Allied health professional

Biomedical research

Case management

Case-mix analysis

Centers for Disease Control and Prevention (CDC)

Centers for Medicare and Medicaid Services (CMS)

Certificate of destruction

Certification

Clinical practice guidelines

Clinical privileges

Confidentiality

Continuous quality improvement (CQI)

Core measures

Corporate negligence

Court order

Credentialing

Data

Demographic data

Diagnostic codes

e-Discovery

Electronic health record (EHR)

Face sheet

Federal Rules of Civil Procedure (FRCP)

Financial data

Health Insurance Portability and Accountability Act (HIPAA)

Health Level Seven (HL7)

Health record

Healthcare Integrity and Protection Data Bank (HIPDB)

ICD-10-CM© and ICD-10-PCS

Incident

Incident report

Information

Informed consent

Liability

Licensure

Master patient index (MPI)

Medical necessity

Medical staff bylaws

National Practitioner Data Bank (NPDB)

National Vital Statistics System (NVSS)

Notifiable diseases

Performance improvement (PI)

Population-based statistics

Privacy

Privileged communication

Procedural codes

Quality improvement organizations (QIOs)

Redisclosure

Reimbursement

Risk management (RM)

Statute of limitations

Subpoena

Subpoena duces tecum

Systematized Nomenclature of Medicine–Clinical Terms® (SNOMED CT®)

Third-party payers

Transcriptionist

Unique identifier

Utilization management (UM)

Utilization review (UR)

World Health Organization (WHO)

Introduction

The health records created and maintained by hospitals contain large amounts of clinical documentation stored as data and information. That documentation must be readily accessible for legitimate healthcare functions and yet protected from unauthorized access, damage, and loss.

The terms *data* and *information* are often used interchangeably, but there are distinct differences in meaning between the two terms when they are used in reference to health records. **Data** represent objective descriptions of processes, procedures, people, and other observable things and activities. Data are collected in the form of dates, numbers, symbols, images, illustrations, texts, lists, charts, and equations. The analysis of data for a specific purpose results in **information**. Data represent facts; information conveys meaning. In other words, data themselves have no meaning until they are considered in the context of a specific purpose or function.

For example, a chart showing a series of columns with times, dates, initials, numbers, and symbols would have little meaning unless it were put in the context of patient care. Then, the numbers and symbols would represent observations of the vital signs of a specific patient, and the times, dates, and initials would constitute authentication for the health record documentation of those observations. Taken further, the data on the patient's temperature, pulse rate, respirations, and blood pressure would have even more specific meaning if it were considered in the context of the patient's age and medical condition.

Before the widespread use of computer technology in healthcare, all of the information in healthcare records was collected and stored in paper format. Each record was a compilation of handwritten progress notes, paper forms, photographs, graphic tracings, and typewritten reports. Many of the typewritten reports of medical findings and operative procedures were originally dictated by physicians and surgeons and subsequently converted into written format by medical **transcriptionists** (specially trained typists who understand medical terminology).

The paper record was organized in a paper folder called a chart. When an episode of care was complete, the paper record was moved from the patient-care unit and stored in a large file room. After a predetermined amount of time, the record might be moved to a more remote storage facility or converted to a film image (called microfiche) that consumed much less space in storage. Eventually, the paper records were destroyed.

Many healthcare organizations, including hospitals, continue to use paper-based health record systems. Most combine handwritten documentation with computer printouts and documents generated in other media, such as digital images, e-mail communications, and video images.

Hospitals and other large healthcare organizations have been slow to adopt new information technologies. The high cost of developing and implementing computer-based health record systems and the reluctance of clinical professionals to learn new documentation processes account for some of the resistance. Another factor has been the lack of national standards on electronic record content, which has hampered the commercial development of health record systems. In addition, the federal government, the largest healthcare payer in the United States, had been silent on the issue until President Bush's state of the union address in January 2004.

The movement toward **electronic health record (EHR)** systems has gained momentum since the implementation of the **Health Insurance Portability and Accountability Act (HIPAA)** in 1996. Similarly, the future adoption of the new diagnostic and procedural coding system (**ICD-10-CM© and ICD-10-PCS**) and the standardized definitions from the **Systematized Nomenclature of Medicine–Clinical Terms (SNOMED CT)** are likely to spur the inevitable change from paper and mixed media to electronic health record systems (AHIMA 2003).

Health Level Seven (HL7) began working on a functional model for EHRs in 2003. (HL7 is a standards development organization that addresses issues at the applications [or seventh] level of healthcare system interconnections.) When HL7 and industry stakeholders adopted the functional model, it provided momentum to develop new technology to support the interoperability of the EHR. The HL7 standards are a very useful tool for evaluating the function of an organization's EHR. HIM professionals play a vital role in evaluating the effectiveness of the EHR by analyzing workflow and daily needs for producing copies or information from the patient's record (Quinsey 2006).

Health information management requires health information management (HIM) professionals who possess solid knowledge of data sets. Obtaining consensus on what data elements should be collected and their definitions in the development of an EHR system with an eye on the HL7 functional model requires HIM professionals to work with those who set standards (Giannangelo 2007).

Principal Functions of the Health Record

Regardless of storage format, the functions of the health record remain the same. The **health record** serves as the principle repository for clinical documentation relevant to the care and treatment of one specific patient. The principle functions are related to specific healthcare encounters between providers and patients. The ancillary functions are related to the environment in which healthcare services are provided.

Administrative Information and Demographic Data

For elective hospital admissions, the patient or the admitting physician's office staff often provide administrative information and demographic data before the patient comes to the hospital. Alternatively, the patient may provide the information to the hospital's registration staff on the day of admission. When patients are admitted through the emergency department, the patient or the patient's representative provides administrative information for unplanned admissions.

Admitting and Registration Information

The registration staff collects personal details about the patient as well as information about the patient's health insurance coverage at the time of admission. Practically all hospitals use a computer-based registration system linked to a database called the **master patient index (MPI)**. When patients are readmitted to a healthcare facility, registration personnel check the patient's personal information against the data in the database to ensure that it is current and correct. The patient's administrative information is then recorded on an identification sheet, which is often called a **face sheet**. In paper-based record systems, a printout of the face sheet is used as the front page in the patient's record. It identifies the patient and contains demographics, original date of admission, insurance coverage or payment source, referral information, hospital stay dates, physician information, and discharge information. It also contains the names of the responsible party, emergency contacts, additional contacts, and the patient's diagnosis.

In an electronic format, data collected from the face sheet may be captured on several screens but displayed in a logical manner to those who need it. For instance, clinical staff caring for the patient should be able to quickly identify the patient by name, health record number, and account number, as well as locate emergency contacts for the patient; whereas the billing office needs the patient's name, account number, and insurance information. While electronic health record systems may display information differently, all the information gathered for the health record is available onscreen on a need-to-know basis (James 2007).

Demographic Data

The term *demographics* refers to the study of statistical data about human populations. In the context of healthcare, **demographic data** includes basic factual details about the individual patient. The demographic data collected from the patient include the following:

- Last, first, and middle name
- Address
- Telephone number
- Gender
- Date of birth
- Place of birth
- Race or ethnic origin
- Marital status
- Name and address of next of kin
- Social Security number

The main purpose of collecting demographic data is to confirm the identity of the patient. Hospitals and other healthcare-related organizations use the demographic data collected from patients as the basis of statistical records, research, and resource planning.

Social Security numbers are often used to help positively identify patients because they are one type of **unique identifier**; that is, it is a number that represents one and only one individual. Hospitals assign unique identifiers to individual health records to make sure information in the records is easily retrievable and not misplaced or lost. Due to the growing issue of identity theft, the collection and use of Social Security numbers as a unique identifier is controversial. Healthcare providers are finding alternative solutions to uniquely identify their patients (AHIMA e-HIM Work Group on Regional Health Information Organizations 2006). (See appendix B on the accompanying CD.)

Financial Data

Details about the patient's occupation, employer, and insurance coverage are collected at the time of treatment. Healthcare providers use this data to complete claims forms submitted to third-party payers. **Financial data** include the following:

- Patient's name
- Name of the insured party and his or her relationship to the patient if the patient is a dependent of the insured party
- Insured party's member identification number
- Name of the insurance company and the group policy number
- Employer's name and address

Clinical Data

Basic clinical data are collected and recorded during the intake process. From this, the treating or admitting physician can provide the patient's preliminary diagnosis and the reason the patient is seeking treatment.

Accurate clinical data collection is important because it becomes the basis of care plans and helps determine medical necessity.

Patient-Care Delivery

The health record combines information about the patient's illness with documentation of the services provided. Clinical observations of the patient, results of physical examinations and diagnostic tests, details of medical-surgical procedures, and descriptions of therapeutic outcomes are all compiled in one record. This record is accessible to all of the clinical professionals and **allied health professionals** who provide services to the patient.

The **health record** serves as a documentation tool that constitutes a permanent account of services the patient received. Communication between the patient's caregivers is very important, and the health record is an effective communication tool that ensures the continuity of customer services. Information recorded in the patient's health record helps physicians make informed decisions about the patient's current condition and treatment requirements. The health record assists with patient assessment and care planning. Nursing assessments document the level of nursing assistance and personal care needed by the patient. To facilitate continuity of customer care, the health record serves as the basis for discharge planning. The purpose of discharge planning is to ensure that the patient will receive appropriate follow-up care.

Information documented in the health record forms the basis for evaluations of potential threats to the welfare of individual customers or the healthcare organization. Using the health record as a risk assessment tool helps manage the risk of the organization.

Because electronic health records are based on sophisticated information processing technology, they offer clinical functions that conventional paper-based records cannot, such as the following:

- The electronic health record performs as an **advanced decision support** instrument. Advanced decision support makes the latest clinical guidelines and research findings available to physicians at a click.

- Medication errors can be easily detected in the electronic health record, which can be considered a medical error prevention tool. Drug interaction and dosage warnings are issued automatically when conflicting medication orders are entered into the record. Other reminders for clinicians can be issued automatically.

- Discharge planning is enhanced because EHR systems can be linked to clinic schedules so that follow-up appointments can be made for patients before they leave the hospital. EHRs can automatically provide patient-specific aftercare or discharge instructions.

Patient-Care Management and Support

Patient-care management encompasses activities related to the management of services provided directly to patients. Many of these activities require an analysis of health records to determine the financial health of an organization and relevance of its services or to develop clinical guidelines.

To determine Medicare reimbursement, a hospital will analyze its case mix. **Case-mix analysis** is a method of grouping patients according to a predefined set of characteristics.

Health record information provides the basis for case management. **Case management** is the ongoing review of clinical care conducted during the patient's hospital stay. The purpose of case management is to ensure the necessity and quality of the services provided to the patient.

Clinicians use health record information to develop clinical pathways and other types of **clinical practice guidelines**. Clinical practice guidelines help clinicians make knowledge- and experience-based decisions on medical treatment. These guidelines make it easier to coordinate multidisciplinary care and services.

To support the patient-care function, the healthcare organization must allocate the necessary resources. An analysis of health record information helps determine appropriate staffing, plan new service lines, and forecast future demand for services or equipment acquisitions.

Quality Management and Performance Improvement

Accreditation organizations and licensing bodies expect hospitals and other healthcare organizations to strive for the highest possible quality in customer care. **Third-party payers** review the quality of care their members receive.

Quality Management
The Joint Commission (2006) uses the concept of **core measures** to assess the quality management efforts of healthcare organizations. Hospitals submit data on core patient-care areas (for example, heart failure and myocardial infarction), and the Joint Commission compares the hospital's results with those of similar facilities.

The Medicare program first established a system of quality review in 1982. Today, local **quality improvement organizations (QIOs)** work under contract with the **Centers for Medicare and Medicaid Services (CMS)**, the federal agency that administers the Medicare and Medicaid programs. QIO contracts set related targets at the state level based on a focused set of publicly reported quality measures. Healthcare organizations submit patient information collected from health records to the QIOs, which then review the appropriateness of delivered care. The QIO launched its 8th Statement of Work (SOW) in August 2005 (the 9th SOW is being readied for released in July 2008). The 8th SOW is a comprehensive document that describes the requirements for QIOs over a three-year cycle (CMS 2005). Based on these requirements, the document describes the national quality improvement projects led by CMS. These deliverables and data submission requirements assist providers in developing the capacity for achieving excellence in healthcare. The statement of work has specific tasks for providers in settings such as nursing homes, home health, hospitals, critical-access hospitals/rural PPS hospitals, and physicians' practices. In the physician practice setting, tasks are further defined to include underserved populations and pharmacies.

The mission of the program is to improve the effectiveness, efficiency, economy, and quality of services delivered to beneficiaries. For example, special projects in the hospital setting focus on acute myocardial infarction, heart failure, pneumonia, and surgical care. All these projects intend to improve patient outcomes.

Managed-care organizations and other third-party payers review information on services provided to their beneficiaries. The appropriateness and quality of care provided to customers is the focus.

Another element of quality management in the healthcare setting is the medical staff credentialing process. Credentialing is the process of reviewing and validating the qualifications of physicians who have applied for permission to treat patients in the facility. The Joint Commission (2006) established credentialing standards to guide hospitals and other healthcare organizations in the process.

Performance Improvement

Healthcare organizations systematically review processes and outcomes to ensure quality services. Many hospitals employ quality management professionals that work directly with clinical and ancillary staff to identify patient-care issues and develop process improvements. Historically, quality assurance efforts concentrated on the identification of mistakes and substandard individual performance. In contrast, present-day **performance improvement (PI)** efforts emphasize the importance of identifying the shortcomings of processes and systems rather than individuals.

Hospitals use a number of different PI models, and the models tend to go in and out of fashion rather quickly. Regardless of the chosen model, PI processes driven by patient-care information are the most effective. Currently, most healthcare organizations utilize some form of **continuous quality improvement (CQI)**. The CQI philosophy emphasizes the critical importance of three factors:

1. Knowing and meeting customer expectations

2. Reducing variation within processes

3. Relying on data to build knowledge for process improvement

CQI entails a continuous cycle of planning, measuring, and monitoring performance and making periodic knowledge-based improvements. Quality managers use a number of tools to monitor performance and identify areas for improvement. Many hospitals use a model originally developed by the Hospital Corporation of America® (LeBlanc 2006). The model is known as FOCUS-PDCA® and is based on five steps:

1. **F**ind a clinical process to improve.

2. **O**rganize a team made up of people who understand the process.

3. **C**larify the team's current knowledge of the process.

4. **U**nderstand the causes of the undesired variation.

5. **S**elect the improvement to be made in the process.

Like other CQI models, FOCUS-PDCA subsequently applies the plan–do–check–act process, which is basically a cycle of trial, measurement, and learning. During the planning phase, the PI team analyzes the process to be improved. The team identifies the process, how it currently works, who is involved, and other performance factors. Then they develop a proposed change to address the identified problem. Team members develop a system for measuring the outcomes of the proposed change to determine whether the change will actually represent an improvement. In the doing phase, the proposed improvement is implemented for a trial period, and data are collected. The checking phase involves analyzing the data that were collected. If the proposed change actually did result in a measurable improvement in the process, the cycle moves on to the action step. The change is adjusted based on the knowledge gained and/or implemented. If the proposed change had no observable effect, the team develops another solution and repeatedly goes through the entire PDCA cycle until a solution that works is identified.

Utilization Management

The process of **utilization management (UM)** focuses on how healthcare organizations use their resources. Hospital utilization management programs ensure that customers receive appropriate levels of services and that the services are performed in an efficient and cost-effective way. State and federal government regulations require hospitals to conduct utilization management reviews. Most commercial health insurance plans conduct their own UM reviews for both inpatient and outpatient services. Health record information is used as the basis for utilization management review of a healthcare organization's resources.

Utilization review (UR) is a formal process conducted to determine the medical necessity of the services provided to, or planned for, an individual patient. Determinations of **medical necessity** are based on whether the services can be expected to have a reasonably beneficial effect on the patient's physical needs and quality of life.

The Medicare *Conditions of Participation for Hospitals* specifically require acute-care facilities to perform utilization reviews for Medicare and Medicaid patients to determine the medical necessity of hospital admissions, lengths of stay, and professional services including drugs and biological substances. This process uses preestablished, objective screening criteria. The criteria are based on the severity of the patient's illness and the intensity of the services needed to effectively treat the patient's illness. Hospitals may conduct utilization review at several points before, during, and after the patient's stay to determine whether the patient's condition and need for services necessitates inpatient treatment. In most cases, the Medicare regulations permit hospitals to conduct utilization for a sample of patients rather than for every Medicare or Medicaid patient.

Risk Management

Health record information is used in risk management activities. The main purpose of risk management (RM) is prevention of situations that might put hospital patients, caregivers, or visitors in danger. Risk management includes investigating reported incidents, reviewing liability claims, and working with the hospital's legal counsel. Hospitals employ professional risk managers, who may manage the hospital's safety programs and disaster planning, depending on size and complexity of the organization.

Billing and Reimbursement

Healthcare **reimbursement** is based on the documentation contained in the health record. By referring to the records of individual patients, coding specialists identify the patients' diagnoses as well as the therapeutic procedures they underwent and the services they received. Using this information, coding specialists assign appropriate **diagnostic** and **procedural codes**. The coded information is then used to generate a patient bill and/or a claim for reimbursement to a third-party payer, such as a commercial health insurance company or government-sponsored health program such as Medicare.

Some third-party payers require billers to submit copies of portions of the health record along with the claims. The health record documentation substantiates the need for services and the fact that such services were provided (Homan 2007, 32).

A traditional principle among health information managers—"if it wasn't documented, it didn't happen"—reflects the importance of complete, timely, and accurate clinical documentation. The quality of the information in health records is especially critical because of the complexity of patient care and the potentially serious consequences incorrect or incomplete information can have for patients and caregivers. Less obvious is the effect poor quality documentation can have on the facility's ability to claim appropriate reimbursement from patients and third-party payers. This, in turn, can damage the short-term and long-term financial stability of healthcare facilities and affect their continued ability to provide high-quality patient care.

Documentation must accurately reflect the healthcare services rendered to the patient. According to Bowman (2008):

> Claims should be submitted only when appropriate documentation supporting them is present in the health record and available for audit and review. Processes for ensuring that health record documentation is adequate and appropriate to support the coded diagnoses and procedures need to be in place.

See figure 3.1 for a list of questions to challenge and improve documentation for reimbursement purposes and to help ensure compliance with federal regulations.

Ancillary Functions of the Health Record

The ancillary functions of the health record are not associated with specific patients and specific healthcare encounters, but to the environment in which patient care is provided. Accreditation, certification, and licensure processes are linked to how healthcare organizations operate, and these processes require health record information. State and federal regulations require a number of specific operational and informational reporting requirements. Biomedical research and clinical education use information in the health record, which is another example of an ancillary function.

Figure 3.1. Questions to ask when evaluating documentation.

- Is the chief complaint and/or reason for the patient encounter or hospitalization documented?
- Do the initial orders for patient care reflect the level of care to be provided?
- Is there an appropriate history and physical examination?
- Are all services that were provided documented?
- Does documentation clearly explain why support services, procedures, and supplies were provided?
- Is assessment of the patient's condition included in the documentation?
- Does documentation include information on the patient's progress and treatment outcome?
- Is there a documented treatment plan?
- Does the plan for care include, as appropriate, treatments and medications (including frequency and dosage), any referrals and consultations, patient and family education, and follow-up instructions?
- Are changes to the treatment plan, including rationale, documented?
- Is there documentation of the medical rationale for services rendered?
- Does documentation support standards for medical necessity?
- Are abnormal test results addressed in the physician documentation? If abnormal test results are returned after discharge, are they documented in an addendum, along with the action taken?
- Are relevant health risk factors identified?
- Does documentation support intensity of patient evaluation and/or treatment, including thought processes and complexity of decision making?
- Are significant changes in the patient's condition and action taken documented?
- Is the status of unresolved problems documented?
- Is planned follow-up care documented?
- Is the hospital discharge status, including transfers to another hospital or to postacute care, clearly documented? Are any plans for home health services clearly documented?
- Does documentation support the level of care provided?
- Does documentation meet the criteria for the evaluation and management code billed?
- Does the documentation for the patient encounter include an assessment, clinical impression, or diagnosis?
- Are all diagnoses and procedures documented as specifically as possible?
- Are all complications and comorbidities documented?
- Do clinical reports include all elements required by regulatory and accreditation agencies?
- Are health record entries appropriately dated and authenticated?
- Is the documentation legible?
- Is surgery done in the emergency department documented in the final progress note?
- Are symptoms used when etiologic factors are known?
- Is there a summation of the visit or hospitalization in the final progress note?
- Is the source identified for patients admitted with pathologic factors?
- Are indications for transfusions clearly documented?
- Are all cancer sites identified as primary or secondary? If there is metastasis, has the site it has spread to been documented?
- Do all diagnoses on the final progress note agree with those on the discharge summary?
- Are surgical procedures that were omitted from the final progress note on the operative record?
- Do pathology reports have findings that do not appear in the health record?
- Do medication sheets often show administration of medication without an associated diagnosis clearly documented in the health record?
- Do diagnoses on the outpatient referral form relate to the ordered test or service?
- Do physicians write "rule out" of certain conditions as the reason for the visit?

Source: Adapted from Bowman 2008, 39.

Health record data are the basis of morbidity and mortality (vital statistics) reports and healthcare-related indexes, registries, and databases. (*Morbidity* refers to illness, and *mortality* refers to death.) Much of the statistical data collected in hospital reports, indexes, registries, and databases are submitted to state, federal, and international agencies. These agencies are responsible for policy making on healthcare delivery, services, research, and education. For example, the World Health Organization, a component of the United Nations, uses record-based statistics to track the incidence of disease worldwide and to plan public health initiatives accordingly.

Accreditation, Licensure, and Certification

Hospitals and other healthcare organizations are subject to a number of practice standards. The purpose of the standards is to ensure the safety of patients and the quality of medical care. The accreditation, licensure, and certification processes that hospitals undergo are based on these standards.

Because hospitals are large, complex organizations, the processes of accreditation, licensure, and certification are complex (Shaw et al. 2003, 243–50). **Accreditation** is the process of granting formal approval to a healthcare organization. Approval is based on whether the organization meets a set of voluntary standards developed by the accrediting organization. The Joint Commission (2006) publishes operational standards for several types of healthcare organizations. The purpose of accreditation is to confirm the quality of the services provided in participating healthcare organizations. After an organization receives initial accreditation by the Joint Commission, periodic surveys further assess whether the facility continues to meet the accreditation standards. Accreditation has a number of benefits for hospitals and other healthcare organizations. After a hospital receives accreditation by the Joint Commission, Medicare automatically allows the hospital to participate in the Medicare and Medicaid programs for reimbursement purposes.

Licensure is the process of granting an organization the right to provide healthcare services. State governments establish licensure requirements. Unlike accreditation, which is a voluntary process, licensure is mandatory. Some individual healthcare practitioners are subject to state licensure requirements. For example, physicians, dentists, and nurses must obtain a license in an individual state in order to practice in that state. Specific licensure requirements are determined by state regulations and vary from state to state. However, it is illegal in all fifty states to operate healthcare facilities and practice medicine without a license.

Certification is the process of granting an organization the right to provide healthcare services to a specific group of individuals. For example, healthcare organizations must meet certain federal regulations to receive funding through the Medicare program. These regulations are published in the Medicare *Conditions of Participation* (COP).

Many individual healthcare practitioners undergo a voluntary certification process. Clinical and ancillary professional certifications are based on requirements established by specialized professional organizations. The requirements usually specify the level of education that must have been achieved, and most involve passing certification examinations. In addition, most certified professionals are required to meet continuing education requirements to maintain their credentials. For example, a physician specializing in dermatology would seek certification from the American Academy of Dermatologists. Health information management technicians and administrators are certified through the American Health Information Management Association (AHIMA).

Biomedical Research

Biomedical research is the process of systematically investigating subjects related to the functioning of the human body. Biomedical research often leads to a greater understanding of disease processes and the development of new or improved treatments and medical technologies. For example, research conducted over the past thirty years has led to the development of new drugs that control several debilitating mental illnesses, such as clinical depression and schizophrenia. Similarly, the development of endoscopic technology has revolutionized the way many surgical procedures are performed.

The goal of scientific research is to prove or disprove theoretical explanations of observable phenomena. To be valid, the results of research must be based on findings that can be reproduced in subsequent studies conducted by different research teams. The general purpose of biomedical research studies is to develop or improve treatment interventions that benefit people. Such developments are the cumulative result of multiple studies conducted over many years.

Biomedical research is usually conducted at large, urban hospitals affiliated with universities and medical schools. Funding for biomedical research comes from a number of different sources, including the federal government, pharmaceutical and medical equipment manufacturers, and charitable foundations. Many acute-care facilities are not involved in long-term research projects, although they often participate in clinical trials.

Biomedical research studies explore the safety and effectiveness of drugs, diagnostic procedures, therapeutic procedures, and disease prevention approaches. A large portion of biomedical research is conducted on the microscopic level or with nonhuman subjects. However, many biomedical research studies involve human subjects directly, or they study clinical cases gleaned from health records.

Studies that involve human subjects must meet federal and international ethical guidelines. The guidelines are intended to protect the welfare of human subjects. In the United States, the *Belmont Report: Ethical Principles and Guidelines for the Protection of Human Subjects of Biomedical and Behavioral Research*, first released in 1979, is still applicable. Internationally, the Declaration of Helsinki represents the ethical principles to be followed in biomedical studies involving biological specimens or medical data that come from an identifiable human source (Osborn 2006).

Federal regulations require that researchers provide human subjects with specific information before biomedical studies are initiated. The information is meant to make it possible for the subjects to give their **informed consent** to participation. (See figure 3.2.) This information must include at least the following:

- A statement that the study involves research, describes the purpose of the research, the expected duration of the subject's participation, a description of the procedures to be followed, and identification of any experimental procedures involved

- A description of any reasonably foreseeable risks or discomforts

- A description of the possible benefits to the subject or others

- A disclosure of any alternative procedures or courses of treatment that might benefit the subject

- A statement that describes the level of **confidentiality** that will be applied to any records that identify the subject

- An explanation of the compensation or medical treatment available to address possible injuries during the study if the study involves more than minimal risk for the subject

- An explanation of where information is available if the subject is injured during the study and a contact who will answer questions about the research or the subject's rights

- A statement explaining that participation is voluntary, that refusal to participate will involve no penalties or loss of benefits, and that the subject may discontinue participation at any time (FDA 2006)

Figure 3.2. Template for informed consent for research involving human subjects.

Consent to Investigational Treatment or Procedure

I, _____ , hereby authorize or direct _____
or associates of his/her choosing to perform the following treatment or procedure (describe in general terms), upon _____ (myself).

The experimental (research) portion of the treatment or procedure is:

This is part of an investigation entitled:

1. Purpose of the procedure or treatment:

2. Possible appropriate alternative procedure or treatment (not to participate in the study is always an option):

3. Discomforts and risks reasonably to be expected:

4. Possible benefits for subjects/society:

5. Anticipated duration of subject's participation (including number of visits):

I hereby acknowledge that _____ has provided information about the procedure described above, about my rights as a subject, and he/she answered all questions to my satisfaction. I understand that I may contact him/her at phone no. _____ should I have additional questions. He/she has explained the risks described above, and I understand them; he/she has also offered to explain all possible risks or complications.

I understand that, where appropriate, the U.S. Food and Drug Administration may inspect records pertaining to this study. I understand further that records obtained during my participation in this study that may contain my name or other personal identifiers may be made available to the sponsor of this study. Beyond this, I understand that my participation will remain confidential.

I understand that I am free to withdraw my consent and participation in this project at any time after notifying the project director without prejudicing future care. No guarantee has been given to me concerning this treatment or procedure.

I understand that in signing this form that, beyond giving consent, I am not waiving any legal rights that I might have, and I am not releasing the investigator, the sponsor, the institution, or its agents from any legal liability for damages that they might otherwise have.

In the event of injury resulting from participation in this study, I also understand that immediate medical treatment is available at _____ and that the costs of such treatment will be at my expense; financial compensation beyond that required by law is not available. Questions about this should be directed to the Office of Research Risks at _____ .

I have read and fully understand the consent form. I sign it freely and voluntarily. A copy has been given to me.

_____   _____
Signature   Date

Source: Osborn 2006, 524.

The Joint Commission has specific standards related to research and clinical trials conducted in hospitals. Joint Commission standards are similar to the federal regulations on human research. To meet the accreditation standards, the consent form must include the name of the person who provided the information, date signed, and an acknowledgment of the patient's right to **privacy**, confidentiality, and safety. Any information given to the patient along with the informed consent form must be documented in the patient's health record or research file (Joint Commission 2006).

Education

Health records are used as educational tools by medical schools, dental schools, nursing schools, and allied health training programs. The case studies derived from health record information provide real-world experience for students. Case studies are useful for in-service training for all of the health professions, including health information management.

Medical Staff Appointments and Privileges

Physicians directly perform or manage the medical/surgical care provided to patients in an acute-care setting. Except in teaching hospitals, most of the physicians who provide medical or surgical services in hospitals are independent practitioners. This means they are not employees or agents of the hospital. However, hospitals assume accountability for the quality of all medical treatment provided to inpatients and outpatients in their facilities. For example, presume a physician who is not qualified to perform orthopedic surgery treats a patient with a broken leg in the emergency department of a hospital. If the physician injures the patient by providing substandard care, both the physician and hospital have joint liability for the patient's injury. This case represents an example of **corporate negligence**, a legal doctrine that was established by a judicial decision handed down in a 1965 court case.

In *Darling v. Charleston Community Hospital* (1965), the court ruled specifically that hospital governing boards have a "duty to establish mechanisms for the medical staff to evaluate, counsel, and when necessary, take action against an unreasonable risk of harm to a patient arising from the patient's treatment by a personal physician" (Pozar 1999, 198). The court's ruling established the hospital's obligation to appoint only highly qualified practitioners to the medical staff. Owing to that obligation, hospitals may be held liable when a member of the medical staff fails to meet established standards of patient care.

Most states have statutes that regulate the medical staff appointment processes. In addition, accreditation programs generally require hospitals to confirm the qualifications of practitioners before clinicians are given the right to practice in the facilities.

Hospital governing boards (sometimes called boards of directors or trustees) are legally responsible for the overall operation of a hospital. Every hospital's governing board has a duty to establish medical staff policies to ensure that unqualified practitioners do not provide medical services in the facility. These policies establish a hospital's medical staff qualification criteria and process.

Physicians and other clinical practitioners who wish to practice in a hospital must first become members of that hospital's medical staff. Although the governing board considers the recommendations of medical staff leaders in making medical staff appointments, the ultimate responsibility for such decisions rests with the board.

The governing board generally relies on the hospital's medical staff leaders to manage independent clinical practitioners by implementing medical staff bylaws. **Medical staff bylaws** describe the rights and responsibilities of individual members and the means by which medical staff leaders govern the conduct of members.

Credentialing Process

Before making medical staff appointments and reappointments, hospitals evaluate the qualifications of physicians, surgeons, podiatrists, dentists, clinical psychologists, and other practitioners through a systematic process called credentialing. **Credentialing** involves the review and validation of an individual practitioner's qualifications to practice medicine. (See figure 3.3.)

Initial credentialing reviews typically include the following types of information:

- Verifications of the applicant's undergraduate, medical, and postdoctoral education
- Verifications of the applicant's residency and fellowship training as well as continuing medical education
- Past and current medical staff appointments at other facilities
- Current state licenses to practice medicine
- Current specialty board certifications
- Current Drug Enforcement Administration registration
- Documentation of professional liability insurance
- References and recommendations from the applicant's professional peers
- Information on the applicant's health status
- Past and current liability status

As part of every medical staff appointment process, hospitals and other healthcare organizations are required by federal law to send inquiries to two national databases: the **National Practitioner Data Bank (NPDB)** and the **Healthcare Integrity and Protection Data Bank (HIPDB)**. The NPDB collects information on medical malpractice settlements, clinical privilege actions, and medical society actions taken against licensed healthcare providers in the United States. The HIPDB collects information on legal actions taken against licensed healthcare providers, including both civil judgments and criminal convictions.

The hospital's medical staff executive committee reviews a practitioner's application after verifying credentials and determining that the practitioner meets established medical staff qualification criteria. The committee subsequently submits its recommendation to the governing board for final action.

Privileging Process

With the board's approval, the hospital grants the practitioner medical staff privileges. These **clinical privileges** authorize the practitioner to provide patient services in the hospital, but only those specific services that fall within his or her area of medical expertise. For example, a cardiovascular surgeon's clinical privileges would allow him or her to perform cardiac bypass surgery but not cataract surgery. Medical staff members typically must submit applications for reappointment to the medical staff every two years.

Reappointments include a review of the practitioner's current qualifications and require new queries to the NPDB and HIPDB. Hospitals consider how often the practitioner used his or her privileges during the preceding period to determine whether the practitioner is still proficient in the clinical services for which he or she is seeking privileges. Outcome data reviewed for the practitioner's patients along with peer review information help determine continuing privileges.

Figure 3.3. Credentialing and privileging processes.

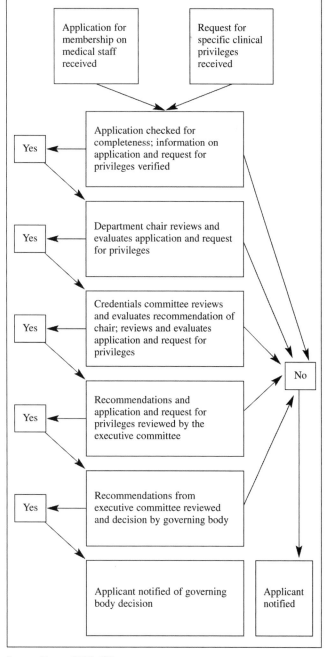

Source: Zeman 2006, 506.

Reappointment decisions consider whether the practitioner fulfilled his or her administrative responsibilities as specified in the hospital's medical staff bylaws. For example, medical staff bylaws may require members to attend a specific percentage of medical staff meetings or participation on medical staff committees.

Medical staff reappointments review the practitioner's medical record delinquency status. Practitioners who have consistently high delinquency rates may lose their medical staff privileges as a result.

Risk Management and Incident Reporting

Although hospitals and caregivers make every effort to ensure the safety of patients, visitors, and staff, unforeseen events can occur. Whether the consequence of accidents or mistakes, some of these unforeseen events inevitably result in serious and sometimes fatal injuries.

Hospitals devise systems for responding to such events and taking steps to prevent similar problems in the future. Several terms are used to describe unforeseen events that lead to injuries and other losses, including *incidents, adverse events, potentially compensable events,* and *adverse occurrences.* The Joint Commission (2006) uses the term *sentinel event* to describe such events and requests that the most serious events be reported to the Joint Commission as well as to government agencies as required by federal or state law. Hospitals develop internal reporting processes to help identify risks within the organization. Internal and external reporting procedures are part of every hospital's risk management program.

Risk management (RM) is the process of overseeing the hospital's internal medical, legal, and administrative operations with the goal of minimizing the hospital's exposure to liability. In this context, *risk* is a formal insurance term referring to situations that may lead to liability claims. **Liability** is the legal responsibility to compensate individuals for injuries and losses sustained as the result of negligence.

Medical records constitute the hospital's legal record of the services provided to individual patients from the time they are admitted until they are discharged. Health record documentation must be objective and based on actual observations rather than on opinions and conjecture.

Like other events and outcomes during the patient's stay in the hospital, adverse events must be completely and accurately described in the patient's health record. However, it is extremely important that the health record documentation of adverse events remains entirely objective, with no comments from caregivers that suggest blame or speculate on causation.

Hospital internal risk management policies usually define the circumstances that constitute a reportable **incident** (an event that is considered to be inconsistent with accepted standards of care). Policies should address the steps to be taken in response to an incident. Most hospitals institute policies that require the preparation of incident reports. Some facilities use the terms *occurrence* and *occurrence report* in this context.

An **incident report** describes the occurrence (time, date, and location); identifies the individual(s) involved (patients, visitors, and/or staff); and the current condition of the individual(s) who were affected. The report should include statements from witnesses and be completed as soon as possible after the incident to ensure accuracy and completeness.

Incident reports are prepared for risk management, performance improvement, and staff education purposes but not for direct patient care. The report contains subjective information from witnesses and individuals involved in the incident. For these reasons, incident reports must never be included or mentioned in a patient's legal health record. Instead, incident reports should be stored in separate, secure databases or files in the facility's risk management or performance improvement department. In anticipation of future court action, incident reports should be marked as confidential and addressed to the hospital's attorney. Incident reports should not be disseminated internally or externally to anyone other than the individuals designated by the hospital's risk management policies (McWay 2002, 181–182). Incident reports are not disseminated because of the risk of copies being filed in another file, which would cause them to become discoverable. When kept as discussed, incident reports are generally not discoverable.

Health Records as Legal Documents

The health record is generally considered a business record, and as such, its contents are admissible as evidence in legal proceedings. Patients who have been treated for injuries related to automobile accidents or violent crimes often become involved in private liability lawsuits or criminal court cases. Patients suffering from employment-related injuries or illnesses may file workers' compensation claims. Sometimes malpractice lawsuits are filed against physicians, hospitals, and other healthcare providers by patients or their families who believe they have been harmed by medical mistakes. Information documented in the health record plays a critical part in the decisions eventually handed down by judges and juries. Because many court cases do not go to trial until years after the original events, the written documentation in health records may be the only reliable information available. For this reason, the importance of complete and accurate health records cannot be overemphasized.

In order for healthcare information to be considered admissible in court, it must represent the health record of one of the persons involved in the legal proceedings. In other words, the contents of the record must be relevant to the issue being decided. Patient authorization or notification is not required for disclosures related to legal proceedings when the proper subpoena or court order is presented.

Legal Proceedings

The contents of health records constitute the healthcare organization's legal business record. In order for a health record to be admissible as evidence, four basic principles must be met.

1. The record must be documented in the normal course of business.

2. The record must be kept in the regular course of business.

3. The record must be created at or near the time that the events occurred.

4. The record must be created by a person within the business with knowledge of the acts, events, conditions, and observations described in the record.

Generally, statements made outside the court by a party in a lawsuit are considered hearsay and not admissible as evidence. Documentation in the health record is technically hearsay; however, Federal Rules of Evidence (803[6]) and the Uniform Business and Public Records Act adopted by most states allow exception to the hearsay rule for records maintained in the regular course of business, including health records. All records must be identified and authenticated prior to admissibility in court (AHIMA e-HIM Work Group 2005a). (See appendix D on the accompanying CD.)

These conditions apply to both paper-based health records and electronic health records as long as the records are shown to be accurate and trustworthy. To be considered trustworthy, records must be secured in a manner that protects them from tampering. The health record is admissible because it passes the business rule of evidence and is not considered hearsay in a court of law. (See figure 3.4 for additional guidelines.)

Personal injury lawsuits and other legal proceedings are often conducted long after the original events take place. Oftentimes, eyewitness testimony is contradictory and written evidence is more reliable. The patient's health record usually provides reliable evidence to substantiate the care and treatment that the patient receives. Incomplete or illegible documentation can lead to judgments against the facility and caregivers.

Figure 3.4. General documentation guidelines for legal purposes.

- The organization's health record policies must stipulate the persons who are authorized to make entries in the health record.
- Every page or screen in the health record must be identified with the patient's name and health record number.
- Health record entries must be made as soon as possible after the observation or event occurred.
- Health record entries must indicate the actual time and date (month, day, and year) when each entry was made. (Predating and postdating are both unethical and illegal.)
- The language used in health record entries must be specific, factual, and objective. (Opinions and speculations must not be included.)
- Health record entries must include all of the pertinent facts and information related to the observation or event being described.
- Health record policy must include a list of the abbreviations that may be used in the health record. The list must include definitions for the abbreviations, and only acceptable abbreviations must be allowed in the documentation.
- Health record entries must be legible and permanent whether they are handwritten, computer generated, or electronic. Policies must be in place to protect health records from alteration, tampering, and loss.
- In paper-based health records, entries must be continuous (no gaps or extra spacing between entries). Blank lines in forms must be crossed out.
- All of the data fields on assessments, flowsheets, and checklists must be completed even when one or more of the fields does not apply to the patient. (Dashes or the abbreviation NA, for not applicable, can be entered in blanks to prevent tampering.)
- Entries must be consistent with previous entries. Any contradictions must be explained.
- Every change in the patient's condition and all significant treatment issues must be noted until the patient's condition becomes stable or the treatment issue is resolved. Documentation must provide evidence of follow through.
- The patient's informed consent for procedures and treatment must be documented in the health record.
- The patient's initial admission note and discharge summary must fully and accurately describe the patient's condition at that time.
- All communications and attempts at communication with the patient's family and personal physician must be documented.
- The charge nurse or nurse manager must ensure the consistency and completeness of all health record entries made by patient care technicians and other clinical staff with delegated responsibilities.
- The facts behind any adverse incidents must be documented in the progress notes. However, no mention of an incident report should be made in the health record.
- The authors of health record documentation must create and sign their own entries in both paper-based and electronic health record systems. Authors must never create or sign entries on behalf of another author.
- Health record entries must contain nothing other than documentation that pertains to the direct care of the patient (no personal statements or complaints).
- When it is necessary to refer to another patient in describing an event, the other patient's health record number must be used in place of his or her name.
- Every health record entry must be authenticated. The healthcare organization's health record authentication policy must stipulate the manner in which handwritten signatures, electronic signatures, fax signatures, or rubber-stamp signatures are to be used.
- When countersignatures are required by state regulations, only qualified persons must countersign health record entries.
- The healthcare organization's health record policies must stipulate the process that is to be followed to correct errors in health record entries.
- Late entries must include the time and date the late entry was entered into the health record, not the date when the entry should have been made.
- Health records must never be removed from the healthcare facility except in response to a legitimate court order or subpoena.

Source: Dougherty 2002.

Subpoenas and Court Orders

When the court has determined that a health record is relevant to a particular case, the judge will issue a subpoena or a court order to the owner of the record. A **subpoena** is a direct command that requires an individual or a representative of an organization to appear in court and/or to present an object to the court. In the healthcare context, a **subpoena duces tecum** directs a hospital's representative (usually the director of health information management) to submit a specific health record or other business record to the court that holds jurisdiction over the pending proceedings. With the advice of legal counsel, an HIM director may decide that it is inappropriate for the hospital to release a subpoenaed record. In such cases, a **court order** must be issued in place of a subpoena when the disclosure of the material would otherwise be prohibited by state or federal statutes or regulations (McWay 2002, 139, 142).

The method used to respond to subpoenas and court orders depends on the regulations in force for the state in which the court is located. Some states allow hospitals to make certified copies of the health records in question and mail the copies to the clerk of the court or to another designated individual. In other states, a representative of the hospital must deliver the original records in person and then testify to their authenticity.

e-Discovery

This section was adapted from Kimberly Baldwin-Stried Reich's article "Developing a Litigation Response Plan," originally published in the October 2007 issue of the *Journal of American Health Information Management Association*.

The e-discovery amendments to the **Federal Rules of Civil Procedure (FRCP)** (updated in 2006) and the Uniform Rules Relating to the Discovery of Electronically Stored Information (2007) (approved in August 2007 at the National Conference of Commissioners on Uniform State Laws) are creating new responsibilities for legal counsel and HIM professionals. Organizations must begin thinking about how they will respond to e-discovery requests for information. The process by which electronic information is produced in response to threatened or impending litigation is changing, and those closely involved with it must be knowledgeable on the requirements for producing information.

The Advisory Committee on the Rules of Civil Procedure amended the FRCP to specifically address **e-discovery**, or the discovery and production of electronically stored information. Congress established the legal rules that dictate allowable methods for discovery at the federal court level. The FRCP, state legislative efforts regarding e-discovery, and the Uniform Rules Related to the Discovery of Electronically Stored Information (2007) will soon define the e-discovery process for all healthcare organizations. Legal counsels throughout the country are becoming educated about e-discovery, information systems, and records management, all in an effort to protect organizations and their information. As a result, discussion of HIM operations has moved to the boardroom, and HIM professionals are in a unique position to help shape and design their organizations' e-discovery processes.

In general terms, *discovery* is the formal pretrial legal process used by parties in a lawsuit to obtain information. Discovery helps ensure that neither party is subjected to surprises at trial. The scope of information that can be obtained through discovery is broad and is not limited to what will be used at trial. Federal courts and most state courts allow a party to discover any information relevant to the claim. Because of the broad nature of this standard, parties often disagree about what information must be exchanged and what is considered "privileged." These disputes are resolved through court rulings on discovery motions.

Historically, discovery encompassed the production of relevant information or paper documents. This information is generally produced after a subpoena or subpoena duces tecum has been served upon an individual or organization. Other common discovery devices include depositions, interrogatories, requests for admissions, document production requests, and requests for inspection of records. The legal process involving the discovery of electronically stored information varies significantly from the discovery process that legal HIM professionals know today. Federal Rules of Civil Procedure sections 16, 26, and 34 compel parties and their counsel to enter into early discussion of key issues about discovery of electronically stored information. As a result, it is incumbent upon legal counsel and HIM and information technology (IT) professionals to evaluate how their roles and responsibilities will change with regard to the production and discovery of electronically stored information.

The basic principles regarding preservation of relevant electronically stored information are essentially the same as those governing the preservation of relevant paper-based business records. That is, at the moment when litigation is reasonably anticipated (known, threatened, or pending), the normal disposition and processing of information in either format should be suspended. The duty to preserve relevant electronically stored information also supersedes an organization's record retention and management policies that would normally result in the destruction of electronically stored information.

Once litigation can be reasonably anticipated, an organization should establish a legal (litigation) hold, and reasonable measures should be taken to identify and preserve all information relevant to the claim. A legal hold (also known as a preservation order) may or may not be issued by a court. An organization's key determination in establishing a legal hold is when litigation is "reasonably anticipated." For example, once an individual or organization is served with a complaint, subpoena, subpoena duces tecum, or receives notice of a government investigation, litigation can be reasonably anticipated. A legal hold should then be immediately established and reasonable measures taken to identify and preserve relevant information. The duty to preserve could arise well before an individual or organization is served with any of these documents or notices. Determining when the legal hold should be established is not a rote decision. When faced with potential litigation, the facts of each situation must be carefully weighed.

Morbidity and Mortality Reporting

In the United States, official vital statistics are maintained under the **National Vital Statistics System (NVSS)**. The NVSS is a federal agency that operates within the **Centers for Disease Control and Prevention (CDC)**. The CDC is a group of federal agencies that oversee health promotion and disease control and prevention activities in the United States. Vital statistics include data on the number of births and deaths that occur during a calendar year. Hospitals and other healthcare providers report the births and deaths in their facilities to designated state authorities. Most states have their own reporting requirements for vital statistics. State authorities report the required statistics to the NVSS. State and federal agencies collect and report other types of morbidity and mortality data submitted by healthcare providers. The source of all this data is the health record.

To ensure consistency in data collection, standard forms and procedures are provided by the NVSS. Data collection forms are revised about every ten years. Standard forms include the U.S. Standard Certificate of Live Birth (figure 3.5), the U.S. Standard Certificate of Death (figure 3.6), and the U.S. Standard Report of Induced Termination of Pregnancy (1988) (figure 3.7). The U.S. Standard Report for Fetal Deaths is very similar to the certificate of live birth (CDC 2003).

Figure 3.5.   U.S. standard certificate of live birth.

U.S. STANDARD CERTIFICATE OF LIVE BIRTH

LOCAL FILE NO.   BIRTH NUMBER:

CHILD

| 1. CHILD'S NAME (First, Middle, Last, Suffix) | 2. TIME OF BIRTH (24 hr) | 3. SEX | 4. DATE OF BIRTH (Mo/Day/Yr) |

5. FACILITY NAME (If not institution, give street and number)   6. CITY, TOWN, OR LOCATION OF BIRTH   7. COUNTY OF BIRTH

MOTHER

8a. MOTHER'S CURRENT LEGAL NAME (First, Middle, Last, Suffix)   8b. DATE OF BIRTH (Mo/Day/Yr)

8c. MOTHER'S NAME PRIOR TO FIRST MARRIAGE (First, Middle, Last, Suffix)   8d. BIRTHPLACE (State, Territory, or Foreign Country)

9a. RESIDENCE OF MOTHER-STATE   9b. COUNTY   9c. CITY, TOWN, OR LOCATION

9d. STREET AND NUMBER   9e. APT. NO.   9f. ZIP CODE   9g. INSIDE CITY LIMITS?   □ Yes □ No

FATHER

10a. FATHER'S CURRENT LEGAL NAME (First, Middle, Last, Suffix)   10b. DATE OF BIRTH (Mo/Day/Yr)   10c. BIRTHPLACE (State, Territory, or Foreign Country)

CERTIFIER

11. CERTIFIER'S NAME: _____

TITLE: □ MD   □ DO   □ HOSPITAL ADMIN.   □ CNM/CM   □ OTHER MIDWIFE

  □ OTHER (Specify)_____

12. DATE CERTIFIED   ____/____/____   MM DD YYYY

13. DATE FILED BY REGISTRAR   ____/____/____   MM DD YYYY

INFORMATION FOR ADMINISTRATIVE USE

MOTHER

14. MOTHER'S MAILING ADDRESS: 9 Same as residence, or: State: City, Town, or Location:

Street & Number: Apartment No.:   Zip Code:

15. MOTHER MARRIED? (At birth, conception, or any time between)   □ Yes   □ No
IF NO, HAS PATERNITY ACKNOWLEDGEMENT BEEN SIGNED IN THE HOSPITAL? □ Yes   □ No

16. SOCIAL SECURITY NUMBER REQUESTED FOR CHILD?   □ Yes   □ No

17. FACILITY ID. (NPI)

18. MOTHER'S SOCIAL SECURITY NUMBER: 19. FATHER'S SOCIAL SECURITY NUMBER:

INFORMATION FOR MEDICAL AND HEALTH PURPOSES ONLY

MOTHER

20. MOTHER'S EDUCATION (Check the box that best describes the highest degree or level of school completed at the time of delivery)	21. MOTHER OF HISPANIC ORIGIN? (Check the box that best describes whether the mother is Spanish/Hispanic/Latina. Check the "No" box if mother is not Spanish/Hispanic/Latina)	22. MOTHER'S RACE (Check one or more races to indicate what the mother considers herself to be)
□ 8th grade or less	□ No, not Spanish/Hispanic/Latina	□ White
□ 9th - 12th grade, no diploma	□ Yes, Mexican, Mexican American, Chicana	□ Black or African American
□ High school graduate or GED completed	□ Yes, Puerto Rican	□ American Indian or Alaska Native (Name of the enrolled or principal tribe)_____
□ Some college credit but no degree	□ Yes, Cuban	□ Asian Indian
□ Associate degree (e.g., AA, AS)	□ Yes, other Spanish/Hispanic/Latina	□ Chinese
□ Bachelor's degree (e.g., BA, AB, BS)	(Specify)_____	□ Filipino
□ Master's degree (e.g., MA, MS, MEng, MEd, MSW, MBA)		□ Japanese
□ Doctorate (e.g., PhD, EdD) or Professional degree (e.g., MD, DDS, DVM, LLB, JD)		□ Korean
		□ Vietnamese
		□ Other Asian (Specify)_____
		□ Native Hawaiian
		□ Guamanian or Chamorro
		□ Samoan
		□ Other Pacific Islander (Specify)_____
		□ Other (Specify)_____

FATHER

23. FATHER'S EDUCATION (Check the box that best describes the highest degree or level of school completed at the time of delivery)	24. FATHER OF HISPANIC ORIGIN? (Check the box that best describes whether the father is Spanish/Hispanic/Latino. Check the "No" box if father is not Spanish/Hispanic/Latino)	25. FATHER'S RACE (Check one or more races to indicate what the father considers himself to be)
□ 8th grade or less	□ No, not Spanish/Hispanic/Latino	□ White
□ 9th - 12th grade, no diploma	□ Yes, Mexican, Mexican American, Chicano	□ Black or African American
□ High school graduate or GED completed	□ Yes, Puerto Rican	□ American Indian or Alaska Native (Name of the enrolled or principal tribe)_____
□ Some college credit but no degree	□ Yes, Cuban	□ Asian Indian
□ Associate degree (e.g., AA, AS)	□ Yes, other Spanish/Hispanic/Latino	□ Chinese
□ Bachelor's degree (e.g., BA, AB, BS)	(Specify)_____	□ Filipino
□ Master's degree (e.g., MA, MS, MEng, MEd, MSW, MBA)		□ Japanese
□ Doctorate (e.g., PhD, EdD) or Professional degree (e.g., MD, DDS, DVM, LLB, JD)		□ Korean
		□ Vietnamese
		□ Other Asian (Specify)_____
		□ Native Hawaiian
		□ Guamanian or Chamorro
		□ Samoan
		□ Other Pacific Islander (Specify)_____
		□ Other (Specify)_____

Mother's Name

Mother's Medical Record No.

26. PLACE WHERE BIRTH OCCURRED (Check one)	27. ATTENDANT'S NAME, TITLE, AND NPI	28. MOTHER TRANSFERRED FOR MATERNAL MEDICAL OR FETAL INDICATIONS FOR DELIVERY? □ Yes □ No
□ Hospital	NAME: _____ NPI:_____	IF YES, ENTER NAME OF FACILITY MOTHER TRANSFERRED FROM:
□ Freestanding birthing center		
□ Home Birth: Planned to deliver at home? 9 Yes 9 No	TITLE: □ MD □ DO □ CNM/CM □ OTHER MIDWIFE	_____
□ Clinic/Doctor's office	□ OTHER (Specify)_____	
□ Other (Specify)_____		

REV. 11/2003

Figure 3.5. *(continued)*

MOTHER	29a. DATE OF FIRST PRENATAL CARE VISIT ___ / ___ / ___ M M D D YYYY □ No Prenatal Care	29b. DATE OF LAST PRENATAL CARE VISIT ___ / ___ / ___ M M D D YYYY	30. TOTAL NUMBER OF PRENATAL VISITS FOR THIS PREGNANCY _____ (If none, enter "0".)

31. MOTHER'S HEIGHT _____ (feet/inches)	32. MOTHER'S PREPREGNANCY WEIGHT _____ (pounds)	33. MOTHER'S WEIGHT AT DELIVERY _____ (pounds)	34. DID MOTHER GET WIC FOOD FOR HERSELF DURING THIS PREGNANCY? □ Yes □ No

35. NUMBER OF PREVIOUS LIVE BIRTHS (Do not include this child)		36. NUMBER OF OTHER PREGNANCY OUTCOMES (spontaneous or induced losses or ectopic pregnancies)	37. CIGARETTE SMOKING BEFORE AND DURING PREGNANCY For each time period, enter either the number of cigarettes or the number of packs of cigarettes smoked. IF NONE, ENTER "0".	38. PRINCIPAL SOURCE OF PAYMENT FOR THIS DELIVERY
35a. Now Living Number _____ □ None	35b. Now Dead Number _____ □ None	36a. Other Outcomes Number _____ □ None	Average number of cigarettes or packs of cigarettes smoked per day. # of cigarettes # of packs Three Months Before Pregnancy _____ OR _____ First Three Months of Pregnancy _____ OR _____ Second Three Months of Pregnancy _____ OR _____ Third Trimester of Pregnancy _____ OR _____	□ Private Insurance □ Medicaid □ Self-pay □ Other (Specify) _____

35c. DATE OF LAST LIVE BIRTH ___ / ___ MM Y Y Y Y	36b. DATE OF LAST OTHER PREGNANCY OUTCOME ___ / ___ MM Y Y Y Y	39. DATE LAST NORMAL MENSES BEGAN ___ / ___ / ___ M M D D YYYY	40. MOTHER'S MEDICAL RECORD NUMBER

MEDICAL AND HEALTH INFORMATION	41. RISK FACTORS IN THIS PREGNANCY (Check all that apply)
	Diabetes
	  □ Prepregnancy (Diagnosis prior to this pregnancy)
	  □ Gestational (Diagnosis in this pregnancy)
	
	Hypertension
	  □ Prepregnancy (Chronic)
	  □ Gestational (PIH, preeclampsia)
	  □ Eclampsia
	
	□ Previous preterm birth
	
	□ Other previous poor pregnancy outcome (Includes perinatal death, small-for-gestational age/intrauterine growth restricted birth)
	
	□ Pregnancy resulted from infertility treatment-If yes, check all that apply:
	  □ Fertility-enhancing drugs, Artificial insemination or Intrauterine insemination
	  □ Assisted reproductive technology (e.g., in vitro fertilization (IVF), gamete intrafallopian transfer (GIFT))
	
	□ Mother had a previous cesarean delivery
	  If yes, how many _____
	
	□ None of the above
	
	42. INFECTIONS PRESENT AND/OR TREATED DURING THIS PREGNANCY (Check all that apply)
	
	□ Gonorrhea
	□ Syphilis
	□ Chlamydia
	□ Hepatitis B
	□ Hepatitis C
	□ None of the above
		43. OBSTETRIC PROCEDURES (Check all that apply)
		
		□ Cervical cerclage
		□ Tocolysis
		
		External cephalic version:
		  □ Successful
		  □ Failed
		
		□ None of the above
		
		44. ONSET OF LABOR (Check all that apply)
		
		□ Premature Rupture of the Membranes (prolonged, ∃12 hrs.)
		
		□ Precipitous Labor (<3 hrs.)
		
		□ Prolonged Labor (∃ 20 hrs.)
		
		□ None of the above
		
		45. CHARACTERISTICS OF LABOR AND DELIVERY (Check all that apply)
		
		□ Induction of labor
		□ Augmentation of labor
		□ Non-vertex presentation
		□ Steroids (glucocorticoids) for fetal lung maturation received by the mother prior to delivery
		□ Antibiotics received by the mother during labor
		□ Clinical chorioamnionitis diagnosed during labor or maternal temperature ≥38°C (100.4°F)
		□ Moderate/heavy meconium staining of the amniotic fluid
		□ Fetal intolerance of labor such that one or more of the following actions was taken: in-utero resuscitative measures, further fetal assessment, or operative delivery
		□ Epidural or spinal anesthesia during labor
		□ None of the above
			46. METHOD OF DELIVERY
			
			A. Was delivery with forceps attempted but unsuccessful?
			  □ Yes □ No
			
			B. Was delivery with vacuum extraction attempted but unsuccessful?
			  □ Yes □ No
			
			C. Fetal presentation at birth
			  □ Cephalic
			  □ Breech
			  □ Other
			
			D. Final route and method of delivery (Check one)
			  □ Vaginal/Spontaneous
			  □ Vaginal/Forceps
			  □ Vaginal/Vacuum
			  □ Cesarean
			    If cesarean, was a trial of labor attempted?
			    □ Yes
			    □ No
			
			47. MATERNAL MORBIDITY (Check all that apply) (Complications associated with labor and delivery)
			□ Maternal transfusion
			□ Third or fourth degree perineal laceration
			□ Ruptured uterus
			□ Unplanned hysterectomy
			□ Admission to intensive care unit
			□ Unplanned operating room procedure following delivery
			□ None of the above

NEWBORN INFORMATION

NEWBORN	48. NEWBORN MEDICAL RECORD NUMBER
	
	49. BIRTHWEIGHT (grams preferred, specify unit)
	
	_____ 9 grams 9 lb/oz
	
	50. OBSTETRIC ESTIMATE OF GESTATION:
	
	_____ (completed weeks)
	
	51. APGAR SCORE:
	Score at 5 minutes: _____
	If 5 minute score is less than 6,
	Score at 10 minutes: _____
	
	52. PLURALITY - Single, Twin, Triplet, etc.
	
	(Specify) _____
	
	53. IF NOT SINGLE BIRTH - Born First, Second, Third, etc. (Specify) _____
		54. ABNORMAL CONDITIONS OF THE NEWBORN (Check all that apply)
		
		□ Assisted ventilation required immediately following delivery
		
		□ Assisted ventilation required for more than six hours
		
		□ NICU admission
		
		□ Newborn given surfactant replacement therapy
		
		□ Antibiotics received by the newborn for suspected neonatal sepsis
		
		□ Seizure or serious neurologic dysfunction
		
		□ Significant birth injury (skeletal fracture(s), peripheral nerve injury, and/or soft tissue/solid organ hemorrhage which requires intervention)
		
		9 None of the above
			55. CONGENITAL ANOMALIES OF THE NEWBORN (Check all that apply)
			
			□ Anencephaly
			□ Meningomyelocele/Spina bifida
			□ Cyanotic congenital heart disease
			□ Congenital diaphragmatic hernia
			□ Omphalocele
			□ Gastroschisis
			□ Limb reduction defect (excluding congenital amputation and dwarfing syndromes)
			□ Cleft Lip with or without Cleft Palate
			□ Cleft Palate alone
			□ Down Syndrome
			  □ Karyotype confirmed
			  □ Karyotype pending
			□ Suspected chromosomal disorder
			  □ Karyotype confirmed
			  □ Karyotype pending
			□ Hypospadias
			□ None of the anomalies listed above

56. WAS INFANT TRANSFERRED WITHIN 24 HOURS OF DELIVERY? 9 Yes 9 No IF YES, NAME OF FACILITY INFANT TRANSFERRED TO: _____	57. IS INFANT LIVING AT TIME OF REPORT? □ Yes □ No □ Infant transferred, status unknown	58. IS THE INFANT BEING BREASTFED AT DISCHARGE? □ Yes □ No

Mother's Name   *Mother's Medical Record No.* _____

Source: CDC 2003.

Figure 3.6.   U.S. standard certificate of death.

U.S. STANDARD CERTIFICATE OF DEATH

LOCAL FILE NO.   STATE FILE NO.

NAME OF DECEDENT — For use by physician or institution

To Be Completed/ Verified By: FUNERAL DIRECTOR:

1. DECEDENT'S LEGAL NAME (Include AKA's if any) (First, Middle, Last)	2. SEX 3. SOCIAL SECURITY NUMBER

4a. AGE-Last Birthday (Years) | 4b. UNDER 1 YEAR — Months / Days | 4c. UNDER 1 DAY — Hours / Minutes | 5. DATE OF BIRTH (Mo/Day/Yr) | 6. BIRTHPLACE (City and State or Foreign Country)

7a. RESIDENCE-STATE | 7b. COUNTY | 7c. CITY OR TOWN

7d. STREET AND NUMBER | 7e. APT. NO. | 7f. ZIP CODE | 7g. INSIDE CITY LIMITS? ☐ Yes ☐ No

8. EVER IN US ARMED FORCES? ☐ Yes ☐ No | 9. MARITAL STATUS AT TIME OF DEATH ☐ Married ☐ Married, but separated ☐ Widowed ☐ Divorced ☐ Never Married ☐ Unknown | 10. SURVIVING SPOUSE'S NAME (If wife, give name prior to first marriage)

11. FATHER'S NAME (First, Middle, Last) | 12. MOTHER'S NAME PRIOR TO FIRST MARRIAGE (First, Middle, Last)

13a. INFORMANT'S NAME | 13b. RELATIONSHIP TO DECEDENT | 13c. MAILING ADDRESS (Street and Number, City, State, Zip Code)

14. PLACE OF DEATH (Check only one: see instructions)

IF DEATH OCCURRED IN A HOSPITAL: ☐ Inpatient ☐ Emergency Room/Outpatient ☐ Dead on Arrival | IF DEATH OCCURRED SOMEWHERE OTHER THAN A HOSPITAL: ☐ Hospice facility ☐ Nursing home/Long term care facility ☐ Decedent's home ☐ Other (Specify):

15. FACILITY NAME (If not institution, give street & number) | 16. CITY OR TOWN, STATE, AND ZIP CODE | 17. COUNTY OF DEATH

18. METHOD OF DISPOSITION: ☐ Burial ☐ Cremation ☐ Donation ☐ Entombment ☐ Removal from State ☐ Other (Specify): | 19. PLACE OF DISPOSITION (Name of cemetery, crematory, other place)

20. LOCATION-CITY, TOWN, AND STATE | 21. NAME AND COMPLETE ADDRESS OF FUNERAL FACILITY

22. SIGNATURE OF FUNERAL SERVICE LICENSEE OR OTHER AGENT | 23. LICENSE NUMBER (Of Licensee)

ITEMS 24-28 MUST BE COMPLETED BY PERSON WHO PRONOUNCES OR CERTIFIES DEATH | 24. DATE PRONOUNCED DEAD (Mo/Day/Yr) | 25. TIME PRONOUNCED DEAD

26. SIGNATURE OF PERSON PRONOUNCING DEATH (Only when applicable) | 27. LICENSE NUMBER | 28. DATE SIGNED (Mo/Day/Yr)

29. ACTUAL OR PRESUMED DATE OF DEATH (Mo/Day/Yr) (Spell Month) | 30. ACTUAL OR PRESUMED TIME OF DEATH | 31. WAS MEDICAL EXAMINER OR CORONER CONTACTED? ☐ Yes ☐ No

To Be Completed By: MEDICAL CERTIFIER

CAUSE OF DEATH (See instructions and examples)

32. **PART I.** Enter the chain of events—diseases, injuries, or complications—that directly caused the death. DO NOT enter terminal events such as cardiac arrest, respiratory arrest, or ventricular fibrillation without showing the etiology. DO NOT ABBREVIATE. Enter only one cause on a line. Add additional lines if necessary.

Approximate interval: Onset to death

IMMEDIATE CAUSE (Final disease or condition ----→ resulting in death)   a. _____
Due to (or as a consequence of): _____

Sequentially list conditions, if any, leading to the cause listed on line a. Enter the UNDERLYING CAUSE   b. _____
Due to (or as a consequence of): _____

(disease or injury that initiated the events resulting in death) LAST   c. _____
Due to (or as a consequence of): _____

d. _____

PART II. Enter other significant conditions contributing to death but not resulting in the underlying cause given in PART I

33. WAS AN AUTOPSY PERFORMED? ☐ Yes ☐ No

34. WERE AUTOPSY FINDINGS AVAILABLE TO COMPLETE THE CAUSE OF DEATH? ☐ Yes ☐ No

35. DID TOBACCO USE CONTRIBUTE TO DEATH? ☐ Yes ☐ Probably ☐ No ☐ Unknown

36. IF FEMALE: ☐ Not pregnant within past year ☐ Pregnant at time of death ☐ Not pregnant, but pregnant within 42 days of death ☐ Not pregnant, but pregnant 43 days to 1 year before death ☐ Unknown if pregnant within the past year

37. MANNER OF DEATH ☐ Natural ☐ Homicide ☐ Accident ☐ Pending Investigation ☐ Suicide ☐ Could not be determined

38. DATE OF INJURY (Mo/Day/Yr) (Spell Month) | 39. TIME OF INJURY | 40. PLACE OF INJURY (e.g., Decedent's home; construction site; restaurant; wooded area) | 41. INJURY AT WORK? ☐ Yes ☐ No

42. LOCATION OF INJURY: State: City or Town: Street & Number: Apartment No.:   Zip Code:

43. DESCRIBE HOW INJURY OCCURRED: | 44. IF TRANSPORTATION INJURY, SPECIFY: ☐ Driver/Operator ☐ Passenger ☐ Pedestrian ☐ Other (Specify)

45. CERTIFIER (Check only one):
☐ Certifying physician-To the best of my knowledge, death occurred due to the cause(s) and manner stated.
☐ Pronouncing & Certifying physician-To the best of my knowledge, death occurred at the time, date, and place, and due to the cause(s) and manner stated.
☐ Medical Examiner/Coroner-On the basis of examination, and/or investigation, in my opinion, death occurred at the time, date, and place, and due to the cause(s) and manner stated.

Signature of certifier: _____

46. NAME, ADDRESS, AND ZIP CODE OF PERSON COMPLETING CAUSE OF DEATH (Item 32)

47. TITLE OF CERTIFIER | 48. LICENSE NUMBER | 49. DATE CERTIFIED (Mo/Day/Yr) | 50. **FOR REGISTRAR ONLY**- DATE FILED (Mo/Day/Yr)

To Be Completed By: FUNERAL DIRECTOR

51. DECEDENT'S EDUCATION-Check the box that best describes the highest degree or level of school completed at the time of death.
☐ 8th grade or less
☐ 9th - 12th grade; no diploma
☐ High school graduate or GED completed
☐ Some college credit, but no degree
☐ Associate degree (e.g., AA, AS)
☐ Bachelor's degree (e.g., BA, AB, BS)
☐ Master's degree (e.g., MA, MS, MEng, MEd, MSW, MBA)
☐ Doctorate (e.g., PhD, EdD) or Professional degree (e.g., MD, DDS, DVM, LLB, JD)

52. DECEDENT OF HISPANIC ORIGIN? Check the box that best describes whether the decedent is Spanish/Hispanic/Latino. Check the "No" box if decedent is not Spanish/Hispanic/Latino.
☐ No, not Spanish/Hispanic/Latino
☐ Yes, Mexican, Mexican American, Chicano
☐ Yes, Puerto Rican
☐ Yes, Cuban
☐ Yes, other Spanish/Hispanic/Latino (Specify) _____

53. DECEDENT'S RACE (Check one or more races to indicate what the decedent considered himself or herself to be)
☐ White
☐ Black or African American
☐ American Indian or Alaska Native (Name of the enrolled or principal tribe) _____
☐ Asian Indian
☐ Chinese
☐ Filipino
☐ Japanese
☐ Korean
☐ Vietnamese
☐ Other Asian (Specify) _____
☐ Native Hawaiian
☐ Guamanian or Chamorro
☐ Samoan
☐ Other Pacific Islander (Specify) _____
☐ Other (Specify) _____

54. DECEDENT'S USUAL OCCUPATION (Indicate type of work done during most of working life. DO NOT USE RETIRED).

55. KIND OF BUSINESS/INDUSTRY

REV. 11/2003

Source: CDC 2003.

Figure 3.7. U.S. standard report of induced termination of pregnancy.

TYPE/PRINT IN PERMANENT BLACK INK FOR INSTRUCTIONS SEE HANDBOOK

U.S. STANDARD
REPORT OF INDUCED TERMINATION OF PREGNANCY

STATE FILE NUMBER

1. FACILITY NAME (If not clinic or hospital, give address)	2. CITY, TOWN, OR LOCATION OF PREGNANCY TERMINATION	3. COUNTY OF PREGNANCY TERMINATION
Merrywood Clinic	Louisville	Jefferson

4. PATIENT'S IDENTIFICATION	5. AGE LAST BIRTHDAY	6. MARRIED?	7. DATE OF PREGNANCY TERMINATION (Month, Day, Year)
25466	23	☐ YES ☒ NO	November 20, 1997

8a. RESIDENCE-STATE	8b. COUNTY	8c. CITY, TOWN, OR LOCATION	8d. INSIDE CITY LIMITS? (Yes or No)	8e. ZIP CODE
Ohio	Hamilton	Cincinnati	☒ YES ☐ NO	45202

9. OF HISPANIC ORIGIN? (Specify No or Yes - If yes, specify Cuban, Mexican, Puerto Rican, etc.)	10. RACE	11. EDUCATION (Specify only highest grade completed) Elementary/Secondary (0-12)	College (1-4 or 5+)
☐ No ☒ Yes Specify: Puerto Rican	☐ American Indian ☐ Black ☒ White ☐ Other (Specify) ______	12	

12. DATE LAST NORMAL MENSES BEGAN (Month, Day, Year)	13. CLINICAL ESTIMATE OF GESTATION (Weeks)	14. PREVIOUS PREGNANCIES (Complete each section) LIVE BIRTHS: 14a. Now Living	14b. Now Dead	OTHER TERMINATIONS: 14c. Spontaneous	14d. Induced (Do not include this termination)
September 5, 1997	10 weeks	Number ____ ☒ None	Number ____ ☒ None	Number ____ ☒ None	Number ____ ☒ None

15. TYPE OF TERMINATION PROCEDURE (Check only one)

☒ Suction Curettage
☐ Medical (Nonsurgical), Specify Medication(s) ______
☐ Dilation and Evacuation (D&E)
☐ Intra-Uterine Instillation (Saline or Prostaglandin)
☐ Sharp Curettage (D&C)
☐ Hysterotomy/Hysterectomy
☐ Other (Specify) ______

16. NAME OF ATTENDING PHYSICIAN (Type/Print)	17. NAME OF PERSON COMPLETING REPORT (Type/Print)
Edmund Matthew Stone, M.D.	Julia Lynn Koval

7-0725

U.S. DEPARTMENT OF HEALTH AND HUMAN SERVICES — CENTERS FOR DISEASE CONTROL AND PREVENTION — NATIONAL CENTER FOR HEALTH STATISTICS — 1997 REVISION

Source: CDC 1998, 19.

Individual states maintain public health databases to manage data on the incidence of communicable diseases. The CDC maintains a database that contains similar data. The **World Health Organization's (WHO)** international health regulations require incidence reporting from participating nations so that the organization can track potential worldwide epidemics. The WHO is the United Nations' agency that oversees global health initiatives. The SARS epidemic that spread from China to Europe, Canada, and the United States in 2003 is an example of how quickly communicable diseases can be carried from continent to continent via international transportation systems.

A number of communicable illnesses must be reported to the CDC, as shown in figure 3.8. National data on these diseases (classified as **notifiable diseases**) are reported weekly. Case-specific information is included in the CDC's reports. The CDC investigates cases where the cause of an illness or the source of an epidemic cannot be determined at the local level.

Hospitals calculate population-based health statistics at the local level. **Population-based statistics** represent estimates of the incidence of a disease as a percentage of the total population that could have been affected. For example, the crude birth rate for a community can be calculated by dividing the number of live births in the community during a specified time period by the estimated population of that community during the same time.

Figure 3.8. Infectious diseases that require notification.

• Acquired Immunodeficiency Syndrome (AIDS)	• Meningococcal disease
• Anthrax	• Mumps
• Arboviral neuroinvasive and non-neuroinvasive diseases	• Novel influenza A virus infections
– California serogroup virus disease	• Pertussis
– Eastern equine encephalitis virus disease	• Plague
– Powassan virus disease	• Poliomyelitis, paralytic
– St. Louis encephalitis virus disease	• Poliovirus infection, nonparalytic
– West Nile virus disease	• Psittacosis
– Western equine encephalitis virus disease	• Q Fever
• Botulism	• Rabies
– Botulism, foodborne	– Rabies, animal
– Botulism, infant	– Rabies, human
– Botulism, other (wound & unspecified)	• Rocky Mountain spotted fever
• Brucellosis	• Rubella
• Chancroid	• Rubella, congenital syndrome
• *Chlamydia trachomatis,* genital infections	• Salmonellosis
• Cholera	• Severe Acute Respiratory Syndrome-associated Coronavirus (SARS-CoV) disease
• Coccidioidomycosis	• Shiga toxin-producing *Escherichia coli* (STEC)
• Cryptosporidiosis	• Shigellosis
• Cyclosporiasis	• Smallpox
• Diphtheria	• Streptococcal disease, invasive, Group A
• Ehrlichiosis	• Streptococcal toxic-shock syndrome
– Ehrlichiosis, human granulocytic	• *Streptococcus pneumoniae,* drug resistant, invasive disease
– Ehrlichiosis, human monocytic	• *Streptococcus pneumoniae,* invasive in children <5 years
– Ehrlichiosis, human, other or unspecified agent	• Syphilis
• Giardiasis	– Syphilis, primary
• Gonorrhea	– Syphilis, secondary
• *Haemophilus influenzae,* invasive disease	– Syphilis, latent
• Hansen disease (leprosy)	– Syphilis, early latent
• Hantavirus pulmonary syndrome	– Syphilis, late latent
• Hemolytic uremic syndrome, post-diarrheal	– Syphilis, latent, unknown duration
• Hepatitis, viral, acute	– Neurosyphilis
– Hepatitis A, acute	– Syphilis, late, non-neurological
– Hepatitis B, acute	– Syphilitic Stillbirth
– Hepatitis B virus, perinatal infection	• Syphilis, congenital
– Hepatitis, C, acute	• Tetanus
• Hepatitis, viral, chronic	• Toxic-shock syndrome (other than Streptococcal)
– Chronic Hepatitis B	• Trichinellosis (Trichinosis)
– Hepatitis C Virus Infection (past or present)	• Tuberculosis
• HIV infection	• Tularemia
– HIV infection, adult(≥13 years)	• Typhoid fever
– HIV infection, pediatric (<13 years)	• Vancomycin—intermediate *Staphylococcus aureus* (VISA)
• Influenza-associated pediatric mortality	• Vancomycin—resistant *Staphylococcus aureus* (VRSA)
• Legionellosis	• Varicella (morbidity)
• Listeriosis	• Varicella (deaths only)
• Lyme disease	• Vibriosis
• Malaria	• Yellow fever
• Measles	

Source: CDC 2007.

Morbidity statistics are calculated as incidence rates (the number of people who contracted the same disease during a specific time period compared to the number of people who could have contracted the disease). Incidence rates usually include race, gender, and age data so that the relative incidence rates among different populations can be compared. Examples of commonly computed mortality statistics include the following:

- Crude death rate
- Neonatal mortality rate
- Postneonatal mortality rate
- Infant mortality rate
- Crude mortality rate
- Cause-specific mortality rate
- Maternal mortality rate

Management of the Healthcare Delivery System

CMS collects data from reimbursement claims in a national database. This database is used as the basis for decision making related to the effectiveness of healthcare delivery systems and reimbursement systems. Federal and state governments use the data reported by hospitals and other healthcare organizations to develop public health policies.

Professional and trade organizations use information reported from health records to develop professional practice standards. They base their support for public actions on healthcare policy issues on clinical information derived from health records. Professional health organizations include the American Medical Association and the American College of Surgeons. The largest trade organization in the healthcare industry is the American Hospital Association.

Form and Content of Health Records

State laws and regulations establish legal requirements related to the form and content of health records for facilities located within the covered geopolitical area. Health record regulations are usually developed by the state administrative agency responsible for licensing hospitals and other healthcare organizations. Some state regulations have minimal standards for maintaining clinical records. Other state regulations require clinical records be complete and accurate. In a few states, health record regulations interpret the specific categories of information that hospitals must collect. In addition, some state regulations integrate the health record requirements of the Medicare *Conditions of Participation* or pertinent accreditation standards (McWay 2002, 69).

Public health regulations in many states require hospitals to routinely report specific confidential, health-related information collected directly from health records. Most public health regulations require the reporting of vital statistics data such as births and deaths. Many states require the collection and reporting of information about the public's health, safety, and welfare. The required reporting of communicable diseases and injuries that resulted from a violent crime would fit in this category. In addition, many states require that hospitals and other healthcare providers report cases of suspected child abuse or neglect to the appropriate legal authorities.

Failure to comply with state health record or public health regulations may result in some type of penalty for noncompliant hospitals. Examples include forfeiture of operating licenses, fines, and criminal sanctions.

Consumer's Right to Health Record Access

More than half of the states have statutes that address the patient's right to view, copy, and/or correct his or her health record. The Medicare *Conditions of Participation for Hospitals* establish the individual's right to access his or her health information. As noted in chapter 2, the HIPAA privacy act describes the limited situations in which patient access is available. Hospital policies should encompass state regulations, the HIPAA privacy act, and *Conditions of Participation* to ensure all applicable state and federal requirements address the patient's right to access his or her record.

Release and Disclosure of Confidential Health Information

Before the HIPAA (2003) privacy standard was implemented, there generally were no applicable federal statutes or regulations to protect the confidentiality of health records. The privacy rights of patients and the confidentiality of health records were addressed in a patchwork of state and federal regulations, professional practice standards, and individual facility policies.

When the Medicare program was established in the late 1960s, the *Conditions of Participation* included a requirement regarding the confidentiality of health records for Medicare beneficiaries. In the 1970s, federal legislation was implemented to ensure the privacy of patients in some types of treatment programs operated or supported by the federal government. However, the regulations applied exclusively to federally supported or operated programs. The drug and alcohol treatment legislation passed in 1970 and amended in 2000 established strict confidentiality requirements for substance-abuse treatment records, but only for records maintained by facilities that receive federal funding. Similarly, the provisions of the Privacy Act of 1974 apply only to facilities operated by the federal government.

In contrast, the HIPAA (2003) privacy standard is widely applicable. It has established a consistent set of rules that apply to virtually every healthcare facility, healthcare professional, healthcare information clearinghouse, and health plan in the United States. The standard supersedes state regulations that permitted less stringent privacy practices.

Although the federal privacy standard has preempted some state health record regulations, many state regulations are still relevant. The federal regulations constitute a minimum standard for protecting confidential records. When state regulations require stricter privacy practices, hospitals and other healthcare organizations must continue to follow state regulations in addition to the federal privacy standard. Healthcare organizations must continue to comply with public health reporting regulations and licensure/certification requirements in their geopolitical area (Hughes 2002b).

Many states base the confidentiality rights of patients on the concept of **privileged communication**. According to this concept, medical practitioners, like lawyers and other professionals, are not allowed to disclose the confidential information that they learn in their capacity as professional service providers. There are very few exceptions to this basic rule for medical practitioners.

The HIPAA (2003) privacy standard does not require healthcare organizations to obtain the patient's formal consent to use health information for treatment, reimbursement, operational, and reporting purposes. However, some state regulations may still require hospitals and other healthcare providers to obtain a written consent from the patient or the patient's legal representative before sharing the patient's confidential health information with external healthcare providers and third-party payers.

Even in the absence of state and federal requirements, many hospitals choose to document the patient's consent for routine uses and disclosures of confidential information. Patients are usually asked to sign general consents during the admissions process. (See figure 3.9 for an example of a general consent form.) Consents relevant to information are treated as separate

Figure 3.9.   Example of a general consent for use and disclosure of health information.

**Consent to the Use and Disclosure of Health Information
for Treatment, Payment, or Healthcare Operations**

I understand that as part of my healthcare, this organization originates and maintains health records describing my health history, symptoms, examination and test results, diagnoses, treatment, and any plans for future care or treatment. I understand that this information serves as:

- A basis for planning my care and treatment

- A means of communication among the many health professionals who contribute to my care

- A source of information for applying my diagnosis and surgical information to my bill

- A means by which a third-party payer can verify that services billed were actually provided

- A tool for routine healthcare operations such as assessing quality and reviewing the competence of healthcare professionals

I understand and have been provided with a Notice of Information Practices that provides a more complete description of information uses and disclosures. I understand that I have the right to review the notice prior to signing this consent. I understand that the organization reserves the right to change its notice and practices and prior to implementation will mail a copy of any revised notice to the address I've provided. I understand that I have the right to object to the use of my health information for directory purposes. I understand that I have the right to request restrictions as to how my health information may be used or disclosed to carry out treatment, payment, or healthcare operations and that the organization is not required to agree to the restrictions requested. I understand that I may revoke this consent in writing, except to the extent that the organization has already taken action in reliance thereon. Therefore, I consent to the use and disclosure of my healthcare information.

☐ I request the following restrictions to the use or disclosure of my health information.

Signature of Patient or Legal Representative

_____

Witness _____

Date Notice Effective _____

Date or Version _____

☐ Accepted   ☐ Denied

Signature _____

Title _____

Date _____

---

documents rather than as elements of the general consent to treatment, which is obtained at admission (Hjort and Hughes 2002).

State regulations governing the release and disclosure of confidential health information take a variety of approaches. Implicitly or explicitly, however, all grant patients or their legal representatives two basic rights: the right to limit access to their records under certain circumstances and to waive their confidentiality rights when they choose.

In general, healthcare facilities and practitioners are required to obtain the patient's explicit, written permission before disclosing information for any purpose not related to treatment, reimbursement, operations, or public health reporting. Federal and state regulations, accreditation standards, and professional practice guidelines dictate the specific form and content of such consents and authorizations.

Redisclosure of Confidential Health Information

Health records sometimes include clinical data originally collected by other healthcare providers. For example, surgeons often supply copies of preadmission laboratory test results for patients scheduled to undergo elective surgery in the hospital. Such documents become a permanent part of the patient's acute-care record only when used during the patient's course of treatment in the hospital.

The process of disclosing health record documentation originally created by a different provider is called **redisclosure**. Federal and state regulations provide specific redisclosure guidelines; however, when in doubt, follow the same principles as the release and disclosure guidelines for other types of health record information (Rhodes and Hughes 2003).

Retention of Health Records

Hospitals and other healthcare facilities develop health record retention policies to ensure that health records comply with all applicable state and federal regulations and accreditation standards as well as meeting future patient-care needs. Establishing and following consistent record retention and destruction policies helps control the cost of record storage space and equipment as well as labor.

Most states have established regulations that address how long health records and other healthcare-related documents must be maintained before they can be destroyed. Although the Medicare *Conditions of Participation for Hospitals* (2006) stipulate a five-year minimum, many states require longer retention periods. Some states base their retention guidelines on the type of services represented in the record. A few state laws specify the length of time that health records must be retained in their original form before converting to a different storage media such as microfilm. In many states, retention guidelines require facilities to retain the records of infants and children longer than the records of adults. For example, the state of South Carolina includes the following health record retention requirements in its hospital licensure regulations:

> The records shall be treated as confidential and shall not be disposed of under 10 years. Records may be destroyed after 10 years provided that: (1) Records of minors must be retained until after the expiration of the period of election following achievement of majority as prescribed by statute. (2) The hospital retains an index, register, or summary cards providing such basic information as dates of admission and discharge, name of responsible physician, and record of diagnoses and operations for all records so destroyed. (SC DHEC 1992)

In states that do not stipulate the retention period of health records, the healthcare providers generally maintain records for the period established by the state's statute of limitations

(Rhodes and Fletcher 2002). A **statute of limitations** is a law that dictates the maximum period of time that may elapse between an event (for example, an injury or a crime) and any consequent legal action. In most states, the statute of limitations requires legal action in less than ten years. Therefore, in the absence of other state retention guidelines, hospitals and other healthcare providers may decide to maintain health records for a minimum of ten years (Kiger 2002, 218).

Similarly, the AHIMA recommends retention of health records for a minimum period of ten years. It recommends a permanent retention period for several other types of patient-care records such as the following (Rhodes and Fletcher 2002):

- Master patient index

- Register of births

- Register of deaths

- Register of surgical procedures

See table 3.1 for more information on the retention standards recommended by AHIMA.

Although the Medicare *Conditions of Participation for Hospitals* (2006) and various accreditation standards provide some guidance, every hospital should establish its own health record retention policies to reflect its unique regulatory climate. As a matter of law, retention policies must comply with the local, state, and federal regulations that apply to the facility. However, hospital retention policies must consider the facility's internal information needs because hospitals use health records for a number of purposes in addition to patient care (for example, in medical staff credentialing and performance improvement activities). Hospital health record retention policies should take into account the advice of the facility's malpractice insurance carrier and legal counsel.

In addition to patient-care records, hospitals and other healthcare organizations maintain huge amounts of administrative information. The hospital's board of directors, executive staff, legal counsel, and medical staff should work together to develop retention guidelines for all of the facility's records, and not just patient records. State and federal regulations on taxation and business reporting must be considered in drafting information retention policies.

Table 3.1   Recommended retention standards

Health Information	Recommended Retention Period
Diagnostic images (such as x-ray film)	5 years
Disease index	10 years
Fetal heart monitor records	10 years after the infant reaches the age of majority
Master patient/person index	Permanently
Operative index	10 years
Patient health records (adults)	10 years after the most recent encounter
Patient health records (minors)	Age of majority plus statute of limitations
Physician index	10 years
Register of births	Permanently
Register of deaths	Permanently
Register of surgical procedures	Permanently

Destruction of Health Records

Because of cost and space limitations, permanently storing paper and microfilm-based health record documents is not an option for most hospitals. The question of how to dispose of original records in a way that protects their confidentiality usually comes up in one of four situations.

1. The retention period for a set of paper-based or micrographic records has elapsed, and the healthcare organization needs to free up storage space for current records.

2. The healthcare organization routinely copies paper-based records onto microfiche or optical disks for long-term storage and needs to dispose of the original paper documents.

3. The healthcare organization is in the process of implementing a new electronic health record system and needs to dispose of paper records that are scanned and loaded onto the new system.

4. The healthcare organization is being sold or is closing permanently and needs to arrange for the disposition of its health records.

The destruction of patient-identifiable clinical documentation should be carried out in accordance with relevant federal and state regulations and organizational policy. Health records related to any open investigations, audits, or court cases should not be destroyed for any reason (Hughes 2002a).

Some states require hospitals and other providers to complete certain preparatory activities before health records are destroyed. Examples include creating health record abstracts or notifying patients so that they have enough time to request copies before the destruction of original records. Some states establish specific requirements for the method of destruction.

According to AHIMA practice standards, acceptable destruction methods include the following (Hughes 2002a):

- **Paper documents**: burning, shredding, pulping, and pulverizing

- **Micrographic film**: recycling and pulverizing

- **Optical disks**: pulverizing

- **Electronic documents**: magnetic degaussing (demagnetizing)

- **Magnetic tapes**: magnetic degaussing (demagnetizing)

Some facilities engage record destruction services to process obsolete health records. In such cases, the facility's contract with the vendor must fulfill the requirements of the HIPAA (2003) privacy standard.

Appropriate documentation of health record destruction must be maintained permanently no matter how the process is carried out. This documentation usually takes the form of a **certificate of destruction** (Hughes 2002a), which should include the following details:

- Date of destruction

- Method of destruction

- Description of the record(s) destroyed, including health record number(s)

- Statement that the record(s) was destroyed during the normal course of business

- Signatures of the individuals who authorized and witnessed the destruction

Maintaining such documentation in a permanent file provides the facility with legal protection in any future liability actions (McWay 2002, 78–80). (See figure 3.10 for an example of a certificate of record destruction.)

State and federal record retention requirements continue to apply to health records maintained by facilities that have been sold or closed permanently. Before a sale or closure, the organization should develop plans for ensuring that the health records of former patients will

Figure 3.10. Example of a certificate of record destruction.

Anytown General Hospital

**CERTIFICATE OF HEALTH
RECORD DESTRUCTION**

PATIENT LABEL

The information described below was destroyed in the normal course of business pursuant to a proper retention schedule and destruction policies and procedures.

Date of destruction: _____

Description of records or record series disposed of:_____

_____

_____

Inclusive dates covered: _____

Method of destruction:_____

☐ Burning   ☐ Shredding   ☐ Pulping
☐ Demagnetizing   ☐ Overwriting   ☐ Pulverizing
☐ Other: _____

Records Destroyed By: _____
                        Signature   Date

Witness Signature:_____
                        Signature   Date

Department Manager: _____
                        Signature   Date

CERTIFICATE OF HEALTH RECORD DESTRUCTION
0943217 (08/2003)

continue to be stored appropriately and made available for legitimate access over the required retention period. (An AHIMA practice brief provides specific guidance on handling patient information after a facility closure [Rhodes and Brandt 2003].)

Summary

The primary functions of the health record can be grouped into four categories: patient-care delivery, patient-care management, patient-care support, and billing and reimbursement. In examining these functions, this chapter focused on the concept that data represent facts but information conveys meaning. Primary users of the health record include nurses, physicians, allied health professionals, and administrative personnel, as well as patients and their family members or legal representatives.

The ancillary functions of the acute-care health record are related to the care environment. Ancillary functions include accreditation, licensure, and certification; biomedical research; clinical education; and morbidity and mortality reporting.

The principal functions of the health record use primary, patient-identifiable information. Most ancillary functions use secondary, de-identified health record information, usually in an aggregate form that protects the confidentiality of patient records.

References

AHIMA e-HIM Work Group on Maintaining the Legal EHR. 2005a. Update: Maintaining a legally sound health record—paper and electronic. *Journal of American Health Information Management Association* 76(10): 64A–L.

AHIMA e-HIM Work Group on Regional Health Information Organizations (RHIOs). 2006. Using the SSN as a patient identifier. *Journal of American Health Information Management Association* 77(3): 56A–D.

American Health Information Management Association. 2003. Press Release: AHIMA urges Secretary Thompson to adopt ICD-10. July 25, 2003. Available online from www.ahima.org.

Bowman, Sue, 2008. Policies and procedures. Chapter 3 in *Health Information Management Compliance: Guidelines for Preventing Fraud and Abuse,* 4th ed., edited by Sue Bowman, 38. Chicago: AHIMA.

Bush, George W. Address before a Joint Session of the Congress on the State of the Union, January 20, 2004. *Public Papers of the Presidents of the United States.* Washington, D.C.: Government Printing Office, 2004.

Centers for Disease Control and Prevention. 1998. *Handbook on the Reporting of Induced Termination of Pregnancy,* revised edition. HHS Publication No. (PHS) 98-1 117. Hyattsville, MD: National Center for Health Statistics. Available online from www.cdc.gov/nchs/data/misc/hb_itop.pdf.

Centers for Disease Control and Prevention. 2003. *2003 Revisions of the U.S. standard certificates of live birth and death and the fetal death.* Hyattsville, MD: National Center for Health Statistics. Available online from www.cdc.gov/nchs/vital_certs_rev.htm.

Centers for Disease Control and Prevention. 2007. *Nationally notifiable infectious diseases, United States, 2007 revised.* Available online from www.cdc.gov/epo/dphsi/phs/infdis2007r.htm.

Centers for Medicare and Medicaid Services. 2005. Eighth Statement of Work for quality improvement organizations. Available online from www.cms.hhs.gov.

DHEC. 1992. Minimum Standards For Licensing Hospitals and Institutional General Infirmaries, 16 SCR, R61-16 § 601.007. Available online from www.scdhec.gov/administration/regs/docs/61-16.pdf.

Food and Drug Administration. 2006 (April 1). Protection of human subjects. 21 CFR 50. Available online from www.access.gpo.gov/nara/cfr/waisidx_06/21cfr50_06.html.

Giannangelo, Kathy. 2007. Unraveling the data set, an e-HIM essential. *Journal of American Health Information Management Association* 78(2): 60–61.

Health Insurance Portability and Accountability Act (HIPAA) of 1996. Public Law 104-191. Available online from www.gpoaccess.gov/cfr/index.html.

Hjort, B., and G. Hughes. 2002. Practice brief: Consent for uses and disclosures of information. *Journal of American Health Information Management Association* 73(10).

Homan, Cheryl. 2007. Functions of the health record. Chapter 2 in *Health Information Management Technology,* 2nd ed., edited by Merida Johns, 32. Chicago: AHIMA.

Hughes, Gwen. 2002a. Practice brief: Destruction of patient health information. *Journal of American Health Information Management Association* 73(10).

Hughes, Gwen. 2002b. Practice brief: Laws and regulations governing the disclosure of health information. *Journal of American Health Information Association* 73(10).

James, Ella. 2007. *Documentation and Reimbursement for Long-term Care,* 2nd ed. Chicago: AHIMA.

Joint Commission on Accreditation of Healthcare Organizations. 2006. *2006 Comprehensive Accreditation Manual for Hospitals; The Official Handbook.* Oakbrook Terrace, IL: Joint Commission.

Kiger, Linda. 2002. Preservation of health records. Chapter 11 in *Health Information Management: Principles and Organization for Health Information Services,* 5th ed., edited by Margaret Skurka. San Francisco: Jossey-Bass.

LeBlanc, M., and A. W. White. 2006. Work design and performance improvement. Chapter 23 in *Health Information Management: Concepts, Principles, and Practice,* 2nd ed., edited by Kathleen LaTour and Shirley Eichenwald-Maki. Chicago: AHIMA.

McWay, Dana. 2002. *Legal Aspects of Health Information Management,* 2nd ed. Clifton Park, New York: Delmar Learning.

National Conference of Commissioners on Uniform State Laws. 2007. *Uniform Rules Relating to the Discovery of Electronically Stored Information.* Available online from www.law.upenn.edu/bll/archives/ulc/udoera/2007_final. htm.

Osborn, Carol. 2006. Biomedical and research support. Chapter 18 in *Health Information Management: Concepts, Principles, and Practice,* 2nd ed., edited by Kathleen LaTour and Shirley Eichenwald–Maki, 522-523. Chicago: AHIMA.

Pozar, G. 1999. *Legal Aspects of Health Care Administration.* Gaithersburg, MD: Aspen Publishers.

Quinsey, Carol Ann. 2006. Using HL7 standards to evaluate an EHR. *Journal of American Health Information Management Association* 77(4): 64A–C.

Reich, Kimberly Baldwin-Stried. 2007. Developing a litigation response plan. *Journal of American Health Information Management Association* 78(9): 76–78, 86.

Rhodes, H., and M. Brandt. 2003. Practice brief: Protecting patient information after a facility closure. *Journal of American Health Information Management Association* 74(10): 64A–C.

Rhodes, H., and D. Fletcher. 2002. Practice brief: Retention of health information. *Journal of American Health Information Management Association* 73(6).

Rhodes, H., and G. Hughes. 2003. Practice brief: Redisclosure of patient health information. *Journal of American Health Information Management Association* 74(4): 56A–C.

Shaw, Patricia, et al. 2003. *Quality and Performance Improvement in Healthcare: A Tool for Programmed Learning,* 2nd ed. Chicago: AHIMA.

Chapter 4

Documentation for Statistical Reporting and Public Health

Barbara Odom-Wesley, PhD, RHIA, FAHIMA

Learning Objectives

- Study how statistics are used in healthcare

- Distinguish between primary and secondary data

- Compare and contrast patient-identifiable data with aggregate data

- Relate how health record data are used for research and statistics

- Define healthcare databases in terms of purpose and content

- Explain the use of health record data in clinical trials

- Identify the role of health record documentation in public health reporting

- Define vital statistics

- Trace the flow of information in reporting vital statistics

- Identify data quality issues to yield statistical information for administrative and clinical decisions

- Describe the role and content of a master patient index

- Recognize secondary data sources

- Identify facility-specific indexes

- List routine healthcare databases

- Identify data elements in standardized clinical data sets

Key Terms

Agency for Healthcare Research and Quality (AHRQ)

Aggregate data

Census

Centers for Disease Control and Prevention (CDC)

Clinical trial

Consolidated Health Informatics (CHI) Initiatives

Data sets

Database

Department of Health and Human Services (HHS)

Disease index

Enterprise master person index (EMPI)

Facility-specific index

Facility-specific registry

Food and Drug Administration (FDA)

Health services research

Incidence

Index

Master patient index (MPI)

National Alliance for Health Information Technology (NAHIT)

National Center for Health Statistics (NCHS)

National Committee on Vital and Health Statistics (NCVHS)

Office of the National Coordinator for Health Information Technology (ONC)

Operation index

Patient-specific/identifiable data

Physician index

Population-based registry

Prevalence

Primary data

Primary data source

Protocol

Public health

Registry

Research

Secondary data

Secondary data source

Vital statistics

Introduction

The primary purpose of healthcare documentation is to chronicle customers' health history over time. Although this benefits consumers by ensuring the continuity of their care, the information compiled from healthcare documentation can reveal trends and contribute to improving healthcare for everyone. Health record documentation is the source data for statistical reports that guide decisions in a local facility. By reporting this data to public health agencies, these decisions can influence the health of a state and even a nation. This chapter provides information on facility-specific, state, and national indexes, registries, and **databases**.

Research and Statistics

Data contained in the health record are required for **research**, statistical reporting, cancer registries, trauma registries, and birth certificate registration to name a few public health uses. Documentation needed for research ranges from identification of candidate health records for projects to actual review of selected records and abstract preparation or collection of data from them for the physician or clinical researcher.

Providing research assistance to clinicians and medical staff committees is a function within the HIM department. Aggregate statistical data are also useful for clinical and administrative decision support. **Indexes** are used to sort data in a variety of ways to assist study of certain data elements. Additionally, HIM departments collect and calculate various statistics about the operations of the healthcare facilities and clinical practices they serve. Many of these statistics are provided electronically; however, the HIM department provides quality control for accuracy of calculations and statistical reports.

The HIM professional may be called upon to assist research by providing information for a clinical trial. Using health record data to guide these studies and document results can lead to new medical discoveries and treatment modalities. A **clinical trial** is a research project in which new treatments and tests are investigated to determine whether they are safe and effective. The trial proceeds according to a **protocol**, which is the list of rules and procedures to be followed. A clinical trials database provides the data that enable patients and practitioners to determine which clinical trials are available and applicable to the patients. The **Food and Drug Administration (FDA)** Modernization Act of 1997 mandated that a clinical trials database be developed. The National Library of Medicine has developed the database, called Clinical Trials, for use by both consumers and practitioners. It is available on the Internet at http://clinicaltrials.gov. Information in the database includes the following (Bowman 2006b, 298–299):

- Study identification number
- Study sponsor
- Brief title
- Brief summary
- Location of trial
- Recruitment status
- Contact information
- Eligibility criteria
- Study type
- Study design
- Study phase
- Condition

- Intervention
- Data provider
- Date last modified

Public Health Reporting

The health of populations in geopolitical locations is the domain of **public health**. One of the duties of public health agencies is surveillance of the health status of the population within their jurisdictions.

Centers for Disease Control and Prevention WONDER Database

The **Centers for Disease Control and Prevention (CDC)** WONDER database is an integrated information and communication system for public health. Its purposes are twofold (CDC 2007):

1. To promote information-driven decision making by placing timely, useful facts in the hands of public health practitioners and researchers

2. To provide the general public with access to specific and detailed information from the CDC

CDC WONDER furthers the CDC's mission of health promotion and disease prevention by speeding and simplifying access to public health information for state and local health departments, the U.S. Public Health Service, and the academic public health community. CDC WONDER is valuable in public health research, decision making, priority setting, program evaluation, and resource allocation (CDC 2007).

Collection and calculation of various healthcare statistics are also dependent on record documentation. Statistics are needed to describe the operation of a healthcare facility. Among these are ratios and percentages (for example, percentage of occupancy, death and autopsy rates; hospital **census** reports). Where the institution has integrated computer information systems, many of these types of statistics are generated automatically. However, data entry and other errors often produce incorrect results, so it is typically the function of the HIM department to verify the accuracy of many of the statistics calculated about institutional operations.

National Center for Health Statistics

The **National Center for Health Statistics (NCHS)** compiles statistical information to guide actions and policies to improve health. NCHS (2007) uses health statistics to

- document the population's and subgroups' health status,
- identify differences in health status and use of healthcare by demographics (such as race/ethnicity, socioeconomic status, or region),
- describe NCHS's experiences with the healthcare system,
- monitor health status and delivery trends,
- identify health problems,

- support medical and HIM research,

- suggest changes in public policies and programs, and

- evaluate the impact of health policies and programs.

The NCHS collaborates with the health community and uses a variety of approaches to obtain information. Data are collected from birth and death records, health records, interview surveys, and through direct physical exams and laboratory testing. NCHS monitors the national public health infrastructure and provides information to identify and address critical health problems (NCHS 2007).

Health record documentation is required for developing the databases used by public health departments to provide information on the **incidence** and **prevalence** of diseases, possible high-risk populations, survival statistics, and trends over time. Data elements for the databases may be collected using a variety of methods, including interviews, physical examinations of individuals, and review of health records. The HIM manager may have input in these databases through information provided from health records (Bowman 2006b, 297).

Department of Health and Human Services Data Council

The **Department of Health and Human Services (HHS)** established a Data Council to coordinate and integrate data collection and analysis activities within HHS. HHS has taken a number of steps to address key data needs, promote a coordinated HHS-wide strategy on data issues, and strengthen collaboration with private sector entities, state and local governments, and other partners (HHS 2005). The Data Council also supports HHS-wide implementation of the Health Insurance Portability and Accountability Act Administrative Simplification, an initiative to adopt national standards for electronic healthcare transactions.

The Data Council assists in decision making, analysis, and dissemination of information within HHS as well as to public and private sector entities with common data interests. In addition, HHS plays a national leadership role in health and human services information policy, including national data standards, privacy policy, and national health information infrastructure issues (HHS 2005).

National Health Care Survey

The National Health Care Survey is one of the major national public health surveys. It relies on data from patients' health records and includes information on several practice areas (Bowman 2006a, 415). (See table 4.1.)

Vital Statistics

Vital statistics include data on births, deaths, fetal deaths, marriages, and divorce. Responsibility for the collection of vital statistics rests with the states. The states share information with the NCHS. The state serves as the official repository for birth and death certificates and provides vital statistics information to the NCHS. From the vital statistics collected, states and the national government develop a variety of databases (Bowman 2006a, 415). For example, one national database links birth certificates and death certificates for infants who die before reaching age one. Such information is useful to analyze patterns of infant deaths.

The **National Committee on Vital and Health Statistics (NCVHS)** provides help in connecting the interests of the U.S. government, the health industry, and research and public

Table 4.1   Databases included in the National Health Care Survey

Database	Type of Setting	Content	Data Source	Method of Data Collection
National Ambulatory Medical Care Survey	Office-based physician practice	Data on the patient and the visit	State discharge databases Office-based physician records	Abstract
National Nursing Home Survey	Nursing home	Data on the facility, current and discharged residents	Administrator Nurse caregiver	Interview
National Hospital Ambulatory Medical Care Survey	Hospital emergency departments and outpatient clinics	Data on the patient, the visit, and the method of payment	Emergency department and outpatient clinic records	Abstract
National Home and Hospice Care Survey	Home health and hospice	Facility data and patient data	Administrator Caregiver	Interview
National Electronic Disease Surveillance System (NEDSS)	Public health departments	Possible bioterrorism incidents	Local and state public health departments	Electronic surveillance

Source: Bowman 2006a, 415.

health entities as well as connecting to those working on health information policy in other countries (Kanaan 2000). The mission of the NCVHS, which was formed in 1949, is to advise the federal government on the information needs underlying health policy. It designs and coordinates improvements in national and international vital and health statistics.

Facility-specific Indexes

Facility-specific indexes are established by healthcare facilities to meet their individual, specific needs for customer care or other reporting requirements. These indexes make it possible to retrieve health records in a variety of ways including by disease, physician, operation, or other data element. Prior to computerization in healthcare, these indexes were kept on cards. Today, most are compiled from databases routinely developed by the facility.

Master Patient Index

The **master patient index (MPI)** is a database of patients within a facility or associated group of facilities (enterprise). The MPI, whether in paper or electronic format, may be considered the most important resource in a healthcare facility because it tracks patient activity across customer-care settings. The MPI identifies all patients who have been treated in a facility or enterprise and lists the health records or identification numbers associated with the names. An index can be maintained manually or as part of a computerized system. Retention of entries depends upon the MPI's use. Typically, entries for healthcare facilities are retained permanently, while those for insurers, registries, or others may have different retention periods.

Data Elements

Data elements included in the MPI should:

- accurately match persons being registered for care with their MPI records,
- minimize duplicate records within a facility and across customer-care settings,

- facilitate merging MPIs to create enterprise MPIs, and

- facilitate access to longitudinal health records.

Complying with these guidelines will speed access to patient information, resulting in significant benefits for customers and healthcare providers. To achieve this, AHIMA (2004) recommends that the core data elements listed in table 4.2 be included in MPIs. Optional data elements are detailed in table 4.3.

The need to identify patients across departments within a facility has lead to the development of the **enterprise master person index (EMPI)**. The EMPI consolidates information from registration, scheduling, financial, and clinical software systems. EMPIs may also assist organizations in maintaining HIPAA patient identification and tracking requirements, as listed in table 4.4.

See appendix E on the accompanying CD for AHIMA's practice brief on building an enterprise master person index.

Physician Index

The **physician index** categorizes patients by primary physician. It guides the retrieval of cases treated by a particular physician. Creating the index simply involves sorting patients by physician. Facilities can designate which physician(s) are recorded as the data element. Information required in a physician index include the physician's name or code, health record number, diagnosis, operations, and disposition of the patients the physician treated, the dates of admission and discharge, patient's gender and age, and other demographic data deemed useful by the facility (Roberts 2006, 377).

For example, a facility could retrieve all of Dr. Anderson's patients with melanoma and compare their treatment with Dr. Bradford's patients with the same diagnosis. The quantity and quality of care by a physician is considered in credentialing and assignment of privileges procedures.

Disease and Operation Indexes

Disease and **operation indexes** allow the retrieval of patient information by diagnosis or surgical procedure. The index is arranged by diagnostic or procedure codes facilitating the study of patients with the same or similar conditions or treatment. This sorting guides the locating of health records to conduct quality improvement and research studies, as well as for monitoring quality of care. The index is also useful for retrieving records for research studies. The following data elements from the health record are essential for this index (Roberts 2006, 376):

- Principal diagnosis and relevant secondary diagnoses with codes

- Associated procedures and codes

- Patient's health record number

- Patient's gender, age, and race

- Attending physician's code or name

- Service rendered to the patient

- The disposition following service

- Dates of encounter

Table 4.2   Recommended core data elements for MPIs

Data Element	Definition	Data Type[a]
Internal patient identification	Primary identifier used by the facility to identify the patient at admission (for example, the health record number)	Extended composite ID with check digit
Person name	Legal name of patient or person, including surname, given name, middle name or initial, name suffixes (such as, Junior, IV), prefixes (for example, Father, Doctor)	Extended person name
Date of birth	Patient's or person's date of birth: enter the year, month, and day using four digits for the year (YYYY), two digits for the month (MM), and two digits for the day (DD) (so that the information is entered as YYYYMMDD). It is essential that the year of birth be recorded as four numbers, not just the last two numbers.	Time stamp
Date of birth qualifier	An indication of whether the date of birth is the actual date or an estimate. This will distinguish what is known from what is approximated (for example, actual, estimate).	Text data
Gender	Gender of patient (male, female, unknown, or not stated)	Coded value
Race	Race of patient. Race is a concept used to differentiate population groups largely on the basis of physical characteristics transmitted by descent. Races currently used by the federal government for statistical purposes are American Indian and Alaska Native, Asian, Native Hawaiian and Other Pacific Islander, Black or African American, White, and unknown.	Coded value
Ethnicity	Ethnicity of the patient. Ethnicity is a concept used to differentiate population groups on the basis of shared cultural characteristics or geographic origins. Ethnic designations currently used by the federal government for statistical purposes are Hispanic origin, not of Hispanic origin, and unknown.	Coded value
Address	Address or location of patient's residence. Components include the street address, other designation (such as the apartment number), city, state/province, zip or postal code, country, type of address (for example, permanent, mailing)	Extended address
Alias/previous name	Any names by which the patient has been known other than the current legal name; including nicknames, maiden name, previous name that was legally changed, etc.	Extended person name
Social Security number	Personal identification number assigned by the U.S. Social Security Administration	String data
Facility identification	The unique identification number of a facility where patients seek care. (The Health Care Financing Administration is developing a universal identifier system for healthcare facilities. Alternately, the American Hospital Association [AHA] numbering system may be used to identify facilities. The AHA numbering system is maintained centrally, updated frequently, covers private sector and federal hospitals, and contains historical data on institutions even if they cease to exist.)	Person location
Universal patient identifier (when established)	Not yet established	Not yet established
Account number	Number assigned by the facility billing or accounting office for all charges and payments for this encounter	Extended composite ID with check digit
Admission or encounter date	Date the patient actually arrived for care (entered in YYYYMMDD format)	Time stamp
Discharge or departure date	Date the patient actually left the facility or died (entered in YYYYMMDD format)	Time stamp
Encounter or service type	A categorization of the encounter such as emergency, inpatient, outpatient, home care, or electronic (such as e-mail, Internet, telemedicine)	Coded value
Patient disposition	Patient's intended care setting following discharge. Examples include discharge to home (not to home health service), to acute-care hospital, to nursing facility, to home to be under the care of a home health service, or to other healthcare facility; left against medical advice; alive, other, or alive, not stated; died; admitted to hospital; admitted to observation; transferred to skilled nursing facility, intermediate care facility, other facility; or other disposition as dictated by type of MPI	Coded value

[a]Data types correspond to those described in Health Level 7 Version 2.3 (HL7 1996) and E1238.94 (ASTM 1994).
Source: AHIMA MPI Task Force 1997.

Table 4.3   Optional data elements for MPIs

Optional Data Element	Definition
Marital status	Marriage status of the patient (such as, never married, married, separated, widowed, divorced, or unknown)
Telephone number	Telephone number at which patient can be contacted. This may be a home or business telephone number or the telephone number of a friend, neighbor, or relative.
Mother's maiden name	The maiden name of the patient's mother. The maiden name is the given, family, or last name of the mother.
Place of birth	The city, state, and country of the patient's birth
Advance directive and surrogate decision making	An advance directive describes an individual's current preferences about treatment should the person become incompetent or unable to communicate these preferences to medical personnel. Surrogate decision making is an alternative method for medical decision making on the individual's behalf; it is invoked in the absence of an advance directive when the individual is not competent to make an informed decision.
Organ donor status	An indication whether the patient has consented to donate his/her organ(s) in the event of death
Emergency contact	The name, address, telephone number, and relationship of the person whom the patient wishes to be the primary contact if notification is necessary
Allergies/reactions	Delineation of the patient's history of an allergic reaction to a medication based on information provided by the patient or a responsible informant, including the reaction manifestation
Problem list	Master list of all the patient's health problems or diagnoses

Source: AHIMA MPI Task Force 1997.

Table 4.4   Recommended EMPI data elements for HIPAA patient identification

Data Element	Definition
Enterprise identification number	Primary identifier used by the enterprise to identify the patient across facilities (for example, the enterprise number or corporate number)
Facility identifier	Primary identifier used by the enterprise to identify the facility contributing data to the EMPI (for example, the facility code)
Internal patient identification	Primary identifier used by the facility to identify the patient at admission (for example, the health record number)
Person name	Legal name of patient or person, including surname, given name, middle name or initial, name suffixes (such as, Junior, IV), prefixes (for example, Father, Doctor)
Date of birth	Patient or person's date of birth: enter the year, month, and day using four digits for the year (YYYY), two digits for the month (MM), and two digits for the day (DD) (so that the information is entered as YYYYMMDD). It is essential that the year of birth be recorded as four numbers, not just the last two numbers.
Gender	Gender of patient (male, female, unknown, or not stated)
Race	Race of patient. Race is a concept used to differentiate population groups largely on the basis of physical characteristics transmitted by descent. Races currently used by the federal government for statistical purposes are American Indian and Alaska Native, Asian, Native Hawaiian and Other Pacific Islander, Black or African American, White, other, and unknown or not stated.
Ethnicity	Ethnicity of the patient. Ethnicity is a concept used to differentiate population groups on the basis of shared cultural characteristics or geographic origins. Ethnic designations currently used by the federal government for statistical purposes are Hispanic origin, not of Hispanic origin, and unknown.
Residence	Address or location of patient's usual residence. Components include the street address, other designation (such as apartment number), city, state/province, zip or postal code, country, type of address (for example, permanent, mailing)
Alias/previous/ maiden name	Any names by which the patient has been known other than the current legal name; including nicknames, maiden name, previous name that was legally changed, etc.
Social Security number	Personal identification number assigned by the U.S. Social Security Administration
Telephone number	Telephone number at which the patient can be contacted. This may be a home or business telephone number or the telephone number of a friend, neighbor, or relative.

AHIMA MPI Task Force 2004.

Most facilities today have an automated index with predetermined data elements captured from the health records. Standard and special reports are then available from the information system. Frequently, the responsibility for entering the index data is assigned to the HIM department.

Registries

A **registry** is a chronological listing of patients with a common characteristic. Registries usually maintained by healthcare facilities are listed in figure 4.1. Creation and maintenance of these registries is often a responsibility of the HIM department.

Registries are different from indexes because they contain information that is more extensive. These reports are typically generated from a facility's existing database. Registries are also used for patient follow-up as well as aggregate studies.

Registry maintenance consists of the following activities.

- **Case definition**: Describing the patients that are to be included

- **Case finding**: Identifying patients that are to be included

- **Case abstracting**: Extracting the information to be included from health records

The **Agency for Healthcare Research and Quality (AHRQ)**, an agency within HHS, aims to improve the quality, safety, efficiency, and effectiveness of healthcare for all Americans. One of its functions is to support **health services research**. In 2007, AHRQ and CMS published a handbook to help providers set up registries, including recommendations for design and data source access and suggestions on ways to encourage participation in registries.

Healthcare Databases

Individual health records are a rich source of data about an individual patient. However, it is not easy to see trends in a population of patients by looking at individual records. To reveal patterns, data must be extracted from individual records and entered into databases. These data may be used in a **facility-specific** or **population-based registry** for research and improvement in customer care. In addition, they may be reported to the state and become part of state and federal databases used to inform health policy and improve healthcare (Bowman 2006b, 288).

The HIM professional can play a variety of roles in managing secondary records and databases including setting up databases. This task includes determining the content of the database and ensuring compliance with the laws, regulations, and accreditation standards that affect its content and use. All data elements included in the database or registry must be defined in a data dictionary. The HIM professional may oversee the completeness and accuracy of the data abstracted for inclusion in the database or registry (Bowman 2006b, 288).

Figure 4.1.   Registries maintained by healthcare facilities.

Standard registries	Specialty registries
• Admissions	• Trauma
• Discharges	• Disease-specific (for example, cancer, AIDS, diabetes)
• Operating/surgical	• Birth defects
• Births	• Implants
• Deaths	• Transplants
	• Immunizations

Data Quality Issues

Indexes, registries, and databases are only helpful when the data they contain are accurate. Decisions concerning new treatment methods, healthcare policy, and physician credentialing and privileging are based on these databases. Incorrect data will likely result in serious errors in decision making (Bowman 2006b, 301). Considerations for protecting the quality of data in indexes, registries, and databases is summarized in table 4.5.

Primary and Secondary Data Sources

Data are categorized as either **primary** or **aggregate data**. The health record consists entirely of **patient-specific/identifiable data** or primary data. Aggregate data (also referred to as **secondary data**) includes compiled information on groups of people or patients without identifying any particular patient individually.

The health record is considered a **primary data source** because it contains patient-specific data and information about a patient that has been documented by the professionals who provided care or services to that patient. Data taken from the health record and entered into registries and databases are considered a secondary data source (Bowman 2006b, 288–289).

Secondary data sources provide information that is not easily available by looking at individual health records. Data taken from health records and entered into disease-oriented databases can help researchers determine the effectiveness of alternate treatment methods. They can also quickly demonstrate survival rates at different stages of diseases. Types of secondary data sources are listed in table 4.6.

There are both internal and external users of secondary data sources. Internal users are located within the healthcare facility. External users are individuals and institutions outside the facility, such as the CDC, NCHS, and NCVHS. Some diseases must be reported to the state department of health. See chapter 3 and figure 3.8 (p. 63) for additional information. The federal government collects data from the states on vital events such as births and deaths (Bowman 2006b, 288–289).

Standardized Clinical Data Sets

Data and information pertaining to individuals who use healthcare services are collected in virtually every setting where healthcare is delivered. These data elements, representing facts, usually describe specific characteristics of individual patients. In healthcare settings, data are stored in the individual's health record whether that record is in paper or electronic format. The numerous data elements in the health record are then combined, analyzed, and interpreted by the patient's physician and other clinicians.

Table 4.5 Strategies to protect the quality of data in indexes, registries, and databases

Data Quality Element	Description	Method to Ensure Quality
Validity	Accuracy of data	Incorporate edits
Reliability	Consistency of data	Have more than one person abstract data for the same case
Completeness	Avoid missing data	Look at a variety of sources Don't allow blanks
Timelines	Up-to-date data	Set targets for abstract completion

Source: Adapted from Bowman 2006a, 421–423.

Table 4.6 Types of secondary data sources

Facility-specific Indexes	Healthcare Databases
Master Patient Index (MPI) and **Enterprise Master Person Index** Alphabetic file	Disease Registries (specific diagnoses)
Disease and **Operation Indexes** (arranged by code number)	Cancer Registries (trends in cancer incidence)
Physician's Index (cases of a physician)	Trauma Registries (injuries caused by external physical force)
	Birth Defects Registries (newborns with defects)
National, State, and County Public Health Databases	Diabetes Registries (patient follow up)
National Healthcare Survey	Implant Registries (device tracking by **FDA**)
National Hospital Discharge Survey	Transplant Registries (donor organs and recipients)
National Employer Health Insurance Survey	Immunization Registries (required childhood immunizations)
National Health Provider Inventory	HIV/AIDS Registries
National Ambulatory Medical Care Survey	Cardiac Registries
National Nursing Home Survey	
National Hospital Ambulatory Medical Care Survey	**National and Administrative Databases**
National Home and Hospice Care Survey	Medicare Provider Analysis and Review File (MEDPAR)— acute care and SNF claims data
	National Practitioner Database (NPDB) —medical malpractice payments and sanctions by boards of medical examiners
	Healthcare Integrity and Protection Data Bank (fraud and abuse information)
Other Databases	
Health Services Research Databases—**Agency for Healthcare Research and Quality (AHRQ)** (efficiency and effectiveness of healthcare delivery system)	
Healthcare Cost and Utilization Project (HCUP) • Nationwide Inpatient Sample (NIS) • State Inpatient Database (SID) • State Ambulatory Surgery Database (SASD) • Kids Inpatient Database (KID)	
National Library of Medicine • MEDLINE • Unified Medical Language System (UMLS)	

The data sets originally developed to support uniform data collection are inadequate for an electronic environment, and many public and private organizations have been actively engaged in the process of developing healthcare information standards to support EHR development and information exchange.

The idea of data standardization became widely accepted during the 1960s. Under the leadership of the NCHS and the NCVHS in collaboration with other organizations, data sets were developed for a variety of healthcare settings. Data sets for acute care, long-term care, and ambulatory care were the first to be created. Standardizing data elements and definitions makes it possible to compare the data collected at different facilities. The **National Alliance for Health Information Technology (NAHIT)** has compiled a comprehensive list of current health-related standards in its Alliance Standards Directory. Available online at www.hitsdir.org, the directory overviews the extent of the many standards used in the healthcare industry (LaTour 2006, 162).

Healthcare **data sets** have two purposes:

1. To identify data elements that should be collected for each patient
2. To provide uniform definitions for common terms

Characteristics of several healthcare data sets are detailed in table 4.7.

Table 4.7   Characteristics of data sets

Data Sets	Characteristics
Uniform Hospital Discharge Data Set (UHDDS)	**Patient-specific** data items on every inpatient
	Collected by all short-term general hospitals in the United States
	Incorporated into federal regulations (Medicare and Medicaid)
Uniform Ambulatory Care Data Set (UACDS)	Used in every facility for outpatient care
	Includes optional data items
	Voluntary
Minimum Data Set for Long-term Care Resident Assessment **Protocols**	Residential facilities, nursing home residents
	Federally mandated
	Collected on admission and at designated reassessment points
	Uses structured lists
	Used for patient assessment
Outcomes Assessment Information Set (OASIS)	Home health industry
	Gathered for Medicare beneficiaries
	Measures patient outcomes
	Assesses quality of care
	Basis for reimbursement
Data Elements for Emergency Department Systems (DEEDS)	Emergency and trauma care
	Hospital-based emergency departments
	Reduces incompatibilities in ER records
	Incorporates national standards for electronic data interchange (EDI)
Essential Medical Data Set (EMDS)	Complement to DEEDS
	Part of NHIN
	Used for emergency encounters
	Past medical history
Health Plan Employer Data and Information Set (HEDIS)	Data to compare performance of managed care plans
	Sponsored by NCQA
	Administrative, claims, health record review data
	Used to develop physician profiles
	Population-based data collection tool
ORYX	Performance measurement
	To promote a comprehensive, continuous, data-driven Joint Commission accreditation process
National Health Information Network (NHIN)	Allow electronic exchange among healthcare facilities
	Increase patient safety, reduce medical errors, increase efficiency and effectiveness
	Contain costs

The main trend in collecting secondary data seems to be the increased use of automated data entry. Registries and databases are more commonly using data already available in electronic form rather than manually abstracting all data. As the electronic health record becomes more common, separate databases for various diseases and conditions will be unnecessary. The patient health record itself will be a database that can be queried for information currently obtained from specialized registries.

Healthcare information standards development is a dynamic process that evolves on a continuous basis as key players in the standards development community negotiate, refine, and revise standards. The critical importance of healthcare information standards has been recognized in recent federal initiatives including the **Consolidated Health Informatics (CHI) Initiatives** as well as efforts of the **Office of the National Coordinator for Health Information Technology (ONC)**.

According to the NCVHS in its initial 2000 report titled *Toward a National Health Information Infrastructure*, if information in multiple locations is to be searched, shared, and synthesized when needed, we will need agreed-upon information guardians that can exchange data with each other. We will need equitable rules of data exchange so that competitors will be willing to connect and share data.

Summary

Health record information is valuable to individual patients for continuity of care and documenting evidence of episodes of care. The information is also valuable in an aggregate form to report incidence of disease and effectiveness of care. Statistical reporting of healthcare trends in a variety of indexes, registries, and databases is another common function of the HIM services. The HIM professional is responsible for developing, maintaining, and ensuring the accuracy of this aggregate data. An additional responsibility is for the transmission of required reports to local, state, and national agencies as well as providing statistics to the local facility that guide administrative and clinical decisions.

References

Agency for Healthcare Research and Quality. 2007. *Registries for Evaluating Patient Outcomes: A User's Guide.* Rockville, MD: AHRQ. Available online from http://effectivehealthcare.ahrq.gov/reports/topic.cfm?topic=0&sid=2&rType=11&selection=9.

AHIMA MPI Task Force. 2004. Practice brief: Building an enterprise master person index. *Journal of American Health Information Management Association* 75(1): 56A–D.

Bowman, Elizabeth. 2006a. Secondary data sources. Chapter 9 in *Health Information Management Technology: An Applied Approach*, 2nd ed. Edited by Merida Johns. Chicago: AHIMA.

Bowman, Elizabeth. 2006b. Secondary records and healthcare databases. Chapter 12 in *Health Information Management: Concepts, Principles, and Practice,* 2nd ed. Edited by Kathleen M. LaTour and Shirley Eichenwald-Maki. Chicago: AHIMA.

Centers for Disease Control and Prevention. 2007. *CDC WONDER Database.* Available online from http://wonder.cdc.gov/.

Department of Health and Human Services. 2005. *Office of the Assistant Secretary for Planning and Evaluation: The HHS Data Council.* Available online from http://aspe.hhs.gov/datacncl.

Kanaan, Susan Baird. 2000. *The National Committee on Vital and Health Statistics, 1949–1999: A history.* Available online from www.ncvhs.hhs.gov/50history.htm.

LaTour, Kathleen M. 2006. Healthcare data sets. Chapter 5 in *Health Information Management Technology: An Applied Approach*, 2nd ed. Edited by Merida Johns. Chicago: AHIMA.

National Center for Health Statistics. 2007. About NCHS. Available online from www.cdc.gov/nchs/about.htm.

National Committee on Vital and Health Statistics (NCVHS). 2000. Toward a national health information infrastructure. Washington, D.C.: HHS.

Roberts, Jane. 2006. Health information technology functions. Chapter 8 in *Health Information Management Technology: An Applied Approach,* 2nd ed. Edited by Merida Johns. Chicago: AHIMA.

Chapter 5

Clinical Information and Observations

Barbara Odom-Wesley, PhD, RHIA, FAHIMA

Learning Objectives

- List the types of demographic data collected in health records and explain the purpose of each element

- List the types of administrative information collected in health records and explain the purpose of each element

- Identify the types of clinical information collected in health records and explain the purpose of each element

- List the data elements collected in the report of history and physical examination and explain their relevance to patient treatment

- Describe the types of services covered in physicians' orders

- List the various types of documentation authored by physicians and explain their content and functions

- Explain the conditions under which medical consultations should be ordered

- List the various types of documentation authored by nurses and explain their content and functions

- Explain the functions of general and special consents

- List the data elements that must be included in laboratory reports

- List the data elements that must be included in imaging reports

- Explain the purpose and content of anesthesia assessments and reports

- List the data elements that must be included in operative reports

- List the data elements that must be included in pathology reports

- List the data elements that should be collected in implant and transplantation records

- Explain the function and content of discharge summaries

- Explain the function and content of patient instructions

- List the various types of specialty documentation maintained in acute-care records

- List the data elements that must be collected in emergency and trauma records
- List the standard clinical data sets that are collected for hospital patients and describe their content

Key Terms

Activities of daily living (ADL)

Administrative information

Advance directive

Agency for Healthcare Research and Quality (AHRQ)

Ancillary services

Autopsy report

Cardiology reports

Care plan

Case management

Charting by exception

Clinical information

Clinical pathways

Clinical practice guidelines

Clinical protocols

Commission on Accreditation of Rehabilitation Facilities (CARF)

Comorbidities

Complication

Computerized physician order entry (CPOE)

Consent to treatment

Consultation reports

Data Elements for Emergency Department Systems (DEEDS)

Demographic data

Discharge summary

Do-not-resuscitate (DNR) order

Dumping

Emergency Medical Treatment and Active Labor Act (EMTALA)

Encounter note

Essential Medical Data Set (EMEDS)

Expressed consent

Financial data

Flow charts

History

Hospitalist

Imaging reports

Implied consent

Interval note

Intraoperative anesthesia record

Labor and delivery record

Laboratory reports

Master patient index (MPI)

Medication record

National Guideline Clearinghouse (NGC)

Neurology reports

Notice of privacy practices

Nursing assessment

Nutritional assessment

Operative report

Pathology report

Patient assessment instrument (PAI)

Patient's rights

Physician's orders

Postoperative anesthesia record

Preoperative anesthesia evaluation

Principal diagnosis

Principal procedure

Progress notes

Recovery room record

Transfer records

Transfusion record

Uniform Ambulatory Care Data Set (UACDS)

Uniform Hospital Discharge Data Set (UHDDS)

Unique identifier

Visit note

Introduction

A separate health record is maintained for every patient who receives services in a healthcare facility. The content of the record reflects the patient's reason for seeking services, diagnosed illnesses, and the types of services that are planned and provided to the patient during his or her treatment.

The services provided by hospitals and other providers are separated into two broad categories: medical and surgical. Categories such as pediatrics, obstetrics, and neonatal may also exist if the facility is large enough to have separate and distinct units for each individual service. The category for each admission is determined by the specialty of the admitting physician in addition to the nature of the patient's illness. For example, a patient with a diagnosis of myocardial infarction could be admitted as a medical patient either to the internal medicine service or to the cardiology service, depending on the specialty of the admitting physician. Another patient with a history of cardiac ischemia who requires cardiac bypass surgery would be admitted as a surgical patient to the cardiovascular surgery service. In this case, the admitting physician would be a cardiovascular surgeon.

The documentation in healthcare records includes both administrative and clinical information. **Administrative information** includes personal information about the patient, such as name, address, birth date, and age. It includes consents for treatment and use of healthcare information. Administrative information also describes the nature of the patient's admission, or chief complaint, and the patient's health insurance coverage. Administrative information is usually collected before or during the admissions process.

The **clinical information** in healthcare records documents the patient's condition and course of treatment. The following types of information are documented in the healthcare record:

- The patient's physical condition upon initial examination and the reason why the patient's condition required treatment

- The patient's medical history

- The diagnostic and therapeutic orders given by the patient's physician(s)

- The observations made by clinicians over the course of the patient's treatment (progress notes)

- The outcomes of diagnostic and therapeutic services, including surgical interventions

- The patient's final diagnosis and condition at discharge

The same administrative and clinical information is collected in both paper-based and electronic health record systems. Only the data collection, storage, authentication, and security technologies differ. This chapter provides examples of both paper and electronic data collection tools.

In addition to fulfilling operational and clinical information requirements, the content of health records must comply with various state and federal regulations, accreditation standards, and professional practice guidelines. (Standards and regulations are discussed in detail in chapter 3.)

The data in hospital records must also conform to one of two uniform healthcare data sets: the **Uniform Hospital Discharge Data Set (UHDDS)** for inpatient services and the **Uniform Ambulatory Care Data Set (UACDS)** for outpatient services. A third data set has been developed for emergency and trauma departments in hospitals, but the use of **Data Elements for Emergency Department Systems (DEEDS)** is voluntary. (See figures 5.1 through 5.3.)

Uniform data sets have two purposes, as follows:

1. They ensure that the same types of data are collected for every patient.

2. They provide standardized definitions of the data to be collected.

Thus, the data sets collected by different hospitals can be compared, and the data can be combined for national analysis and healthcare delivery planning.

Administrative Information and Demographic, Financial, and Clinical Data

For elective services, administrative information and demographic data are often collected prior to the scheduled services, which could include preauthorization and/or precertification from the insurance company. Alternatively, the patient may provide the information to registration staff on the day of the service. Administrative information for unplanned services is often provided by the patient or the patient's representative in the hospital's emergency department or other point of intake.

Admitting and Registration Information

The registration staff collects personal information about the patient as well as information about the patient's health insurance coverage at the time of admission. Virtually all healthcare organizations currently use a computer-based registration system tied to a database called the **master patient index (MPI).** When the patient has been treated in the facility in the past, registration personnel check the patient's current information against the information in the database to ensure that it is current and correct. The patient's administrative information is then recorded on an identification sheet (often called a face sheet). In paper-based record systems, a printout of the identification sheet is used as the front page in the patient's record.

Demographic Data

The term *demographics* refers to the study of statistical information about human populations. In the context of healthcare, **demographic data** includes basic factual information about the individual patient, including the following:

- Patient's full name
- Patient's address
- Patient's telephone number
- Patient's gender
- Patient's date and place of birth
- Patient's race or ethnic origin
- Patient's marital status
- Name and address of the patient's next of kin
- Patient's Social Security number
- Patient account number
- Patient medical record number
- Admission date
- Primary-care physician
- Admitting physician

The main purpose of collecting demographic data is to confirm the unique identity of the patient. Hospitals and other healthcare-related organizations also use the demographic data collected from patients as the basis of statistical records, research, and resource planning.

Figure 5.1.   UHDDS data elements.

Data Element	Definition/Descriptor
01. Personal identifier	The unique number assigned to each patient within a hospital that distinguishes the patient and his or her hospital record from all others in that institution.
02. Date of birth	Month, day, and year of birth. Capture of the full four-digit year of birth is recommended.
03. Sex	Male or female

04. Race and ethnicity	04a. Race
	    American Indian/Eskimo/Aleut 04b. Ethnicity
	    Asian or Pacific Islander Spanish origin/Hispanic
	    Black Non-Spanish origin/Non-Hispanic
	    White Unknown
	    Other race
	    Unknown

05. Residence	Full address of usual residence Zip code (nine digits, if available) Code for foreign residence
06. Hospital identification	A unique institutional number used across data collection systems. The Medicare provider number is the preferred hospital identifier.
07. Admission date	Month, day, and year of admission.
08. Type of admission	Scheduled: Arranged with admissions office at least 24 hours prior to admission Unscheduled: All other admissions
09. Discharge date	Month, day, and year of discharge
10 & 11. Physician identification • Attending physician • Operating physician	The Medicare unique physician identification number (UPIN) is the preferred method of identifying the attending physician and operating physician(s) because it is uniform across all data systems.
12. Principal diagnosis	The condition established, after study, to be chiefly responsible for occasioning the admission of the patient to the hospital for care.
13. Other diagnoses	All conditions that coexist at the time of admission or that develop subsequently or that affect the treatment received and/or the length of stay. Diagnoses that relate to an earlier episode and have no bearing on the current hospital stay are to be excluded.
14. Qualifier for other diagnoses	A qualifier is given for each diagnosis coded under "other diagnoses" to indicate whether the onset of the diagnosis preceded or followed admission to the hospital. The option "uncertain" is permitted.
15. External cause-of-injury code	The ICD-9-CM code for the external cause of an injury, poisoning, or adverse effect (commonly referred to as an E code). Hospitals should complete this item whenever there is a diagnosis of an injury, poisoning, or adverse effect.
16. Birth weight of neonate	The specific birth weight of a newborn, preferably recorded in grams.
17. Procedures and dates	All significant procedures are to be reported. A significant procedure is one that is: • Surgical in nature, or • Carries an anesthetic risk, or • Carries a procedural risk, or • Requires specialized training. The date of each significant procedure must be reported. When more than one procedure is reported, the principal procedure must be designated. The principal procedure is one that is performed for definitive treatment rather than one performed for diagnostic or exploratory purposes or was necessary to take care of a complication. If two procedures appear to be principal, the one most closely related to the principal diagnosis should be selected as the principal procedure. The UPIN must be reported for the person performing the principal procedure.

18. Disposition of the patient	• Discharged to home (excludes those patients • Discharged to other healthcare facility
	  referred to home health service) • Left against medical advice
	• Discharged to acute-care hospital • Alive, other; or alive, not stated
	• Discharged to nursing facility • Died
	• Discharged home to be under the care of a
	  home health service (including a hospice)

19. Patient's expected source of payment	Primary source Other sources All categories for primary and other sources are: • Blue Cross/Blue Shield • Health maintenance organization (HMO) • Other health insurance companies • CHAMPUS • Other liability insurance • CHAMPVA • Medicare • Other government payers • Medicaid • Self-pay • Worker's Compensation • No charge (free, charity, special research, teaching) • Self-insured employer plan • Other
20. Total charges	All charges billed by the hospital for this hospitalization. Professional charges for individual patient care by physicians are excluded.

Figure 5.2.   UACDS data elements.

Data Element	Definition/Descriptor
Provider identification, address, type of practice	Provider identification: Include the full name of the provider as well as the unique physician identification number (UPIN). Address: The complete address of the provider's office. In cases where the provider has multiple offices, the location of the usual or principal place of practice should be given. Profession: • Physician, including specialty or field of practice • Other (specify)
Place of encounter	Specify the location of the encounter: • Private office • Clinic or health center • Hospital outpatient department • Hospital emergency department • Other (specify)
Reason for encounter	Includes, but is not limited to, the patient's complaints and symptoms reflecting his or her own perception of needs, provided verbally or in writing by the patient at the point of entry into the healthcare system or in the patient's own words recorded by an intermediary or provider at that time.
Diagnostic services	All diagnostic services of any type.
Problem, diagnosis, or assessment	Describes the provider's level of understanding and the interpretation of the patient's reasons for the encounter and all conditions requiring treatment or management at the time of the encounter.
Therapeutic services	List, by name, all services done or ordered: • Medical (including drug therapy) • Surgical • Patient education
Preventive services	List, by name, all preventive services and procedures performed at the time of encounter.

Disposition	The provider's statement of the next step(s) in the care of the patient. At a minimum, the following classification is suggested:
	
	1. No follow up planned
	2. Follow up planned
	   • Return when necessary
	   • Return to the current provider at a specified time
	   • Telephone follow up
	   • Return to referring provider
	   • Refer to other provider
	   • Admit to hospital
	   • Other

Figure 5.3.   Example of a DEEDS data element.

 4.06 **CHIEF COMPLAINT**

PART OF THE CHIEF COMPLAINT GROUP (4.06 AND 4.07)*

Definition

Patient's reason for seeking care or attention, expressed in terms as close as possible to those used by patient or responsible informant.

Uses

Data collected on the patient's chief complaint are pivotal to the clinical process and provide an important resource for measuring and evaluating health care services. The chief complaint figures prominently in triage decision making and is a key determinant of the direction and extent of history taking, physical examination, and diagnostic testing in the ED. When ED data on chief complaint are aggregated and linked with process, diagnosis, and financial data, they take on added value for clinical and epidemiologic research, practitioner training, quality management, and health care administration and finance.

Discussion

Chief complaints encompass more than reports of symptoms or complaints. A chief complaint may also be a request for:
- a diagnostic, screening, or preventive procedure;
- treatment or compliance with a practitioner's instructions to seek a specific treatment, procedure, or medication;
- test results;
- an examination required by a third-party;
- a referral, such as follow-up initiated from this ED or elsewhere; or
- intervention for a stated diagnosis or disease.

Although data describing the chief complaint are routinely and often repetitively recorded during a single ED visit, the data generally are not classified, coded, and stored in a form that facilitates aggregate analysis. Several established systems are candidates for classifying and coding ED chief complaints, but modifications or adaptations are likely to be needed for routine ED use. Among the candidate systems are the *International Classification of Primary Care* (ICPC), *Reason for Visit Classification and Coding Manual* (RVC), *Systematized Nomenclature of Human and Veterinary Medicine—(SNOMED) International*, *Read Codes Version 3*, and the *International Classification of Diseases, 9th Revision, Clinical Modification* (lCD-9-CM). In the interim, text descriptions or local codes can be used.

Data Type (and Field Length)

CE—coded element (200).

Repetition

Yes; if there is more than one chief complaint, the Chief Complaint Group repeats.

---

*The Chief Complaint Group includes data elements 4.06 and 4.07. A single iteration of this group is used to report each chief complaint.

Figure 5.3. (continued)

Field Values

Component 1 is the chief complaint code.

Component 2 is the chief complaint descriptor.

Component 3 is the coding system identifier.

Components 4–6 can be used for an alternate code, descriptor, and coding system identifier.

For example, to encode headache using the *International Classification of Primary Care* (ICP):

Component 1 = N01

Component 2 = Headache

Component 3 = ICP

Text data also can be entered without an accompanying code, as follows:

Component 1 = ""

Component 2 = Headache

If the chief complaint is unknown, enter data in the following manner:

Component 1 = Unknown

Data Standards or Guidelines

None.

Other References

ICPC (Lamberts and Wood 1987), *RVC* (National Center for Health Statistics 1994), *SNOMED International* (Cote et al. 1993), *Read Codes Version 3: A User Led Terminology* (O'Neill et al. 1995), and *ICD-9-CM* (U.S. Department of Health and Human Services 1995).

Social Security numbers are often used to help identify patients. Healthcare facilities assign **unique identifiers** to individual health records to ensure that the information in the records is not misplaced, lost, or confused with another person. For most facilities, the health record (often called a medical record) remains constant for each patient. Each time the patient presents to the facility, the same medical record number is utilized; this allows communication between past and present admissions and course of treatment to be passed along in a consistent manner. The account number changes with each admission to provide an account of the current course of treatment.

Financial Data

Details about the patient's occupation, employer, and insurance coverage are also collected at the time of admission/intake. These data are used to complete the claims forms that will be submitted by the provider to third-party payers. It is not unusual to include a copy of the insurance card to verify information. Financial data also provide the beginning of the revenue cycle by identifying those patients who may need follow-up contact with the insurance company by the case manager. **Financial data** include the following:

- Patient's name
- Name of the insured party and his or her relationship to the patient if the patient is a dependent of the insured party
- Insured party's member identification number
- Name of the insurance company and the group policy number
- Employer's name and address

Clinical Data

Basic clinical data are also recorded during the admissions process. The reason for the patient's admission and the patient's preliminary diagnosis should be provided or confirmed by the admitting physician. The accuracy of this information is important because it becomes the basis of care plans and determinations of medical necessity.

Consents, Authorizations, and Acknowledgments

Hospitals and other healthcare organizations are required to obtain written consents and authorizations before they provide treatment or release confidential patient information. Acknowledgments usually apply to the patient's confirmation that he or she has received specific information. All consents, authorizations, and acknowledgments that have been signed by patients or their legal representatives in connection with services to be provided in a hospital should be stored in the patients' health records.

Consents Related to Clinical Care

The need to obtain the patient's consent before performing medical and surgical procedures is based on the legal concept of battery. Battery is the unlawful touching of a person without his or her implied or expressed consent.

Implied consent is assumed when a patient voluntarily submits to medical treatment. The rationale behind this conclusion is that it is reasonable to assume that patients must understand the nature of the medical care or they would not submit to it. **Expressed consent** is permission that is either spoken or written. Although the courts recognize both spoken and written forms of consent, spoken consent is more difficult to prove in a legal proceeding.

Most healthcare providers ask patients or their legal representatives to sign a general **consent to treatment**. By signing a general consent to treatment, the patient agrees to submit to routine clinical procedures and medical and nursing care while he or she is a patient. Except in emergency situations, patients are usually asked to sign a general consent form during the admissions process. More specific consents are required for procedures that involve significant risk, such as invasive diagnostic tests, transfusions, and surgery. These specific consents are completed in addition to the general consent forms. (See figure 5.4.)

Consents Related to Confidential Health Information

Since the implementation of the Health Insurance Portability and Accountability Act (HIPAA) (1996), hospitals and other healthcare organizations have been required to provide information to patients about the facilities' use of confidential health information. The explanation must be provided in the form of a **notice of privacy practices**. The notice must describe how the patient's health information will be used, and it must provide examples of those uses in hospital treatment and operations as well as reimbursement. (See figure 5.5.)

Acknowledgments

Several types of administrative information are provided or collected by admissions staff. Patients are asked to sign forms to verify that they have received the required information. The acknowledgments then become part of the patient's health record.

Advance Directives

The admissions staff is required by law to ask patients whether they have established advance directives and to inform patients that they have the right to accept or refuse medical treatment. An **advance directive** is a written document that describes the patient's healthcare preferences in the event that he or she is unable to communicate directly at some point in the future. Advance directives include such items as living wills and statements of the patient's wishes in case of a critical illness, such as life support, ventilator support, and food and hydration.

Hospitals are also required to provide written information to patients explaining hospital policies regarding advance directives. The information must describe the treatment decisions that patients may make and any related hospital policies.

When the patient has executed such a document, federal law also requires that fact to be noted in the patient's health record. A copy of the document may be included in the record, but it is not required. Evidence that the patient's physician has discussed the patient's wishes with the patient or the patient's next of kin constitutes sufficient health record documentation.

Patient's Rights Information

The Medicare *Conditions of Participation* (2006) require hospitals to provide patients with a **patient's rights** statement at the time of admission. The patient's healthcare rights include the following:

- The right to know who is providing treatment
- The right to confidentiality

Figure 5.4.   Combined consent to treatment and consent to the use and disclosure of protected health information.

University of Anystate Hospitals

**CONSENT FOR TREATMENT AND DISCLOSURE
OF PROTECTED HEALTH INFORMATION**
PAGE 1 OF 2

PATIENT LABEL

To the Patient (or his/her parent, guardian, or legal representative):

Before University of Anystate Hospitals and Clinics or any of its departments can provide inpatient or outpatient services to you, you will need to understand the services you are to receive, give the hospital your consent to perform those services, and agree to pay for them. You will also need to understand the ways the hospital uses the information in your health record and agree to allow the hospital to use that information.

Part I of this form covers your consent to treatment and explains other important matters related to your healthcare. Part II explains the use of your personal health information. You may ask a member of the admissions staff to read this form to you, and we encourage you to ask any questions you may have about it. When you fully understand the form's content, please sign it in the place indicated on the back of the form. Thank you very much for helping us to fulfill the hospital's responsibility to you and the rest of the community we serve.

Part I: Treatment-Related Information

Consent to the Treatment

You authorize your physician and/or other qualified medical providers to perform medical treatments and services on your behalf. You also consent to all of the hospital medical and/or diagnostic services ordered for you during your outpatient visit or inpatient stay in the hospital. This consent includes testing for infections such as hepatitis B and HIV and providing blood or body fluids for such tests in order to protect you and/or those who care for you.

Payment for Services and Insurance

You are directly responsible for paying for the services provided during your hospital visit or stay. The hospital will work directly with the third parties who provide coverage of your medical expenses, including health insurance companies, Medicare, Medicaid, Workers' Compensation, and various types of liability, accident, and disability insurance providers. By signing this form, you attest that your insurance coverage is current, valid, and effective and that you will promptly pay any required copayment amounts and unpaid deductibles. If your stay qualifies for Medicare coverage, the benefits you will receive include coverage for the physician services that were performed as part of your hospital care.

You guarantee payment to the hospital for all noncovered services and any unpaid, billed amounts not covered by insurance benefits when your insurance plan allows the hospital to bill you for any unpaid balances. You understand and accept that your physician's orders may include services not paid by insurance plans but will be provided to you by the hospital. Also, you accept that insurance plans may deny payment for what you believed were covered services, resulting in your responsibility for paying for these services. You may be billed for the professional component of any hospital services, such as the professional component for clinical laboratory tests.

Valuables

You accept full responsibility for your valuables, especially money or jewelry. The hospital does not accept any liability for your valuables. The hospital expects you will entrust any valuables to family or friends for safekeeping. Alternatively, you may deposit them in the safe that the hospital provides for that purpose. This is especially important when you are an inpatient, but this responsibility also extends to when you are an outpatient and must change into a hospital gown, remove jewelry, or undergo sedation during a medical procedure.

Special Note for Medicare or CHAMPUS Beneficiaries

You acknowledge and certify by your signature that all of the information you have provided to the hospital for Medicare or CHAMPUS benefits is correct. You also agree to allow the hospital or others who have information on your Medicare or CHAMPUS benefits claim to provide this information to Medicare or CHAMPUS or their agents in order for them to determine your eligibility for benefits. To carry out this activity, the hospital may use a copy rather than the original of this consent form. You also acknowledge that you have received a copy of the *Important Message from Medicare* or the *Important Message from CHAMPUS* form. This acknowledgement does not waive your rights for a review or make you liable for payment.

Figure 5.4. (continued)

University of Anystate Hospitals

**CONSENT FOR TREATMENT AND DISCLOSURE
OF PROTECTED HEALTH INFORMATION**
PAGE 2 OF 2

PATIENT LABEL

Part II: Health Record-Related Information

Consent to the Use and Disclosure of Protected Health Information

You agree to honestly, completely, and correctly provide all requested information. You also agree to permit the hospital to share your health record as applicable under the law with your physician, your insurers, Medicare, Medicaid, or their designated agents. They may review your record and copy it in full or in part in order to obtain billing and payment information. Insurers (private or government) may also use your health record to determine whether they cover your services. You agree to allow the hospital to use the record created during this visit to meet any reporting requirements related to your care and to collect payment for the services you received. You agree to allow your physicians to send copies of your health records to other physicians, hospitals, and healthcare facilities as they deem necessary for continuity of care. You also agree to have your name posted on scheduling boards and outside your hospital room.

Specific Uses of Your Protected Information

The hospital originates and maintains health records describing your health history, symptoms, examination and test results, diagnoses, treatment, and any plans for future care or treatment. This information serves as:

- The basis of care planning and treatment

- A means of communication among the many healthcare professionals who contribute to your care

- A source of information for applying diagnosis and surgical information to your bill

- A means by which a third-party payer (usually your insurance company or a government healthcare program) can verify that the services billed were actually provided

- A tool for routine healthcare operations, such as assessing quality and reviewing the competence of healthcare professionals

Your signature acknowledges that you received the *Notice of Information Practices,* which provides a description of information uses and disclosure practices. You accept and understand that:

- You have the right to review the notice prior to signing this consent.

- The hospital reserves the right to change the notice and its information practices, for past, current, or future information. The new notice will contain the effective date on its first page and be made available on our Web site.

- You have the right to object to the use of your health information for the hospital's patient directory.

- You have the right to request restrictions on the use or disclosure of your health information to carry out treatment, payment, or healthcare operations and to correct error(s) in your record. The hospital, however, is not required to agree to the restrictions requested.

- You may revoke in writing the consent that you provide to the hospital. The revocation does not apply to any uses of your information made by the hospital in reliance upon this consent form and on the belief that your consent was still effective.

I certify that I have read (or had read to me) both parts of this form and fully understand and agree to the content.

Patient/Agent: _____ Date: _____

If you are signing as the patient's agent, please state your relationship to the patient (parent, guardian, or legal representative): _____

Witness (when form is accepted verbally,
by telephone, or by electronic means): _____ Date: _____

CONSENT FOR TREATMENT AND DISCLOSURE
000002 (11/2002)

Figure 5.5.   Acknowledgment of notice of privacy practices.

Anytown Community Hospital

**ACKNOWLEDGMENT OF NOTICE
OF PRIVACY PRACTICES**

PATIENT LABEL

I understand that as part of my healthcare, this organization originates and maintains health records describing my health history, symptoms, examination and test results, diagnoses, treatment, and any plans for future care or treatment. I understand that this information serves as:

- A basis for planning my care and treatment
- A means of communication among the many health professionals who contribute to my care
- A source of information for applying my diagnosis and surgical information to my bill
- A means by which a third-party payer can verify that services billed were actually provided
- And a tool for routine healthcare operations such as assessing quality and reviewing the competence of healthcare professionals

I understand and have been provided with a *Notice of Information Practices* that provides a more complete description of information uses and disclosures. I understand that I have the right to review the notice prior to signing this consent. I understand that the organization reserves the right to change their notice and practices and prior to implementation will mail a copy of any revised notice to the address I've provided. I understand that I have the right to object to the use of my health information for directory purposes. I understand that I have the right to request restrictions as to how my health information may be used or disclosed to carry out treatment, payment, or healthcare operations and that the organization is not required to agree to the restrictions requested. I understand that I may revoke this consent in writing, except to the extent that the organization has already take action in reliance thereon.

☐ I request the following restrictions to the use or disclosure of my health information:

_____

_____

Signature of Patient or Legal Representative	Date

Witness	Date

Notice Effective Date or Version

☐ Accepted   ☐ Denied

Signature	Title	Date

ACKNOWLEDGMENT OF PRIVACY NOTICE
100093 (1/2002)

- The right to receive information about treatment

- The right to refuse treatment

- The right to participate in care planning

- The right to be safe from abusive treatment

Some hospitals ask patients to sign an acknowledgment that they have received patient's rights information. The signed acknowledgment then becomes a permanent part of the patient's record. State regulations often require similar explanations and stipulate additional patient's rights, such as the right to privacy in treatment.

Other Administrative Information

Some hospitals ask patients to sign a release that absolves the facility from any responsibility for the loss or damage of personal property. This form is signed during the admissions process and then becomes part of the patient's health record.

Birth and death certificates are not considered part of the legal health record, although copies may be stored in patients' records. Hospital personnel often prepare this administrative documentation and submit it to state and local departments of health.

Clinical Information

The most important function of the health record is the collection of information on the patient's medical condition and progress throughout his or her treatment. Physicians, surgeons, and nurses are the main authors of clinical documentation. Most states outline requirements for clinical documentation within their hospital rules and regulations; in addition, facilities will address clinical entries made in the medical record in their medical staff bylaws.

Allied health professionals who provide direct patient care also document their services and author health record entries. Allied health professionals who provide patient care include respiratory, physical, occupational, and speech therapists.

Depending on facility policy, social workers, psychologists, and dietitians may also document their services directly in the health record. Dietitians write nutritional assessments and nutrition plans. Psychologists report the results of developmental assessments and behavioral tests. Social workers report assessments related to psychosocial functioning, living arrangements, and postacute care requirements.

Many other healthcare specialists provide information that becomes part of the patient's record, such as the following:

- Pharmacists provide information on the formulation of intravenous medications and nutritional substances for parenteral administration.

- Medical technologists and bacteriologists provide documentation of the results of blood tests and other laboratory analyses.

- Audiologists provide documentation of the results of hearing tests.

- Other technicians provide copies of tracings from electrocardiographs (EKGs) and electroencephalographs (EEGs).

Physicians working in ancillary service departments report on the results of many diagnostic procedures. Pathologists issue reports on their examinations of specimens collected during diagnostic and surgical procedures. Radiologists document the results of x-ray examinations, computed tomography (CT) examinations, and magnetic resonance imaging (MRI) procedures. Radiologists who specialize in nuclear medicine document radiation therapy services.

Medical History

The **history** is a summary of the patient's illness from his or her point of view. The purpose of documenting the patient's medical history is to gather background information about the patient's condition before he or she is admitted to the facility. In most cases, the history is documented in the patient's record by the admitting physician. In teaching hospitals, the history may be collected and documented by a resident in the hospital. In other facilities, assigned personnel are responsible for collecting this initial information. Increasingly, patients have the responsibility of responding to questionnaires (on paper or electronically) to create this history. (See figures 5.6 and 5.7.)

When a patient is unable to communicate and the history is provided by a second party, that fact should be recorded in the health record. Similarly, documentation should note that no history could be taken in cases where the patient is alone and unable to communicate. However, history can be obtained from exam records from physicians who previously treated the patient.

The physician bases his or her approach to assessing and treating the patient on the information provided by the patient or the patient's representative. The physician gathers this information by asking a series of questions about the patient's current and past health-related problems and circumstances, such as the following:

- What brought you to the hospital/office today?

- How long have you had these symptoms?

- What were you doing when you first experienced the problem?

- Have you ever had this problem before?

- What medications are you taking?

- Are you experiencing any other symptoms?

The physician attempts to record the patient's responses in the patient's own words to create a subjective account of the illness. Health record documentation of the patient's medical history usually includes the following elements:

- **Chief complaint:** a subjective description of the reason the patient is seeking medical treatment

- **Present illness:** a subjective description of the development of the patient's illness

- **Past medical history:** a subjective account of current and past illnesses, injuries, surgeries, and hospitalizations, including information on current medications and allergies

- **Social and personal history:** a subjective description of the patient's occupation, marital status, personal habits, and living conditions

- **Family medical history:** a subjective description of illnesses that occurred among close family members

- **Review of systems:** a subjective description of other symptoms or illnesses organized by body system

Figure 5.6.   History report in paper format.

University of Anystate Hospitals and Clinics

HISTORY

Order of Recording:

1. Chief complaint
2. History of present illness
3. History of past illness
4. Family history
5. General history
6. System review:
   Skin
   HEENT
   Neck and thyroid
   Lymphatics
   Respiratory
   Cardiovascular
   Gastrointestinal
   Genitourinary
   Neuropsychological
   Musculoskeletal
   Endocrine
7. Allergies (medications and drugs)

For Children and Adolescents:

8. Evaluation of developmental age
9. Immunization status

PATIENT LABEL

Physician Signature: _____   Date:_____

HISTORY
000005 (11/2002)

Figure 5.7. History report in electronic format.

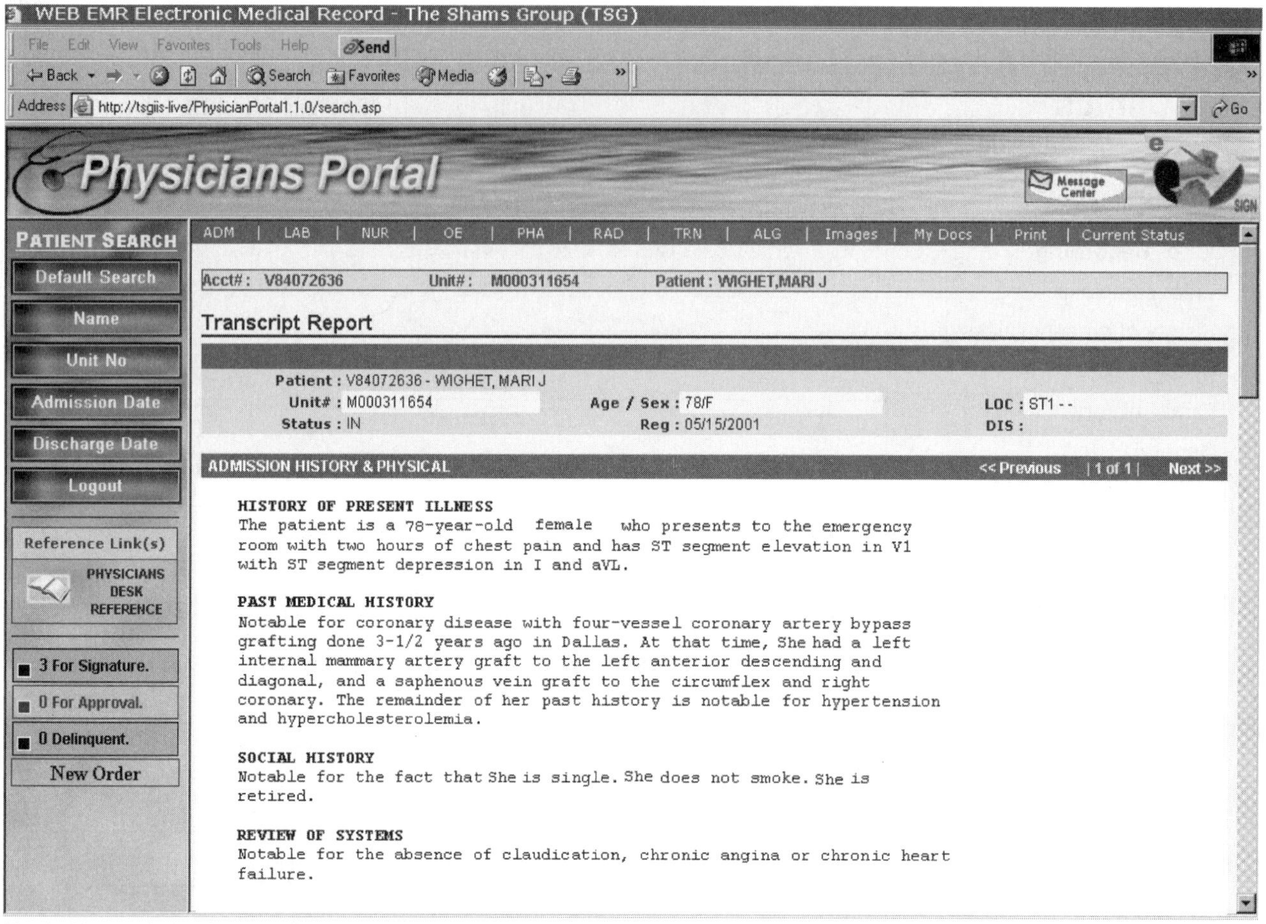

Table 5.1 provides examples of the information collected in a complete medical history.

The expectation that patients provide this medical history information underscores the value of accurate and up-to-date personal health records (PHR). In order to provide a complete and accurate account, the patient should maintain a personal health record. The PHR is a valuable resource to the patient, family, and the healthcare professionals who provide treatment and care. In most cases, a complete record of all of personal health information cannot be found in any single location or consistent format. The various elements of any one person's health information are likely scattered across several healthcare providers, possibly in different cities, states, or even countries, and are kept in various combinations of paper-based and electronic record-keeping formats. Figure 5.8 lists suggested content for a PHR.

Keeping a PHR allows consumers to provide valuable information that can help improve the quality of care. A PHR can help reduce or eliminate duplicate tests and facilitate faster, safer treatment and care in an emergency. The PHR empowers the individual. The information provides knowledge that assists preparation for appointments and establishes a resource (more accurate than memory) for a customer's health history. Overall, it gives consumers more intimate knowledge of their health information and prepares them to play an active role in preventive care and care management. In this way, customers are more involved in their own care.

Table 5.1 Information typically included in a complete medical history

Components of the History	Complaints and Symptoms
Chief complaint	Nature and duration of the symptoms that caused the patient to seek medical attention as stated in his or her own words
Present illness	Detailed chronological description of the development of the patient's illness, from the appearance of the first symptom to the present situation
Past medical history	Summary of childhood and adult illnesses and conditions, such as infectious diseases, pregnancies, allergies and drug sensitivities, accidents, operations, hospitalizations, and current medications
Social and personal history	Marital status; dietary, sleep, and exercise patterns; use of coffee, tobacco, alcohol, and other drugs; occupation; home environment; daily routine; and so on
Family medical history	Diseases among relatives in which heredity or contact might play a role, such as allergies, cancer, and infectious, psychiatric, metabolic, endocrine, cardiovascular, and renal diseases; health status or cause and age at death for immediate relatives
Review of systems	Systemic inventory designed to uncover current or past subjective symptoms that includes the following types of data: • *General:* Usual weight, recent weight changes, fever, weakness, fatigue • *Skin:* Rashes, eruptions, dryness, cyanosis, jaundice; changes in skin, hair, or nails • *Head:* Headache (duration, severity, character, location) • *Eyes:* Glasses or contact lenses, last eye examination, glaucoma, cataracts, eyestrain, pain, diplopia, redness, lacrimation, inflammation, blurring • *Ears:* Hearing, discharge, tinnitus, dizziness, pain • *Nose:* Head colds, epistaxis, discharges, obstruction, postnasal drip, sinus pain • *Mouth and throat:* Condition of teeth and gums, last dental examination, soreness, redness, hoarseness, difficulty in swallowing • *Respiratory system:* Chest pain, wheezing, cough, dyspnea, sputum (color and quantity), hemoptysis, asthma, bronchitis, emphysema, pneumonia, tuberculosis, pleurisy, last chest X-ray • *Neurological system:* Fainting, blackouts, seizures, paralysis, tingling, tremors, memory loss • *Musculoskeletal system:* Joint pain or stiffness, arthritis, gout, backache, muscle pain, cramps, swelling, redness, limitation in motor activity • *Cardiovascular system:* Chest pain, rheumatic fever, tachycardia, palpitation, high blood pressure, edema, vertigo, faintness, varicose veins, thrombophlebitis • *Gastrointestinal system:* Appetite, thirst, nausea, vomiting, hematemesis, rectal bleeding, change in bowel habits, diarrhea, constipation, indigestion, food intolerance, flatus, hemorrhoids, jaundice • *Urinary system:* Frequent or painful urination, nocturia, pyuria, hematuria, incontinence, urinary infections • *Genitoreproductive system:* Male—venereal disease, sores, discharge from penis, hernias, testicular pain, or masses; female—age at menarche, frequency and duration of menstruation, dysmenorrhea, menorrhagia, symptoms of menopause, contraception, pregnancies, deliveries, abortions, last Pap smear • *Endocrine system:* Thyroid disease; heat or cold intolerance; excessive sweating, thirst, hunger, or urination • *Hematologic system:* Anemia, easy bruising or bleeding, past transfusions • *Psychiatric disorders:* Insomnia, headache, nightmares, personality disorders, anxiety disorders, mood disorders

Figure 5.8. Content of a personal health record (PHR).

• Personal identification information
• Emergency contacts
• Contact information for healthcare providers
• Health insurance information
• Advance directives, living will, durable power of attorney
• Organ donor authorization
• Problem list for all conditions being treated
• Medical and surgical history
• Description and dates of significant illnesses and surgeries
• Family health history
• Health and wellness information
• Immunizations and dates
• Allergies
• Important events, dates, and hereditary conditions in the family
• Recent physical examination report
• Records from visits to specialists
• Important test results
• Eye and dental records
• Correspondence with providers
• Permission forms to release information or for treatment
• Medication records
• Copies of reports from provider medical records
• Any information relevant to your health

Report of Physical Examination

A physician usually records the patient's medical history as part of the initial physical examination. The physical examination provides objective information on the patient's condition. Most hospital policies require that admitting physicians perform an initial physical examination within twenty-four hours of admission. Documentation of medical history, consents, and the physical examination must be available in the patient's record before any surgical procedures may be performed (McCain 2006, 182). To ensure that a facility is meeting all of the time requirements of a history and physical examination, the health information professional should check the state regulations, federal regulations, and medical staff bylaws. Reviewing agencies will hold a facility to the strictest time frame.

For planned admissions, the physical examination may also be performed before admission. However, the Medicare *Conditions of Participation for Hospitals* (2006) require that the examination must be performed no more than seven days before admission. In addition, a legible copy of the results of the preadmission physical examination must be included in the patient's medical record.

The initial physical examination includes an assessment of the main body systems. The physician gathers this information by observing the patient's physical condition and behavior, palpating (touching) the patient's body, tapping the patient's chest and abdomen, listening to the patient's breath and heart sounds, and taking the patient's vital signs. Table 5.2 shows the types of information usually documented for a physical examination. (See also figures 5.9 and 5.10.)

Patients are sometimes readmitted to the same hospital for treatment of the same condition. When the readmission occurs within thirty days after the previous discharge, the admitting physician may add an interval note to the patient's record in place of a complete history and physical. An **interval note** includes information about the patient's current complaint, any relevant changes in his or her condition, and the physical findings since the last admission. However, when the patient is admitted for treatment of a different condition, a complete history and physical must be performed and documented. If a patient is admitted more than thirty days after the previous discharge for the same condition, a complete history and physical must be obtained.

Diagnostic and Therapeutic Orders

Hospital-based diagnostic and therapeutic services are provided under the direction of the patient's physician or physicians. **Physician's orders** are the instructions that the physician gives to the other healthcare professionals who perform diagnostic and therapeutic procedures,

Table 5.2 Information typically documented in the report of a physical examination

Report Components	Content
General condition	Apparent state of health, signs of distress, posture, weight, height, skin color, dress and personal hygiene, facial expression, manner, mood, state of awareness, speech
Vital signs	Pulse, respiration, blood pressure, temperature
Skin	Color, vascularity, lesions, edema, moisture, temperature, texture, thickness, mobility and turgor, nails
Head	Hair, scalp, skull, face
Eyes	Visual acuity and fields; position and alignment of the eyes, eyebrows, eyelids; lacrimal apparatus; conjunctivae; sclerae; corneas; irises; size, shape, equality, reaction to light, and accommodation of pupils; extraocular movements; ophthalmoscopic exam
Ears	Auricles, canals, tympanic membranes, hearing, discharge
Nose and sinuses	Airways, mucosa, septum, sinus tenderness, discharge, bleeding, smell
Mouth	Breath, lips, teeth, gums, tongue, salivary ducts
Throat	Tonsils, pharynx, palate, uvula, postnasal drip
Neck	Stiffness, thyroid, trachea, vessels, lymph nodes, salivary glands
Thorax, anterior and posterior	Shape, symmetry, respiration
Breasts	Masses, tenderness, discharge from nipples
Lungs	Fremitus, breath sounds, adventitious sounds, friction, spoken voice, whispered voice
Heart	Location and quality of apical impulse, trill, pulsation, rhythm, sounds, murmurs, friction rub, jugular venous pressure and pulse, carotid artery pulse
Abdomen	Contour, peristalsis, scars, rigidity, tenderness, spasm, masses, fluid, hernia, bowel sounds and bruits, palpable organs
Male genitourinary organs	Scars, lesions, discharge, penis, scrotum, epididymis, varicocele, hydrocele
Female reproductive organs	External genitalia, Skene's glands and Bartholin's glands, vagina, cervix, uterus, adnexa
Rectum	Fissure, fistula, hemorrhoids, sphincter tone, masses, prostate, seminal vesicles, feces
Musculoskeletal system	Spine and extremities, deformities, swelling, redness, tenderness, range of motion
Lymphatics	Palpable cervical, axillary, inguinal nodes; location; size; consistency; mobility and tenderness
Blood vessels	Pulses, color, temperature, vessel walls, veins
Neurological system	Cranial nerves, coordination, reflexes, biceps, triceps, patellar, Achilles, abdominal, cremasteric, Babinski, Romberg, gait, sensory, vibratory
Diagnosis(es)	

Figure 5.9. Physical examination report in paper format.

University of Anystate Hospitals and Clinics

PHYSICAL EXAMINATION

PATIENT LABEL

Date: _____ Age: _____ Sex: _____ Height: _____ Weight: _____

T: _____ P: _____ R: _____ BP: _____

Order of Recording:
1. General appearance
2. Skin
3. HEENT
4. Lymph glands
5. Neck
6. Breasts
7. Chest
8. Heart
9. Abdomen
10. Genitalia
11. Musculoskeletal
12. Neurological
13. Rectal
14. Vaginal

Impression: _____

_____

_____

_____

Course of Action Planned: _____

_____

_____

Physician Signature:_____ Date: _____

PHYSICAL EXAMINATION
000006 (11/2002)

Figure 5.10. Physical examination report in electronic format.

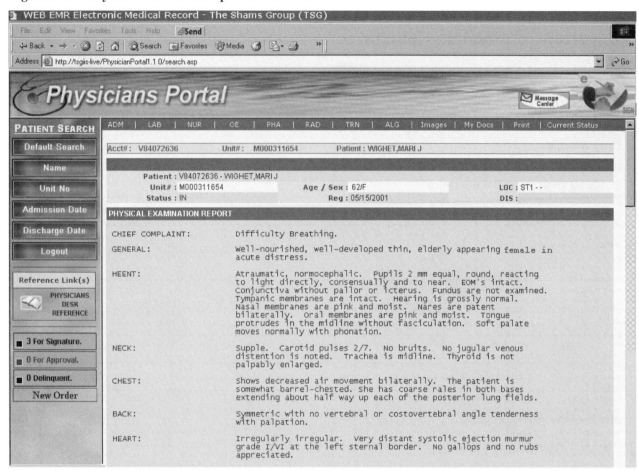

provide nursing care, formulate and administer medications, and provide nutritional services to the patient. (See figures 5.11 and 5.12.) Orders are changed and updated often as the patient's condition progresses.

In most states, only licensed physicians are allowed to issue orders for the medications, diagnostic tests, therapeutic services, ancillary medical services, and medical devices to be provided to patients. They may also order the use of seclusion or restraints when required. In some states, however, psychologists, physician's assistants, and certified nurse-practitioners are also allowed to write orders under limited conditions. In all cases, health record documentation must support the medical necessity of the services and materials ordered.

State regulations and hospital medical staff policies also stipulate which healthcare professionals may receive and execute physicians' orders. For example, only licensed nurses and pharmacists are allowed to receive and fulfill medication orders in most states. However, most allied health professionals are allowed to accept physicians' orders for services within their area of practice. Examples include nurse-anesthetists, physical therapists, and respiratory therapists.

In paper-based health record systems, it is vital that physicians submit orders that are legible and complete. This includes the elimination of abbreviations defined as serious or easily misunderstood. The orders must include the physician's signature and the date the orders were entered into the patient's record. Many hospitals also permit physicians to communicate verbal

Figure 5.11. Physician's order sheet in paper format.

University of Anystate Hospital

PHYSICIAN ORDERS

PATIENT LABEL

Drug Allergies

Date and Time	RN Signature	

PHYSICIAN ORDERS
000122 (02/2003)

Figure 5.12. Physician's order in electronic format.

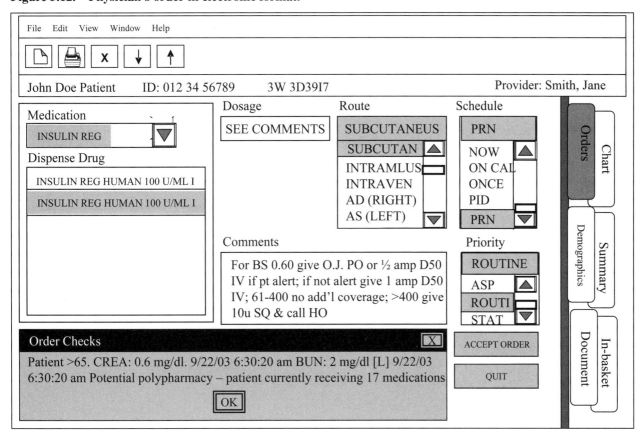

orders via telephone. In such cases, state regulations and the hospital's medical staff bylaws stipulate which healthcare practitioners are allowed to accept and carry out verbal orders and how such orders are to be authenticated.

Many hospitals use electronic order-entry systems. The systems include safeguards that ensure the authenticity, accuracy, and completeness of physicians' orders. Such computer-based order-entry systems are an integral part of electronic health record systems. **Computerized physician order entry (CPOE)** systems are gaining acceptance in the medical community; however, many healthcare facilities face resistance from physicians who are reluctant to use the new technology.

Standing orders are routine physicians' orders that have been established by individual physicians or by the hospital's medical staff. (See figure 5.13.) Each standing order applies to a specific diagnosis or procedure. For example, a standing order might be established for the postoperative care to be provided to all patients who have undergone an appendectomy. Some facilities allow nurses to implement standing orders that have been previously approved by the medical staff. Others require physicians to specifically order the implementation of standing orders for their patients, and others may allow a registered nurse to initiate standing orders preapproved by medical staff (McCain 2006, 180).

Authentication Requirements

State and federal regulations require that physicians sign, date, and note the time of their orders for diagnostic and therapeutic services. The authentication requirements for physicians' orders

Figure 5.13.   Physician's standing order in paper format.

Midwest Medical Center

HEPARIN ORDER: REGULAR UNFRACTIONATED HEPARIN FOR ADULTS

PATIENT LABEL

Diagnosis: _____

Allergies:_____

Total Body Weight: _____lb = _____kg

Warning: Due to an increased risk of serious bleeding, patients should not receive both regular heparin and low-molecular-weight heparin.

Patients should also be evaluated for continuance of other medications such as aspirin, clopidogrel, and NSAID therapy.

1. Check baseline PTT, PT/INR, heme panel

2. Check the appropriate bolus regimen according to diagnosis/disease
   a. ☐ No initial bolus
   b. ☐ Acute coronary syndrome—heparin bolus 75 units/kg = _____ units IV
      (round to the nearest 1000 units—maximum bolus = 10,000 units)
   c. ☐ In combination with thrombolytic therapy for acute MI (TNKase, Retavase, TPA)
      ☐ 5000 units bolus if 65 kg or greater
      ☐ 4000 units bolus if less than 65 kg
   d. ☐ Treatment of DVT/PE—heparin bolus 80 units/kg = _____ units IV
      (round to the nearest 1000 units—maximum bolus = 10,000 units)

3. Following bolus, begin IV heparin infusion (check the appropriate regimen):
   • Premixed IV bag contains heparin 25,000 units in 250 ml of D5W (100 units/ml)
   • Maximum initial infusion rate not to exceed 2000 units/h
   ☐ All cardiology regimens: 16 units/kg/h = _____ ml/h
   ☐ Treatment of DVT or PE: 18 units/kg/h = _____ ml/h

4. Check PTT 6 hours after initiation of heparin infusion

5. Adjust heparin based on guidelines below
   (document all changes on MAR and physician's orders sheet):

PTT (seconds)	Bolus Dose	Rate Changes	Repeat PTT after Each Dosage Change
PTT <35	Bolus 4000 units	Increase rate 200 units/h	6 h
PTT 35–45	Bolus 3000 units	Increase rate 200 units/h	6 h
PTT 46–70	No bolus	No rate change	Next a.m.
PTT 71–90	No bolus	Decrease rate 100 units/h	6 h
PTT 91–100	No bolus	Hold infusion 1 h, then decrease rate by 200 units/h	6 h
PTT >100	No bolus	Hold infusion 1 h, then decrease rate by 300 units/h	6 h

6. Check PTT and heme panel every morning (while patient is on heparin protocol).

7. Check stools daily for occult blood and notify physician if positive.

8. Notify physician for bleeding, hematoma, or heart rate above 120 bpm.

Physician Signature: _____   Date/Time:_____

RN Signature: _____   Date/Time:_____

HEPARIN ORDER
000013 (11/2002)

are the same in paper-based and electronic health record systems. Only the mechanism for authentication is different.

Special Orders

Two types of special orders are relatively common in healthcare facilities: do-not-resuscitate orders and orders for restraint and seclusion. **Do-not-resuscitate (DNR) orders** are issued when it has been decided that the patient is near death and that no resuscitation attempts should be made when the patient stops breathing. In addition to the order, health record documentation must indicate that the decision to withhold resuscitation efforts was discussed with the patient or the patient's legal representative, when the decision was made, and who took part in making the decision.

See chapter 12 for information about restraints and seclusion.

Discharge Orders

Only the patient's physician can decide when the patient is ready to be discharged from the hospital. Discharge orders must be made in writing. When a patient leaves the hospital against medical advice, a note describing the situation should be included in the patient's health record. Similarly, when a patient dies, a note should be added to the health record in lieu of a discharge order. (See figure 5.14.)

Clinical Observations

In healthcare facilities, the records of clinical observations are usually referred to as **progress notes**. In the ambulatory setting, the terms *encounter* or *visit note* are used. The purpose of this type of interdisciplinary documentation is to create a chronological record of the patient's condition and response to treatment during his or her entire hospital stay or episode of care. The progress notes also allow clinicians to communicate their observations to other members of the healthcare team.

The collection of information on the patient's progress is also required for reimbursement purposes. This information serves to justify the patient's continued stay and treatment, and it supports the medical necessity of the services provided to the patient. Specifically, the progress notes should indicate why the intervention of medical professionals was required and why that intervention needed to be performed in a specific type of setting. In addition, the notes should support the logic behind the patient's care and demonstrate how the services were planned and coordinated.

The rules of the hospital's medical staff specify which healthcare professionals are allowed to enter clinical documentation into the health record. Typically, the patient's principal physician, consulting physicians, house medical staff, nurses, dietitians, social workers, and clinical therapists are authorized to create and access health record documentation. Like physicians, nurses and allied health professionals sign and date all of their record entries and include their credentials after their names. (See table 5.3.) Depending on the record format used by the hospital, each discipline may maintain a separate section of the health record. Alternatively, all of the observations may be combined in the same chronological report.

Progress notes include the following types of information:

- Patient's health status on admission and discharge
- Findings of physical examinations

Figure 5.14. **Discharge order in paper format.**

University of Anystate Hospitals

PHYSICIAN ORDERS

PATIENT, PETUNIA P.
000000001
DOB: 08/14/1949

Drug Allergies: *Codeine*

Date/Time	RN Signature	Physician Order/Physician Signature
10/11/200x 6:00 a.m.	Claire Barton, RN	(1) Admit via surgery (2) NPO (3) CBC, urinalysis (4) BCP 8 (5) Prothrombin time, PTT (6) Type and screen (7) PA chest X-ray (8) EKG (9) Prep abdomen (10) Start IV fluids: 1000 cc D5LR at 125 cc/h via 18g Jelco (11) Mefoxin 2 g IV at 7:45 a.m. Myron P Gynasurg MD 10/11/200x
10/11/200x 10:00 a.m.	Claire Barton, RN	(12) Morphine sulfate 2 mg PCA IV RR q.1.0-1.5.h. (13) Mefoxin 2 g IV in 8 h then discontinue (14) D5LR 1000 cc at 125 cc/h (15) Liquid diet (16) Bed rest (17) Vital signs every 4 h Myron P Gynasurg MD 10/11/200x
10/11/200x 2:00 p.m.	Nancy Nurse, RN	Telephone order from Dr. Gynesurg: (18) Morphine sulfate 2 mg IV push Myron P Gynasurg MD 10/12/200x
10/11/200x 3:00 p.m.	Nancy Nurse, RN	Telephone order from Dr. Gynesurg: (19) Temporarily discontinue PCA pump until vital signs return to normal (20) Vital signs every hour Myron P Gynasurg MD 10/12/200x
10/12/200x 12:05 p.m.	Nancy Nurse, RN	(21) Remove Foley (22) Begin to ambulate (23) Soft diet (24) Vital signs every 4 h Myron P Gynasurg MD 10/12/200x
10/13/200x 12:15 p.m.	Nancy Nurse, RN	(25) Discontinue morphine (26) Darvacet-N 100 mg. one or two tablets q.4h. as needed for pain (27) Solid diet Myron P Gynasurg MD 10/13/200x
10/14/200x 8:00 a.m.	Nancy Nurse, RN	(28) Discontinue IVs (29) Discharge to home—see discharge instruction sheet Myron P Gynasurg MD 10/12/200x

PHYSICIAN ORDERS
000010 (11/2002)

Table 5.3   Clinical credentials of healthcare professionals who author health record documentation

Credential	Abbreviation	Health Record Documentation
Registered nurse	RN	Nursing assessments, progress notes, medication records, vital signs, care plans, transfer records, flow charts
Licensed practical nurse or licensed vocational nurse	LPN or LVN	Nursing assessments, progress notes, medication records, vital signs, transfer records, flow charts
Nurse-anesthetist	CRNA	Anesthesia records
Nurse-midwife	CRNM	Obstetrical records
Nurse-practitioner	NP	Records associated with specialized nursing practice (pediatric, geriatric, obstetric, and others)
Clinical social worker	LSW	Psychosocial assessments, progress notes
Respiratory therapist	CRT	Records of respiratory therapy, progress notes
Occupational therapist	OT	Records of occupational therapy, progress notes
Speech therapist or speech–language pathologist	SLP	Records of speech therapy, progress notes
Physical therapist	PT	Records of physical therapy, progress notes
Dietitian	RD	Nutritional assessments and plans
Physician assistant	PA	Records of assessments and patient education
Surgeon assistant	SA	Records of assessments and patient education
Pharmacist	RPh	Records of pharmaceuticals and intravenous solutions formulated and dispensed
Clinical psychologist	PhD	Reports of psychological assessments, progress notes
Medical physician	MD	Records of history and physical, orders, progress notes, discharge summaries
Surgeon	MD	Reports of history and physical, orders, progress notes, discharge summaries, and preoperative, intraoperative, and postoperative reports
Radiologist	MD	Records of radiotherapy (nuclear medicine) and imaging results
Pathologist	MD	Records of pathology results and laboratory results and blood bank records
Osteopathic physician	DO	Reports of history and physical, orders, progress notes, and discharge summaries
Oral surgeon	MD/DDS	Records of oral surgery (preoperative, intraoperative, and postoperative), orders, progress notes, and discharge summaries

- Observations of vital signs, including pain assessments

- Chronological record of the patient's course, including his or her response to treatment

- Results of laboratory and imaging procedures along with interpretations and plans for follow-up

- Requests for consultations and reasons for the requests

- Records of patient and family education

- Postoperative progress notes

Documentation of Physicians' Services

In teaching hospitals affiliated with university medical schools, resident physicians and house staff provide medical services to patients as part of their postgraduate medical training. They work under the supervision of attending physicians who are fully qualified in their medical specialties and are members of the faculty for the medical school affiliated with the hospital.

In the past, resident physicians worked long hours and were responsible for providing much of the patient care in teaching hospitals. Starting in the 1980s, however, several highly publicized cases of patients dying while under the care of overworked and underqualified residents created significant concern about the way teaching hospitals operate. Recent changes in federal regulations now limit the number of hours residents may work and require teaching hospitals to employ fully qualified physicians to coordinate patient care. These changes have resulted in the development of a new category of physician known as a *hospitalist*. When patients enter the hospital under the care of emergency physicians or medical faculty, **hospitalists** play the role that admitting physicians fulfill in hospitals that are not affiliated with resident-training programs.

Physicians' Progress Notes

The physician who is primarily responsible for the patient's care performs an initial assessment of the patient's condition early in the hospitalization or episode of treatment. The physician's report of the patient's history and physical examination describes the patient's condition on admission and constitutes the first progress note in the patient's record. Subsequently, the physician's clinical decision making is documented in additional progress notes. Physicians' orders for diagnostic tests, medications, and other therapeutic services are usually documented on a separate order sheet in paper-based records or in a separate section in computer-based records.

The patient's daily progress and reactions to therapeutic interventions are documented by the patient's principal physician. The physician also notes the results of diagnostic tests and documents his or her interpretation of the results and plans for follow-up care.

Physicians' progress notes report conversations with the patient and the patient's family. Progress notes are also used to document discharge planning and instructions for posthospital care. The physician's final progress note usually describes the patient's status upon discharge.

Consultation Reports

Physicians often seek the advice of other physicians before making final diagnostic and therapeutic decisions. The patient's principal physician documents the request for a consultation in the patient's record. The consulting physician then documents his or her examination of the patient as a progress note. The consultant may discuss the case with the patient's physician to arrive at a mutual diagnostic decision or treatment plan. The consultant's findings and recommendations may also be documented as a progress note in the patient's record or supplied to the physician who requested the consultation in the form of a written report. The consultant's report then becomes part of the patient's record.

Consultation reports usually contain the following types of information (see figure 5.15 for an example):

- Name of the physician who requested the consultation and the reason for the consultation
- Date and time the consultant examined the patient
- Pertinent findings of the examination
- Consultant's opinion, diagnosis, or impression
- Recommendations for diagnostic tests and/or treatment
- Signature, credentials, and specialty of the consultant

The Medicare *Conditions of Participation* (2006) require the hospital's medical staff to set rules regarding consultations. Some hospitals have very specific requirements that define the circumstances under which a consultation is or is not required. For example, consultations may be required on every patient who is critically ill. Physicians responsible for the following types of cases usually choose to request consultations:

- Patients who are not good risks for surgery
- Patients whose diagnoses are unclear
- Patients whose physicians are not sure which treatment regimen would have the most favorable results
- Patients whose illnesses or injuries may be the result of criminal activities

Medical staff rules may also categorize the types of consultations. For example, consultations that allow the consultant to write orders may be considered materially different than consultations that do not allow the consultant to write orders. Medical staff rules also determine whether partners in multispecialty group practices may provide care to each other's patients without going through a formal consultation process (Glondys 1999, 59–61).

Physicians who are routinely involved in providing inpatient care are not considered consultants. Examples include radiologists who interpret imaging results, cardiologists who interpret electrocardiograms, neurologists who interpret electroencephalograms, and pathologists who examine tissue specimens.

Documentation of Nursing Services

Registered nurses (RNs) and licensed practical (or vocational) nurses (LPNs or LVNs) maintain chronological records of the patient's vital signs (blood pressure, heart rate, respiration rate, and temperature) and level of discomfort throughout the patient's hospital stay. They also maintain medication records, write progress notes, and document patient assessments. In hospitals that employ patient-care technicians and nursing assistants, registered nurses verify any information provided by unlicensed patient-care staff before it becomes part of the permanent health record.

Figure 5.15. Consultation report.

# Anytown Community Hospital **CONSULTATION REPORT** PAGE 1 OF 2	PATIENT, BLUTO P. 070095111 DOB: 04/01/1930

I was asked by Dr. Doctor to evaluate Mr. Patient for consideration of left VATS talc pleurodesis.

CHIEF COMPLAINT: Shortness of breath

HISTORY OF PRESENT ILLNESS: Mr. Patient is a 73-year-old male who has a history of metastatic pancreatic cancer. He was found to have left pleural effusion and underwent thoracentesis. He returned with a recurrent effusion. He was admitted on 05/12/200x and underwent left chest tube thoracostomy and an attempt at talc pleurodesis through the chest tube. He has had residual pneumothorax and continues to drain from the left chest tube. He was referred for the purpose of left VATS talc pleurodesis.

PAST SURGICAL HISTORY: His past surgical history is remarkable for Whipple procedure.

PAST MEDICAL HISTORY: His past medical history is remarkable for prostate cancer and pancreatic cancer.

MEDICATIONS: Avalide and pancrease

ALLERGIES: He has no known drug allergies.

FAMILY/SOCIAL HISTORY: Remarkable for being married. He drinks socially.

REVIEW OF SYSTEMS: Remarkable for no history of seizure or stroke, no history of previous pneumonia, no history of previous myocardial infarction, no history of previous liver failure, renal failure. He has had no swelling in his legs.

PHYSICAL EXAMINATION: He is 5 feet 6 inches tall. He weighs 158 pounds. His blood pressure is 126/70. His pulse is 62. His respiratory rate is 20. His temperature is 97.1. His neurological exam is remarkable for a normal affect. He is oriented × 3. His gross motor examination is 5/5 in all four extremities. His head and neck exam is remarkable for no icteric sclerae. He has no oral lesions. His neck demonstrates no cervical or supraclavicular adenopathy. He has no carotid bruits. His chest exam is remarkable for no use of accessory muscles, no dullness to percussion. He has a left chest tube in place with no air leak. He has serous-appearing drainage from his left chest tube. His breath sounds are remarkable for a slight decrease in breath sounds in the left lateral lung. His cardiovascular exam is remarkable for no lift, heave, or thrill. He has a normal S1, S2 without murmurs. Abdomen is remarkable for well-healed Whipple incision. His abdomen is nontender, nondistended without evidence of masses or organomegaly. His extremities are without clubbing, cyanosis, or edema.

His chest CT shows a loculated left pneumothorax with small residual effusion. He has chest tube in place. This is a small caliber tube. His chest X-ray shows loculated left pneumothorax.

Figure 5.15 (continued)

Anytown Community Hospital

CONSULTATION REPORT
PAGE 2 OF 2

PATIENT, BLUTO P.
070095111
DOB: 04/01/1930

His laboratory studies are further remarkable for urinalysis that is normal, an EKG that is normal sinus rhythm, sodium of 133, potassium 3.8, chloride 95, BUN 19, creatinine 1.1, PPTT of 11.8, INR of 0.9, PTT of 29.

My impression is that Mr. Patient is a 73-year-old male with metastatic pancreatic cancer status post Whipple. He has a recurrent left pleural effusion. He has undergone previous tube thoracostomy and pleurodesis and now has a residual left pneumothorax and residual chest tube drainage from his malignant effusion.

I have recommended to Mr. Patient that we proceed with left VATS talc pleurodesis today. He understands that his risks include, but are not limited to, death (1–2%), bleeding requiring blood transfusion, infection, prolonged air leak from the cut surface of his lung, and a 30% chance of recurrent effusion. Understanding these risks as well as the alternative of continued drainage, he wishes to proceed today with left VATS talc pleurodesis.

Thank you very much for allowing me to participate in his care.

Signature:

James V Medman   _5/17/200x_
_____   _____
James W. Medman, MD   Date

d: 05/17/200x
t: 05/20/200x
JWM, MD/mc

Nursing Assessments

An initial **nursing assessment** is always performed to obtain clinical and personal information about the patient shortly after he or she has been admitted to the nursing unit. State, Joint Commission, and federal guidelines now require nursing assessments within 24 hours. At a minimum, the initial nursing assessment summarizes the date, time, and method of admission as well as the patient's current condition, symptoms (including level of pain), and vital signs. Most hospitals develop and use a nursing assessment instrument to collect additional information about the patient's physical condition and psychosocial status at admission. The instruments are designed to solicit the following types of information (see figure 5.16):

- Patient's reason for being in the hospital

- Patient's current and past illnesses

- Patient's current medical condition, including the condition of his or her skin and the level of pain

- Patient's current cognitive status, including his or her ability to communicate and to understand and follow instructions

- Patient's current functional status, including his or her level of physical activity and ability to walk, move, and perform personal care

- Patient's current psychosocial status, including his or her marital status, living arrangements, personal habits (such as smoking, alcohol consumption, and use of illegal drugs), and occupation

- Patient's family history, including information about his or her parents, children, and siblings and their current health status or cause of death

- Patient's current nutritional status, including his or her ability to feed himself or herself and any special dietary requirements or food allergies

- Patient's known drug allergies, including any sensitivity to latex products

- Patient's current medications

- Patient's need for special discharge planning

Care Plans

Current accreditation standards and the Medicare *Conditions of Participation* (2006) require hospitals to develop patient-specific care plans. A **care plan** is a multidisciplinary tool for organizing the diagnostic and therapeutic services to be provided to a patient. Care plans are also required in the long-term care setting and other inpatient environments. The purpose of the care plan is to ensure the efficacy and efficiency of patient services and the quality of patient outcomes. Care plans usually include the following elements (see figure 5.17):

- Initial assessment (medical and nursing) of the patient's immediate and long-term needs

- Statement of treatment goals based on the patient's needs and diagnosis

- Description of the activities planned to meet the treatment goals

- Patient education goals

- Discharge planning goals

Figure 5.16.   Initial nursing assessment in paper format.

Midwest Medical Center

INITIAL NURSING ASSESSMENT

PATIENT LABEL

Baseline Information

Date:	Time:	Age:	Arrived: AMB WC Stretcher EMS Carried Other:		Primary MD:

Initial/Chief Complaint/History of Present Illness:

T: PO R TM	P:	R:	BP: R L	$\oplus$ O$_2$ Sats %	Sex: M F	Height:	Weight: Actual: Stated:

$\oplus$ Tetanus/Immunizations:	Pneumococcal Vaccine ☐ No ☐ Yes Most Recent Date:
$\oplus$ Pregnant ☐ No ☐ Yes LNMP:	Influenza Vaccine ☐ No ☐ Yes Most Recent Date:

Allergies: ☐ None   ☐ Medications   ☐ Latex   ☐ Food   ☐ Anesthesia   ☐ Other

List Names and Reactions:

TB Assessment (Initiate airborne isolation if 4 or more criteria are checked yes)

Persistent Cough > 2 weeks ☐ No ☐ Yes	Abnormal Chest X-Ray	☐ No ☐ Yes	Respiratory Isolation
Fever > 100.4 (night sweats) ☐ No ☐ Yes	Physician Order for AFB (smear/culture)	☐ No ☐ Yes	Ordered ☐ No ☐ Yes
Unexplained Weight Loss ☐ No ☐ Yes	Recent Exposure to Person with Suspected TB or +PPD	☐ No ☐ Yes	

RN/LPN Signature: _____

☐ See Home Medication Orders   Medication/Over the Counter/Herbal History   ☐ Investigation Drugs/Devices

Medication	Dose	Freq	Last Dose	Medication	Dose	Freq	Last Dose

Hospitalizations/Surgeries:

Medical History

Neurological	☐ No	☐ Yes		Sensory Impairment	☐ No	☐ Yes	
Cardiovascular	☐ No	☐ Yes		Endocrine	☐ No	☐ Yes	
Hypertension	☐ No	☐ Yes		Blood Disorder	☐ No	☐ Yes	
Respiratory	☐ No	☐ Yes		Cancer	☐ No	☐ Yes	
Gastrointestinal	☐ No	☐ Yes		Psychological	☐ No	☐ Yes	
Renal/Urological	☐ No	☐ Yes		Tobacco Use	☐ No	☐ Yes	
Gynecological	☐ No	☐ Yes		Alcohol/Drug Use	☐ No	☐ Yes	
Musculoskeletal	☐ No	☐ Yes		Infectious Disease	☐ No	☐ Yes	
Integumentary	☐ No	☐ Yes		Cough/Cold Past 2 Weeks	☐ No	☐ Yes	
EENT	☐ No	☐ Yes		Anesthesia	☐ No	☐ Yes	

Source of Information   ☐ Patient   ☐ Family   ☐ Unable to Obtain   ☐ Other | ☐ Medications Sent Home with Patient: _____

Arrival Date:	Arrival Time:	T: PO R TM	P:	R:	BP: R L	O$_2$ Sats %: (If applicable)

RN Initial: _____   **RN Signature:** _____   **Date:** _____   **Time:** _____   **Unit:** _____

RN Initial: _____   **RN Signature:** _____   **Date:** _____   **Time:** _____   **Unit:** _____

INITIAL NURSING ASSESSMENT
000039 (10/2002)

- Timing of periodic assessments to determine progress toward meeting the treatment goals

- Indicators of the need for reassessing the plan to address the patient's response to treatment and/or the development of complications

Clinical Practice Guidelines and Protocols

Several types of clinical tools are available to support clinical decision making, ensure clinical quality, and facilitate interdisciplinary-care planning. Clinical tools include the following (Willner 2006, 503–504):

- **Clinical practice guidelines**: Detailed step-by-step guides used by healthcare practitioners to make knowledge-based clinical decisions directly related to patient care. Clinical practice guidelines are developed with the goal of standardizing clinical decision making. Practice guidelines are based on scientific evidence and research and are issued by authoritative organizations such as medical societies, professional associations, and government agencies. See figure 5.18 for an example (U.S. Department of Health and Human Services 1996).

- **Clinical protocols**: Treatment recommendations that are often based on clinical practice guidelines.

- **Clinical pathways**: Structured plans of care that help organizations implement clinical guidelines and protocols. Sometimes known as critical paths, care paths, and/or care maps, they are widely used by institutions hoping to reduce costs and improve quality through decreased variation in practices. See figure 5.19 for an example.

The Institute of Medicine and other public and private organizations concerned with the quality of healthcare actively support the development of evidence-based clinical tools. For example, the **National Guideline Clearinghouse (NGC)** is an initiative of the **Agency for Healthcare Research and Quality (AHRQ).** The NGC is a comprehensive database of evidence-based clinical practice guidelines and related documents. The purpose of the NGC is to provide physicians, nurses, and other healthcare professionals; healthcare facilities and networks; health insurance plans; and healthcare consumers with an accessible source for objective, authoritative, and detailed information on effective clinical practices. The NGC's mission also includes facilitating the dissemination, implementation, and use of clinical guidelines in the United States (National Guideline Clearinghouse 2007).

Case Management Reports

In many hospitals, registered nurses called case managers prepare patient assessments and care plans. Most clinical case managers are highly experienced nurses, many of whom hold advanced degrees. In some hospitals, clinical social workers are responsible for case management functions. **Case management** involves a process of ongoing and concurrent review performed to ensure the medical necessity and effectiveness of the clinical services being provided to the patient, specifically:

Case managers review the condition of patients to identify each patient's care needs and to integrate patient data with the patient's course of treatment. . . . [In many organizations] the case manager [compares] the patient's course [to] a predetermined optimal course (known as a care map, critical path, or practice guideline) for the patient's condition. [The case manager] identifies the actions to be taken when the patient's care is not proceeding optimally. (Shaw et al. 2007, 109)

Figure 5.17.   Patient care plan in paper format.

University of Anystate Hospital

PATIENT CARE PLAN
PAGE 1 OF 2

PATIENT LABEL

Admitting Physician:

Admission Date:	Diagnosis:	Isolation:

Operative/Special Procedures:	Date:	Allergies:

Vital Signs	**Activity**	**Bladder/Bowel**	**Treatments**

☐ TPR _____
 ☐ BP _____
 ☐ Neuro checks _____
 ☐ Circ. checks _____
 ☐ Weight _____
 ☐ Telemetry _____
 ☐ Transport S Tele _____
	☐ Bedrest _____
	 ☐ BRP _____
	 ☐ Up in Chair _____
	 ☐ Ambulate _____
	
	 ☐ Up Ad Lib _____
	 ☐ Head of Bed _____
	 ☐ Foot of Bed _____
	 ☐ TCDB _____
	 ☐ Leg Exercises _____
	 ☐ Others _____
		Bladder:
		 ☐ Strain Urine
		 ☐ Check Voiding _____
		 ☐ Cath PRN _____
		 ☐ Foley Cath
		   ☐ Date Inserted _____
		 ☐ S.P. Cath
		 ☐ Condom Cath
		 ☐ Irrigate Cath q. ____ h.
		   with: _____
		 ☐ Bladder Irrigation _____
		 ☐ IDEO Conduit _____
		 ☐ Incontinent _____
			☐ S&A _____
			   ☐ Self _____
			 ☐ NG _____
			 ☐ Gomco _____
			   ☐ Clamp _____
			   ☐ Irrigate _____
			 ☐ Chest Tube _____
			 _____
			 ☐ Wound _____
			
			 ☐ Others: _____
			 _____

Diet and Fluids			

Diet:
 ☐ NPO _____
 ☐ Regular _____
 ☐ Other _____
 ☐ Snack _____
 ☐ Tube Feedings _____
 ☐ Supplemental _____
 ☐ Restrict _____
 ☐ Force _____
 ☐ Ice Chips _____
 Fluids:
 ☐ Intake _____
 ☐ Output _____
 ☐ Others _____
	Hygiene
	 ☐ Self
	 ☐ Assist
	 ☐ Complete
	 ☐ Tub/Shower
	 ☐ Mouth/Denture Care
	 _____
	 ☐ Shampoo _____
	 ☐ Skin Care _____
	 ☐ Others _____
		Bowel:
		 ☐ Check BMs _____
		 ☐ Suppository _____
		 _____
		 ☐ Enema _____
		 ☐ Ostomy _____
		 ☐ Incontinent _____
		 ☐ Others _____
		 _____
		 _____
			Respiratory
			 ☐ Ventilator _____
			 _____
			 ☐ O$_2$ _____
			   ☐ Mask
			   ☐ Nasal Cannula
			   ☐ AMT
			 ☐ Suction
			 ☐ Triflow
			 ☐ IPPB/HHN _____
			
			 ☐ Others _____

Tube Feeding

Type of Tube	Type and Strength of Feeding	Rate	Count	Irrigation	Bag ▲

Safety Measures
☐ Siderails
  ☐ Upper _____
  ☐ Lower _____
☐ Restraints
☐ Seizure Precautions
☐ High Risk for Falls
☐ Self-Injury Precautions

IV Therapies					**Site Care/Tubing Change**				
#	Solution	Additives	Rate	Count	Start/Date				
					Type/Size				
					Blood Transfusions				

Figure 5.17. (continued)

University of Anystate Hospital

PATIENT CARE PLAN
PAGE 2 OF 2

PATIENT LABEL

Date	Daily Lab Work	Date	Lab Work	Date	X-Ray/Special Procedures

Date	Preps for Procedures

Special Equipment	Miscellaneous
☐ Traction _____	
☐ Trapeze _____	
☐ _____Bed	
☐ _____Mattress	
☐ Sheepskin	
☐ Crutches	
☐ Walker	
☐ Teds	
☐ Others_____	
_____	

Therapies	
☐ Physical _____	
☐ Speech _____	
☐ OT _____	

Transportation	
☐ Wheelchair	
☐ Stretcher	
☐ Ambulatory	
☐ Bed	

Consultations	
_____	
_____	
_____	

PATIENT CARE PLAN
000072 (10/2002)

Figure 5.18. Example of a clinical practice guideline.

TITLE:	Recognition and initial assessment of Alzheimer's disease and related dementias
SOURCE(S):	Rockville (MD): U.S. Department of Health and Human Services, Public Health Service, AHCPR; 1996 Nov. 128 (Clinical practice guidelines number 19)
ADAPTATION:	Not applicable: Guideline was not adapted from another source
DATE:	November 1996

MAJOR RECOMMENDATIONS:	Triggers for Recognition and Initial Assessment for the Presence of Dementia
	Initiation of an Assessment for Alzheimer's Disease and Related Dementias
	    An initial clinical assessment should be performed . . . (strength of evidence = B)
	    A focused history is critical . . . (strength of evidence = C)
	    The history should be obtained from the patient and a reliable informant
	      (strength of evidence = C)
	      The Functional Activities Questionnaire . . . (strength of evidence = A)
	      . . . Mental status test is clearly superior . . . (strength of evidence = A)
	      . . . Visual impairment, sensory impairment, and physical disability . . .
	        (strength of evidence = B)
	Assessment for Delirium and Depression
	Interpretation of Findings and Recommended Actions
	    . . . Normal . . . reassessment in 6–12 months . . . referral for second opinion
	      (strength of evidence = C)
	    Further clinical evaluation . . . if abnormal . . . mental . . . functional status
	      (strength of evidence = C)
	    . . . Neuropsychological, neurological, or psychiatric . . . if mixed results
	      (strength of evidence = C)
	    Confounding factors . . . should be . . . considered in the interpretation
	      (strength of evidence = B)
	Neuropsychological Testing

CLINICAL ALGORITHMS(S):	Algorithms are provided for the clinical assessment of dementia
DEVELOPER(S):	Agency for Healthcare Research and Quality (AHRQ)
COMMITTEE:	Alzheimer's Disease and Related Dementias Guideline Panel
GROUP COMPOSITION:	AHCPR solicited nominations for an expert panel . . . AHCPR appointed 18 panel members, including 5 psychologists, 3 psychiatrists, 2 neurologists, 2 nurses, 1 internist, 2 geriatricians, 1 social worker, and 2 consumer representatives . . .
ENDORSEMENT(S):	Not stated
GUIDELINE STATUS:	This is the current release of the guideline. An update is not in progress at this time.
GUIDELINE AVAILABILITY:	Electronic copies: Available from the National Library of Medicine's HSTAT database Print copies: Information regarding the availability of these publications can be found in the Agency for Healthcare Research and Quality's publications catalog
COMPANION DOCUMENTS:	The following documents are available . . .
PATIENT RESOURCES:	
NGC STATUS:	
COPYRIGHT STATUS:	The contents of these clinical practice guidelines are in the public domain within the United States only and may be used and reproduced without special permission in America, except for those copyrighted materials noted for which further reproduction, in any form, is prohibited without the specific permission of copyright holders. Citation as to source is requested.

Figure 5.19.   Example of a clinical pathway.

University of Anystate Hospitals

CLINICAL PATHWAY:
CESAREAN SECTION DELIVERY
PAGE 1 OF 3

PATIENT LABEL

This document should be considered a *guideline*. Outcomes will vary depending on the patient's severity of illness and other factors/conditions that affect or alter expected outcomes.

Key: Fill in appropriate location for nursing unit. Initial completed intermediate and discharge outcomes. Circle any variances and document on variance log. Once variance is resolved, date and initial clinical pathway.

Expected Discharge Outcomes	Preop Date _____ Time _____	Operative/Recovery Date _____ Time _____
	Nursing Unit _____	Nursing Unit _____

Cardiovascular
• Hemodynamically stable
• Chest clear to auscultation bilaterally
	Stable BP (< 140/90 or no increases
	    > 30 mm systolic or
	    > 15 mm diastolic) _____
	Chest clear _____
		Stable BP (< 140/90 or no increases
		    > 30 mm systolic or
		    > 15 mm diastolic) _____

Gastrointestinal • Bowel sounds present • Tolerates regular diet • Passing flatus	NPO	
Genitourinary • Normal bladder function		Foley patent, draining clear yellow urine _____ UOP ≥ 30 cc/h _____

Reproductive
• Delivery of well newborn
• Involution progressing
• Minimal physical discomfort
• Breast: Skin and nipples intact
	Adequate prenatal care _____
	Reassuring father _____
	No signs/symptoms of
	    uterine/vaginal bleeding _____
		Fundus firm, lochia small
		    to moderate _____
		Pain control initiated _____
		EBL ≤ 1000 cc _____
		Delivery of well newborn _____

Integumentary • Incision intact with evidence of healing • No signs/symptoms of infection		Abdominal dressing dry and intact _____
Psychosocial • Patient/family demonstrates adjustment to parental role		

Education
• Patient/family able to identify problems
    that require immediate medical attention
• Patient/family able to verbalize under-
    standing of care needs (wound, etc.)
	States/understands
	plan of care _____	

Discharge Planning
• Patient/family able to verbalize support
    system(s) and/or support system for
    home care established
• Patient/family able to manage
    continuing care needs
• Patient discharged
	Patient/family identifies
	support system
	for home care _____	

Date	Initials	Signature	Date	Initials	Signature	Date	Initials	Signature

Figure 5.19.   (continued)

University of Anystate Hospitals

CLINICAL PATHWAY:
CESAREAN SECTION DELIVERY
PAGE 2 OF 3

PATIENT LABEL

This document should be considered a *guideline*. Outcomes will vary depending on the patient's severity of illness and other factors/conditions that affect or alter expected outcomes.

Key: Fill in appropriate location for nursing unit. Initial completed intermediate and discharge outcomes. Circle any variances and document on variance log. Once variance is resolved, date and initial clinical pathway.

Expected Discharge Outcomes	Postoperative Day Date _____ Time _____	Postop Day #1 Date _____ Time _____
	Nursing Unit _____	Nursing Unit _____
Cardiovascular • Hemodynamically stable	Able to turn, cough, and deep-breathe every 2 h _____ Chest clear _____	Ambulates with assistance _____ Chest clear _____
Gastrointestinal • Bowel sounds present • Tolerates regular diet • Passing flatus	Tolerates clear liquids, no nausea or vomiting _____	Bowel sounds present _____ Tolerates regular diet _____
Genitourinary • Normal bladder function	Foley patent, draining clear yellow urine _____ UOP > 240 cc/8 h _____	Normal bladder function _____ UOP < 240 cc/8 h _____

Reproductive
• Delivery of well newborn
• Involution progressing
• Minimal physical discomfort
• Breast: Skin and nipples intact
	Fundus firm, lochia small
	  to moderate _____
	Pain controlled _____
		Fundus firm, lochia small
		  to moderate _____
		Pain controlled _____

Integumentary
• Incision intact with evidence of healing
• No signs/symptoms of infection
	Abdominal dressing dry
	  and intact _____
	Afebrile (<100.4ºF) _____
		Wound edges approximated,
		  no signs/symptoms
		  of infection _____
		Afebrile (<100.4ºF)

Psychosocial
• Patient/family demonstrate adjustment
  to parental role
	Demonstrates appropriate
	  parent/infant interaction _____
		Demonstrates appropriate
		  parental/infant interaction _____

Education
• Patient/family able to identify problems
  that require immediate medical attention
• Patient/family able to verbalize under-
  standing of care needs (wound, etc.)
	States/understands postop
	  plan of care _____
	Initiates breast-feeding _____
		Establishes infant feeding _____

Discharge Planning
• Patient/family able to verbalize support
  system(s) and/or support system for
  home care established
• Patient/family able to manage continu-
  ing care needs
• Patient discharged
		Discusses plan for discharge _____

Date	Initials	Signature	Date	Initials	Signature	Date	Initials	Signature

Figure 5.19. (continued)

University of Anystate Hospitals

CLINICAL PATHWAY:
CESAREAN SECTION DELIVERY
PAGE 3 OF 3

PATIENT LABEL

This document should be considered a *guideline*. Outcomes will vary depending on the patient's severity of illness and other factors/conditions that affect or alter expected outcomes.

Key: Fill in appropriate location for nursing unit. Initial completed intermediate and discharge outcomes. Circle any variances and document on variance log. Once variance is resolved, date and initial clinical pathway.

Expected Discharge Outcomes	Postop Day #2 Date _____ Time _____	Postop Day # 3/Discharge Outcomes Date _____ Time _____
	Nursing Unit _____	Nursing Unit _____
Cardiovascular • Hemodynamically stable	Participates in self-care _____ Ambulates in hall _____ Chest clear _____ Stable BP (<140/90 or no increases > 30 mm systolic or > 15 mm diastolic _____	Responsible for self-care _____ Vital signs within normal _____ Chest clear _____
Gastrointestinal • Bowel sounds present • Tolerates regular diet • Passing flatus	Active bowel sounds _____ Passing flatus _____ Tolerates regular diet _____	Active bowel sounds _____ Passing flatus _____ Tolerates regular diet _____
Genitourinary • Normal bladder function	Bladder function normal _____ UOP >240 cc/8 h	Normal bladder function _____
Reproductive • Delivery of well newborn • Involution progressing • Minimal physical discomfort • Breast: Skin and nipples intact	Fundus firm, lochia small to moderate Pain controlled _____	Delivery of well newborn _____ Involution progressing _____ Minimal physical discomfort _____ Breasts and nipples intact _____
Integumentary • Incision intact with evidence of healing • No signs/symptoms of infection	Wound edges approximated, no signs/symptoms of infection _____ Remains afebrile (<100.4ºF) _____	Incision intact with evidence of healing _____ No signs/symptoms of infection _____
Psychosocial • Patient/family demonstrates adjustment to parental role	Parental adjustment progressing _____ Demonstrates appropriate parental–infant interaction _____ Patient/family verbalizes thoughts/ feelings about childbirth _____	Patient/family demonstrates adjustment to parental role _____
Education • Patient/family able to identify problems that require immediate medical attention • Patient/family able to verbalize under- standing of care needs (wound, etc.)	Verbalizes/demonstrates self-care knowledge and skills _____ Demonstrates infant feeding _____	Patient/family able to identify problems that require immediate medical attention _____ Patient/family able to verbalize understanding of care needs (wound, infant feeding) _____
Discharge Planning • Patient/family able to verbalize support system(s) and/or support system for home care established • Patient/family able to manage continu- ing care needs • Patient discharged	Support system for home care established _____	Patient/family able to verbalize support system(s) and/or support system for home care established _____ Verbalizes understanding of follow-up care _____ Discharged home _____

Date	Initials	Signature	Date	Initials	Signature	Date	Initials	Signature

CLINICAL PATHWAY: C-SECTION
300111 (5/2004)

Case management follows a five-step process that is documented in the patient's medical record (Shaw et al. 2003, 109–111):

1. **Perform preadmission care planning**. The case manager reviews the patient's needs with the admitting physician or emergency department physician. The case manager may also contact the patient or the patient's insurance carrier to confirm that the patient is covered for the planned hospital services. The case manager can also be helpful in determining the correct patient status, such as inpatient or observation.

2. **Perform care planning at the time of admission**. The case manager reviews the patient's health record shortly after admission to confirm that the patient meets intensity of service and severity of illness requiring acute-care admission. The case manager then consults the treatment guidelines for the patient's diagnosis and verifies that all of the necessary services have been ordered. The case manager may also initiate communication with the patient's insurance company to ensure that the insurance company is aware of the admission, patient's diagnosis, and expected length of stay.

3. **Review the progress of care**. The case manager reviews the patient's progress throughout the period of hospitalization. When progress is slower than expected, the case manager coordinates interventions among clinicians. The case manager also provides patient-status reports to the insurance company and facilitates communication between the payer and physician regarding the plan of care and expected length of stay.

4. **Conduct discharge planning**. Once the patient's progress ensures his or her recovery, the case manager finalizes the discharge plan. The patient and the patient's family as well as his or her primary-care physician are included in the process.

    Postdischarge medications and medical equipment and supplies are ordered, and follow-up appointments are scheduled. Arrangements for transporting the patient to a subacute facility are made, if necessary, as are arrangements for home care or hospice services.

5. **Conclude postdischarge planning**. After the patient has been discharged, the case manager provides information about the patient's hospital course to the clinicians who will continue the patient's care in nonacute-care settings.

Nurses' Progress Notes

The nursing staff begins writing progress notes in the patient's health record soon after the patient is admitted to the nursing unit. Because nurses have frequent contact with patients, the progress notes written by nurses provide a complete record of the patient's care and response to treatment. Nurses also ensure the continuity of patient care by confirming that all physicians' orders have been carried out and appropriately documented.

Nurses usually record the patient's vital signs at least every shift. (See figure 5.20.) Intensive-care nurses provide continuous patient monitoring. A complete assessment of the patient's condition is performed every time the nursing shifts change (McCain 2006, 181). When problems are noted, a member of the nursing staff contacts the patient's physician and recommends appropriate action.

Nursing notes are written in a narrative style. (See figures 5.21 and 5.22 for examples.) The notes are recorded in a handwritten format in paper-based health records. Many hospitals that have implemented electronic health records provide bedside computer terminals to make the process of documentation more efficient and timely. Some intensive-care monitoring systems record vital signs automatically.

Figure 5.20.   Vital signs documentation in graphic format.

University of Anystate Hospitals

GRAPHIC VITAL SIGNS

PATIENT LABEL

Date																											
Hospital Day/Postop																											

Temperature

°C	°F	a.m. / p.m. (12–8, times repeated across five days)
40.0	104	
39.5	103	
38.9	102	
38.4	101	
37.8	100	
37.2	99	
36.7	98	
36.1	97	
35.6	96	

Hour columns: 12 (2400) · 4 (0400) · 8 (0800) · 12 (1200) · 4 (1600) · 8 (2000) repeated for a.m./p.m. across each hospital day.

P	
R	
BP	

S&As	a.m.
(time/results)	p.m.

Height: _____   Weight: _____   _____ Bed/Chair/Stand   _____ Bed/Chair/Stand   _____ Bed/Chair/Stand   _____ Bed/Chair/Stand   _____ Bed/Chair/Stand

Stool				24-H				24-H				24-H				24-H				24-H
Shift	7-3	3-11	11-7	**Total**	7-3	3-11	11-7	**Total**	7-3	3-11	11-7	**Total**	7-3	3-11	11-7	**Total**	7-3	3-11	11-7	**Total**

Intake

- Tube Feedings
- Oral
- Intravenous
- Piggyback
- Blood
- Shift Total

Output

- Voided
- Catheter
- Gastric
- Emesis
- Shift Total

GRAPHIC VITAL SIGNS
000029 (11/2002)

Figure 5.21. Nursing progress notes in paper format.

University of Anystate Hospitals

PROGRESS NOTES
PAGE 1 OF 2

	Date	Time	Discipline	PROGRESS NOTES

Barriers to Patient Education

☐ No Barriers   ☐ Language
☐ Physical   ☐ Reading Difficulties
☐ Cognitive   ☐ Lacks Readiness
☐ Emotional   ☐ Lacks Motivation
☐ Other _____

Patient/Family Instructions		Outcome	Initials	Discipline
☐ Nutrition	P/F			
☐ Medications	P/F			
☐ Activity/Rehabilitation	P/F			
☐ Safety	P/F			
☐ Signs/Symptoms	P/F			
☐ Wound/Skin Care	P/F			
☐ Pre/Postop Care	P/F			
☐ Equipment	P/F			
☐ Procedures	P/F			
☐ Treatments	P/F			
☐ Pain Management	P/F			
☐ PEARLS	P/F			
☐ Other	P/F			

Outcome Key:
1. Able to state understanding and/or return demonstration.
2. Unable to state understanding and/or return demonstration. Continue to reinforce. (See progress notes.)

Figure 5.21.   (continued)

University of Anystate Hospitals

PROGRESS NOTES
PAGE 2 OF 2

PATIENT LABEL

Date	Time	Discipline	PROGRESS NOTES

Key

CM = Case Manager
CR = Cardiac Rehabilitation
DTC = Diabetes Treatment Center
ETN = Enterostomal Nurse
FSR = Financial Services Representative
HCC = Home Care Coordinator

NSG = Nursing
NSPY = Neuropsychology
OT = Occupational Therapy
PC = Pastoral Care
PHM = Pharmacy
PT = Physical Therapy

RD = Registered Dietitian
RT = Respiratory Therapy
SLP = Speech/Language Pathologist
SW = Social Worker
TR = Therapeutic Recreation

Figure 5.22.   Nursing progress notes in electronic format.

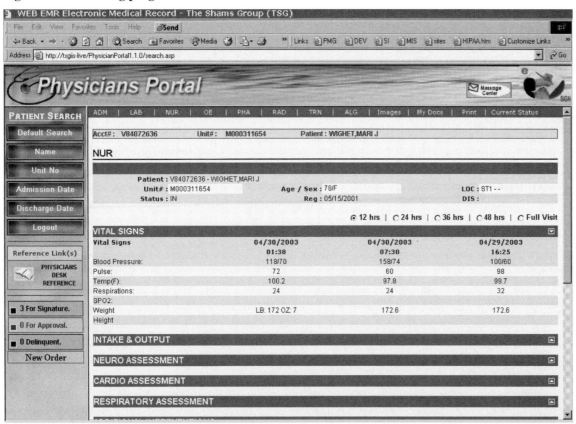

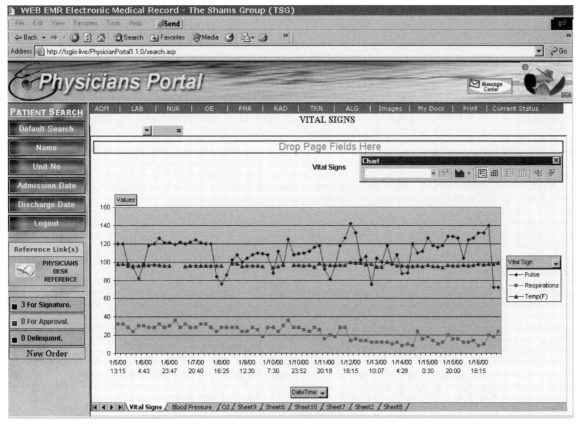

Documentation in nursing notes has expanded to include other members of the healthcare team. In many settings, the term has been changed to *interdisciplinary notes,* indicating these entries are not restricted to nurses.

Some hospitals follow a system called **charting by exception** or focus charting. Under this system, only abnormal or unusual findings are documented. Progress notes focus on abnormal events and describe any interventions that were ordered and the patient's response. The purpose of charting by exception is to reduce the amount of routine record keeping required.

Medication Records

Nurses keep a separate log for each patient's medications. The **medication record** includes all of the medications administered to the patient while the patient is in the nursing unit. The surgery department and ancillary departments that perform diagnostic and therapeutic procedures also maintain records of the medications administered to patients under their care.

The medication record indicates the date and time each drug was administered, the name of the medication, the form of administration, and the medication's dosage and strength. The entry for each medication is signed or initialed and dated by the person who administered the drug.

Surgical patients and others who experience severe levels of pain are sometimes treated with patient-controlled analgesics such as morphine. The medications are administered through a pump that delivers continuous doses controlled manually by the patient. Monitoring equipment automatically records the patient's respiration rate, level of sedation, and pain level as well as pump volume, dose received, and cumulative dosage since the beginning of the monitoring period. (See figure 5.23.)

Medication errors are not uncommon in healthcare facilities, and such mistakes can have serious consequences. Every medication error must be described fully in the patient's health record. The time the incorrect medication was administered and the names of the correct and incorrect medications involved must be included in the documentation. The patient's response to the incorrect medication must also be documented, as well as any treatment interventions performed to address the effects of the medication and the patient's response to the interventions.

Adverse reactions to drugs administered correctly or incorrectly must be documented in a progress note and reported to the patient's principal physician. Most hospitals have policies that dictate when adverse reactions and medication errors should also be reported to the risk management and performance improvement departments.

New requirements from the Joint Commission (2007) focus on medication reconciliation within the medical record. Medications must be reconciled on admission to include name of medication, route, and dosage. Medication reconciliation must include any over-the-counter medications the patient may be taking in addition to those medications prescribed by a physician. In addition, medications must be reconciled upon moving from one level of care to another, such as from ICU to a step down unit and on discharge.

Flow Charts

Flow charts are graphic illustrations of data and observations. Flow charts make it easy to visualize patterns and identify abnormal results. Flow charts are often used in addition to narrative progress notes for recording the patient's fluid consumption (input) and elimination (output) patterns. Input and output records are especially important in pediatric patients because medications are often based on the patient's weight and may affect input and output. Blood glucose records for diabetic patients are also maintained as flow charts. Pain assessments can be charted as well. (See figure 5.24 for an example of a flow chart.)

Figure 5.23. Patient-controlled analgesia record in paper format.

Midwest Medical Center

PATIENT-CONTROLLED ANALGESIA
FLOW CHART

PATIENT LABEL

Physician Order:

_____ Morphine   1 mg/ml = 50 mg/50 ml
_____ Mependine   10 mg/ml = 500 mg/50 ml
_____ Hydromorphone   1 mg/ml = 50 mg/50 ml
Customized

_____   _____ mg/ml = ___ /50 ml
     List Medication   List Concentration

Order Date	Dose		Delay	Basal	1-H Limit	Load	Bolus		Physician
		mg	mg	mg	mg	mg	mg	q. ____ h.	
		mg	mg	mg	mg	mg	mg	q. ____ h.	
		mg	mg	mg	mg	mg	mg	q. ____ h.	
		mg	mg	mg	mg	mg	mg	q. ____ h.	
		mg	mg	mg	mg	mg	mg	q. ____ h.	

Start Date: _____   Signature (MD/RN): _____
Time: _____ a.m./p.m.   Cosignature: (RN): _____

☐ Check if syringe change only.   **Initial Baseline Vital Signs:**   BP: _____ P: _____ R: _____   15 min. after administration: BP: _____ P: _____ R: _____

Date	Time	R	Sedation Level	Pain Level (greater than or equal to 5 × 2 requires documented intervention)	O₂ Sat. (peds required; adults only if ordered)	Total Given	Syringe Volume Infused	Syringe Infused (syringe volume Infused × concentration)	Loading or Bolus Dose	Initials
	a.m.									
	p.m.					mg	cc	mg	mg	
	a.m.									
	p.m.					mg	cc	mg	mg	
	a.m.									
	p.m.					mg	cc	mg	mg	
	a.m.									
	p.m.					mg	cc	mg	mg	
	a.m.									
	p.m.					mg	cc	mg	mg	

Vital Signs: Date: _____ Time: _____ BP: _____ P: _____ R: _____   *Document additional boluses on BP graphic sheet.*
15 Min. after Rebolus: Date: _____ Time: _____ BP: _____ P: _____ R: _____

Initials	Signature	Initials	Signature	Initials	Signature	Initials	Signature	Initials	Signature

Pain Scale: For the Conscious Patient

   0   5   10
no pain   bad pain   worse pain

For Adult Patients: Stop infusion and call physician for respiratory rate of 10/minute or less.
For Pediatric Patients: Stop infusion and call physician for oxygen saturation less than 94% and/or respiratory rate of 14/minute or less.

Pain Scale: For the Pediatric Patient
Wong-Baker FACES Pain Rating Scale

0 NO HURT	2 HURTS LITTLE BIT	4 HURTS LITTLE MORE	6 HURTS EVEN MORE	8 HURTS WHOLE LOT	10 HURTS WORST

Pain Scale: For the Cognitively Limited

Observe	Criteria	Points	Observe	Criteria	Points
Emotion	Smiling	0	Facial Cues	Relaxed, calm expression	0
	Anxious/ irritable	1		Drawn around mouth and eyes	1
	Almost in tears	2		Facial frowning, wincing	2
Movement	None	0	Positioning/Guarding	Relaxed body	0
	Restless/slow or decreased movement	1		Guarding/tense	
	Immobile, afraid to move	2		Fetal position/jumps if touched	1
Verbal Cues	States no pain	0			2
	Whining/whimper-ing/moaning	1			
	Screaming, crying out	2			

Sedation Level: Modified Ramsay Scale
1. Patient anxious, agitated, or restless
2. Patient cooperative, oriented, and tranquil
3. Patient responds to commands only
4. Patient responds to gentle shaking
5. Patient responds to noxious stimulus
6. Patient has no response to firm nail bed pressure or other noxious stimuli

PATIENT-CONTROLLED ANALGESIA FLOW CHART
000031 (10/2002)

Figure 5.24. Example of a flow chart.

Midwest Medical Center

VASCULAR FLOW CHART

PATIENT LABEL

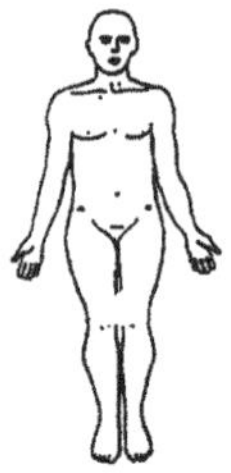

Use diagram to identify graft site

Key	RL/LL = Right Leg/Left Leg	**Date**													
	RA/LA = Right Arm/Left Arm	**Time**													
	Graft Site = A, B, C	**Extremities**													
Pain	Pain Level (0–10)														
	Homan's Sign (+ or −)														
Sensation	N = Normal NB = Numbness T = Tingling A = Absent														
P	0 = No Pulse 1+ = Diminished 2+ = Normal 3+ = Bounding DM = Doppler Monophasic DB = Doppler Biphasic														
Color	R = Red PK = Pink PL = Pallor MOT = Mottled CY = Cyanotic														
T	H = Hot W = Warm C = Cool CD = Cold														
Capillary Refill	N = Normal (1–3 sec) S = Sluggish (>3 sec) B = Brisk (<1 sec)														
Edema	A = Absent 1+, 2+, 3+, 4+														
Two-Pt. Discrim.	1–10 mm (normal = 3–5 mm)														
Vital Signs	T														
	P														
	R														
	BP														
		Initials													

Initial	Signature

Comments
Signature: ______________________ Date/Time: __________

VASCULAR FLOW CHART
000032 (10/2002)

Transfer Records

Nurses maintain records of patient transfers from one hospital department to another, for example, from their rooms to the surgery department. They also document any instances when the patient leaves the facility for a physician's appointment or a procedure to be performed outside the hospital. (See figure 5.25.) **Transfer records** are important to the continuum of care because they document communication between caregivers in multiple settings. It is important that a patient's treatment plan be consistent as the patient moves through the healthcare delivery system.

Diagnostic and Therapeutic Reports

Patients usually undergo a variety of diagnostic and therapeutic procedures, depending on the nature of their illnesses. Some procedures are performed as a part of general patient management; for example, basic blood and urine analyses. Other procedures, such as brain scans, are performed to determine the extent and nature of a patient's illness. Surgical interventions are performed to determine the extent and nature of the patient's disease as well as to provide definitive treatment; breast cancer surgery would be one example.

The most common diagnostic and management procedures performed by hospitals include routine laboratory analyses of blood and other bodily fluids, x-ray examinations, and other imaging procedures. Surgical procedures such as biopsies, endoscopic examinations, surgical explorations, excisions, and resections are performed for both inpatients and outpatients. The circumstances and findings of these procedures require precise documentation in the form of reports to be placed in the patient's health record.

Special Consents

Special consents are required for procedures that involve a significant risk for the patient, such as invasive diagnostic tests, transfusions, and surgical procedures. Medical staff rules and/or hospital policies usually list which types of services always require written documentation of the patient's expressed consent. In general, the following types of procedures usually require special consent:

- Procedures that involve the use of anesthetics

- Treatments that involve the use of experimental drugs

- Surgical procedures that involve the manipulation of organs and tissues

- Procedures that involve a significant risk for complications

- Use of blood and blood products

In addition, some states require documentation of the patient's written consent for specific types of diagnostic procedures; for example, human immunodeficiency virus (HIV) testing.

It is primarily the responsibility of the patient's physician or surgeon to explain the nature of the specific procedure to be performed. The physician should make sure that the patient or the patient's legal representative understands the procedure's potential risks, complications, and benefits. Patients or their representatives should also be made aware of the comparative risks and benefits of any alternative treatments that are available. Only then should the patient or the patient's representative be asked to sign and date the consent form.

Special consents become a permanent part of the patient's health record. The content of the consent form varies according to the type of procedure to be performed, but most include at least the following information:

- Patient identification, including name and record number

- Name of the procedure to be performed

Figure 5.25.   Interdepartmental transfer record in paper format.

Anycity General Hospital

INTERDEPARTMENTAL TRANSFER RECORD

PATIENT LABEL

Admit/Transfer to Room #: _____ From: _____ Via ☐ Stretcher ☐ Wheelchair
Date: _____ Diagnosis: _____
Vital Signs (within 30 min):   T: _____ P: _____ R: _____ BP: _____
Valuables: ☐ N/A   ☐ Given to Patient   ☐ Given to Family   ☐ Other: _____

Time Report Given: _____
☐ Falls prevention protocol
must be initiated on unit.
Pain Scale: _____

Assessment

Cardiovascular
Rhythm: _____
Edema: ☐ Yes   ☐ No
　　　Where: _____
　　　Amt.: _____
Pulses   × 4 3 2 1
☐ Other: _____
_____

Respiratory
☐ Lungs Clear
☐ Lung Sounds Abnormal
Explain: _____
_____
Oxygen Sat. _____ % on room air
Oxygen at _____ liters/min via:
☐ N/C   ☐ Mask   ☐ Other: _____
☐ Other: _____

Neurological
Responds: ☐ Alert/Oriented × 3 2 1
　　　　　☐ Verbal
　　　　　☐ Pain
　　　　　☐ Unresponsive
Pupils: ☐ ERLA   ☐ Other: _____
Weakness: ☐ Yes   ☐ No
Where: Right: _____
　　　　Left: _____
☐ Other: _____

Gastrointestinal
Abd: ☐ Soft, nontender
　　　☐ Distended
　　　☐ Tender
Bowel Sounds:
　　　☐ All quadrants
　　　☐ Absent
　　　☐ Other: _____
☐ Other: _____

Renal
☐ Incontinent
☐ Foley   Size: _____
☐ Dialysis
　　Type: _____
Intake: _____
Output: _____
☐ Other: _____
_____

Musculoskeletal
☐ Fracture: _____
☐ Dislocation: _____
Immobilization:
　　☐ Cast　　　☐ Splint
　　☐ Traction
Neurovascular Status:
　　☐ Intact
　　☐ _____
☐ Other: _____

Integumentary
☐ Intact   ☐ Ecchymosis/Redness: _____   ☐ Decubitus/Breakdown: _____   ☐ Wounds: _____
_____ _____ _____

Interventions

IV Access   ☐ N/A
☐ INT   ☐ IV   ☐ Implanted Port
Size: _____ Site: _____
Fluid: _____ Amount: _____ Rate: ____
Other: _____

Drip Infusions   ☐ N/A
_____ Rate: _____
_____ Rate: _____
_____ Rate: _____
_____ Rate: _____

Medications   ☐ N/A
_____ @ _____
_____ @ _____
_____ @ _____
_____ @ _____

Labs   ☐ N/A
☐ CBC　　　☐ Heme Panel
☐ B/CMP　　☐ Fingerstick Glucose
☐ CIP　　　☐ PT/PTT
☐ UA　　　☐ Urine Dip   ☐ HCG
☐ Hemoccult   ☐ Amylase   ☐ Lipase

Other: _____
Abnormals: _____
_____

Procedures   ☐ N/A
☐ EKG
☐ X-rays   ☐ CXR   ☐ KUB
　　　　　☐ Other: _____
☐ Tube Insertion
Type: _____ Size: ____ Location: ___
Type: _____ Size: ____ Location: ___
Other: _____

Miscellaneous   ☐ N/A
_____
_____

Infection Control   ☐ N/A
☐ Contact   ☐ Droplet   ☐ Airborne

Equipment Needed in Room ☐ N/A
☐ Oxygen   ☐ IV Pump   ☐ Suction
☐ Monitor   ☐ Other: _____

Nurse Preparing Report

Unit Phone #: _____

Nurse Receiving Patient

☐ Agree with Above Assessment
☐ See Nurses' Notes

INTERDEPARTMENTAL TRANSFER RECORD
000102 (10/2002)

- Name of the person who is to perform the procedure, if applicable

- Description of the procedure to be performed

- Date the procedure is to be performed

- Patient's or representative's signature (with a note on the representative's relationship to the patient)

- Date the consent was signed

Ancillary Services

The results of every diagnostic procedure performed on the patient's behalf must be permanently documented in the patient's health record. In healthcare facilities, laboratory and imaging procedures are performed in separate departments and are known collectively as **ancillary services**.

Laboratory Reports: Clinical laboratories routinely examine samples of blood, urine, spinal fluid, and other fluids and substances collected from patients. Laboratory tests require a physician's order. The samples for testing are usually collected from patients by nurses or phlebotomists (technicians specially trained to draw blood samples) and then delivered to the laboratory.

When the samples are received in the laboratory, a medical technologist or another laboratory specialist performs the standardized testing procedures ordered. Medical technologists receive training in four-year college programs, where they learn a combination of manual and automated biochemical analysis techniques. Large clinical laboratories may also employ bacteriologists, biologists, and other scientists to conduct more complex analyses, such as genetic testing.

In hospitals, the results of most routine laboratory procedures are generated automatically by electronic testing equipment. Laboratory computer systems generate reports on the test results, which are returned to the physician who ordered the tests. Paper or electronic copies of the results are also placed in the patient's health record. (See figures 5.26 and 5.27.) Reports of laboratory results include the following information:

- Patient identification, including name and record number

- Name of the test performed

- Date the test was performed and time in/time out of the laboratory

- Signature of the laboratory technologist or scientist who performed the test

- Name of the laboratory where the test was performed

- Results of the test

In hospitals with clinical computer systems, laboratory test results are available to physicians and nurses as soon as the results are generated by the laboratory reporting system. A laboratory summary is available electronically throughout the patient's hospital stay, and a final summary of laboratory results is available soon after the patient's discharge. Copies of the summaries are placed into paper-based records.

Imaging Reports: Scans and x-ray images of various parts of the body and organs are frequently performed by inpatient and outpatient imaging departments. Most hospital imaging departments are equipped to perform x-ray examinations and CT scans. Many large, urban hospitals also provide more advanced imaging services including MRI and

Figure 5.26.   Example of a laboratory report in paper format.

Midwest Medical Center

**LABORATORY SERVICES REPORT:
COAGULATION**

PATIENT, WYLIE C.
090241237
DOB: 10/10/1918

ADMISSION DATE: 05/14/03

ADMITTING PHYSICIAN: M. D. Doctor

SPECIMEN DATE: 05/20/03

COLLECTED TIME: 4:55 p.m.

WEEKDAY: Tuesday

——ROUTINE COAGULATION——		UNITS	REFERENCE	
PT	**17.6 H**	SEC	11.2–13.8	
INR	1.9			(1)
PTT	32.0	SEC	22.1–32.5	(2)

H = High

Footnotes

(1) The INR therapeutic range (1.5–4.0) for patients on warfarin therapy will depend on the clinical disorder being treated.

(2) Effective August 19, 2002, the suggested therapeutic range may vary from 40.9–68.3 sec for inpatients on heparin therapy.

Figure 5.27. Example of a laboratory report in electronic format.

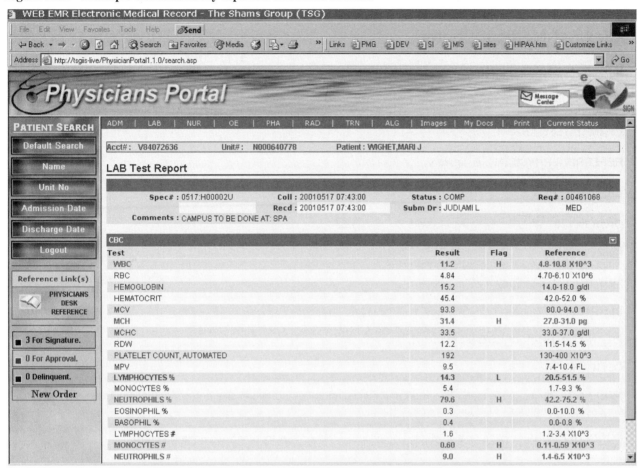

positron-emission tomography (PET). Some imaging procedures require the administration of radiopharmaceuticals, radioactive contrast media administered to the patient before or during the procedure to make it possible to visualize physiological processes and tissues more clearly.

Imaging procedures require a physician's order. Most imaging procedures are performed by specially trained radiology technicians. However, the interpretation of scans and images must be performed by physicians specially trained in radiology. The radiologist's written report, signed and dated, becomes part of the patient's permanent record. (See figure 5.28.) The original scans and images are generally stored in the radiology department rather than in patient records. However, most electronic health record systems are capable of storing copies of diagnostic scans and images for easy reference.

Imaging reports generally include the following information:

- Patient identification, including name and record number

- Image identification data including image number and hospital number

- Physician's order for the examination, signed and dated

- Name of the examination performed

Figure 5.28.   Example of an imaging services report in paper format.

Midwest Medical Center

IMAGING SERVICES REPORT

OUTPATIENT, OLIVE O.
121212000
DOB: 02/27/1942

EXAM DATE: 5/12/200x

REFERRING PHYSICIAN: B. Interary

Check-in #: 62

Order #: 1201

Exam #: 36080

FXR: Chest Single View

DIAGNOSIS: V72.84

PA AND LATERAL CHEST: 5/12/200x

COMPARISON: 6/8/98

FINDINGS: The lungs are clear. The heart and mediastinum are normal in size and configuration. There are minor degenerative changes of the lower thoracic spine.

CONCLUSION: Minor degenerative change of the lower thoracic spine; otherwise negative chest.

Signature:

Norman D. Radiol, MD

Norman D. Radiol, MD

5/12/200x

Date

d: 05/12/200x
t: 05/14/200x
NDR, MD/na

- Date the examination was performed

- Type and amount of radiopharmaceutical administered, if applicable

- Radiologist's interpretation of the images, authenticated by date and signature

Hospital imaging departments perform a number of routine diagnostic tests that do not require sedation in most cases. Examples of routine diagnostic tests include mammograms, fetal ultrasounds, and preoperative chest x-rays. These procedures carry a very low risk of adverse events and complications, and so recordkeeping requirements are minimal.

Invasive diagnostic examinations such as angiocardiography and image-guided surgical procedures require recordkeeping and special consents similar to those required for regular surgical procedures. Procedures that involve conscious sedation require documentation of the sedatives administered and the patient's period of recovery. The physicians who perform the procedures must author short discharge progress notes in addition to full reports of the procedures and any findings. For procedures performed under general anesthesia, documentation is required for the entire perioperative period. The facility should establish a list of the imaging procedures that require special consents and documentation.

Specialty Diagnostic Services

Several diagnostic tests are performed by clinical specialists rather than as ancillary services. The most common are tests related to cardiac and neurological functioning.

Cardiology Reports: Cardiologists perform and/or report on a number of different cardiac diagnostic tests performed in the hospital on both inpatients and outpatients. Many patients being treated primarily for noncardiac diagnoses may also have preexisting cardiac conditions that need monitoring through routine electrocardiography. (See figures 5.29 through 5.31.) Other specialized tests performed and/or interpreted by cardiologists include the following:

- Exercise and pharmacological stress tests

- Tilt-table tests

- Holter monitoring

- Pacemaker checks

- Electrocardiography

- Echocardiography

- Cardioradionucleide imaging

- Myocardial imaging

- Cardiac catheterization

Cardiac catheterizations may also include treatment interventions such as the insertion of stents and balloons.

Neurology Reports: Neurologists are often called upon to evaluate the neurological status of patients being treated for other types of illnesses. For example, neurological dysfunction is common among patients suffering from systemic disorders such as alcoholism, cancer, cerebrovascular and cardiovascular disease, and autoimmune disease. It can be difficult to distinguish neurological impairment from psychiatric illness; so psychiatrists sometimes ask for neurological evaluations of patients with ambiguous symptoms. In addition, because critically

Figure 5.29.   Example of a cardiac catheterization report in paper format.

Midwest Medical Center

CARDIAC CATHETERIZATION REPORT
PAGE 1 OF 2

PATIENT, SYLVESTER Q.
00999067
DOB: 01/03/1960

DATE: 05/17/200x

REFERRING PHYSICIAN(S): M. D. Doctor

PROCEDURES PERFORMED:

1. Left heart catheterization
2. Selective coronary artery study
3. Left ventriculography
4. Insertion of an intra-aortic balloon pump

DESCRIPTION OF PROCEDURE: The patient was brought over from Anyplace General Hospital, where he had been admitted last week with acute respiratory failure. It was felt that it was on the basis of an acute myocardial event. The above procedures were performed. He was taken to the cardiac diagnostic unit at Midwest Medical Center, where the right groin was prepped and draped in the usual sterile manner. One percent Xylocaine was instilled in the region surrounding the right femoral artery. An 18-gauge needle was advanced into the right femoral artery area. Using exchange guide wire technique, a #5 French sheath was placed. This was later exchanged for a #8 French sheath when the intra-aortic balloon pump was placed.

Hemodynamic Data: (1) ascending aortic pressure was 188/62; (2) left ventricle was 188/23-35.

With the patient in the right anterior oblique position, 12 cc of Isovue was injected into the left ventricular chamber. The ejection fraction is approximately 50–55%.

Selective coronary arteriography was performed of both the right and left coronary arteries in multiple oblique projections.

Left Main Coronary Artery: The left main coronary artery was markedly narrowed. The ostium was very significantly obstructed. As the catheter tip barely entered the main coronary artery, the pressure dipped to near 0%. This was confirmed on two further very careful positionings of the catheter. Direct injection into the left main coronary artery was not possible.

Left Anterior Descending Artery: The very proximal portion of the left anterior descending artery shows very high-grade near-total occlusion. The distal vessel is irregular, however, free of high-grade occlusions. There is a large intermediate branch.

Left Posterior Circumflex Coronary Artery: The left posterior circumflex coronary artery was nearly totally occluded at its origin. Minor disease is noted throughout the system.

Right Coronary Artery: The right coronary artery was irregular; however, there was no evidence of significant obstructive disease.

Figure 5.29.   (continued)

Midwest Medical Center

CARDIAC CATHETERIZATION REPORT
PAGE 2 OF 2

PATIENT, SYLVESTER Q.
00999067
DOB: 01/03/1960

At the conclusion of the procedure, Dr. Surgeon was contacted regarding the possibility of urgent surgery. With Dr. Doctor and Dr. Surgeon consulting by phone, it was elected to place an intra-aortic balloon pump.

The intra-aortic balloon pump was placed without difficulty. Its position was confirmed by fluoroscopy. It appeared to be functioning normally.

During the procedure when the intra-aortic balloon pump was put in, the patient was given 5000 units intravenous heparin and will be on an intravenous heparin drip.

IMPRESSIONS:

1. Relative preservation of left ventricular systolic function at rest with ejection fraction of approximately 50%.

2. Coronary artery disease—three vessels involved
    a. Near-total occlusion of left main coronary artery
    b. High-grade near-total occlusion of the left anterior descending artery proximally
    c. High-grade near-total occlusion of the left posterior circumflex coronary artery proximally
    d. Mild diffuse disease, right coronary artery, as described above

3. Placement of intra-aortic balloon pump in patient with left main coronary artery disease and history of flash pulmonary edema.

Signature:

M. Dennis Heartmann (signature)

M. Dennis Heartmann, MD

5|17|200x

Date

d: 05/17/200x
t: 05/18/200x
MDH, MD/dq

Figure 5.30. Example of an echocardiography report in paper format.

Anytown Community Hospital

ECHOCARDIOGRAPHIC REPORT

TEST, PATIENT
009999999
DOB: 04/01/1930

DATE: 06/02/200x

REFERRING PHYSICIAN: Dr. Doctor

INDICATION FOR STUDY: Murmur

TAPE: House 528

Outpatient Study

Two-dimensional and M-mode echocardiograms were performed

The left atrium is at the upper limits of normal size at 3.7 cm compared to an aortic root diameter of 2.9 cm. The left ventricle is at the upper limits of normal size with a normal internal dimension of 5.6 cm in diastole and 3.3 cm in systole. There is normal wall thickness. There is hyperdynamic left ventricular systolic performance. The ejection fraction is estimated at greater than 70%. No specific regional wall motion abnormalities were identified. The cardiac valves appear structurally normal. No intracardiac masses were identified and a pericardial effusion was not visualized.

Conventional as well as color-flow Doppler imaging was performed. There are findings of mitral regurgitation which is estimated to be at least moderate to severe, if not severe. There is tricuspid regurgitation with peak right ventricular systolic pressure of 31 mmHg. No other significant valvular stenoses or regurgitation were identified.

IMPRESSION:

1. The left atrium and left ventricle at the upper limits of normal size with a hyperdynamic left ventricular systolic performance.

2. There is evidence of mitral regurgitation which is at least moderate to severe. Would consider transesophageal echocardiography to further assess the severity of the mitral regurgitation as well as potentially its etiology.

Signature: _Philip Default_   _6/2/200x_
_____   _____
Philip Default, MD   Date

d: 06/02/200x
t: 06/02/200x

Figure 5.31. Example of an electrocardiography report in paper format.

University of Anystate Hospitals

GRAPHIC EKG REPORT

PATIENT, PETUNIA P.
000000001
DOB: 08/14/1949

NAME: Patient, Petunia

TECHNICIAN: SKH

PROCEDURE DATE/TIME: 10/06/200x 9:59:02

CARDIOLOGIST: Julius W. Cardiolini, MD

SEX/RACE: Female, White

REPORT DATE: 10/08/200x

REQUESTED BY: M. Gynesurg, MD

RESULTS: Normal EKG
PR   200   Normal sinus rhythm rate: 59
QRST   73
QT   407
QTc   403
Axes
P   28
QRS   36
T   35

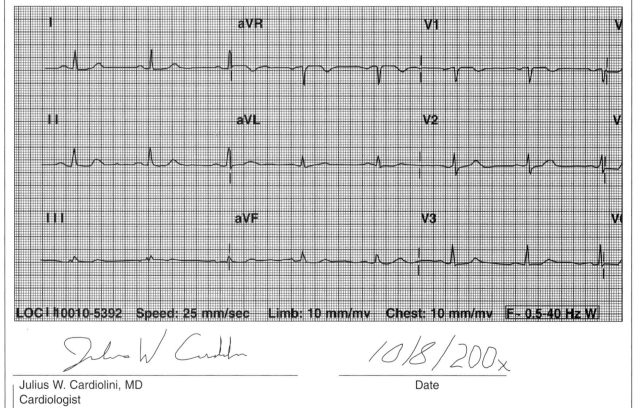

Julius W. Cardiolini, MD
Cardiologist

Date

ill patients can be maintained indefinitely on cardiopulmonary support after their other systems have shut down, neurologists may be called upon to perform an examination to confirm brain death. (See figure 5.32.)

Common diagnostic tests that must be performed or interpreted by neurologists include the following:

- Mental status examinations

- Electroencephalography

- Echoencephalography

- Cerebral angiography

- Myelography

- Lumbar puncture

Surgical Services

Hospital-based surgery departments provide services to both inpatients and outpatients, although many hospitals maintain separate preoperative and recovery areas for outpatients. The documentation requirements for outpatient surgery (also called ambulatory surgery and same-day surgery) are exactly the same as the requirements for inpatient surgical procedures.

Consents for Surgery

Except in emergency situations, surgeons or their representatives must receive written documentation of the patient's consent to surgery before the operation can begin. After the surgery is complete, surgical consent forms become part of the surgical section of the patient's permanent health record.

In day-surgery clinics, patients are usually asked to sign consent forms during the admissions process. The assumption is that the patient's surgeon explained the benefits and risks of the procedure before the surgery was scheduled. Similarly, in inpatient settings, patients about to undergo planned, elective surgery should already understand the nature of the surgery since it would have been discussed during preadmission office visits with the surgeon. Prior to an unplanned inpatient surgery, however, the surgeon or the patient's principal physician must explain the nature of the procedure before asking patients or their legal representatives to sign the consent forms. (See figure 5.33 for an example of a surgical consent form.)

Preoperative History and Physical Reports

Except in emergency situations, every surgical patient's chart must include a report of a complete history and physical conducted no more than seven days before the surgery is to be performed. This requirement is the same for inpatient and outpatient procedures. The report of the history and physical must be present in the patient's chart before surgery can begin. Ideally, advance directives and organ donation forms should also be placed in the chart before surgery. (These documents are discussed in "Advance Directives" earlier in this chapter.)

Anesthesia Evaluations and Records

The anesthesia and/or sedation administered to patients during surgical procedures represent a significant risk independent of the risks involved in the surgery itself. Regulations and accreditation standards require anesthesiologists (who are physicians) and certified nurse-anesthetists (advanced practice nurses who work under the direction of anesthesiologists) to perform and

Figure 5.32. Example of a neurological assessment in paper format.

University of Anystate Hospitals

**NEUROLOGICAL ASSESSMENT
AND REASSESSMENT**

PATIENT LABEL

Date and Time																		
Glasgow Coma Scale																		
Eye Opening	Spontaneous	=	4															**C =** Eyes Closed by Swelling
	To Voice	=	3															
	To Pain	=	2															
	None	=	1															
Verbal Response	Oriented	=	5															**T =** Endotracheal Tube or Tracheostomy
	Confused	=	4															
	Inappropriate Words	=	3															
	Incomprehensible Words	=	2															**A =** Aphasia
	None	=	1															
Motor Response	Obeys Command	=	6															
	Localizes Pain	=	5															
	Withdraws	=	4															Record Best Arm Response
	Flexion	=	3															
	Extension	=	2															
	None	=	1															
Total Score		3–7 = Severe 8–13 = Moderate 13+ = Mild																

Limb Movement Grade limb movement either spontaneous or to command. Do not rate reflex movement. Use scale below.	RA															
	RL															
	LA															
	LL															

Limb Movement Scale: 0 = No Response 1 = Flicker or Trace of Movement 2 = Active Movement without Gravity
3 = Active Movement against Gravity 4 = Active Movement against Gravity with Limited Resistance 5 = Normal Power

Pupils	**Reaction**																
Size	C = Closed by swelling B = Brisk S = Sluggish F = Fixed	Size	R														
1 mm 6 mm 2 mm 3 mm 7 mm 4 mm 5 mm 8 mm			L														
		Reaction	R														
	Shape		L														
	R = Round O = Oval K = Keyhole I = Irregular	Shape	R														
			L														

Ventriculostomy Data Key: CL = Clear R = Red Y = Yellow PK = Pink CLO = Cloudy	ICP																
	CSF Output																
	Color																
	Character																

Vital Signs	Temperature																
	Pulse																
	Respirations																
	Blood Pressure																

Other:

Other:

Comments: _____

Signature: _____ Date/Time: _____

NEUROLOGICAL ASSESSMENT
000080 (10/2002)

Figure 5.33. Example of an informed consent for operation with blood products.

University of Anystate Hospitals

**INFORMED CONSENT FOR OPERATION/
PROCEDURE/ANESTHESIA INCLUDING
BLOOD AND BLOOD PRODUCTS**

PATIENT LABEL

1. I give permission to Dr.(s) _____ to perform

   the following procedure(s): _____

   _____

   _____ on _____ (patient's name).

2. I understand that during the procedure(s), new findings or conditions may appear and require an additional procedure(s) for proper care.

3. My physician has explained the following items:
   • the nature of my condition
   • the nature and purpose of the procedure(s) that I am now authorizing
   • the possible complications and side effects that may result, problems that may be experienced during recuperation, and the likelihood of success
   • the benefits to be reasonably expected from the procedure(s)
   • the likely result of no treatment
   • the available alternatives, including the risks and benefits
   • the other possible risks that accompany any surgical and diagnostic procedure (in addition to those already discussed). I acknowledge that neither my physician nor anyone else involved in my care has made any guarantees or assurances to me as to the result of the procedure(s) that I am now authorizing.

4. I know that other clinical staff may help my physician during the procedure(s).

5. I understand that the procedure(s) may require that I undergo some form of anesthesia, which may have its own risks.

6. Any tissue or specimens taken from my body as a result of the procedure(s) may be examined and disposed of, retained, preserved, or used for medical, scientific, or teaching purposes by the hospital.

7. I understand that my procedure(s) may be photographed or videotaped and that observers may be present in the room for the purpose of advancing medical care and education.

8. I understand that during or after the procedure(s) my physician may find it necessary to give me a transfusion of blood or blood products. My physician has explained the alternatives to, and possible risks of, transfusion.

9. I understand what my physician has explained to me and have had all my questions fully answered.

10. Additional comments: _____

    _____

After talking with my physician and reading this form, I give my consent to the procedure(s) described above.

Signature of Patient or
Legal Representative: _____ Date: _____ Time: _____

If Legal Representative, Relationship to Patient:_____

Witness: _____

Verbal or Telephone Consent

Name of Legal Representative:_____ Date: _____ Time: _____

Relationship to Patient: _____

Witness:_____ Witness: _____

I have explained the risks, benefits, potential complications, and alternatives of the treatment to the patient and have answered all questions to the patient's satisfaction, and he/she has granted consent to proceed.

Physician Signature: _____ Date: _____ Time: _____

INFORMED CONSENT FOR OPERATION
000015 (11/2002)

document their own **preoperative anesthesia evaluations**. The evaluation collects information on the patient's medical history and current physical and emotional condition. The evaluation becomes the basis for an anesthesia plan that stipulates the type of anesthesia to be used; addresses the patient's risk factors, allergies, and drug usage; and considers the patient's general medical condition. (See figures 5.34 and 5.35.)

The professional who is to administer anesthesia to the patient must also perform a reevaluation of the patient's condition immediately before the procedure. The purpose of the reevaluation is to confirm that it is safe to begin the operation. The timing and dosage of any preanesthesia medications should also be documented at this point.

The professional administering anesthesia during the procedure must also maintain an **intraoperative anesthesia record**. The intraoperative record is created while the procedure is being performed. (See figures 5.36 and 5.37.) The record describes the entire surgical process and includes the following information:

- Patient identification, including name and record number

- Name of the anesthesiologist or nurse-anesthetist

- Type and amount of anesthesia administered

- Induction mechanisms

- Medication log, including medical gases and fluid administration

- Usage of blood products

- Placement of lines and monitoring devices

- Patient's reaction to anesthesia

- Results of continuous patient monitoring, including vital signs and oxygen saturation levels

The **postoperative anesthesia record** contains information on any unusual events or complications that occurred during surgery. The postoperative anesthesia record also documents the patient's condition at the conclusion of surgery and after recovery from anesthesia. (See figures 5.38 and 5.39.)

Transfusion Records

Surgical and emergency patients sometimes require transfusions of whole blood and/or blood products. Blood transfusions carry an inherent risk for complications. Except in emergency situations, the patient's physician should discuss the relative risks and benefits with the patient and/or the patient's family before the procedure is performed. This discussion and patient consent must be documented in the patient's health record.

A **transfusion record** includes information on the type and amount of blood products the patient received, the source of the blood products, and the patient's reaction to the transfusion. The record also documents the blood group and Rh status of the patient and the donor, the results of cross-matching tests, and a description of the transfusion process. Every adverse reaction to a transfusion must be fully documented in the patient's health record.

Occasionally, hospitals receive information from area blood banks that a specific batch of blood products may have been contaminated with disease-causing organisms. In such cases, the Medicare *Conditions of Participation* (2006) require hospitals to notify the patients who received the tainted blood products and/or their physicians of the potential contamination.

Figure 5.34. Preprocedure record in paper format.

University of Anystate Hospitals

PREPROCEDURE RECORD
PAGE 1 OF 2

PATIENT LABEL

Preprocedure Care (Day of Procedure)

Date: _____ Time: _____
☐ NPO Since: _____ Voided? ☐ Yes ☐ No
Valuables (check if present, put O if removed)?
☐ Clothing ☐ Dentures ☐ Glasses ☐ Contact
☐ Hearing aid ☐ Hair piece/wig ☐ Jewelry Lenses
☐ Other: _____
☐ Patient was informed hospital is not responsible for lost
  valuables
Signature of Person Responsible for Valuables

Disposition if no one is present: _____
☐ Responsible adult available to accompany patient at discharge
☐ TED Hose ☐ SCDs/plexi pulse
☐ Skin prep: _____ By: _____

Medication Given Prior to Procedure:

_____ Time: _____ Initials: ____
_____ Time: _____ Initials: ____
_____ Time: _____ Initials: ____
_____ Time: _____ Initials: ____
_____ Time: _____ Initials: ____
_____ Time: _____ Initials: ____
_____ Time: _____ Initials: ____
Douche/Enema: _____ Time: _____ Initials: ____
☐ IV gauge #: ____ Site: ____ Fluid: ____ Rate: ____ Initials: ____
☐ IV gauge #: ____ Site: ____ Fluid: ____ Rate: ____ Initials: ____

Completed by _____

Operating Room Checklist (initial when completed)
_____ ID Bracelet Correct
_____ Informed Consent
_____ H&P
_____ Operative Plan
_____ Site/Procedure Verified with Schedule/MD Order, Consent, and Patient/Representative
_____ Procedure Site Marked
_____ Procedure and Site Verified with Available Imaging Studies by MD, if Applicable (procedure
      staff)
_____ Patient, Procedure, and Site Verified Verbally Immediately prior to Start by Procedural Team
      (final "time out") (procedure staff)

For Moderate Sedation and Anesthesia Patients:
_____ Preanesthesia Assessment
_____ Anesthesia Plan of Care

Completed by: _____

Diagnostic Studies
(O if ordered, checkmark if on chart)
☐ CBC   ☐ Sed. Rate   ☐ Heme
☐ Chemistry ☐ Urine C&S   ☐ Potassium
☐ PT, PTT   ☐ U/A   ☐ Creatinine
☐ EKG   ☐ X-rays   ☐ T+S
☐ T&C _____ Units Available

☐ Pregnancy ☐ _____

Bedside Glucose: _____

☐ Abnormal Results Called to MD

Completed by: _____

Assessment | Nursing Assessment (Inpatient) Initiated

Alert and Oriented: ☐ Yes ☐ No (see supplemental nurses' notes)
Suspected Abuse: ☐ No ☐ Yes (see supplemental nurses' notes)
Learning Barriers: ☐ No Barriers ☐ Physical ☐ Religious ☐ Cultural ☐ Cognitive ☐ Emotional ☐ Language (see supplemental nurses' notes)
Pain: ☐ No Pain ☐ Yes, Location: _____ ☐ Onset: _____ ☐ Duration: _____ ☐ Intensity: ____ (1–10) Qual/Characteristics/Pattern: _____
  Alleviating Factors: _____ Aggravating Factors: _____ Effects on ADL: _____ Relieved by: _____
Diabetic/Special Diet? ☐ No ☐ Yes (see supplemental nurses' notes)
Recent Mobility Limitation? ☐ No ☐ Yes (see supplemental nurses' notes)

Completed by: _____ **RN**

Plan of Care | Clinical Pathway Initiated

Potential for Fear and/or Anxiety **Goal: Reduction of Fear and Anxiety** ☐ **Goal Met**
☐ Procedures Explained to Patient and Family
☐ Patient and Family Encouraged to Verbalize Concerns and Questions
☐ Patient and Family's Questions Answered
☐ Age-Appropriate Emotional Support Provided
Knowledge Deficit Relating to Procedure **Goal: Demonstrates and/or Verbalizes Knowledge** ☐ **Goal Met**
☐ Patient's Level of Learning Assessed and Instructions Modified to Meet Needs
☐ Reviewed Printed Discharge Instructions with Patient and Family
☐ Cough, Turn, Deep-Breathe
☐ PRN Pain Medications/Pain Scale
☐ Patient/Family Verbalize Understanding of Instructions
☐ Age-Appropriate Approach Used in Education

Initials/Signature:
_____
_____

Potential for Injury
Goal: Patient Is Free from Injury ☐ **Goal Met**
Side Rails Up: ☐ × 2 ☐ × 4   Bed Position: ☐ Low ☐ High
☐ Instructed Patient to Call for Assistance
Potential for Alteration in Fluid Volume
Goal: Fluid Volume Is within Normal Limits ☐ **Goal Met**
☐ IV Access Present, No Infiltration Noted
Privacy/Confidentiality
Goal: Privacy/Confidentiality Maintained ☐ **Goal Met**
☐ Confidentiality of Patient Records, Diagnosis, Procedure Maintained
☐ Patient Minimally Exposed during Preparation
Potential Alteration in Cardiovascular Function
Goal: Hemodynamically Stable ☐ **Goal Met**
☐ Continuous Cardiac Monitoring ☐ Continuous Heart Rate Monitoring
Potential Alteration in Gas Exchange
Goal: Adequate Air Exchange ☐ **Goal Met**
☐ Continuous Pulse Oximetry in Use ☐ Oxygen Therapy Initiated as Ordered

Initials/Signature:
_____
_____

PREPROCEDURE RECORD
000019 (11/2002)

Figure 5.34. (continued)

University of Anystate Hospitals

PREPROCEDURE RECORD
PAGE 2 OF 2

> PATIENT LABEL

Pediatrics (Neonate through 17 Years of Age)

☐ Grade in School _____   Feeding   ☐ Breast   ☐ Bottle/Formula   ☐ Solids
☐ Developmental Milestones Appropriate for Age   Type of Formula _____
    ☐ Yes   ☐ No
☐ Security Object/Toys _____   Primary Caregiver _____
☐ Immunizations Current   ☐ Yes   ☐ No
Signature: _____

Interaction between Caregiver and Child _____   Head Circumference _____
☐ Calming   ☐ Agitative   (infants under 1 year of age only)
Signature: _____

Further Assessment

Cardiac Rhythm:

Preprocedure Peripheral Pulses (Absent, 1+, 2+, 3+, 4+, Doppler)
R DP: _____ L DP: _____ R PT: _____ L PT: _____ R Rad.:_____ L Rad.: _____ Other: _____

Other: _____
Signature: _____
Supplemental Nurses' Notes: _____
_____
_____
_____

Preprocedure Preparation

Type of Procedure: _____ Date Called: _____ Time Called: _____
Date of Procedure: _____ Time of Procedure: _____ Arrival Time: _____
Instructions Given To: _____
Via: ☐ Phone   ☐ Appointment   ☐ Left Phone Message   ☐ Unable to Reach
☐ No Makeup, Jewelry, Perfume, Nail Polish, or Valuables   ☐ Medications A.M. of Procedure with a Sip of Water
☐ NPO Status/Time _____   _____
☐ Instructions for: _____
_____   ☐ Bring Medications/Inhalers/List to Hospital
_____   ☐ Preadmission Diagnostic Tests Done:
_____   Date: _____ Location: _____
_____   ☐ Date/Location Previous CXR: _____
_____   ☐ Date/Location Previous EKG: _____
☐ Informed that responsible adult must accompany patient to hospital, transport home, and remain with patient after the procedure
Name of Responsible Person after Procedure: _____
Signature: _____ RN/LPN

PREPROCEDURE RECORD
000019 (11/2002)

Figure 5.35. Preoperative checklist.

University of Anystate Hospitals

PREOPERATIVE CHECKLIST

> PATIENT LABEL

(It is the responsibility of the unit nurse to see that this is completed before the patient goes to the operating room.)

Vital Signs Taken prior to Transfer

Date:	Time:	BP:	T:	P:	R:	O₂Sat:	Weight:	Height:

	Yes	No	Initials		Yes	No	Initials		Yes	No	Initials
Side Rails Raised?	☐	☐	_____	Instructed Not to Smoke?	☐	☐	_____	Instructed to Stay in Bed?	☐	☐	_____

	Yes	No	N/A	Initials	
Dentures Removed?	☐	☐	☐	____	**Prep Site:** _____
Contact Lens Removed?	☐	☐	☐	____	By Whom: _____ Checked By: _____
Jewelry Removed?	☐	☐	☐	____	**NPO Since:** _____ a.m./p.m.
Jewelry Disposition _____	☐	☐	☐	____	**Voided:** _____ cc Catheter: _____ cc
Hair Piece, Pins, Clamps Removed?	☐	☐	☐	____	**Bedside Glucose:** _____ Time: _____
Hearing Aid(s) Removed?	☐	☐	☐	____	
Hospital Gown?	☐	☐		____	
ID Name Band on Patient?	☐	☐		____	
Fenwal ID Band on Patient?	☐	☐	☐	____	

If Ordered to Operating Room with Patient

	Yes	No	N/A	Initials		Yes	No	N/A	Initials
X-rays?	☐	☐	☐	____	Meds?	☐	☐	☐	_____
Old Charts?	☐	☐	☐	____					_____
SCDs/TEDs	☐	☐	☐	____					_____

On Chart

		Initials
Site/procedure verified with schedule/MD order, consent, and patient/representative		____
Procedure site marked		____

	Yes	No	Initials
Informed Consent?	☐	☐	____
History and Physical?	☐	☐	____
Operative Plan?	☐	☐	____
Patient Labels?	☐	☐	____
MARS?	☐	☐	____
Clinical Pathway, if applicable?	☐	☐	____

OR/Procedure Staff Use Only

	Initials
Procedure and site verified with available imaging studies by MD, if applicable	____
Patient, procedure, and site verified verbally immediately prior to start by procedural team (final "time out")	____
Preanesthesia/moderate sedation assessment completed	____
Anesthesia/moderate sedation plan completed	____

Results on Chart: Preop Diagnostics

	Yes	No	N/A	Initials		Yes	No	N/A	Initials
T&C/T+S ____ Units available	☐	☐	☐	____	EKG	☐	☐	☐	____
CBC	☐	☐	☐	____	X-ray reports	☐	☐	☐	____
Chemistry	☐	☐	☐	____	PT/PTT	☐	☐	☐	____
Urinalysis	☐	☐	☐	____	Physician notified of abnormal results?	☐	☐	☐	____

Preop Medications/IV Therapy

☐ IV gauge # _____ Site _____ Fluid _____ Rate _____ Initials _____

☐ IV gauge # _____ Site _____ Fluid _____ Rate _____ Initials _____

Preop Meds	**Time Given/Initials**
_____	_____
_____	_____

Plan of Care

Privacy/Confidentiality Goal: Privacy/Confidentiality Maintained	☐ Goal Met
☐ Patient Minimally Exposed during Preparation	

Potential for Fear and/or Anxiety Goal: Reduction of Fear and Anxiety	☐ Goal Met
☐ Procedures Explained to Patient and Family	
☐ Patient and Family Encouraged to Verbalize Concerns and Questions	
☐ Patient and Family's Questions Answered	
☐ Age-Appropriate Emotional Support Provided	

Knowledge Deficit Relating to Procedure Goal: Demonstrates and/or Verbalizes Knowledge	☐ Goal Met
☐ PEARLS for Progress Reviewed with Patient	
☐ Cough, Turn, Deep Breath	
☐ PRN Pain Medications/Pain Scale	
☐ Patient/Family Verbalize Understanding of Instructions	
☐ Age-Appropriate Approach Used in Education	

_____ Initials _____

_____ Initials _____

Clinical Pathway Initiated

Potential for Alteration in Fluid Volume Goal: Fluid Volume Is within Normal Limits	☐ Goal Met
☐ IV Access Present, No Infiltration Noted	

Potential for Injury Goal: Patient Is Free From Injury	☐ Goal Met

Bed Position: ☐ Low ☐ High

Side Rails Up ☐ × 2 ☐ × 4

☐ Instructed to Call for Assistance

Location of Family during Surgery _____

Report Called: Yes ☐ No ☐ N/A ☐ Called to: _____

Miscellaneous Information: _____

Signature of Nurse Transferring Patient to Operating Room

_____ Initials _____

_____ Initials _____

PREOPERATIVE CHECKLIST
000018 (11/2002)

Figure 5.36. Intraoperative anesthesia record in paper format.

University of Anystate Hospitals

INTRAOPERATIVE RECORD

PATIENT LABEL

OR #: _____ ☐ SDA ☐ Outpatient   ☐ **Preoperative Assessment Reviewed**
Date: _____ ☐ Inpatient ☐ Add-On (day of surgery)   ☐ Agree with Assessment   ☐ **Patient Confirms Surgical Site**
                                               ☐ See Additional Notes   ☐ Yes
                                                                           ☐ See Additional Notes

Allergies: _____

Preprocedure Diagnosis: _____

Postprocedure Diagnosis: _____

Procedure Performed: _____

Times: Room In/Room Out_____ / _____   **Transferred to/Discharge:** ☐ PACU ☐ ICU ☐ Room # _____ ☐ Home
Anesthesia Start _____ / _____   Method of Transfer: ☐ Stretcher ☐ Bed ☐ Other: _____ ☐ Report Called: _____
Procedure Start/Stop _____ / _____   Condition on Discharge: ☐ Satisfactory ☐ Other _____

Anesthesia:	**Personnel Role:**
☐ General	MD: _____ _____
☐ MAC	Circ.: _____ Relief: _____ Time: _____
☐ Regional	Scrub: _____
☐ Epidural	Anes.: _____ Relief: _____ _____
☐ Spinal	Other: _____ Rad. Tech.: _____
☐ Axillary Block	Role: _____ Perfusionist: _____
☐ Bier Block	
☐ IV Sedation	
☐ Local	
☐ Other: _____	

☐ **Potential for Fear and Anxiety**   **Goal: Reduction of Fear and Anxiety**

☐ Perioperative Events Explained   ☐ Goal Met
☐ Intraop Family Communication   Time: _____

☐ **Potential for Injury**   **Goal: Patient Free From Injury**

Intraop Position: ☐ Goal Met

☐ Supine	Safety Strap =
☐ Prone	Arm Position →
☐ Lithotomy	ESU Pad ∅
☐ Lateral R	Padding #
☐ Lateral L	Pulse Oximeter ☐
☐ Jackknife	EKG ●
☐ Beach Chair	BP Cuff **X**
☐ Other: _____	

Positional Aids: ☐ None   **Equipment:** ☐ None

☐ Donut	☐ ESU #: _____ PAD #: _____
☐ Pillow	Coagulation: _____ Cut: _____
☐ Eggcrate Pad	Post Op Site: _____
☐ Bean Bag	☐ Bipolar #: _____
☐ Lami Rolls	Setting: _____
☐ Chest Roll	☐ C-Arm/OEC
☐ Axilla Roll	☐ Phaco #: _____
☐ Shoulder Roll	☐ Cryo #: _____
☐ Sand Bag	☐ Laser #: _____
☐ Stirrups	☐ Ultrasound #: _____
☐ Candy Cane	☐ CUSA #: _____
☐ Bierhoff	☐ Bair Hugger #: _____
☐ Allen	☐ Seq. Comp. Mach. #: _____
☐ Knee Holder	Settings _____
☐ Mayfield Headrest	☐ Tourniquet #:_____
☐ Lami-Frame	☐ Arm ☐ Leg ☐ R ☐ L
☐ Shoulder Holder	Applied by: _____
☐ Beach Chair Attachment	Pressure:_____mm Hg
☐ Fracture Table	Time Up: _____
☐ Surgita Headrest	Time Down: _____
☐ Other: _____	

Final Counts:
☐ Correct   ☐ Incorrect

Circ. Signature: _____

☐ **Patient Privacy**   **Goal: Privacy Maintained**

☐ Patient Minimally Exposed during Positioning, Prepping, and Draping

☐ **Potential for Infection**   **Goal: Sterile Technique Maintained**

Skin Preparation: ☐ None   **Prep:**   ☐ Goal Met
☐ Shave _____   ☐ Iodophor Prep
☐ Clip _____   ☐ Iodophor Scrub
                                ☐ Iodophor Gel
                                ☐ Dura-Prep
Skin Condition: ☐ Other: _____
Before Surgery: ☐ Normal ☐ Other:_____
After Surgery: ☐ Normal ☐ Other: _____

Cultures: ☐ None   **Wound Class:**
☐ Aerobic—Site: _____   ☐ I
☐ Anaerobic—Site: _____   ☐ II
☐ AFB—Site: _____   ☐ III
☐ Fungus—Site: _____   ☐ IV

Lines/Drains: ☐ None   **Dressings:** ☐ Yes ☐ No
☐ JP/Hemovac/Blake   _____
☐ Chest Tube
☐ Foley   ☐ Splint _____
☐ Arterial   ☐ Cast _____
☐ CVP/Swanz   ☐ Other: _____
☐ NG Tube   ☐ **Packing:** ☐ Yes ☐ No
☐ Other: _____

☐   **Miscellaneous**

Meds: _____   Irrigation Type: _____
        _____   ☐ Heparin Amount: _____
        _____   ☐ NS Amount: _____
                              ☐ LR Amount: _____
Blood Products: ☐ None   ☐ Triple Amount: _____
☐ PRC _____Units   ☐ H_2O Amount: _____
☐ FFP _____Units   ☐ Glycerin Amount: _____
☐ Cryo _____Units   ☐ Other: _____
☐ Cell Saver _____   CCs Infused:_____
Specimens: ☐ None
☐ Gross Only—Site: _____
☐ Frozen—Site: _____
☐ Fresh—Site: _____
☐ Routine—Site: _____

INTRAOPERATIVE RECORD
000020 (11/2002)

Figure 5.37. **Intraoperative vital signs documentation in graphic format.**

University of Anystate Hospitals

ANESTHESIA RECORD
PAGE 1 OF 2

PATIENT LABEL

Date: _____ Time: _____
Age: ____ Sex: ____ Height: ____ Weight: ____ BP: ____ P: ____ R: ____ T: _____
Lab: _____ Status: _____
Allergies: _____ Last Intake: _____
Premedication: _____

☐ **Patient reassessed immediately prior to induction. Condition satisfactory for planned anesthesia.**

Vital Signs

Time		

Machine Check

Initials

Patient Position

☐ General
☐ Regional
☐ Local
☐ Monitored
☐ IVs (spinal/EPI needle)

Position

Prep

Site

Agent

Paresthesia

Catheter

Sensory Block TO

☐ Heat/Moisture Exchanger
☐ Warming Blanket
☐ Fluid Warmer
☐ Bair Hugger

Endotracheal Tube

Cuff Inflated

Laryngoscope Blade

Stylet

Direct Vision

Blind

Systolic
∨
Diastolic
∧
Pulse
∿
Respiration
○
Spon
●
Assist
☉
Controlled

Surgery
Start/
End
⊗

Anesthesia
Start/End
×

Anesthesia
Start
_____

Anesthesia
End
_____

240
220
200

180

160

140

120

100

80

60

40

20
15
10
5

Figure 5.37. **(continued)**

University of Anystate Hospitals

ANESTHESIA RECORD
PAGE 2 OF 2

PATIENT LABEL

Monitors
- ☐ NIBP ☐ R ☐ L
- ☐ APB ☐ R ☐ L
- ☐ T (site): _____
- ☐ Pulse oximeter (site): _____
- ☐ ECG (lead): _____
- ☐ Airway gas monitor
- ☐ FiO_2 analyzer
- ☐ Pulmonary artery
- ☐ CVP
- ☐ EEG
- ☐ Stethoscope (site): _____
- ☐ SSEP
- ☐ Peripheral nerve stimulator
- ☐ Capnography

Remarks
_____
_____
_____
_____
_____
_____
_____
_____
_____

Fluid		Fluid		Fluid		Fluid		Fluid		Fluid	
Start	Finish	Start	Finish	Start	Finish	Start	Finish	Start	Finish	Start	Finish

Operation	Recovery Room Time: _____
	BP
	P T °F Endotracheal
Surgeon Anesthesiologist Date	In ☐ Out ☐
	Condition SpO_2 %

Preanesthesia Evaluation

Review of Clinical Data

- ☐ Yes ☐ No Patient Medical History Reviewed
- ☐ Yes ☐ No Current Medications Reviewed
- ☐ Yes ☐ No Allergies Reviewed
- ☐ Yes ☐ No ☐ N/A Lab Results Reviewed
- ☐ Yes ☐ No ☐ N/A CXR Results Reviewed
- ☐ Yes ☐ No ☐ N/A EKG Results Reviewed

Pertinent Physical Exam

	Normal	Abnormal	Comments
EENT			
Respiratory			
Cardiac			
Mental Status			

Anesthesia History

- ☐ Yes ☐ No Past Hx of Anesthesia Complications
- ☐ Yes ☐ No Family Hx of Anesthesia Complications
- ☐ Yes ☐ No History of Malignant Hyperthermia

ASA Classification

1   2   3   4   5   E

Airway Evaluation

Dentures:	☐ None ☐ Upper ☐ Lower
Capped Teeth:	☐ None ☐ Yes
Condition of Teeth:	☐ Good ☐ Fair ☐ Poor

Estimated Intubation Difficulty:

☐ Normal ☐ Moderately Difficult ☐ Difficult

Anesthesia Plan

- ☐ General
- ☐ Spinal
- ☐ Epidural
- ☐ Regional Block
- ☐ Rapid Sequence Intubation
- ☐ MAC
- ☐ Epidural for POPM

☐ Alternatives, risks of anesthesia, and potential complications were discussed. Patient and/or guardian state understanding and acceptance of anesthesia plan.

Comments:

_____   _____
Anesthesiologist   Date

ANESTHESIA RECORD
000017 (11/2002)

Figure 5.38. Postoperative anesthesia record in paper format.

Midwest Medical Center

POSTANESTHESIA RECORD
PAGE 1 OF 2

PATIENT LABEL

Date: _____
PACU Admission Time: _____ a.m./p.m.   Anesthesia End Time: _____ a.m./p.m.
Procedure: _____
Surgeon: _____   Anesthetist: _____
Anesthesia: ☐ General ☐ Regional ☐ Local Only ☐ Spinal ☐ Epidural ☐ Local w/Sedation
☐ Chart Orders Checked   Allergies: _____
Admitting Nurse(s): _____

Assessment	Plan of Care/Interventions

Assessment

LOC: ☐ Drowsy ☐ Alert   ☐ Oriented ☐ Sleeping while undisturbed
Respiratory Quality: ☐ Deep   ☐ Shallow ☐ Labored
Circulatory: ☐ Pink   ☐ Warm   ☐ Cool   ☐ Mottled
Circulation Check: ☐ N/A   ☐ Pink   ☐ Warm   ☐ Cool ☐ Mottled
Operative: ☐ Pulse Palpable ☐ Unable to Palpate Due to Dressing
Extremity: ☐ Capillary Refill Adequate ☐ Other (see notes)
Dressing/Operative Site: _____ ☐ Dry and Intact ☐ Other (see notes)
IV Therapy: Fluid: _____ Site: _____ Amt.: _____ cc
☐ Patent, No Redness or Edema Noted ☐ Other (see notes)
Level of Pain: _____ Init. _____

Vital Signs

Time	BP	Pulse	Resp.	Pain Level	Time	BP	Pulse	Resp.	Pain Level

Dressing Check: ☐ Time: ☐ Dry and Intact ☐ Other (see supplemental notes)
☐ Time: ☐ Dry and Intact ☐ Other (see supplemental notes)

Medications

Medicine	Dosage	Route	Time Given	Initials

PACU Scoring

Time						
Activity						
R						
Circulation						
LOC						
Skin T						
Total						

Discharge Evaluation

☐ Vital Signs at Preoperative Level
☐ Meets PACU Score of 10 OR ☐ Return of Preoperative Level
☐ Minimal or No Pain
☐ Minimal or No Nausea
☐ Dressing Dry and Intact
☐ Ambulates with Minimal Assistance
☐ Responsible Adult Present to Accompany Patient Home
Initials: _____ Signature: _____
Initials: _____ Signature: _____
Initials: _____ Signature: _____

Plan of Care/Interventions

Potential Alteration in Mental Status   **Goal: Return to Pre-Op Status**
☐ Reoriented to time and place   ☐ Goal Met
☐ Other: _____

Potential for Fear and/or Anxiety   **Goal: Reduction of Fear and Anxiety**
☐ Oriented to Environment   ☐ Goal Met
☐ Encouraged to Verbalize Concerns
☐ Age-Appropriate Emotional Support Provided
☐ Family at Bedside
☐ Patients and/or Family's Questions Answered
☐ Other: _____

Potential Alteration in Comfort   **Goal: Decrease Level of Pain**
☐ Patient Repositioned for Comfort   ☐ Goal Met
☐ Pain Scale Used According to Verbal Communication Level
☐ Medication Given as Ordered
☐ Other: _____

Potential for Injury   **Goal: Create a Safe Environment**
☐ Siderails Elevated   ☐ Goal Met
☐ Ambulated with Assistance
☐ Family at Bedside
☐ Other: _____

Potential Alteration in Fluid Volume   **Goal: Adequate I/O**
☐ PO Fluids Given ☐ IV Discontinued ☐ Voided   ☐ Goal Met
☐ Antiemetic Medication Administered
☐ Other: _____

Knowledge Deficit/Potential for Postop Complications at Home   **Goal: Exhibits Knowledge of Postop Care**
☐ Need for Home Care Assistance Assessed   ☐ Goal Met
Assistance Needed:
☐ No ☐ Yes If Yes: ☐ Physician ☐ Case Management Notified
☐ Written Discharge Instructions Given
☐ Prescriptions Given to Patient/Family
☐ Other: _____

Other Problems/Needs
_____
_____
_____

Discharge to	Phase II Recovery

Discharge _____ MD
Discharge to ☐ Home ☐ Room #: _____ Postop Contact #: _____
Discharged @: _____ Via ☐ Wheelchair ☐ Ambulance ☐ Stretcher
☐ Other _____
RN Signature: _____

Figure 5.38.   (continued)

Midwest Medical Center

POSTANESTHESIA RECORD
PAGE 2 OF 2

PATIENT LABEL

PACU Scoring Guide

Activity
2 = Able to move 4 extremities
1 = Able to move 2 extremities
0 = Able to move 0 extremities

Respirations
2 = Clear, unsupported
    (strong cry, if pediatric)
1 = Obstructed, supported
    (spontaneous respiration may
    be shallow or slow)
0 = Apneic/mechanical ventilation/
    Ambu

Circulation
(adults and children)
2 = BP ± 20 of preanesthesia level
1 = BP ± 20-50 of preanesthesia
    level
0 = BP ± 50 or more of
    preanesthesia level

Infants
2 = Radial pulse easy to palpate
1 = Axillary pulse palpable, radial
    pulse weak
0 = Carotid is only palpable pulse

Consciousness
2 = Awake—Oriented to time
    and place (preop level)
1 = Drowsy—Able to be aroused
    on name calling or gentle
    stimuli
0 = Unresponsive

Skin Temperature
2 = Warm, dry, pink
1 = Warm, dry, pale
0 = Cool, clammy, mottled

Supplemental Nursing Notes

Postprocedure Followup

Date: _____ Time: _____

☐ Patient Contacted   ☐ No Answer   ☐ Answering Machine

Dressing: ☐ Dry and Intact   ☐ Drainage Present (see comments)
            ☐ Redness Present (see comments)

Comfort: ☐ No Discomfort   ☐ Mild Discomfort
            ☐ Moderate   ☐ Severe Discomfort
              Discomfort   (any discomfort, see comments)

N/V: ☐ None   ☐ Minimal   ☐ Moderate   ☐ Severe

Fever: ☐ No   ☐ Yes:_____°F

Instructions: ☐ Easily Understood   ☐ Further Instructions Needed
                                       (see comments)

Comments: _____

Signature: _____

POSTANESTHESIA RECORD
000024 (11/2002)

Figure 5.39. Postoperative record in paper format.

University of Anystate Hospitals

POSTOPERATIVE RECORD
PAGE 1 OF 2

PATIENT LABEL

Type of Procedure: _____ Date: _____ Time Arrive on Unit: _____
Arrived Via: ☐ Bed ☐ Stretcher ☐ Wheelchair

Postprocedure Assessment

Level of Consciousness	☐ Alert ☐ Drowsy	☐ Responds to Painful/Verbal Stimuli ☐ Unresponsive

IV Therapy
#1 Fluid: _____ Site: _____ Rate: _____
☐ No Redness or Swelling at Site ☐ Other: _____
#2 Fluid: _____ Site: _____ Rate: _____
☐ No Redness or Swelling at Site ☐ Other: _____
#3 Fluid: _____ Site: _____ Rate: _____
☐ No Redness or Swelling at Site ☐ Other: _____

Oxygen ☐ Room Air ☐ Nasal Cannula ☐ Other @ _____ liter/min

Respiratory Quality ☐ Regular ☐ Irregular ☐ Other

Breath Sounds ☐ Clear all Fields ☐ Other: _____

Cardiac ☐ Regular ☐ Irregular ☐ Dysrhythmia

GI ☐ N/A ☐ Hypo Bowel Sound ☐ Hyper Bowel Sound ☐ Absent Bowel Sound
☐ Firm ☐ Distended ☐ Tender ☐ Protuberant

Skin Color ☐ Pink ☐ Pale ☐ Mottled ☐ Cyanotic

Skin Condition ☐ Warm ☐ Dry ☐ Cold ☐ Clammy

Circ. √ Distal to Site ☐ N/A ☐ Warm ☐ Pink
☐ Cyanotic ☐ Mottled ☐ Cool

Peripheral Pulses (absent, +1, +2, +3, +4, Doppler) _____ N/A
_____ R Rad _____ R DP _____ R PT _____ Other
_____ L Rad _____ L DP _____ L PT

Dressing/Operative Site:_____ ☐ Dry and Intact
Dressing/Operative Site:_____ ☐ Dry and Intact
RN Signature: _____

Drainage Tubes: ☐ N/A
Type: _____ ☐ Patency Checked Drainage: _____
Type: _____ ☐ Patency Checked Drainage: _____
Type: _____ ☐ Patency Checked Drainage: _____

Puncture Site: ☐ N/A
Location: _____
Sand Bag Intact: ☐ Yes ☐ No   Bleeding: ☐ Yes ☐ No
Hematoma: ☐ Yes ☐ No   Sheath Sutured: ☐ Yes ☐ No ☐ N/A

Sheath Removal Date: _____ Time: _____ Initials: _____
Assessment Unchanged from Postprocedure ☐ Yes ☐ See Notes
Verbalizes Understanding of Sheath Removal ☐ Yes ☐ See Notes

Site Check Post Sheath Removal
Sandbag Intact	☐ Yes	☐ No
Hematoma	☐ Yes	☐ See Notes
Pain	☐ Yes	☐ See Notes
Loss of Distal Pulse	☐ Yes	☐ See Notes
Compression Device in Use	☐ Yes	☐ See Notes
Uncontrolled Bleeding	☐ Yes	☐ See Notes
Vasovagal Reaction	☐ Yes	☐ See Notes

Plan of Care   Clinical Pathway Continued

☐ **Potential for Alteration and Ventilation**
Goal: Adequate Air Exchange ☐ Goal Met
☐ Continuous Pulse Oximetry in Use
☐ Coughing and Deep Breathing Encouraged
☐ O₂ Therapy Initiated as Ordered
☐ Incentive Spirometry Initiated as Ordered
☐ Other: _____

☐ **Potential Alteration Cardiovascular Function**
Goal: Hemodynamically Stable ☐ Goal Met
☐ Continuous Cardiac Monitoring in Use
☐ Other: _____

☐ **Potential Alteration in Mental Status**
Goal: Return to Preop Status ☐ Goal Met
☐ Reoriented to Time and Place
☐ Other: _____

☐ **Potential for Fear and/or Anxiety**
Goal: Reduction of Fear and Anxiety ☐ Goal Met
☐ Oriented to Environment
☐ Encouraged to Verbalize Concerns
☐ Age-Appropriate Emotional Support Provided
☐ Family at Bedside
☐ Patients/Families Questions Answered
☐ Other: _____

☐ **Potential for Injury**
Goal: Create a Safe Environment ☐ Goal Met
☐ Side Rails Raised
☐ Ambulated with Assistance
☐ Family at Bedside
☐ Call Bell within Reach
☐ Bed in Low Position
☐ Other: _____

☐ **Knowledge Deficit/Potential for Postprocedure Complications at Home**
Goal: Exhibits Knowledge of Postprocedure Care ☐ Goal Met
☐ Need for Home Care Assistance Assessed
☐ If Assistance Needed, Notify: ☐ Physician ☐ Case Manager
☐ Written Discharge Instructions Reinforced. Copy to Patient.
☐ Prescription Given to Patient/Family with Instructions on Usage
☐ Explained Procedure for Transferring to Inpatient Unit
☐ Other:_____

☐ **Potential Alteration in Fluid Volume**
Goal: Adequate I/O ☐ Goal Met
☐ IV Hydration Initiated
☐ Antiemetic Medication Administered
☐ PO Fluids Given without Nausea/Vomiting
☐ Other:_____

☐ **Potential Alteration in Comfort**
Goal: Decrease Level of Pain ☐ Goal Met
☐ Patient Repositioned for Comfort
☐ Pain Level (0–10)
☐ Wong-Baker Face Scale for Pediatrics—Face Score: _____
☐ Reevaluation of Pain after Medication—Level of Pain: _____
☐ Medication Given as Ordered
☐ Other: _____

☐ **Other Problems/Needs** ☐ Goal Met
_____
_____
_____

RN Signature: _____ Date: _____

Figure 5.39. (continued)

University of Anystate Hospitals

POSTOPERATIVE RECORD
PAGE 2 OF 2

PATIENT LABEL

Postprocedure Record (page 2)

IV Site	Date	7–3	3–11	11–7	Date	7–3	3–11	11–7

Date: _____

0 NO HURT	2 HURTS LITTLE BIT	4 HURTS LITTLE MORE	6 HURTS EVEN MORE	8 HURTS WHOLE LOT	10 HURTS WORST

Pain Management (scale 0–10 for adults—Wong/Baker Faces for Pediatrics)

Time	Pain Scale	Medication/Dose	Initials	Response/Pain Scale	Time	Initials

Vital Sign Postprocedure/Sheath Removal

Time	LOC	T	BP	P	RR/O$_2$ Sat.	Pain Level	Peripheral Pulse	Site Check	Initials

Daily Care Record

Shift: Date	7–3	3–11	11–7	7–3	3–11	11–7
Bedrest						
Ambulating						
R or L Leg Straight						
SCD						
Antiembolism Hose						
PCA Pump						
Traction						
Telemetry						
Type of Diet						
Amount Eaten						
Bath/Shower/Bed						
Complete—Self/Assist.						
Oral Care/P.M. Care						
Other:						

Level of Consciousness (LOC) Scale

2 = Awake—Oriented to Preop Time and Place

1 = Drowsy—Able to Arouse with Name Calling or Gentle Stimuli

0 = Unresponsive—Unable to Arouse Except with Painful Stimuli

Date/Time	Notes:

Initials	Signature	Initials	Signature	Initials	Signature

POSTOPERATIVE RECORD
000022(11/2002)

Postoperative Progress Notes

The surgeon primarily responsible for the case must write a brief postoperative progress note in the patient's record immediately after surgery and before the patient leaves the operative suite. The purpose of the note is to communicate postoperative-care instructions to recovery room nurses. The note should also indicate the presence or absence of anesthesia-related complications or other postoperative abnormalities in addition to the patient's vital signs and general condition at the conclusion of the operation. Surgeons may also document postoperative orders in progress notes. (See figures 5.40 and 5.41.) In the absence of, or delay in obtaining, a dictated operative note, the postoperative progress note should serve as the communication between the surgeon and other care providers.

Recovery Room Records

Postsurgery patients are monitored in a dedicated recovery room until the effects of the anesthesia are completely reversed. Recovery room nurses monitor postsurgery patients very carefully until the patients are well enough to be moved to surgical intensive care or their regular rooms. (See figure 5.42.) Same-day surgery patients receive the same level of care and observation as inpatients do until they are ready to leave the hospital.

Most hospitals have developed a **recovery room record** form that is used by nursing staff to document the patient's reaction to anesthesia and condition after surgery. Information on the patient's level of consciousness, overall medical condition, vital signs, and medications and intravenous fluids is documented by nurses when the patient enters the recovery room. The same information is documented when the patient is ready to be transferred or discharged. The status of any surgical dressings, catheters, tubes, and drains is also recorded.

The patient's surgical record should also include documentation that demonstrates that the patient met the facility's discharge criteria before being discharged or transferred. The name of the physician or surgeon who was responsible for the discharge must be included on the discharge order.

Operative Reports

Surgical procedures involve substantial medical, legal, and financial risks for patients, surgeons, and hospitals. For this reason, it is especially important that surgical documentation be complete, accurate, and timely. In addition to anesthesia and recovery room records, an operative report must be prepared for every surgical procedure performed outside the patient's room.

An **operative report** is a formal document prepared by the principal surgeon to describe the surgical procedure(s) performed for the patient. (See figures 5.43 and 5.44.) Each report includes the following information:

- Patient identification, including name and record number

- Patient's preoperative and postoperative diagnoses and indications for surgery

- Descriptions of the procedures performed

- Descriptions of all normal and abnormal findings

- Descriptions of any specimens removed

- Descriptions of the patient's medical condition before, during, and after the operation

- Estimated blood loss

- Descriptions of any unique or unusual events that occurred during the course of the surgery

- Names of the surgeons and their assistants

- Date and duration of the surgery

- Signature of principal physician, credentials, and date the report was written

Figure 5.40. Postoperative progress note in paper format.

Midwest Medical Center

POSTOPERATIVE PROGRESS NOTE

PATIENT LABEL

Procedure(s) Performed:

Name of Primary Surgeon:

Assistant(s):

Findings:

Technical Procedures Used:

Specimens Removed:

Estimated Blood Loss:

Postoperative Diagnosis:

Physician Signature: _____ Date: _____

POSTOPERATIVE PROGRESS NOTE
000025 (11/2002)

Figure 5.41. Postoperative orders in paper format.

Midwest Medical Center

POSTOPERATIVE ORDERS

PATIENT LABEL

Date: _____

Postoperative Diagnosis: _____

Operation: _____

Orders: _____ Allergies: _____

Date/Time	RN Signature	Postop Orders Begin Here
		1. Position of Patient
		2. Ambulate
		3. Leg Exercises
		4. Medication for Pain
		5. Medication for Nausea
		6. Medication for Sleep
		7. Other Medications—Include Previous Orders to Be Continued
		8. Antibiotic
		9. Oral Intake
		10. IV Fluids (include blood)
		11. Tubes to Be Connected
		A. Nasogastric
		B. T Tube
		C. Thoracotomy
		D. Foley
		E. Other
		12. Catheterize
		13. Care of Dressing
		14. Drains
		15. Respiratory Care
		16. IPPB Freq. Duration Pressure Drug
		17. Vital Signs
		18. Intake and Output
		19. Lab Studies
		20. Other:

RN Signature: _____ Date: _____

Physician Signature: _____ Date: _____

POSTOPERATIVE ORDERS
000026 (11/2002)

Figure 5.42.   Postanesthesia nursing record in paper format.

University of Anystate Hospitals

POSTANESTHESIA NURSING RECORD
PAGE 1 OF 4

PATIENT LABEL

Procedure: _____   Date: _____

Surgeon: _____ Anesthetist: _____
Anesthesia: ☐ General   ☐ Regional   ☐ Local Only   ☐ Epidural   ☐ Local w/Sedation
☐ Chart Orders Checked   Allergies: _____

PACU Admission Time: _____ a.m./p.m.

Anesthesia End Time: _____ a.m./p.m.

Phase I Assessment

Arrived Via:	☐ Stretcher	☐ Bed	☐ Infant Carried by Anesthetist	☐ Crib
LOC:	☐ Drowsy	☐ Reacting	☐ Alert ☐ Disoriented	☐ Unresponsive

Circulatory:
  Skin: ☐ Pink   ☐ Warm   ☐ Cool   ☐ Mottled   ☐ Cyanotic
  Extremities: ☐ Pink   ☐ Warm   ☐ Cool   ☐ Mottled   ☐ Cyanotic   ☐ SCD _____
Airway Support: ☐ None   ☐ Oral   ☐ Nasal   ☐ Chin Lift   ☐ Jaw Thrust   ☐ ET Tube   ☐ Tracheostomy
Oxygen Ventilation: ☐ None   ☐ 40%   ☐ _____%   ☐ Mask   ☐ Cannula   ☐ T-Bar   ☐ LMA
                     ☐ Adequate Exchange   ☐ Ambu   ☐ Ventilator   ☐ Other   ☐ Tent
Respiratory Quality: ☐ Deep   ☐ Shallow   ☐ Snoring   ☐ Stridor   ☐ Labored   ☐ Tachypnea
                     ☐ Regular   ☐ Irregular
Breath Sounds: ☐ Clear All Fields   ☐ Equal Bilat.   ☐ Rates   ☐ Rhonchi   ☐ Wheezing   ☐ Other
Cardiac: ☐ Regular Rhythm: _____   ☐ Irregular Rhythm:_____
Abdomen: ☐ Soft   ☐ Firm   ☐ Distended

Dressing/Operative Site: _____ ☐ Dry and Intact   ☐ Other: _____
              ☐ Peripad   ☐ Dry and Intact   ☐ Other: _____
              ☐ Cast   ☐ Dry and Intact   ☐ Damp   ☐ Other: _____
              ☐ Epidural   ☐ Dry and Intact   ☐ Other: _____
              ☐ Packing   Site: _____
Drains: ☐ None   ☐ CBI Fluid: _____ Amt. on Admisssion: _____ ☐ Other: _____
☐ Foley Cath.   ☐ Suprapubic   ☐ Patent   Color of Drainage: _____   ☐ JP   Site: _____   ☐ Patent   Color of Drainage: _____
☐ Hemovac   Site: _____   ☐ Patent   Color of Drainage: _____   ☐ NG   Site: _____   ☐ Patent   Color of Drainage: _____
☐ Chest Tube Site: _____   ☐ Patent   Color of Drainage: _____   ☐ Penrose Site: _____   ☐ Patent   Color of Drainage: _____

IVs: ☐ None #1 Site: _____ Fluid: _____ Amount: _____   ☐ Patent, Dressing Dry and Intact, No Redness or Edema Noted   ☐ Other
           #2 Site: _____ Fluid: _____ Amount: _____   ☐ Patent, Dressing Dry and Intact, No Redness or Edema Noted   ☐ Other
           #3 Site: _____ Fluid: _____ Amount: _____   ☐ Patent, Dressing Dry and Intact, No Redness or Edema Noted   ☐ Other
       ☐ A-Line Site:_____   ☐ Calibrated to Monitor   ☐ Heparin Flush   ☐ Appropriate Waveform   ☐ Other: _____
       ☐ Swan Site:_____   ☐ Calibrated to Monitor   ☐ Heparin Flush   ☐ Appropriate Waveform   ☐ Other:_____

Physician Orders

PACU Orders	**Pain Control**	**As Needed for Pain**

O_2 3 LNC for O_2 Sat. < _____ for 24 hours

_____

_____

_____

Meperidine IV: Dosage   ☐ 6.25 mg   ☐ 12.5 mg   ☐ 25 mg   ☐ Other: _____
                    Frequency   ☐ q.5min.   ☐ q.10min.   ☐ q.15min.   ☐ Other: _____
                    Maximum Dosage: _____ mg

Morphine IV: Dosage   ☐ 1.0 mg   ☐ 2.0 mg   ☐ 5 mg   ☐ Other: _____
                  Frequency   ☐ q.5min.   ☐ q.10min.   ☐ q.15min.   ☐ Other: _____
                  Maximum Dosage: _____ mg

Diagnostic Studies

_____

_____

_____

_____

_____

_____

_____

Antiemetics	**As Needed for Nausea, Vomiting**

Phenergan IV: Dosage   ☐ 6.25 mg   ☐ 12.5 mg   ☐ Other: _____
                   Frequency   ☐ q.5min.   ☐ q.10min.   ☐ Other: _____
                   Maximum Dosage: _____ mg/h

Inapsine IV: Dosage   ☐ 0.25 cc   ☐ Other: _____
                  Frequency: _____   Maximum Dosage: _____

Anzemet: Dosage   ☐ 12.5 meq   ☐ Other: _____
              Frequency: _____

Signature of MD: _____

Discharge after Score (≥) 8

_____MD

Discharge

_____MD

Figure 5.42. **(continued)**

University of Anystate Hospitals

POSTANESTHESIA NURSING RECORD
PAGE 2 OF 4

PATIENT LABEL

Ongoing Assessment/Evaluations/Documentation

Postop V/S: _____

Neurovascular/ Orthopedic Surgery Pulse Checks	R / L

Palpable=1+, 2+, 3+
√ = Yes X = No
B = Brisk S = Sluggish
W = Warm C = Cool
D = Doppler
U = Unable to palpate due to dressing/cast

Time				
Site				
Movement				
Sensation				
T				
Cap Refill				
P				

☐ See vascular flow sheet
☐ See neuro flow sheet

Sensory Chart
T-4 = Nipple line
T-6 = Xiphoid process
T-8 = Costal margin
T-10 = Umbilicus
T-12 = Iliac arrest
L-2, 3 = Thigh
S-2, 5 = Perineum

Site Code
A = L upper arm
B = R upper arm
C = L hip (LUOQ)
D = R hip (RUOQ)
E = L thigh
F = R thigh
G = Abdomen

IV Site Code
1 = R Extremity
2 = L Extremity
3 = Central Line
4 = Other (i.e., scalp)

Time	
Activity	
Respirations	
Circulation	
Consciousness	
Temperature	
Total	
Pulse Oximetry	
Temperature	
CVP	
Pap	
Spinal Level	
Epidural Level	

Cuff ▽
BP △
A-Line ▼▲
NBP ∨∧
Pulse ●
Warm Blanket B

	250
	240
	230
	220
	210
	200
	190
	180
	170
	160
	150
	140
	130
	120
	110
	100
	90
	80
	70
	60
	50
	40
	30
	20
	10
	0

Temperatures
Tympanic, unless indicated:
R = Rectal
O = Oral
A = Axillary

Respirations
Dressing _____

| **Pain Level** | | | | | | | | |

Activity
2 = Able to move 4 extremities
1 = Able to move 2 extremities
0 = Able to move 0 extremities

Respirations
2 = Clear, unsupported (strong cry if pediatric)
1 = Obstructed, supported (spontaneous respiration may be shallow or slow)
0 = Apneic/mechanical (ventilation/ambu)
Mandatory Score = 2 in Respiratory

Circulation
Adults and Children
2 = BP plus or minus 20 of preanesthesia level
1 = BP plus or minus 20-50 of preanesthesia level
0 = BP plus or minus 50 or more of preanesthesia level
Infants
2 = Radial pulse easy to palpate
1 = Axillary pulse palpable, radial pulse weak
0 = Carotid is only palpable pulse

Consciousness
2 = Awake—Oriented to time and place (preop level)
1 = Drowsy—Able to be aroused with name calling or gentle stimuli
0 = Unresponsive

Temperature
2 = Tympanic T > 96° F, R= > 97°, 0= > 96°, A= >96°
1 = Tympanic T 95–96° F, R=96-97°, 0=95–96°, A=94–96°
0 = Tympanic T < 95°, R= < 96°, 0= < 95°, A= < 94°

Dressing
0 = Dry
* = See note

Miscellaneous
* = See note

Medication	Amount	Route	Site	Time / Initials				Time Started	Fluid, Amount, Additives	Initials

Ongoing Assessment Nurse: _____ RN _____ RN _____ RN

Figure 5.42. (continued)

University of Anystate Hospitals

POSTANESTHESIA NURSING RECORD
PAGE 3 OF 4

PATIENT LABEL

Plan of Care/Interventions

☐ **Potential for Alteration in Ventilation**   Goal: Adequate Air Exchange
☐ Continuous pulse oximetry in use   ☐ Goal Met
☐ Coughing and deep breathing encouraged
☐ O_2 therapy initiated as ordered
☐ Airway out @ _____   ☐ Extubated @ _____
☐ O_2 discontinued @: _____
☐ O_2 reapplied @: _____ via mask @ _____ %
☐ O_2 reapplied @ _____ via nasal cannula @ _____ l/m
☐ Other: _____

☐ **Potential Alteration in Cardiovascular Function**   Goal: Hemodynamically Stable
☐ Continuous cardiac monitoring   ☐ Goal Met
☐ Other: _____

☐ **Potential Alteration in Mental Status**   Goal: Return to Preop Status
☐ Reoriented to time and place   ☐ Goal Met
☐ Other: _____

☐ **Potential for Fear and/or Anxiety**   Goal: Reduction of Fear and Anxiety
☐ Oriented to PACU environment
☐ Encouraged to verbalize concerns
☐ Age-appropriate emotional support provided
☐ Family at bedside
☐ Patient's and/or family's questions answered
☐ Other: _____

☐ **Potential for Injury**   Goal: Create a Safe Environment
☐ Side rails elevated   ☐ Goal Met
☐ Family at bedside
☐ Other: _____

☐ **Potential Alteration in Comfort**   Goal: Decrease Level of Pain
☐ Patient repositioned for comfort   ☐ Goal Met
☐ Medication given as ordered
☐ Scale used according to verbal communication level
☐ Other: _____

☐ **Potential Alteration in Body Temperature**   Goal: Return to Preop Status
☐ Bair hugger applied   ☐ Goal Met
☐ Warm blanket applied
☐ Warmed IV fluids given
☐ Other: _____

☐ **Potential Alteration in Tissue Perfusion**   Goal: Adequate Vascular Perfusion
☐ Capillary refill monitored on operative limb   ☐ Goal Met
☐ Circulation of operative limb monitored
☐ Other: _____

☐ **Potential Alteration in Fluid Volume**   Goal: Adequate I/O
☐ IV infusing   Goal Met
☐ Antiemetic medication administered
☐ Other: _____

☐ **Other Problems/Needs**
_____
_____
_____

Phase I Discharge Assessment

Time	Intake				Output				
	IV	Blood	PO	CBI	Urine ☐ Foley ☐ Voided	☐ NG / ☐ CT	Emesis	☐ Hemovac / ☐ JP	Other
OR I/O									
PACU I/O									
Total I/O									

LOC   ☐ Drowsy ☐ Alert ☐ Oriented ☐ Sleeping While Undisturbed
Circulatory:
  Skin   ☐ Pink ☐ Warm ☐ Cool ☐ Mottled
  Extremities ☐ Pink ☐ Warm ☐ Cool ☐ Mottled
Oxygen   ☐ Room Air ☐ O_2 @ _____ % _____ ☐ Vent
Respiratory Quality   ☐ Deep ☐ Regular ☐ Other: _____
Breath Sounds   ☐ Clear All Fields ☐ Equal Bilat. ☐ Rales
        ☐ Rhonchi ☐ Wheezing
Cardiac   ☐ Regular Rhythm ☐ Cardiac Monitoring ☐ Rhythm: _____
Dressing/Operative Site: _____ ☐ Dry and Intact ☐ Other: _____
Drains   ☐ None ☐ Secure and Patent
IV Sites   ☐ Patent, Dressing Dry and Intact, No Redness or Edema Noted
        ☐ Other (see nurses' notes)
   ☐ A-Line: ☐ To Monitor ☐ Heparin Flush ☐ Appropriate Waveform
   ☐ Swan: ☐ To Monitor ☐ Heparin Flush ☐ Appropriate Waveform
Comfort   ☐ Comfortable ☐ Other
Discharged To: ☐ Phase II Recovery ☐ Room #: _____ ☐ Side Rails Up
☐ Prescription on Chart _____
_____
_____

Discharge Time: _____ a.m./p.m.
☐ Family Notified ☐ Unable to Reach
Report Called to: _____ Transported by: _____
RN Signature: _____
☐ Patient Reassessed—Agree with PACU Discharge   V/S: _____
_____ a.m./p.m.
RN Receiving Patient   Time

Discharge IV Fluid

Type: _____   Amount: _____

Type: _____   Amount: _____

Type: _____   Amount: _____

Type: _____   Amount: _____

Figure 5.42.   (continued)

University of Anystate Hospitals

POSTANESTHESIA NURSING RECORD
PAGE 4 OF 4

PATIENT LABEL

Rhythm Strips

Supplemental Nursing Notes

POSTANESTHESIA NURSING RECORD
000023 (11/2002)

Operating room nurses maintain a record of the number of ligatures, sutures, packs, drains, sponges, instruments, and needles used during the procedure. This information may also be included in the surgeon's operative report.

The operative report should be written or dictated immediately after surgery and filed in the patient's health record as soon as possible. Some hospitals may require surgeons to include brief descriptions of the operations in their postoperative progress notes when delays in dictation or transcription are likely. The progress note can then be referred to by other caregivers until the final operative report becomes available.

Pathology Reports

Pathology examinations must be performed on every specimen or foreign object removed or expelled from a patient during a surgical procedure. Each examination includes a microscopic and macroscopic (or gross) evaluation of the specimen, which is fully described in a **pathology report**. Some hospitals have established medical staff rules that exempt some types of specimens from microscopic examination. Examples of such specimens include normal placentas, tonsils, and foreign bodies such as bullets.

Pathology reports must be prepared by pathologists, specialty physicians who analyze surgical specimens, perform autopsies, and supervise other laboratory services. Pathology reports on surgical specimens must be authenticated by the pathologist who performed the examination and then placed in the surgery section of the patient's health record. (See figures 5.45 and 5.46 for examples of pathology reports.) The following basic information is usually included in pathology reports:

- Patient identification, including name and record number

- Date of examination

- Description of the tissue examined

- Findings of the microscopic and macroscopic examination of the specimen

- Diagnosis or diagnoses

- Name, credentials, and signature of the pathologist

Preliminary pathology results are sometimes communicated to the surgical team while the procedure is still in progress. The purpose of the preliminary report is to provide information about the characteristics of any neoplasms or other abnormalities that have been removed for examination. The information allows the surgeons to modify their operative scope when the condition is more or less widespread than originally estimated.

Implant Information

Millions of Americans have undergone surgery for the implantation of artificial joints and heart valves, cardiac pacemakers, ocular lenses, and other types of medical devices in the past few decades. Although most of these devices are safe, there have been periodic product alerts and recalls.

The International Implant Registry was created in 1988. It collects information about patients who have received implants worldwide. Since 1991, federal regulations have required manufacturers to number and track many types of implantable devices so that patients and their physicians can be notified of potential safety concerns. In addition, the Food and Drug Administration (FDA 2006) requires hospitals and other healthcare organizations to report deaths and serious illnesses that appear to have been the result of malfunctioning medical

Figure 5.43. Operative report in paper format.

Midwest Medical Center

OPERATIVE REPORT
PAGE 1 OF 2

PATIENT, TWEETY PYE
00555066
DOB: 02/18/1948

DATE: 06/02/200x

SURGEON: Douglas Default

ASSISTANT: Stanley Cutter

ANESTHETIC: Spinal

PREOPERATIVE DIAGNOSES:

1. Intrauterine pregnancy, term, previous cesarean section, voluntary repeat cesarean section
2. Multiparity, voluntary sterilization

POSTOPERATIVE DIAGNOSES:

1. Intrauterine pregnancy, term, previous cesarean section, voluntary repeat cesarean section
2. Multiparity, voluntary sterilization
3. Delivery of viable unengaged 6 pound 2 ounce female, APGAR 8–9

OPERATION:

1. Low-segment transverse cesarean section
2. Bilateral partial salpingectomy

COMPLICATIONS: None

DRAINS: One Foley catheter in urinary bladder

ESTIMATED BLOOD LOSS: Approximately 500 to 600 cc

PACKS: None

DESCRIPTION OF OPERATION: After satisfactory level of spinal anesthesia was obtained, the patient was placed in the dorsal supine position with mild left lateral uterine displacement. The lower abdominal skin tissues were prepped with a Hibiclens solution. She was then draped with sterile drapes in a sterile manner.

There was a previous transverse skin scar on the lower abdominal skin. A repeat transverse skin incision was made very carefully with sharp dissection. The fascia of the anterior abdominal wall was incised in a lateral crescentic manner exposing the rectus muscles, which were then bluntly divided in the midline exposing the peritoneum, which was then carefully incised in a vertical manner. There was a wetting amount of peritoneal fluid. The peritoneum reflection over the lower anterior uterine segment was then incised in a superficial transverse manner, and the "bladder flap" was gently pushed off the lower segment without difficulty.

Figure 5.43. (continued)

Midwest Medical Center

OPERATIVE REPORT
PAGE 2 OF 2

PATIENT, TWEETY PYE
00555066
DOB: 02/18/1948

A transverse uterine incision was made very carefully with both sharp and blunt dissection. The myometrium was noted to be only 2 to 3 mm in thickness. The amniotic fluid was clear. The unengaged vertex was delivered through the uterine and abdominal incision without difficulty. The nasal and oropharynx were suctioned with bulb suction prior to the newborn's initial inspiration. The remainder of the delivery was accomplished without difficulty. The cord was clamped and severed, and the newborn was handed crying and in good condition to the awaiting nursery personnel.

The placenta was then manually removed from a fundal location showing a central insertion of a three-vessel cord. There were no visible extensions of the uterine incision. Both tubes and ovaries appeared normal for pregnant state. The uterine incision was then closed with a running interlocking #1 chromic suture.

With the patient's strong desire for permanent sterilization, approximately 1 to 1.5 cm segment of the isthmic portion of each fallopian tube was isolated with Babcock clamps, doubly ligated and excised, and sent to the laboratory labeled as portion of left and right fallopian tube, respectively. Hemostasis was deemed adequate. Both tubes appeared occluded.

The abdominal cavity was irrigated with copious amounts of warm normal saline. The first sponge, needle, and instrument counts were correct. The parietal peritoneum was then closed with a running 0 chromic suture. Hemostasis was deemed adequate in the subfascial space. The fascia was then approximated with running 0 PDS suture. Hemostasis was deemed adequate in the subcutaneous tissue. The skin was then approximated with running 3-0 Vicryl subcuticular suture. Sterile dressing was placed upon the incision.

The patient tolerated the procedure quite well and was sent to the recovery room in good condition. The newborn was taken to the nursery by the nursery personnel in good condition. The second and third sponge, needle, and instrument counts were corrected.

Signature:

Douglas D Dpull   6/2/03

Douglas D. Default, MD   Date

d: 06/02/2003
t: 06/04/2003
DDD, MD/sf

Figure 5.44.   Operative report in electronic format.

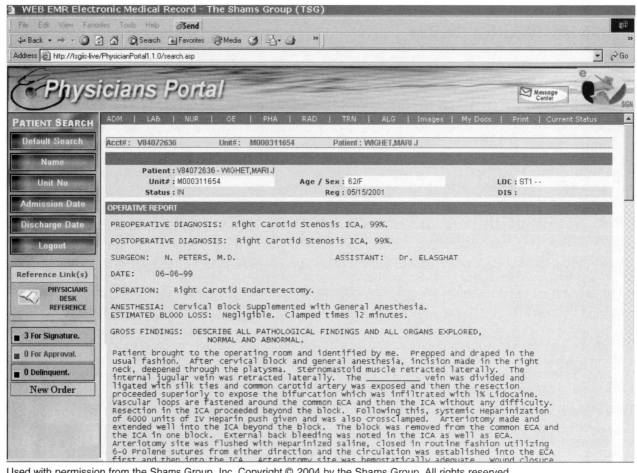

devices. Some hospitals maintain their own implant registries in addition to taking part in the International Implant Registry.

Information about the type of medical device, its manufacturer, and any product numbers on the device should be included in the operative report for the implantation procedure. In addition, for medical devices that require batteries, such as pacemakers, the operative reports should also indicate how often the devices must be replaced to ensure patient safety.

Transplantation and Organ Donation Records

Organ transplants have become increasingly common since the first attempts were made in the 1950s and 1960s. Today, thousands of patients every year receive kidneys, livers, hearts, and lungs salvaged from healthy patients who died from injuries and other causes. Organ donations from live donors have also become quite common, and it is not unusual for a family member to donate a kidney or part of his or her liver to a child or sibling. Bone marrow transplants from live donors have also saved the lives of thousands of cancer patients when other treatments failed.

Living donors must undergo surgery to remove bone marrow, kidneys, and other organs for transplantation to another patient. The surgical teams for the donor and the recipient must prepare operative reports for both patients, and the reports must follow the same standards as any other operative record.

Figure 5.45. Surgical pathology consultation report in paper format.

Midwest Medical Center

SURGICAL PATHOLOGY CONSULTATION

PATIENT, SWEETPEA C.
007770021
DOB: 12/18/1931

ADMITTING PHYSICIAN: M. D. Doctor

CONSULT PHYSICIAN 1:

CONSULT PHYSICIAN 2:

ACCESSIONED IN LAB: 05/20/2003

ACCESSION #: S-03-010101

DATE OF SURGERY: 5/20/2003

SPECIMEN: A-Vag Mucosa

CLINICAL DATA: Cystocele/rectocele, stress incontinence

GROSS: Received are four wrinkled, variegated, pink/tan portions of vaginal mucosa, which are 7 × 6 × 1 cm in aggregate dimension. Representative portions of each are submitted for microscopic evaluation. M/1/pg.

MICROSCOPIC COMMENT: Sections are of squamous mucosa. There are no atypia.

DIAGNOSIS: Squamous mucosa, multiple portions exhibiting no atypia (vaginal)

Signature:

Walter Q. Pathman

_5/20/03_

Walter Q. Pathman, MD

Date

d: 05/20/2003
t: 05/23/2003
WQP, MD/jt

Figure 5.46.   Surgical pathology consultation report in electronic format.

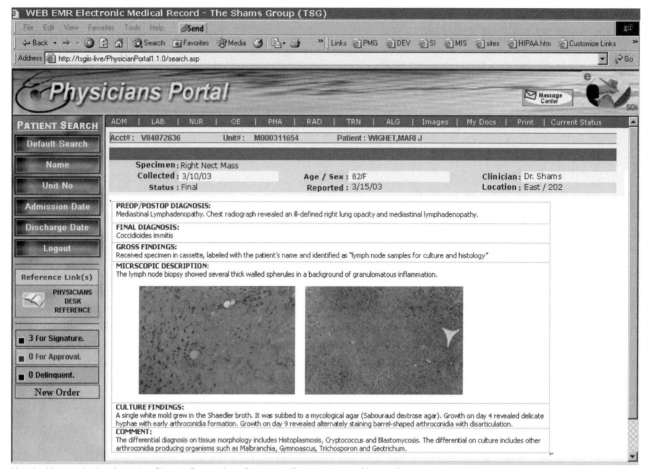

Because of a shortage of transplantable organs and the difficulty of matching donors to recipients, transplantation entails a number of ethical problems. To ensure that the available organs are going to the most suitable recipients, the national Organ Procurement and Transplantation Network was implemented. Patients who need transplants are placed on a national waiting list. The application for the waiting list reports information about the patient, such as race, ethnicity, and geographic location.

The Medicare *Conditions of Participation* (2006) require hospitals to provide organ donation information to the families of potential organ donors. When a patient is near death and the family has decided to donate his or her organs, documentation that shows that the transplantation network has been notified must be placed in the patient's record. Arrangements should be made to harvest the patient's organs soon after death, and those procedures should also be documented in the patient's health record.

Outpatient Services Provided in Acute-Care Facilities

Acute-care hospitals provide outpatient services in several departments. Outpatients receive treatment or undergo diagnostic procedures in hospital-based departments and then leave after the treatment or procedure is complete. A physician's order must accompany the patient to the hospital to provide a diagnosis and medical necessity prior to the service being rendered. The contents of outpatient records depend on the type of procedures provided. Outpatient services include the following examples:

- Sleep lab testing
- Outpatient radiology exams
- Pulmonary function testing
- Radiation therapy
- Physical therapy
- Occupational therapy
- Speech therapy

Emergency and Trauma Care

Hospital emergency departments provide urgent diagnostic and therapeutic services to patients who have potentially life-threatening medical conditions or traumatic injuries that need immediate attention. The patients treated in emergency departments are considered hospital outpatients, although many emergency patients require inpatient care after their conditions have been diagnosed and stabilized in the emergency department. After being evaluated and treated in the emergency department, patients may be admitted to one of the hospital's inpatient units, discharged, or transferred to another facility.

Most states require emergency-care facilities to maintain a chronological record of every patient who was treated at the facility, including those who were dead on arrival or left the facility against medical advice. The records in most states must include at least the patient's name, the date and time of arrival, and the patient's medical record number.

In accordance with the **Emergency Medical Treatment and Active Labor Act (EMTALA)** (CMS 2006), emergency departments must complete a medical screening examination prior to collecting any information regarding the patient's ability to pay for the services.

Records of Emergency Services

The health records maintained for emergency services contain the same basic information as inpatient records. Emergency physicians take a medical history and perform a physical examination soon after each patient is admitted to the department. Nurses also perform a nursing assessment for each new patient. Physicians' orders, progress notes, and reports from ancillary services are documented throughout the patient's stay in the emergency department.

The content of the emergency health record usually includes the following information:

- Patient identification, including name and record number
- Time of arrival
- Means of arrival (ambulance, private automobile, or police vehicle)
- Name of the person or organization that transported the patient to the emergency department
- Consent to treatment
- Pertinent history, including chief complaint and onset of injury or illness
- Significant physical findings

- Laboratory, x-ray, EEG, and EKG findings

- Treatment rendered and results

- Conclusions at termination of treatment

- Disposition of patient, including transfer, admission, or discharge home

- Condition of patient at discharge or transfer

- Diagnosis upon discharge

- Instructions given to the patient or family regarding care and follow-up

- Signatures and credentials of caregivers

Emergency services records may be filed separately or incorporated into the patient's inpatient record when the patient is admitted to the same facility. When the records are filed separately, the emergency record must be made available when the patient is readmitted or appears for care in the future.

Emergency Department Transfer Records
State regulations specifically require emergency facilities to maintain records of the screening examinations performed on patients who were subsequently transferred to other facilities. Similarly, federal legislation passed in 1986 and implemented in 1990 contains provisions intended to curtail the practice known as patient dumping. As stated in EMTALA, **dumping** refers to the once-common practice of private hospitals to transfer indigent patients to the emergency departments of nearby public hospitals with the sole purpose of avoiding the cost of providing emergency treatment to patients who were uninsured or underinsured and could not pay for the services themselves. Basically, state and federal regulations require emergency facilities to thoroughly document the reasons for patient transfers to confirm that the transfers were not related to the patients' ability to pay for treatment or the source of payment.

To avoid the appearance of dumping, it is particularly important that the records of emergency-care patients include enough information to justify each patient's disposition after emergency treatment is complete or deemed unnecessary. In addition, when a decision is made to transfer a patient to another facility, the physician primarily responsible for the patient's care must document in detail the reason for the transfer and the results of the patient's screening examination. Specifically, the patient's record for the encounter must contain documentation that confirms that the following actions were taken (Glondys 1999, 215):

- The physician explained to the patient why the transfer was appropriate and what the risks and benefits of the transfer would be.

- Emergency department nursing and medical staff monitored the patient's medical condition from the time he or she came to the department for treatment until the time he or she was transferred.

- Emergency department staff recorded the patient's time of arrival and time of transfer.

- A screening examination was performed and clinical findings were analyzed to support the physician's initial diagnosis.

- Appropriate treatment was provided to stabilize the patient's medical condition before and during the transfer.

- On-call physicians were consulted as appropriate, the timing of the calls and responses was noted, and the on-call physicians' recommendations were documented.

- The hospital documented the patient's informed consent for the transfer if the patient decided to refuse the screening examination or the recommended care and treatment.

- If the patient requested a transfer, his or her request was documented, and it was specifically noted that the transfer was not requested by a healthcare provider.

- The transferring hospital sent a copy of the patient's emergency record along with the patient to the second facility. The record described the reason the patient sought treatment, the results of any diagnostic examinations or tests, and the treatments provided, including any medications that were administered. The record also included a copy of the patient's informed consent for the transfer or the physician's certification that the transfer was appropriate.

- Prior to transfer, the patient was clinically stable and consented to the transfer. In addition, the transferring hospital contacted the receiving hospital and obtained approval to transfer. This conversation was documented on the transfer form.

Ambulatory Surgery

The records of outpatients who receive surgical services in an ambulatory surgery unit of the hospital must meet the same documentation requirements as inpatient surgical cases. (See "Surgical Services," earlier in this chapter, for the discussion of surgical services.) The outpatient records of patients who require inpatient admission after ambulatory surgery should be combined with the patients' inpatient records.

Diagnostic and Therapeutic Services

Many patients receive diagnostic services in hospital departments on an outpatient basis. Their personal physicians send them to local hospitals for specialized tests such as colonoscopies and MRIs that require equipment that is not available in most physicians' offices. Similarly, because most physicians' offices are not equipped to perform procedures that require the use of anesthesia or sedation, patients go to local hospitals for such services. Physicians may also order diagnostic procedures that must be performed and/or interpreted by hospital specialists. The patient must present the physician's order for each diagnostic test to be conducted.

Many hospital-based therapeutic services can also be provided on an outpatient basis. Examples include renal dialysis, chemotherapy, and radiotherapy, which are discussed later in this chapter (see "Renal Dialysis Services," "Chemotherapy Services," and "Radiotherapy Services").

Accreditation standards require that records of patients receiving ongoing ambulatory-care services in hospital-based outpatient departments include at least a summary page that lists the patient's diagnoses, past procedures, medications, and allergies. The results of outpatient procedures are reported to the physicians who ordered the procedures, and copies of the reports are filed in the patients' outpatient records.

Specialty-Care Documentation

Specialty-care records often include information that is not required in general medical and surgical records. Government regulations, accreditation standards, and professional practice standards dictate unique content requirements for several types of specialty-care records. However, the basic content and documentation guidelines that apply to general health records apply equally to specialty-care records.

Nutritional Services

A nutritional-care plan is based on an initial **nutritional assessment** performed by a registered dietitian. The assessment includes the patient's diet history, weight and height, appetite and food preferences, and information on food sensitivities and allergies. Nutritional-care plans usually include the following information:

- Confirmation that a diet order for the patient was issued within twenty-four hours of admission

- Summary of the patient's diet history and/or the nutritional assessment performed upon admission

- Documentation of nutritional therapy and/or dietetic consultation

- Timely and periodic assessments of the patient's nutrient intake and tolerance of the prescribed diet

- Nutritional discharge plan and patient instructions

- Documentation that a copy of the plan was forwarded to the facility to which the patient was transferred after discharge from the hospital, if applicable

- Dietitian's signature, credentials, and date

Obstetrical Services

The hospital records for pregnant women admitted for labor and delivery contain elements similar to general health records. The obstetrician's records of prenatal care constitute documentation of the patient's preadmission history and physical. At admission, the physician also prepares a note describing the patient's progress since he or she last saw her for prenatal care. (See figure 5.47.) For normal deliveries, a **labor and delivery record** takes the place of an operative report. (See figure 5.48.)

Cesarean deliveries are operative procedures, and as such, they require documentation of the patient's informed consent. Obstetricians who perform Cesarean deliveries must prepare complete operative reports. Similarly, sterilization procedures performed after a Cesarean or normal delivery are considered separate procedures that must be fully documented.

Discharge summaries are not required for normal deliveries. A preprinted discharge form or discharge progress note is considered sufficient discharge reporting for mother and child. Complete discharge summaries, however, are required for surgical and complicated deliveries.

The health records of the mother and her newborn infant or infants must be maintained separately. An exception is made for cases of stillbirth. Information on the stillborn infant can be incorporated into the mother's record.

Every labor and delivery record should contain the following information:

- Patient's married and/or maiden name(s)

- Patient's record number

- Delivery date

- Gender of the infant

- Names and credentials of the physician and any assistants

Figure 5.47.   Maternal/prenatal care summary in paper format.

Anytown Community Hospital

MATERNAL/PRENATAL CARE SUMMARY

PATIENT LABEL

Mother's Name: _____

Mother's Age: _____   Gravida: _____   Term: _____

Premature: _____   Abnormal: _____   Living: _____

Expected Delivery Date: _____

Prenatal Labs:_____

Maternal/Prenatal/Family History:_____

_____

_____

Social Problems:_____

_____

Type of Delivery: ☐ Vaginal

                    ☐ C-Section

Type of Anesthesia: _____

Tubal Ligation: ☐ Yes   ☐ No

Apgars: 1 min __   5 min __   10 min __

Complications of Labor and Delivery: _____

_____

_____

Transfer From: _____

Date: _____

Delivery Weight: _____

Last Weight: _____

Service Notified: _____

Date and Time: _____

Person Notified: _____

Examined:_____

Void: ☐

Stool: ☐

Circumcision: ☐ Yes ☐ No

Done: _____

Date:_____

Metabolic Screen: ☐ Yes ☐ No

Done: _____

Date:_____

Hearing Screen: ☐ Yes ☐ No

Done: _____

Date:_____

Pass/Refer:

Follow-up Appointment
Made: _____

Vitals: _____

Glucoses: _____

Breast: _____

Formula: _____

IVF _____ @ _____

UAC _____ @ _____

UVC _____ @ _____

Mother's Blood Type and RH: _____

Cord Blood: _____

COOMBS: _____

Cord Bili:_____

Baby Safe Signed: ☐

Gift Bags Given: ☐

Hepatitis B Vaccine:
☐ Yes   ☐ No

Orders:

_____

_____

_____

_____

_____

_____

_____

_____

_____

_____

Medications: _____

_____

_____

Messages: _____

_____

Obstetrician	Delivery Date	Delivery Time	Baby's Gender
Mother's Room Number		Pediatrician	

Figure 5.48.   Labor and delivery summary in paper format.

Anytown Community Hospital

LABOR AND DELIVERY SUMMARY
PAGE 1 OF 5

PATIENT LABEL

LABOR SUMMARY

G	T	Pt	A	L	Blood Type and Rh	EDD
						/ /

Prenatal Events ☐ None

☐ No Prenatal Care

☐ Preterm Labor (≤37 Weeks)

☐ Postterm Labor (≥42 Weeks)

☐ Previous Cesarean

☐ Prenatal Complications

☐ Other _____

Maternal Intrapartal Events

☐ None

☐ Febrile (≥100.4ºF/38ºC)

☐ Bleeding—Site Undetermined

☐ Preeclampsia: ☐ Mild   ☐ Severe

☐ Seizure Activity

☐ Medications: ☐ None

Date	Time	Medication	Dose	Route

☐ Transfusion _____ *units*

Blood Component _____

☐ Other _____

Amniotic Fluid

☐ SROM   ☐ AROM   Date ____ Time ____

☐ Premature ROM   ☐ Prolonged ROM

☐ Clear

☐ Meconium-Stained (Describe) _____

☐ Bloody

☐ Foul Odor

   ☐ Cultures Sent _____ Time _____

☐ Polyhydramnios

☐ Oligohydramnios

☐ Other_____

Placenta

☐ Placenta Previa

☐ Abruptio Placenta

☐ Other_____

Labor

☐ Precipitous Labor (<3 h)

☐ Prolonged Labor (≥20 h)

☐ Prolonged Latent Phase

☐ Prolonged Active Phase

☐ Prolonged 2nd Stage (>2.5 h)

☐ Secondary Arrest of Dilatation

☐ Induction:

   ☐ None   ☐ AROM

   ☐ Oxytocin   ☐ Other_____

☐ Augmentation:

   ☐ None   ☐ AROM

   ☐ Oxytocin   ☐ Other_____

Figure 5.48. (continued)

Anytown Community Hospital

LABOR AND DELIVERY SUMMARY
PAGE 2 OF 5

PATIENT LABEL

LABOR SUMMARY (Continued)

Fetus

Gestational Age (Weeks): _____ By Dates _____ By Ultrasound

Presentation: **Position:**

☐ Vertex ☐ Face/Brow

☐ Breech: ☐ Frank ☐ Complete ☐ Single Footing ☐ Double Footing

☐ Transverse Lie: ☐ Back Up ☐ Back Down

☐ Compound

☐ Unknown

☐ Cephalopelvic Disproportion (CPD)

☐ Cord Prolapse

Monitor: ☐ None ☐ External FHR ☐ External UC
☐ Internal FHR ☐ Internal UC

STV: ☐ Present ☐ Absent

☐ LTV _____

☐ Fetal Bradycardia

☐ Fetal Tachycardia

☐ Sinusoidal Pattern

☐ Accelerations: ☐ Spontaneous ☐ Uniform

☐ Decelerations: ☐ Early ☐ Late ☐ Variable ☐ Prolonged

☐ Scalp pH ≤ 7.2

☐ _____

FM Discontinued _____ Time _____

FHR Prior to Delivery _____ bpm Time _____

Signature _____ Date _____

DELIVERY SUMMARY

Support Person Present: ☐ Yes ☐ No

Location: ☐ LDR ☐ LDRP ☐ DR ☐ OR ☐ Birthing Room ☐ Other _____

Method of Delivery: Vaginal

☐ VBAC (Number _____)

☐ Vertex

☐ Spontaneous

☐ Assisted   **Position:**   to   **Position:**

☐ Manual Rotation

☐ Forceps (Type) _____)

☐ Outlet ☐ Low ☐ Mid

☐ Vacuum Extraction Duration ___min.

Degree of Suction _____kg/cm²

☐ Breech (Type _____)

☐ Spontaneous ☐ Partial Extraction (Assisted) ☐ Total Extraction

☐ Forceps Assist

☐ Piper ☐ Other _____

Episiotomy

☐ None ☐ Midline ☐ Mediolateral   L   R

Laceration/Episiotomy Extension:

☐ None ☐ Periurethral ☐ Vaginal ☐ Cervical ☐ Uterine

☐ Perineal ☐ 1" ☐ 2" ☐ 3" ☐ 4"

Repair Agent Used _____

☐ Vagina Free of Sponges

Placenta

☐ Spontaneous ☐ Expressed ☐ Manual Removal

☐ Adherent (Type _____)

☐ Uterine Exploration

☐ Curettage

Configuration

☐ Normal

☐ Abnormal _____

Weight _____ g

Disposition _____

Cord

☐ Nuchal Cord (× _____) ☐ True Knot Length _____ cm

☐ 2 Vessels ☐ 3 Vessels

Cord Blood ☐ To Lab ☐ Refrig ☐ Discard

Lab ☐ Type + Rh ☐ Cultures ☐ COOMBS

☐ pH ☐ _____

Signature _____ Date _____

Figure 5.48. **(continued)**

Anytown Community Hospital

LABOR AND DELIVERY SUMMARY
PAGE 3 OF 5

PATIENT LABEL

DELIVERY SUMMARY (Continued)

Method of Delivery: Cesarean
☐ Scheduled   ☐ Emergency   ☐ Primary   ☐ Repeat (× ————)   ☐ Other _____
Operative Indication: ☐ Previous Uterine Surgery   ☐ Failure to Progress   ☐ Placenta Previa   ☐ Abruptio Placenta
☐ Fetal Malpresentation _____   ☐ Nonreassuring FHR Pattern _____
☐ Other_____

Uterine Incision: ☐ Low Cervical, Transverse   ☐ Low Cervical, Vertical   ☐ Classical

Hysterectomy: ☐ Yes   ☐ No   **Tubal Ligation:**   ☐ Yes ☐ No

Skin Incision: ☐ Vertical   ☐ Pfannenstiel

Surgical Data

Sponge Counts Correct: ☐ NA   ☐ Yes   ☐ No _____

Needle Counts Correct: ☐ NA   ☐ Yes   ☐ No _____

Vaginal Pack Count Correct: ☐ NA   ☐ Yes   ☐ No _____

Estimated Blood Loss _____ *cc*

Anesthesia: ☐ None   ☐ Local   ☐ Pudendal   ☐ General   ☐ Epidural   ☐ Spinal

Date	Time	Medication	Dose	Effect

Complications of Anesthesia: ☐ Yes _____   ☐ None

Medications: ☐ None

Date	Time	Medication	Dose	Route Site	Initials

Chronology

	Date	Time		
EDD				
Admit to Hospital				
Membranes Ruptured				
Onset of Labor			**Total Time H/Min**	
Complete Cervical Dilation				I
Delivery of Infant				II
Delivery of Placenta				III
				Total Labor

Signature _____ Date _____

Figure 5.48.   (continued)

Anytown Community Hospital

LABOR AND DELIVERY SUMMARY
PAGE 4 OF 5

NEONATAL SUMMARY

Birth Data

Time of Birth _____ ☐ Male   ☐ Female

ID Band # _____

Condition: ☐ Alive   ☐ Antepartum Death   ☐ Intrapartum Death   ☐ Neonatal Death

Birth Order _____ of _____

Apgar Score	1 min	5 min	10 min
Heart Rate			
Respiratory Effort			
Muscle Tone			
Reflex Irritability			
Color			
Total			

Signature _____

Airway
☐ Bulb Suction
☐ Suction Catheter   Size _____ Fr
   ☐ Mouth   Pressure _____ mm Hg
   ☐ Nose   ☐ At Delivery
   ☐ Pharynx
☐ Endotracheal Tube Size _____ Fr
   ☐ Meconium Below Cords   Times _____

Breathing
☐ Spontaneous
☐ O$_2$ _____ Liters   Time Initiated
   ☐ Free Flow   _____
   ☐ PPV
     ☐ Bag/Mask   _____
     ☐ ET Tube Size _____ Fr   _____
     ☐ CPAP _____ mm
_____ Minutes to First Gasp
_____ Minutes to Sustained Respiration

Circulation
☐ Spontaneous
☐ External Cardiac Massage
   Time Initiated _____ Time Completed _____
_____ Minutes for HR > 100
   Heart Rate (bpm)
   _____ Time _____
   _____ Time _____
   _____ Time _____

IV Access
☐ Umbilical Catheter
☐ Peripheral Line

Person Managing Reuscitation
_____

Medications: ☐ None

Date	Time	Medication	Dose	Route Site	Initials

Laboratory Data: ☐ None

Blood Gases	Sent	Umb Art	Umb Vein
pH			
pO$_2$			
pCO$_2$			
HCO$_3$			

Test   **Result**
Dextrostix   _____

Figure 5.48. **(continued)**

Anytown Community Hospital

LABOR AND DELIVERY SUMMARY
PAGE 5 OF 5

NEONATAL SUMMARY (Continued)

Initial Newborn Exam

Weight _____ g _____ lb _____ oz ☐ Deferred
Length _____ cm _____ in ☐ Deferred
Head _____ cm _____ in ☐ Deferred
Chest _____ cm _____ in ☐ Deferred
Abdomen _____ cm _____ in ☐ Deferred
T _____ ☐ Rectal   ☐ Axillary
AP _____ R _____ BP _____
☐ No Observed Abnormalities
☐ Abnormalities Noted
☐ Meconium Staining   ☐ Cephalhematoma
☐ Petechiae   ☐ Other
Describe _____
_____
_____

Intake ☐ None
  Breast Feed: ☐ Yes   ☐ No
Output ☐ None
  ☐ Urine   ☐ Stool (Type_____)
  ☐ Gastric Aspirate _____ *cc*
Examined By _____
Transfer: ☐ With Mother
        ☐ To Newborn Nursery
        ☐ To NICU
        ☐ Other_____
Date ___ / ___ / ___ Time _____
Mode of Transport_____

Delivery Personnel
RN   (1)_____
      (2)_____
Anesthesiologist/CRNA _____
CNM _____
Physician—Attending _____
Physician—Assist (1) _____
        (2) _____
Pediatric Provider _____
☐ Notified   ☐ Present at Birth

Remarks

_____   _____
Signature   Date

LABOR AND DELIVERY SUMMARY
200366 (6/2004)

- Descriptions of any complications that developed

- Type of anesthesia

- Name of the person who administered the anesthesia

- Names of other persons who witnessed the delivery

Neonatal Services

The health records of newborn infants are maintained separately from their mothers' records. For normal deliveries, the neonatal record usually duplicates much of the information documented in the mother's record in addition to a general assessment of the newborn's condition at birth. (See figure 5.49.) In some cases, a discharge progress note is acceptable for a normal newborn's record.

Much more extensive documentation is required for premature infants and other infants who require intensive care after birth. Some infants require months of treatment in the neonatal intensive-care unit before they are strong enough to go home with their parents. The records of these babies require full documentation, including admission and discharge assessments, operative reports when applicable, and discharge summaries.

Some hospitals do not offer neonatal intensive-care services. Infants born at these hospitals require immediate transfer to another facility equipped to handle their needs. In such cases, the neonatal record maintained by the hospital where the infant was born should include admission and discharge information and documentation of the reason for the child's transfer to the other facility.

For those newborns who are born and expire shortly after delivery a unique medical record number and account number should be assigned and a separate record generated by the hospital. A common guideline for creating newborn records is to review the APGAR score; if a newborn is born with an APGAR score of one (1) or above, an individual record for the newborn should be generated, regardless of how long the newborn survives.

If a newborn is born with no APGAR score or an APGAR score of zero (0), it is considered a stillbirth. Hospitals may choose in this instance to combine the newborn record with that of the mother and not generate a separate medical record number and account number for the newborn.

Observation Services

Observation patients are considered outpatients, and they generally stay in the hospital for less than twenty-four hours. The health records for observation patients must include a physician's order for admission to an observation bed or unit as well as the time and date of the patient's admission and discharge. Other documentation should include vital signs and medication records as well as physicians' and nurses' progress notes. A discharge summary or note should describe the patient's condition and disposition at discharge.

Third-party payers have strict rules on reimbursement for observation services. Therefore, complete documentation of the medical necessity and length of observation services is particularly important.

Case managers can be of particular assistance in monitoring observation admissions and ensure that medical necessity is met. The case manager can also avoid potential inappropriate observation admissions by communicating with the physician to ensure the patient is placed in appropriate status.

Figure 5.49. Neonatal assessment record in paper format.

Anytown Community Hospital

NEONATAL ASSESSMENT RECORD
PAGE 1 OF 2

PATIENT LABEL

	Within Normal Anatomical Limits	
Development		Birth Date _____ Type of Delivery ☐ Vaginal ☐ C-Section Gender _____ Head Circumference _____ Birth Weight _____ Birth Length _____

Neurological/ Musculoskeletal Pupil Size R ___ L ___	Yes ☐	No ☐	**LOC** ☐ Lethargic ☐ Unresponsive ☐ Irritable ☐ Responds Only to Stimuli **Comments:**	**Movement** ☐ ↓ RA ☐ ↓ RL ☐ ↓ LA ☐ ↓ LL	**Pupils** ☐ Nonreactive ☐ Sluggish ☐ Constricted ☐ Fixed

	Yes	No	**Heart**	**Edema**	**Vascular (0, 1, 3, 4)**
Heart/Vascular	☐	☐	☐ Skips ☐ Palpitations ☐ Valve Click ☐ Murmur **Comments:**	☐ Generalized Location _____ Degree (1–4) _____	R Radial + _____ ☐ Dop ☐ Abs L Radial + _____ ☐ Dop ☐ Abs R Pedal + _____ ☐ Dop ☐ Abs L Pedal + _____ ☐ Dop ☐ Abs R Brach + _____ ☐ Dop ☐ Abs L Brach + _____ ☐ Dop ☐ Abs

	Yes	No	**Respirations**		**Breath Sounds**	**Right**	**Left**
Pulmonary/ Lungs	☐	☐	☐ Orthopnea ☐ Dyspnea ☐ Apnea ☐ Labored ☐ Tachypnea **Comments:**	☐ Retractions ☐ Shallow ☐ Cough ☐ Nasal Flaring	☐ Crackles ☐ Rhonchi ☐ Wheezes ☐ Diminished ☐ Absent	☐ ☐ ☐ ☐ ☐	☐ ☐ ☐ ☐ ☐

	Yes	No	**Bowel Sounds**	**Abdomen**	**Bowel Habits**
Gastrointestinal Last BM _____ Pattern _____	☐	☐	☐ Hypo ☐ Hyper ☐ Absent **Comments:**	☐ Firm ☐ Protuberant ☐ Distended ☐ Tender	☐ Frequency ☐ Diarrhea

Nutritional		☐ Breast Feeding Frequency _____ Feeding Length _____ ☐ Bottle Feeding Frequency _____ Formula _____ Amount _____

	Yes	No	**Urinary**		**Reproductive**
Genitourinary/ Reproductive	☐	☐	☐ Hematuria ☐ Frequency ☐ Oliguria ☐ Dysuria **Comments:**		☐ Undescended testicles R ☐ L ☐

	Yes	No	**Problem**	**Hearing**	**Sight**
EENT	☐	☐	☐ Swallowing ☐ Choking **Comments:**	↓☐ R ↓☐ L	↓☐ R ↓☐ L

Figure 5.49. **(continued)**

Anytown Community Hospital

NEONATAL ASSESSMENT RECORD
PAGE 2 OF 2

PATIENT LABEL

	Within Normal Anatomical Limits		

	Yes	No	
Skin Integumentary	☐	☐	**Problem** **Location** **Problem** **Location** **Problem** ☐ Bruise _____ ☐ Wound _____ ☐ Pale ☐ Burn _____ ☐ Ulcer _____ ☐ Jaundice ☐ Rash _____ ☐ Bleeding _____ ☐ Mottled ☐ Oral Mucosa _____ ☐ Other _____ ☐ Tugor ☐ Dry ☐ Thrush ☐ Lesions ☐ Tenting ☐ Dry Comments:
Emotional/ Mental	Yes ☐	No ☐	☐ Lethargic ☐ Fussy ☐ Withdrawn ☐ Inconsolable Crying Comments:
Sleep Pattern			Bedtime _____ Naptime _____
Family Information			Primary Caretaker _____ Siblings? How many and what are their ages? _____
Pain	Yes ☐	No ☐	

Neonatal/Infant Pain Scale (NIPS) (A score greater than 3 indicates pain)

Observe	Criteria	Points
	Relaxed Muscles—restful face, neutral expression	0
	Grimace—tight facial muscles, furrowed brow, chin, jaw (negative facial expression nose, mouth, and brow)	1
	No Cry—quiet, not crying	0
	Whimper—intermittent	1
	Vigorous Cry—loud scream, rising, shrill, continuous (note: silent cry may be scored if baby is intubated as evidenced by obvious mouth and facial movement)	2
	Relaxed—usual pattern for this infant	0
	Change in Breathing—indrawing, irregular, faster than usual, gagging, breath holding	1
Arms	Relaxed/Restrained—no muscular rigidity, occasional random movements of arms	0
	Flexed/Extended—tense, straight legs, rigid and/or rapid extension, flexion	1
Legs	Relaxed/Restrained—no muscular rigidity, occasional random leg movement	0
	Flexed/Extended—tense, straight legs, rigid, and/or rapid extension, flexion	1
State of Arousal	Sleeping/Awake—quiet, peaceful sleeping or alert random leg movement	0
	Fussy—alert, restless, and thrashing	1
	Total Score	

Or
Nonverbal Assessment

Observe	Criteria	Points
	Anxious/Irritable	1
	Almost in Tears	2
	None	0
	Restless/Slow or Decreased Movement	1
	Immobile	2
Verbal Cues	Whining/Whimpering/Moaning	1
	Screaming, Crying Out	2
Facial Cues	Relaxed, Calm Expression	0
	Drawn Around Mouth and Eyes	1
	Facial Frowning, Wincing	2
Positioning/ Guarding	Relaxed Body	0
	Guarding/Tense	1
	Fetal Position/Jumps If Touched	2
	Total Points	

Comments:

RN Initials: _____ RN Signature: _____ Date: _____ Time: _____ Unit: _____

RN Initials: _____ RN Signature: _____ Date: _____ Time: _____ Unit: _____

NEONATAL ASSESSMENT RECORD
000060 (10/2002)

Psychiatric Services

Inpatient psychiatric hospitals and psychiatric units within acute-care hospitals maintain documentation similar to other inpatient units in addition to documentation unique to psychiatric care. The following list includes the elements of minimum documentation established by accreditation standards, federal regulations, and Medicare *Conditions of Participation* (2006):

- Demographic data

- Source of referral

- Reason for referral

- Patient's legal status

- All appropriate consents for admission, treatment, evaluation, and aftercare

- Admitting psychiatric diagnoses

- Psychiatric history

- Record of the complete patient assessment, including the complaints of others regarding the patient as well as the patient's comments

- Medical history, report of physical examination, and list of medications

- Provisional diagnoses based on assessment that includes other current diseases as well as psychiatric diagnoses

- Written, individualized treatment plan

- Documentation of the course of treatment and all evaluations and examinations

- Multidisciplinary progress notes related to the goals and objectives outlined in the treatment plan

- Appropriate documentation related to special treatment procedures such as the use of physical and chemical restraints and seclusion techniques to control dangerous patient behavior

- Updates to the treatment plan as a result of ongoing assessments detailed in the progress notes

- Records of multidisciplinary case conferences and consultation notes, which include the dates of the conferences or consultations, the recommendations made, and the actions taken

- Information on any unusual occurrences such as treatment complications, accidents or injuries to the patient, death of the patient, and procedures that placed the patient at risk or caused unusual pain

- Correspondence related to the patient, including all letters and dated notations of telephone conversations relevant to the patient's treatment

- Discharge or termination summary

- Plan for follow-up care and documentation of its implementation

- Individualized aftercare or posttreatment plan

See chapter 12 for additional information about behavioral healthcare.

Rehabilitation Services

Rehabilitation services include a number of different therapies designed to build or rebuild the patient's ability to perform the activities of daily living. **Activities of daily living (ADLs)** include the basic activities of self-care, including the ability to communicate with others, feed oneself, bath and dress oneself, use the toilet, and move within one's environment. Rehabilitation services include physical therapy, occupational therapy, and speech therapy as well as treatment by physicians specializing in rehabilitation and the use of orthotics.

Physical therapists help patients to build or rebuild their muscle strength and respiratory and circulatory capacities. Physical therapists work with patients who have been disabled by illnesses (stroke and heart disease are the most common), injuries, and birth defects.

Occupational therapists help patients to restore their ability to read and write and to perform self-care activities after they have been disabled by illness or injury. Similarly, speech therapists conduct dysphasia evaluations and help disabled patients to regain their ability to communicate.

Inpatient rehabilitation hospitals and rehabilitation units within acute-care hospitals are subject to a Medicare prospective payment system that is based on documentation. A standardized assessment tool called the **patient assessment instrument (PAI)** must be completed shortly after the patient's admission and upon discharge. Payment level is based on the patient's medical condition and diagnostic profile as well as the services provided.

The Joint Commission's *Comprehensive Accreditation Manual for Hospitals* (2006) and the Medicare *Conditions of Participation for Hospitals* (2006) both require that the records of rehabilitation services include documentation of a preliminary patient assessment and a written rehabilitation plan. The plan must be developed by qualified professionals on the basis of the patient's needs. (See figure 5.50.)

Many rehabilitation facilities are accredited through the **Commission on Accreditation of Rehabilitation Facilities (CARF).** CARF requires rehabilitation facilities to maintain a single case record for every patient they admit. The documentation standard for health records includes the following requirements:

- Patient identification data
- Pertinent history
- Diagnosis of disability
- Rehabilitation problems, goals, and prognosis
- Reports of assessments and individual program planning
- Reports from referring sources and service referrals
- Reports from outside consultations and laboratory, radiology, orthotic, and prosthetic services
- Designation of a manager for the patient's program
- Evidence of the patient's or family's participation in decision making
- Evaluation reports from every service
- Reports of staff conferences
- Patient's total program plan
- Plans from each service
- Signed and dated service and progress reports

Figure 5.50. Rehabilitation care plan in paper format.

University of Anystate Hospital

REHABILITATION PLAN OF CARE
PAGE 1 OF 4

PATIENT LABEL

Date Developed/Updated:_____ Anticipated Discharge:_____

Rehab Diagnosis:_____ Prognosis:_____

Anticipated Discharge Disposition:_____

Patient/Caregiver Goals:_____

Medical Status:_____

Self-Care/Events	TD	RD	Interventions	Person(s) Responsible
1. Upper extremity dressing with:_____			1. ADL program	OT, Nursing
2. Lower extremity dressing with:_____			2. ADL program	OT, Nursing
3. Bathing with:_____			3. ADL program	OT, Nursing
4. Toileting with:_____			4. ADL program	OT, Nursing
5. Grooming with:_____			5. ADL program	OT, Nursing
6. Eating with:_____			6. ADL program	OT, Nursing, SLP

Discharge Outcome(s): ADLs with:_____

Mobility/Events	TD	RD	Interventions	Person(s) Responsible
1. Transfers with:_____			1. Transfer training	PT, Team
2. Tub/shower transfers with:_____			2. Transfer training	OT, Team
3. Toilet transfers with:_____			3. Transfer training	OT, Team
4. Bed mobility with:_____			4. Rolling, bridging, supine-sit	PT, Team
5. Wheelchair propulsion:_____ ft with:_____			5. Wheelchair skills training	PT, Team
6. Ambulation:_____ ft using:_____ with:_____			6. Gait training	PT, Team
7. Up and down:_____ stairs with:_____			7. Real-life room, flight of stairs	PT, TR
8. Community surfaces/barriers:_____			8. RLR, outing	TR, Team

Discharge Outcome(s): Transfer with:_____ Ambulation with:_____
Wheelchair propulsion with:_____ Up/down stairs with:_____

Figure 5.50. (continued)

University of Anystate Hospital

REHABILITATION PLAN OF CARE
PAGE 2 OF 4

PATIENT LABEL

Communication/Events	TD	RD	Interventions	Person(s) Responsible

Discharge Outcome(s): Effective communication skills with: _____

Bio-Psycho-Social Functioning/Events	TD	RD	Interventions	Person(s) Responsible
Redirect pain complaints with: _____			Peer interaction, relaxation techniques	TR
Interact with peers/staff with: _____			Group and individual socialization	TR

Discharge Outcome(s): Adjust to lifestyle changes and to disability; to participate in community activities at level of functioning

Cognitive/Events	TD	RD	Interventions	Person(s) Responsible
Alert and oriented X: _____			Reorientation	SLP, Team
Adaptive leisure skills with: _____			Assistive devices, resources, body awareness	TR
				SLP, Team

Discharge Outcome(s): Increase cognition to within functional limits for basic self-care with good safety awareness and judgment

Patient/Caregiver Education/Events	TD	RD	Interventions	Person(s) Responsible
1. Patient/caregiver able to relate use and frequency of medications			1. Medication teaching	Nursing
2. Patient/caregiver able to assist patient with activities of daily living and transfers			2. ADL program, transfer training	Team
3. Patient/caregiver able to relate bowel and bladder programs			3. Bowel and bladder programs	Nursing
4. Patient/caregiver able to demonstrate skin care			4. Turning, pressure relief, skin assessment, skin care, signs of infection	Team
5. Patient/caregiver able to relate nutrition and hydration requirements			5. Dietary teaching	Nursing
6. Patient/caregiver able to relate safety issues/ management precautions			6. Demonstration, discussion, activities of daily living, mobility	Team

Discharge Outcome(s): Caregiver able to safely and appropriately assist patient; patient able to manage own care

Figure 5.50. **(continued)**

University of Anystate Hospital

REHABILITATION PLAN OF CARE
PAGE 3 OF 4

```
PATIENT LABEL
```

Environmental/Discharge Planning/Events	TD	RD	Interventions	Person(s) Responsible
Discharge planning			Patient/caregiver teaching, DME assessed and ordered, patient–caregiver conference, home healthcare	Team
Identify resources and complete appropriate applications			Leisure education, transportation resources	TR

Discharge Outcome(s): Safe discharge home with caregiver and support from community resource

Other Areas of Concern/Events	TD	RD	Interventions	Person(s) Responsible
1. Preadmission bowel status			1. Bowel program	Nursing
2. Preadmission bladder status			2. Bladder program	Team
3. Skin free of breakdown			3. Pressure relief measures	Nursing
4. Wound free of infection; facilitate healing			4. Wound care: per MD; D/C staple: per MD; ET consult PRN	Physician, Nursing, ET
5. Pain less than or equal to level 3			5. Medicate prior to therapy and PRN; cold pack PRN; relaxation techniques; position Δ	Team
6. Preadmission nutritional status			6. I&O, dietary consult, monitor caloric intake	Team
7. UE strength:			7. UE exercise program	OT
8. LE strength:			8. LE exercise program	PT
9. Endurance:			9. Endurance activities	Team

Discharge Outcome(s): No fall or injury during rehabilitation stay; reestablish appropriate bowel elimination; reestablish appropriate urinary elimination; skin intact; no signs of infection; patient/caregiver able to manage wound/skin care; adequate management of pain; adequate nutritional status; maximize UE/LE strength to perform ADLs

Figure 5.50. **(continued)**

University of Anystate Hospital

REHABILITATION PLAN OF CARE
PAGE 4 OF 4

Functional Independence Measure

	ADM	CURR		ADM	CURR			
Eating			Transfer: Tub/Shower					
Grooming			Locomotion: Walk		FT	SLS	US	FIM
Bathing			Locomotion: Wheelchair		FT	SLS	US	FIM
Dressing—Upper			Stairs					
Dressing—Lower			Comprehension					
Toileting			Expression					
Bladder Management			Social Interaction					
Bowel Management			Problem Solving					
Transfer: Bed, Chair, Wheelchair			Memory					
Transfer: Toilet								

Communication with patient/caregiver prior to team conference	NSG	OT	PT	PSY	SLP	TR	SW
Progress discussed with patient/caregiver							
Patient/caregiver input for treatment goals given and discussed							
Patient/caregiver input for treatment goals given/discussed; progress related							

N/A = Patient unable to provide input toward goals due to deficit

_____   _____
Physician Signature   Date

_____   _____
Patient/Caregiver Signature   Date

_____ Initials of person reviewing team conference with patient/caregiver

Signature	Date/Time	Signature	Date/Time

REHABILITATION PLAN OF CARE
0000205 (10/2002)

- Correspondence pertinent to the patient
- Release forms
- Discharge report
- Follow-up reports

Renal Dialysis Services

Renal failure is a relatively common illness among older people. The only cure for renal failure is a kidney transplant, but dialysis performed on a regular basis (for example, three times per week) can treat the illness's symptoms. Dialysis is the process of removing toxins from the blood directly or indirectly. Hemodialysis works by gradually removing the patient's blood and pumping it through an external filtering system before the blood is returned to the body via a vascular port. Peritoneal dialysis works by instilling an electrolyte solution into the patient's peritoneum. Periodically, the fluid is drained to remove the fluid and accumulated toxins.

Hemodialysis is performed in hospital-based units as well as in dedicated ambulatory-care centers. Although it is less effective than hemodialysis, peritoneal dialysis is a simpler procedure and may even be performed in the patient's home.

The health records of dialysis patients include the following information (figure 5.51):

- Patient identification, including name and record number
- Diagnosis
- Name of the procedure
- Duration of the procedure
- Dates the procedure was performed
- Findings or results of the procedure
- Names, credentials, and signatures of the nurses or physicians who oversaw the procedure

Respiratory Services

Respiratory therapy is administered by respiratory therapists, nurses, and pulmonologists (physicians who specialize in the diagnosis and treatment of respiratory illness). Patients with acute and/or chronic respiratory conditions such as pneumonia and asthma often require respiratory therapy. Emergency respiratory therapy is often provided in hospital emergency departments when patient-administered treatments are not effective.

Basic treatments include the administration of aerosol medications and humidified oxygen. When breathing problems become life threatening, physicians administer cardiopulmonary resuscitation and/or place the patient on mechanical ventilation.

Hospitals also provide a number of diagnostic services related to respiratory conditions. Common services include pulmonary function testing and blood gas analysis. Respiratory therapists and nurses work directly with patients to provide coughing and breathing exercises and therapeutic percussion and vibration to clear the lungs of fluid and mucus.

Respiratory therapy services must be ordered by the patient's physician. Respiratory assessments and treatment plans contain information about the patient's diagnosis, the services to be provided, and the goals of treatment. (An example of a respiratory therapy report is provided in figure 5.52.)

Figure 5.51. Hemodialysis record in paper format.

Anycity General Hospital

HEMODIALYSIS RECORD

PATIENT LABEL

Machine Serial #: _____

Orders	Duration	Concentrate K+	Cell Type	Heparinization Systemic: _____ ACT Range: _____

Blood Flow	Desired Weight Loss	BP Support		Blood TXM: _____ Transfuse: _____
		Saline	Albumin	

Predialysis Labs: Postdialysis Labs:

_____   _____
_____   _____
_____   _____

Assessment: _____ kg, Weight: _____ Time:

_____
_____
_____
_____
_____
_____
_____

Plan:

_____
_____

Abbreviations

ACT	= Activated clotting time	Pres = Pressure
Art	= Arterial	Seq = Sequential
BF	= Blood flow	TMP = Transmembrane pressure
DLSC	= Dual Lumen subclavian catheter	UF = Ultrafiltration

Vital Signs	Post: ____	Pre: ____	Post: ____
Weight			
BP Supine			
BP Standing			
P			
T			
Edema			
Lungs/R			

Time	BP	Blood Flow	Dialysate Flow	Arterial Pressure	Venous Pressure	Dialysate Pressure	UF / TMP	ACT / Heparin	NS / Albumin	Weight	Interventions/Comments:

Evaluation/Goal Achievement: _____ kg   Weight: ____   Cell: ____   Total Heparin Dose: ____ units   Total Saline: ____ cc   Total Albumin: ____ g

☐ Goals and/or plan of care revised/reviewed with patient/family

Physician Signature: _____ Date: _____ RN Signature: _____ Date: _____

HEMODIALYSIS RECORD
000140 (10/2002)

Figure 5.52.   Respiratory therapy record in paper format.

Midwest Medical Center

VENTILATOR FLOW SHEET

PATIENT LABEL

Diagnoses: _____

Physician: _____

Current Settings: _____

DATE				
TIME				
INITIALS				
MODE				
SET VT				
ACTUAL VT				
PS/SPONT VT				
MINUTE VOLUME				
SET RATE/TOTAL RATE				
WAVE FORM/PF				
FIO$_2$/FIO$_2$ ACTUAL				
PRESSURE SUPPORT				
PEEP/CPAP				
PEAK PRESSURE				
SENSITIVITY				
PIP ALARM				
LIP ALARM				
LOW-PEEP ALARM				
LOW-VT ALARM				
LOW/SET VE ALARM				
HIGH-RR ALARM				
HME				
AMBU BAG/MASK				
HHN/MDI MED				
RESTRAINTS				
HR/PULSE O$_2$				
CUFF PRESSURE				
ET SIZE/PLACE CM				
BREATH SOUNDS R LUNG				
L LUNG				
SUCTION SITE				
SPUTUM AMOUNT				
COLOR				
APNEA ALARMS	Sec/VT	RR/PF/FIO$_2$	PIP/Itime	I:E/H PR

Breath Sounds:	1. Rhonchi	2. Rales	3. Wheezing	4. Diminished	5. Clear	6. Other _____
Sputum Amount:	1. Scant	2. Small	3. Moderate	4. Large	5. Copious	
Sputum Color:	1. Beige	2. Yellow	3. Blood-tinged	4. White	5. Clear	6. Other _____

Therapist Signature: _____   Date: _____

VENTILATOR FLOW SHEET
000035 (10/2002)

Chemotherapy Services

Chemotherapy involves the administration of oral and intravenous pharmaceuticals for the treatment of many forms of cancer. The type of disease determines the exact type of chemotherapeutic agent administered. Chemotherapy is performed as the primary treatment for diseases that are inoperable or cannot be treated surgically, such as leukemia. Chemotherapy is also performed in combination with surgery, radiotherapy, or with surgery and radiotherapy. The treatment goals of chemotherapy, like all treatments for cancer, may be to cure the disease, control it, or relieve its symptoms.

Intravenous forms of chemotherapy are usually performed in hospital oncology departments. Services may be performed on either an inpatient or an outpatient basis. Most patients, however, receive chemotherapy as outpatients either before or after surgical interventions to remove their tumors.

The health records of chemotherapy patients include the following information:

- Patient identification, including name and record number
- Diagnosis
- Name of the agent and method of administration
- Dates the procedure was performed
- Findings or results of treatment procedure
- Date of report and signature of the oncologist who oversaw the treatment

Radiotherapy Services

Like chemotherapy, radiotherapy (also called radiation therapy) is performed as a primary or adjuvant (supporting) treatment for neoplastic disease and many forms of cancer. Physicians specializing in nuclear medicine work with oncologists and other specialty physicians to develop treatment plans targeted to reach specific types of lesions. Radiation therapy equipment is precisely calibrated to deliver radiation to the abnormal tissue while sparing the patient's normal tissue as much as possible. Individual patients may undergo weeks of daily radiation therapy to achieve partial or complete relief of their symptoms. Radiation therapy also prevents the recurrence of the disease in many cases.

Radiotherapy is usually performed in hospital nuclear medicine or radiology departments. Services may be performed on either an inpatient or an outpatient basis. Most patients, however, receive radiotherapy as outpatients either before or after surgical interventions to remove their tumors.

The health records of radiotherapy patients include the following information:

- Patient identification, including name and record number
- Diagnosis
- Name and site of the procedure
- Dates the procedure was performed
- Findings or results of treatment procedure
- Date of report and signature of the radiologist who oversaw the treatment

Other Documentation

Special reports include autopsy reports in the case of death and incident reports in the case of unforeseen events. Certain administrative reports are also required for risk management purposes.

Additionally, facility policies and procedures should outline guidelines for treatment and the release of protected health information of minors. Special documentation procedures are also required for treatment and disclosure in specific psychiatric cases.

Who may grant authority for treatment and the disclosure of protected health information is a matter governed by federal and state laws and regulations. Generally, the authority rests with the following individuals:

- The patient, if the patient is a competent adult or emancipated minor

- A parent or legal guardian on behalf of a minor child or legally incompetent adult

- The executor or administrator of an estate if the patient is deceased

Minors Seeking Services

Additional documentation requirements are in place when the patient is a minor. Consent for treatment or release of information is required from the custodial parent or legal guardian. This applies until the minor reaches the age of majority or becomes emancipated in the eyes of the law. Documentation in the record must establish whether the patient is an emancipated minor. Common conditions of emancipation include evidence that the minor is as follows:

- Married

- On active duty with the U.S. armed forces

- Self-supporting and living away from home

- Unmarried and pregnant

Orders and Treatment in Specific Psychiatric Cases

Generally, the patient and the patient alone decides whether to consent to or forgo treatment. There are two assumptions, however:

1. The patient is competent under the law.

2. An emergency situation is not present.

In the case of a patient declared incompetent by a court of law, state law provides the order of individuals who may serve to authorize treatment and disclosure.

Discharge Summaries

The **discharge summary** is a concise account of the patient's illness, course of treatment, response to treatment, and condition at discharge. (Other terms for this type of documentation include *discharge abstract* and *clinical resume*.) The physician principally responsible for the patient's hospital care writes and signs the discharge summary. The discharge summary must be completed within thirty days after discharge for most patients but within twenty-four hours for patients transferred to other facilities. Discharge summaries are not always required for patients who were hospitalized for less than forty-eight hours. (See figures 5.53 through 5.55.)

The functions of the discharge summary include the following:

- Ensuring the continuity of future care by providing information to the patient's primary-care physician and any consulting physicians

- Providing information to support the activities of the medical staff review committee

- Providing concise information that can be used to answer information requests from authorized individuals or entities

Hospitals are required to collect specific data elements at the time of discharge. (Standardized clinical data sets are discussed in chapter 4.) These data include the following:

- Name of the physician principally responsible for the patient's care

- Date and time of discharge

- Principal and secondary diagnoses

- ICD-9-CM code for the external cause of the patient's injury, if applicable

- Diagnostic and therapeutic procedures and the dates on which the procedures were performed

- Name of the surgeon or surgeons who performed the surgical procedures, if applicable

- Disposition of the patient (for example, transferred to a subacute facility or a rehabilitation facility or discharged to home)

- Medication reconciliation

Accreditation standards and the Medicare *Conditions of Participation* (2006) require that the patient's principal diagnosis be documented by the attending physician in the patient's health record no more than thirty days after discharge. The **principal diagnosis** is the condition established, after study, to have been the main reason for the patient's admission for inpatient treatment. The **principal procedure** is the procedure that was performed for the definitive treatment (rather than the diagnosis) of the main condition or a complication of the condition. A **complication** is defined as a condition that began after the patient was admitted for inpatient care. Preexisting conditions that affected the patient's care are called **comorbidities**.

At patient discharge, hospitals are also required to collect and/or update the demographic and clinical data to be included on reimbursement claims. For inpatient services, as many as eight additional diagnostic codes can be reported in addition to the principal diagnosis. Up to five additional procedural codes can be reported along with the principal procedure. The additional diagnostic codes represent any comorbidities and/or complications that modified the course of the patient's illness and so should be considered in determining the amount of payment. The principal and additional procedural codes represent the most significant actions taken to diagnose and treat the patient's illness. The diagnostic and procedural codes are used

Figure 5.53.   Discharge summary in paper format.

Midwest Medical Center

DISCHARGE SUMMARY

SAYLORMEN, POPEYE T.
333333333
DOB: 02/09/1961

PHYSICIAN/SURGEON: Philip P. Heartstopper, MD

DATE OF DISCHARGE: 05/18/200x

PRINCIPAL OPERATION AND PROCEDURE: OPCAB × 3, left internal mammary artery of the LAD, saphenous vein graft to D-1, and saphenous vein graft to OM-1

HISTORY OF PRESENT ILLNESS: Mr. Saylormen was seen at the request of Dr. Doctor regarding surgical treatment of ischemic heart disease. He is a 42-year-old male with a family history of coronary artery disease. He smokes a pipe and had a previous myocardial infarction approximately three years ago. His current status is postangioplasty. While working on a construction project, he developed anginal-type symptoms and was seen in the emergency room and then admitted to the hospital for further evaluation.

ADMITTING DIAGNOSIS: Coronary artery disease

HOSPITAL COURSE: The patient underwent cardiac catheterization and was found to have significant three-vessel coronary artery disease. It was felt that he would benefit from undergoing an OPCAB procedure. On 05/14/200x, the patient underwent OPCAB × 3 as described above. The patient tolerated the procedure well and returned to the Cardiothoracic Intensive Care Unit hemodynamically stable. On postoperative day one, he was weaned from mechanical ventilation, extubated, and transferred to the Cardiothoracic Step-Down Unit, where he continued on a progressive course of recovery. On postoperative day four, he was up and about in his room and the halls without difficulty. Upon discharge, he was tolerating his diet well. His lungs were clear. His abdomen was soft, and his incisions were unremarkable. His vital signs were stable. He was in normal sinus rhythm. His heart rate was in the 70s and 80s. Blood pressure had been running consistently in the low 110s/60s. He was afebrile. Oxygen saturations on room air were reported at 97%.

LABORATORY DATA AT DISCHARGE: BUN 14, Creatinine 0.9, H&H 8.8 and 25.4

MEDICATIONS AT DISCHARGE: Lisinopril 5 mg q.d.; Lipitor 80 mg q.d.; metoprolol 50 mg q.d.; aspirin 81 mg q.d.; Darvocet-N 100—one to two tablets every 4–6 hours as needed for pain; iron sulfate 325 mg q.d. × 30 days; and Colace 100 mg b.i.d. × 30 days

DIET: He may follow a regular diet.

FINAL DIAGNOSIS: Coronary artery disease

DISPOSITION: No lifting greater than 10 pounds. No driving for 4–6 weeks. He may shower but he should not take a tub bath. Follow up with Dr. Doctor in 1–2 weeks.

_____   5/18/200x
Philip P. Heartstopper, MD   _____
                                                                    Date

d: 05/18/200x
t: 05/19/200x
PPH, MD/mb

Figure 5.54. Discharge summary in electronic format.

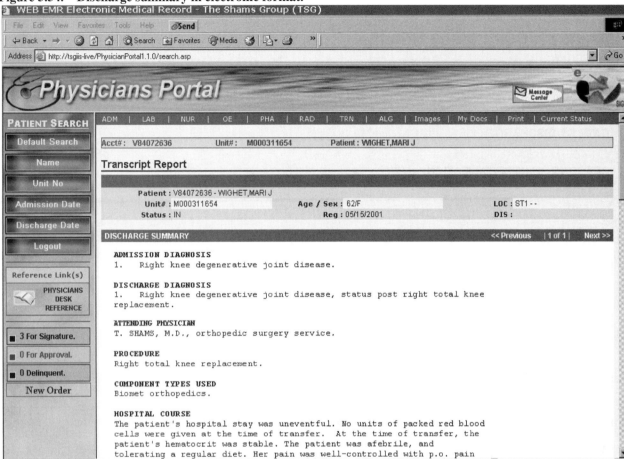

for determining reimbursement for commercial third-party payers and diagnosis-related group assignments for Medicare patients.

Despite the best efforts of hospital caregivers and physicians, some patients die while they are hospitalized. In such cases, the principal physician should add a summary statement to the patient's health record to document the circumstances surrounding the patient's death. The statement can take the form of a final progress note, a discharge summary, or a separate report. The statement should indicate the reason for the patient's admission, his or her diagnosis and course in the hospital, and a description of the events that led to his or her death.

Discharge Instructions

The discharge summary usually includes specific instructions for patient care after discharge. The instructions for aftercare may be given directly to the patient or to his or her caregiver at the time of discharge. Discharge instructions usually include the primary physician's recommendations for diet and activity levels, prescriptions for any needed medications, and referrals for follow-up care. Many hospitals also provide standardized aftercare instructions to patients

Figure 5.55.   Short form discharge summary in paper format.

Anytown Community Hospital

SHORT-FORM DISCHARGE SUMMARY

PATIENT LABEL

DATE OF DISCHARGE: _____

REASON FOR HOSPITALIZATION: _____

_____

_____

SIGNIFICANT FINDINGS: _____

_____

_____

CONDITION/CONCLUSIONS AT DISCHARGE: _____

_____

_____

PROCEDURES AND TREATMENT: _____

_____

_____

INSTRUCTIONS TO PATIENT/FAMILY: _____

_____

_____

DISCHARGE DIAGNOSIS(ES): _____

_____

_____

Physician Signature: _____   Date: _____

SHORT-FORM DISCHARGE SUMMARY
0034632 (02/2002)

who underwent inpatient or outpatient surgical procedures or received other relatively common therapeutic services (for example, chemotherapy).

To ensure patient safety after hospital treatment, it is vital that the patient receive clear, concise discharge instructions. Ideally, patient instructions should be communicated both verbally and in writing. The healthcare professional (usually the patient's primary nurse) who delivers the instructions to the patient or the caregiver should also complete health record documentation that indicates that he or she explained the instructions before the patient left the facility. In addition, the person receiving the instructions should be asked to sign a form verifying that he or she understands the instructions. A copy of the written instructions should then be filed in the patient's health record. (See figure 5.56 for an example of patient instructions.)

When someone other than the patient assumes responsibility for the patient's aftercare, the record should indicate that the instructions were given to the party responsible. Documentation of patient education may be accomplished by using forms that prompt the person providing instruction to cover specific information.

Autopsy Reports

A hospital **autopsy report** is a description of the examination of a patient's body after he or she has died. Autopsies are usually conducted when there is some question about the cause of death or when information is needed for educational or legal purposes. The purpose of the autopsy is to determine or confirm the cause of death or to provide more information about the course of the patient's illness. (See figure 5.57 for an example of an autopsy report.)

When local authorities suspect that a patient's death may have been the result of a crime, a local medical examiner may conduct the autopsy rather than a hospital pathologist. In such cases, the patient's body is generally moved to a county facility for autopsy. In most states, medical examiners are required to issue provisional autopsy reports within three days of the autopsy and final reports within sixty days.

Authorizations for autopsy, signed by the patients' next of kin or by law enforcement officials, should also be filed in the patients' permanent health records. Copies of hospital autopsy reports should also be stored in the patients' records.

Summary

In order for health records to fulfill the purpose of their creation, they must be well documented. This chapter gives widely accepted standards for quality documentation for each report type found in medical records. The content for the most commonly used forms is included along with some specialty requirements.

Documentation is compiled throughout the treatment of a patient. It begins with admission to a service and concludes with discharge from care. The four categories of information are administrative, demographic, financial, and clinical. The required elements can be collected in a paper-based or electronic system. In both cases, it is imperative that complete information be documented to facilitate quality and continuity of care for a patient and to serve the legal, statistical, and reimbursement needs of the facility and healthcare provider.

Figure 5.56.   Example of patient discharge instructions.

University of Anystate Hospitals

PATIENT/FAMILY INSTRUCTIONS
PAGE 1 OF 2

PATIENT LABEL

This is a guide for your care. Call your doctor for any problems or changes that concern you.

Diet

Diet: _____ If on special diet and have questions, call dietitian.

Managing Your Meds Discussed
(Place a checkmark if medication handouts given) ↓

Medications (list all medications)

Name/Dose	How to Take	

Activities/Special Care

Activities (Check as indicated)
- ☐ Crutches/walker
- ☐ Walk with assistance
- ☐ Gradually resume normal activity
- ☐ Bedrest
- ☐ Other _____

Dressing and Wound Care
(Report increased pain, redness, swelling, drainage, or fever)
- ☐ Doctor to change dressing
- ☐ Keep dressing dry
- ☐ If no dressing, keep incision clean and dry
- ☐ Clean wound and change dressing

Additional Instructions (PEARLS)

Follow Up (appointments/equipment/referrals)

Agency	Phone	Arrangements (instructions provided by agency)

Dr. _____   Date/Time _____ ☐ Call for an appointment

Dr. _____   Date/Time _____ ☐ Call for an appointment

Dr. _____   Date/Time _____ ☐ Call for an appointment

I understand the above instructions and have the ability to carry these out after discharge. I am aware of the importance of medical follow up with my doctor.

Patient/Patient Rep. Signature: _____ Date: _____

RN Signature: _____ Date: _____

Figure 5.56. **(continued)**

University of Anystate Hospitals

PATIENT/FAMILY INSTRUCTIONS
PAGE 2 OF 2

PATIENT LABEL

Discharge Date: _____ Time: _____ Mode: _____

Discharged With:

☐ Family member ☐ Friend ☐ By self ☐ Other: _____

Escorted by: ☐ Hospital Attendant ☐ Ambulance Attendant

RN Discharge Assessment

Continuing Care Assessment	Care Plan	☐ All goals resolved on IPOC/clinical path/plan of care. Exceptions documented.
	Discharge with: ☐ Self/family care	• Patient and/or family verbalized an understanding of instructions. Person (s) to assist if needed: _____
	Discharge with: ☐ Support services	• Patient will receive follow-up with a referral agency or extended care facility. See front of form.
	Discharge to: ☐ Home ☐ Home with home health ☐ Extended care facility ☐ Other: _____	

☐ Patient Expired   Date: Time: Valuables Given to: ☐ Family ☐ Funeral Home ☐ Security
☐ Patient Left without Permission   Date: Time:

RN Signature: _____ Date: _____

PATIENT INSTRUCTIONS
5435680 (03/2002)

Figure 5.57.   Autopsy report in paper format.

Lincoln County Hospital

AUTOPSY REPORT
PAGE 1 OF 4

O'PATIENT, RENATA H.
4378802133524
DOB: 02/18/1958

ACCESSION NUMBER: 1-1213200x

DATE OF DEATH: 12/13/200x   **DATE OF AUTOPSY:** 12/15/200x

ADMITTING PHYSICIAN: Nelda Oncodoct, DO   **PATHOLOGIST:**   Frank Reeper, MD

CONSULTING PHYSICIAN #1: Leo Kardiovsky, MD   **PROSECTOR:**   Nelda Oncodoct, DO

CONSULTING PHYSICIAN #2: NA   **ATTENDANT:**   Georges Helper

FINAL ANATOMICAL DIAGNOSES

CLINICAL DIAGNOSES:

1. Metastatic sarcoma

2. Possible sepsis

3. History of thyroid carcinoma

4. Hypocalcemia

5. Hypokalemia

6. Cortical nodules, right adrenal gland

7. Angiolipoma, left kidney

8. Myocardial hypertrophy, left ventricle

9. Diverticulosis, colon

PATHOLOGICAL DIAGNOSES:

1a. Possible primary osteosarcoma of superior sternum/anterior rib cage with superior mediastinal extension

1b. Metastatic osteosarcoma involving lungs extensively and T5 vertebral body with pathologic fracture

2a. Hemorrhagic bronchopneumonia

2b. Premortem sputum culture positive for Staphylococcus aureus (cocci identified in inflamed areas of lung at autopsy)

2c. Diffuse alveolar damage syndrome, lungs (shock lung)

3. No evidence of recurrent thyroid carcinoma, examination of neck not included

4. No anatomic correlate

5. No anatomic correlate

INCIDENTAL FINDINGS:

Signature: _____   12/15/200x
                              PATHOLOGIST   DATE

Figure 5.57. (continued)

Lincoln County Hospital

AUTOPSY REPORT
PAGE 2 OF 4

O'PATIENT, RENATA H.
4378802133524
DOB: 02/18/1958

CASE HISTORY: This 45-year-old, white female was admitted to the Medical ICU at County Hospital on 12/12/2003 after presenting earlier that day at Dr. Oncodoct's office with profound general weakness and difficulty breathing. The patient's past medical history indicated a history of thyroidectomy for tall-cell variant papillary carcinoma. She was treated postthyroidectomy with I-131 and external beam radiation because of multiple lymph node metastases. She had been diagnosed last month with metastatic sarcoma, which presented as a symptomatic T5 vertebral compression fracture. She had also developed progressive swelling of the legs, but a CT scan of the abdomen and pelvis performed several days before admission showed no evidence of venous thrombosis.

On admission, she had a potassium level of 2.5, calcium of 4.8, and phosphorus of 7.3. She was initially treated with two amps of calcium gluconate and potassium chloride administered intravenously. A chest X ray performed upon admission showed extensive masses within the lung fields, consistent with metastatic disease. Other studies performed after admission showed a free T-4 of 4.04 ng per deciliter (0.71 to 1.85). Shortly after admission, the patient was intubated and placed on a ventilator. A cardiology consultant noted pump failure secondary to tumor burden. The patient was febrile at admission, and her hypotension was thought to be secondary to sepsis. She was treated with antibiotics, but despite supportive measures, she died on the second hospital day (12/13) at 3:55 p.m. An autopsy limited to the chest and abdomen was performed on 12/15.

GROSS EXAMINATION

GENERAL INSPECTION: The body was that of a slightly malnourished female who looks like her stated age of 45 years. The body was identified as that of Renata H. O'Patient according to the ID band on her left wrist and the ID tag on her right big toe. The irises were hazel and the hair was brown, with normal female distribution. Oral and nasal tubes were present and in place. There was a single-lumen catheter in the right neck. A 9-cm, well-healed, longitudinal scar was also present on the anterior neck. There was also a full-lumen catheter in the right antecubital fossa. A Foley catheter was present. Postmortem lividity was present posteriorly, and marked edema was noted.

BODY CAVITIES: The organs of the thorax and abdomen were in their normal anatomic relationships. There was 10 ml of straw-colored serous fluid in the right and 15 ml of straw-colored serous fluid in the left pleural cavities. The pericardial sac contained 10 ml of serous fluid. The great vessels and chambers of the heart were in a normal anatomic relationship. Firm areas of gray and tan tumor involved the mediastinum. Tumor was identified and involved the upper sternum, skeletal muscle, anterior rib cage, and mediastinum. There was no fluid within the peritoneal cavity. The cranial cavity and neck organs were not examined due to permit restrictions.

CARDIOVASCULAR SYSTEM: The heart weighed 510 g and was of a normal configuration. The epicardium was normal. The heart was opened in the plan of the atrioventricular groove. Neither ventricle appeared dilated. The myocardium was reddish brown and firm. The right ventricular wall was 0.6 cm in thickness, and the left ventricular wall was 2.1 cm in thickness. The left ventricle appeared hypertrophic. No significant abnormalities were found in the valves, and the endocardium was normal. The coronary arteries had a normal anatomic distribution, with the right coronary artery being predominant. The arteries were sectioned in 0.2- to 0.3-cm intervals. The proximal right coronary artery, the main left coronary artery, the left anterior descending coronary artery, and the left circumflex coronary artery showed no calcific atherosclerosis. The aorta also showed no calcific atherosclerosis, ulceration, or mural thrombi.

RESPIRATORY SYSTEM: The mucosa of the trachea was unremarkable. The right lung weighed 1100 g and the left lung 1050 g. The pleura was glistening and nodular with multifocal gray and tan, firm lesions. The lung was fresh cut. The cut surfaces showed greater than twenty nodules within the parenchyma. The largest nodule was 8 by 6 by 3 cm, and it was located within the base of the left lower lobe. In addition, the parenchyma was congested and hemorrhagic. The bronchial walls were thickened and the mucosa reddened. The pulmonary arteries showed no atherosclerosis or thromboemboli. The hilar and bronchial lymph nodes had tumor and were enlarged.

Figure 5.57. (continued)

Lincoln County Hospital

AUTOPSY REPORT
PAGE 3 OF 4

O'PATIENT, RENATA H.
4378802133524
DOB: 02/18/1958

DIGESTIVE SYSTEM: The esophagus was unremarkable. The stomach contained approximately 10 ml of semi-liquid, tan material. The mucosa was markedly reddened. The small intestine was unremarkable. The large intestine contained brown fecal material, and scant colonic diverticula were noted. The appendix was present and unremarkable. The liver weighed 2300 g, and the capsular surface was smooth and glistening. On section, the parenchyma was reddish brown with central lobular congestion. The gallbladder contained approximately 35 ml of brown-green bile. The mucosa showed prominent yellow streaks. No stones were identified. The common bile duct was unremarkable. The pancreas appeared normal and was normal in consistency.

GENITOURINARY SYSTEM: The right kidney weighed 210 g, and the left kidney weighed 220 g. The capsule was stripped with difficulty, and the underlying cortical surfaces were coarsely granular and pitted. A 0.3-cm, firm, tan-colored nodule was noted on the left kidney. On section, the cortex measured 0.8 cm in thickness. The cortex was markedly hyperemic. The renal arteries showed no atherosclerosis. The urinary bladder showed no mass lesions. Mucosal hemorrhages were absent. The endocervical canal and os appeared unremarkable. The endometrium was pale yellow. No leiomyomas were present. The myometrium was unremarkable. The ovaries were pale yellow and without cysts.

HEMATOPOIETIC SYSTEM: The thymus was not identified. The spleen weighed 250 g and had a dull-gray capsule. On section, the spleen was dark red and firm. Systemic lymph nodes were grayish tan and enlarged. The bone marrow was reddish brown.

ENDOCRINE SYSTEM: The adrenal glands were slightly enlarged. Two separate nodules were present within the right adrenal gland. Each nodule was about 1 cm in diameter.

MUSCULOSKELETAL SYSTEM: The vertebral column showed no osteopenia. A fracture was identified along the vertebral column at T5. The fracture site was surrounded by firm areas of tan to gray tumor.

CASSETTE SUMMARY: (1) Left lung, lower lobe and tumor; (2) left lung, upper and middle lobes and tumor; (3) right lung, upper lobe and tumor; (4) right lung, middle and lower lobes; (5) T5 soft-tissue mass; (6) upper sternum and mediastinal mass; (7) T5 vertebra; (8) liver and gallbladder; (9) spleen; (10) right kidney and adrenal gland with mass; (11) left kidney and adrenal gland with cortical nodule; (12) uterus, cervix, right tube and ovary; (13) pancreas and bladder; (14) stomach, small and large intestines; (15) right and left ventricles of heart.

MICROSCOPIC EXAMINATION

GENERAL TUMOR DESCRIPTION: Sections of the tumor masses show a neoplasm characterized by highly cellular proliferations of spindle cells with generally indistinct cytoplasm and marked nuclear pleomorphism. Best demonstrated in slide A1 from a metastatic site and A6, a possible primary site, there is prominent, irregular osteoid formation characteristic of osteosarcoma. Infiltration of subchondral bone is present in the latter area. Sections of the T5 vertebra show extensive necrosis of the neoplasm within the bone with no morphologically intact residual tumor seen. The adjacent soft-tissue mass, however, shows large zones of intact neoplasm associated with areas of necrosis.

RESPIRATORY SYSTEM: In addition to the metastatic osteosarcoma, the uninvolved lung tissue shows numerous areas of an exudate of neutrophils within the alveolar spaces associated with focal areas of hemorrhage. Numerous colonies of coccoid bacteria are present within these zones of inflammation. In addition to the extensive broncho-pneumonia, other areas show vascular congestion, prominent alveolar lining cells, and focal hyaline membrane formation consistent with shock lung (diffuse alveolar damage syndrome).

Figure 5.57. **(continued)**

Lincoln County Hospital

AUTOPSY REPORT
PAGE 4 OF 4

O'PATIENT, RENATA H.
4378802133524
DOB: 02/18/1958

GENITOURINARY SYSTEM: Sections of the nodule in the left kidney show a lesion composed of spindle cells with a prominent vascular network mixed with fat cells. Spindle cells show fibrillar eosinophilic cytoplasm characteristic of smooth-muscle differentiation. This lesion represents an angiomyolipoma. There is no evidence of metastatic sarcoma. Elsewhere, the kidney shows pigment casts within tubules but no other significant findings.

ENDOCRINE SYSTEM: Sections confirm the presence of adrenal cortical nodules.

GENERAL: Sections of the other organs sampled show no additional significant findings or confirmed the gross impressions.

CASE SUMMARY: This 45-year-old white woman with a history of tall-cell variant of papillary carcinoma had been treated with I-131 and external beam radiation therapy because of multiple lymph node metastases and an aggressive primary tumor. Her course had been complicated by hypoparathyroidism. Recently, she had developed a compression fracture of the T5 vertebral body and on further evaluation was found to have a widely metastatic sarcoma involving the lungs and bones of the chest. Mediastinal tumor was noted on imaging studies. On the day before her death, the patient presented with a febrile illness and hypotension secondary to sepsis. Despite treatment, she died on the second hospital day.

Autopsy documented extensive metastatic sarcoma involving the lungs, and the large samples available at autopsy showed osteoid formation within several areas characteristic of osteosarcoma. A relatively large mass involving the superior sternum, anterior rib cage, and superior mediastinum suggested a possible primary tumor in this site. This finding raised the possibility of a postradiation sarcoma. Autopsy documented extensive pulmonary metastases involving nearly half of the lung parenchyma bilaterally. There was a large soft-tissue extension surrounding the vertebral body metastasis, and there was extensive necrosis of the bone tumor in this site consistent with recent radiation therapy.

The immediate cause of death was hemorrhagic bronchopneumonia secondary to Staphylococcus aureus, which was cultured postmortem from the sputum. Other findings in the lungs were consistent with diffuse alveolar damage syndrome secondary to shock and sepsis (shock lung).

Other findings of an incidental nature are documented in the final diagnoses.

References

American Health Information Management Association. 2005. *Documentation and Reimbursement for Behavioral Healthcare Services.* Chicago: AHIMA.

American Health Information Management Association Ambulatory Care Section. 2001. *Documentation and Reimbursement for Ambulatory Care,* Revised Ed. Chicago: AHIMA.

Centers for Medicare and Medicaid Services. 2006 (Nov. 27). Conditions of participation for hospitals; Final rule. 42 CFR Part 482. *Federal Register* 71(227): 68672–68695. Available online from http://a257.g.akamaitech. net/7/257/2422/01jan20061800/edocket.access.gpo.gov/2006/pdf/E6-19957.pdf.

Centers for Medicare and Medicaid Services. 2006. Provider agreements and supplier approval; Special responsibilities of Medicare hospitals in emergency cases; Final rule. 42 CFR Part 489.24. *Federal Register* 71(160): 48143. Available online from www.access.gpo.gov/nara/cfr/waisidx_06/42cfr489_06.html.

Food and Drug Administration. 1998. Medical device reporting; Final rule. 21 CFR 803. *Federal Register* 63(91): 26069. Available online from http://www.access.gpo.gov/nara/cfr/waisidx_06/21cfr803_06.html.

Glondys, Barbara. 1999. *Documentation Requirements for the Acute Care Patient Record.* Chicago: AHIMA.

Health Insurance Portability and Accountability Act (HIPAA) of 1996. Public Law 104-191. Available online from www.gpoaccess.gov/cfr/index.html.

Joint Commission. 2006. *2006 Comprehensive Accreditation Manual for Hospitals: The Official Handbook (CAMH).* Oakbrook Terrace, IL: Joint Commission.

McCain, Mary. 2006. Paper-based health records. Chapter 8 in *Health Information Management: Concepts, Principles, and Practice,* 2nd ed. Edited by Kathleen LaTour and Shirley Eichenwald-Maki. Chicago: AHIMA.

National Center for Injury Prevention and Control. 1997. Data elements for emergency department systems, release 1.0. Atlanta, GA: CDC. Available online from www.cdc.gov/ncipc/pub-res/pdf/deeds.pdf.

National Guideline Clearinghouse. 2007. *About NGC.* Available online from www.guideline.gov/about/about.aspx.

Shaw, Patricia, et al. 2007. *Quality and Performance Improvement in Healthcare: A Tool for Programmed Learning,* 3rd ed. Chicago: AHIMA.

U.S. Department of Health and Human Services. 1996. Public Health Service, AHCPR. Clinical practice guidelines number 19. Rockville, MD: U.S. Department of Health and Human Services.

Willner, Susan B. 2006. Clinical quality management. Chapter 11 in *Health Information Management Technology: An Applied Approach,* 2nd ed. Edited by Merida Johns. Chicago: AHIMA.

Chapter 6

Format of the Health Record

Barbara Odom-Wesley, PhD, RHIA, FAHIMA

Learning Objectives

- Compare the format, functionality, and features of three different paper-based health record formats

- Describe the format, function, and features of electronic health records

- Explain the types of technological systems that support EHRs

- Explain the functions of clinical decision support systems included in medical records

- Explain the importance of the standardization of forms and views to improve the functionality of health records

- Describe the value of standardization for acronyms, abbreviations, and symbols to improve the functionality of health records

- Link specified components of the health record system as improvements for users of the health records

- Describe the challenges of the hybrid health record

- Describe how paper-based, hybrid, and electronic health record formats affect HIM functions

Key Terms

Agency for Healthcare Research and Quality (AHRQ)

American Society for Testing and Materials (ASTM)

Clinical data repository

Clinical decision support (CDS) systems

Data exchange standards

Database

Database management system

EHR Collaborative

Electronic document management system (EDMS)

Electronic health record (EHR)

Functionality standards

Health information exchange (HIE)

Health Level Seven (HL7)

Integrated health record

Messaging standards

National Committee on Vital and Health Statistics (NCVHS)

National health information infrastructure (NHII)

National Health Information Network (NHIN)

Nationwide network for health data exchange

National Resource Center for Health Information Technology

Office of the National Coordinator for Health Information Technology (ONC)

Problem list

Problem-oriented health record

Prohibited abbreviations

Source-oriented health record

Structure and content standards

Technical standards

Vocabulary standards

Introduction

The main function of the health record is the same, no matter what format is used for documenting, processing, or storage. The health record is the principal repository for the clinical documentation relevant to the care and treatment of one specific patient. Health records also have many additional functions. The principal functions are related to specific healthcare encounters between providers and patients. The ancillary functions are related to the environment in which healthcare services are provided. A complete discussion of health record functions is given in chapter 3.

Health records must include the same patient information and perform the same communications functions without regard for the media used for data capture, process, and storage. This chapter will explore documentation formats of paper, electronic, and hybrid medical records.

Paper-based Health Records

Most healthcare facilities currently follow one of three formats for paper-based health records: the source-oriented health record, the problem-oriented health record, or the integrated health record. It is important to remember, however, that no hard-and-fast rules exist for arranging the elements of a health record. Facilities are free to select the arrangement that best suits their needs as long as their systems fulfill the requirements of state laws, federal regulations, and accreditation standards.

Source-oriented Health Records

In the **source-oriented health record**, documents are grouped together according to their point of origin. That is, laboratory records are grouped together, radiology records are grouped together, clinical notes are grouped together, and so on. Thus, physicians' progress notes for a single episode of patient care are arranged, usually in reverse chronological order, and filed together in the patient's health record. Similarly, notes prepared by nursing services, social services, and other clinical services are grouped according to service and arranged sequentially.

Under this format, the individuals charged with filing reports in paper-based records can do so simply by looking at the source and date of the report. However, the users of information filed in this type of record have more trouble. To follow or document information on the patient's course of treatment, they must search by date of occurrence in each of the sections (that is, laboratory, radiology, and every group of clinical notes). The more departments a hospital has, the more sections the source-oriented health record can have. It is left to the end user to tie together information from the various sections of the record to get a full picture of the patient's course of treatment.

Problem-oriented Health Records

The **problem-oriented health record** is easier for the patient's caregivers to use. The key characteristic of this format is that it is arranged according to a **problem list.** A problem list is an itemized description of the patient's past and present social, psychological, and medical problems. Each problem is indexed with a unique number, and reports and clinical documentation are keyed to the numbers representing the problems they address. The documentation is arranged in chronological or reverse chronological order. (See figure 6.1.)

In addition to the problem list, the problem-oriented health record contains a prescribed set of patient data, an initial care plan, and progress notes. The content of the problem-oriented health record is basically the same as the content of the source-oriented health record. Content includes the following:

- Chief complaint
- Present illness(es)
- Social history
- Medical history
- Physical examination
- Diagnostic test results

The initial care plan serves as an overall guide for addressing each of the patient's problems. The services described in the plan are numbered to correspond to the problems they address.

The patient's caregivers use progress notes to document how the patient's problems are being treated and how the patient is responding to treatment. Each progress note is labeled with the number of the problem it is intended to address. This problem-indexing system allows the clinician to easily follow the patient's course of treatment. Ideally, other elements of the health

Figure 6.1.   Example of a problem list.

Anytown Community Hospital

**INTERDISCIPLINARY PROBLEM LIST
AND PLAN OF CARE**

PATIENT LABEL

Category: Problem List:

Subcategory: ☐

                                                 ☐

Discharge Outcomes

Target Date/ Initials	Key Interventions	Discipline	Start Date/ Initials	Stop Date/ Initials

Initials	Signature	Discipline	Initials	Signature	Discipline

Key

CM = Case Manager   NSG = Nursing   RD = Registered Dietitian
DTC = Diabetes Treatment Center   OT = Occupational Therapist   RT = Respiratory Therapist
ETN = Enterostomal Nurse   PC = Pastoral Care   SLP = Speech/Language Pathologist
FSR = Financial Services Representative   PHM = Pharmacy   SW = Social Worker
HCC = Home Care Coordinator   PT = Physical Therapist

Origin:

INTERDISCIPLINARY PROBLEM LIST
000100 (10/2002)

record (such as physicians' orders) are also numbered according to the problems they address. Information in the progress notes is organized using a sequence referred to as SOAP—an acronym that reminds the provider to address all four areas of patient care:

1. **S**ubjective information (such as patient complaint)

2. **O**bjective data (such as diagnostic test results)

3. **A**ssessment (diagnosis)

4. **P**lan (treatment)

The biggest shortcoming of problem-oriented records is the inconsistent application of problem numbers to every piece of documentation.

Integrated Health Records

The third format used for paper-based acute-care records is the **integrated health record.** The integrated health record is arranged so that the documentation from various sources is intermingled and follows a strict chronological or reverse chronological order. The advantage of the integrated format is that it is easy for caregivers to follow the course of the patient's diagnosis and treatment. The disadvantage is that the format makes it difficult to compare related information. (See figure 6.2 for an example of a progress note from an integrated health record.)

To meet the required function of health records, the format, data structure, and organization are important factors. The traditional paper-based health record has many limitations.

- **Chart order**: Paper-based health records need to adhere to a strict record format, sometimes referred to as "chart order." Because paper-based records are lengthy, it is often challenging to retrieve information when it is needed. Healthcare facilities organize records according to a specific format that must be followed by every user. The greater the number of users, the more important it is that the records follow strict format guidelines.

- **Viewing capability**: Paper-based health records can be viewed by only one user and in only one place at a time. Therefore, the valuable information documented in health records is often unavailable to individual users when and where they need it.

- **Updating**: Paper-based health records are difficult to update. An active record of a patient receiving care moves from provider to provider within the healthcare facility. Individuals responsible for updating record content must hand-deliver paper documents to the record's location or wait until the record is returned to them to file the information. Updates and reports may be delayed or misplaced as a result.

- **Impermanence**: Paper-based health records are fragile. They are susceptible to damage from water, fire, and the effects of daily use. For most hospitals, maintaining duplicate copies as backups for paper records is prohibitively expensive. Consequently, paper-based health records are always at risk for being misplaced, misfiled, or damaged.

Electronic Health Records

A number of different terms are used when referring to health records created and maintained in a digital environment. Computer-based patient record (CPR), electronic medical record

Figure 6.2. **Example of an integrated progress note.**

University of Anystate Hospitals

PROGRESS NOTES
PAGE 1 OF 4

PATIENT LABEL

Barriers to Patient Education

☐ No Barriers   ☐ Language
☐ Physical   ☐ Reading Difficulties
☐ Cognitive   ☐ Lacks Readiness
☐ Emotional   ☐ Lacks Motivation
☐ Other _____

Patient/Family Instructions		Outcome	Initials	Discipline
☐ Nutrition	P/F			
☐ Medications	P/F			
☐ Activity/Rehabilitation	P/F			
☐ Safety	P/F			
☐ Signs/Symptoms	P/F			
☐ Wound/Skin Care	P/F			
☐ Pre/Postop Care	P/F			
☐ Equipment	P/F			
☐ Procedures	P/F			
☐ Treatments	P/F			
☐ Pain Management	P/F			
☐ Other	P/F			

Outcome Key:
1. Able to state understanding and/or return demonstration.
2. Unable to state understanding and/or return demonstration. Continue to reinforce. (See progress notes.)

Date	Time	Discipline	PROGRESS NOTES

Figure 6.2. (continued)

University of Anystate Hospitals

PROGRESS NOTES
PAGE 2 OF 4

PATIENT LABEL

Date	Time	Discipline	PROGRESS NOTES

Key

CM = Case Manager	NSG = Nursing	RD = Registered Dietitian
CR = Cardiac Rehabilitation	NPSY = Neuropsychology	RT = Respiratory Therapy
DTC = Diabetes Treatment Center	OT = Occupational Therapy	SLP = Speech/Language Pathologist
ETN = Enterostomal Nurse	PC = Pastoral Care	SW = Social Worker
FSR = Financial Services Representative	PHM = Pharmacy	TR = Therapeutic Recreation
HCC = Home Care Coordinator	PT = Physical Therapy	

Figure 6.2.   (continued)

University of Anystate Hospitals

PROGRESS NOTES
PAGE 3 OF 4

	PATIENT LABEL

DAILY RN REASSESSMENT

	Within Normal Anatomical Limits		

	Yes	No	
Neurological/ Musculoskeletal	☐	☐	**Level of Consciousness** ☐ Disoriented ☐ Lethargic ☐ Unresponsive ☐ Respond Only to Stimuli **Speech** ☐ Slurred ☐ Impediment ☐ Aphasic **Movement** ☐ ↓RA ☐ ↓RL ☐ ↓LA ☐ ↓LL **Sensation** ☐ Tingling ☐ Numbness **R/L Pupils** R ☐ L ☐ Nonreactive ☐ ☐ Sluggish ☐ ☐ Constricted ☐ ☐ Fixed ☐ ☐ Dilated Comments:
Heart/Vascular	☐	☐	**Heart** ☐ Skips ☐ Palpitations ☐ Valve Click ☐ Murmur ☐ Irreg. Rhythm ☐ Tachycardia ☐ Bradycardia **Edema** ☐ Generalized Location ___ Degree (1–4) ___ **Vascular (0,1,3,4)** R Radial + ___ ☐ Dop R Pedal + ___ ☐ Dop L Radial + ___ ☐ Dop L Pedal + ___ ☐ Dop Comments:
Pulmonary/ Lungs	☐	☐	**Respirations** ☐ Orthopnea ☐ Sputum Prod. ☐ Apnea ☐ Labored ☐ Shallow ☐ Retractions ☐ Snoring ☐ Irregular **Breath Sounds** ☐ Crackles ☐ Rhonchi ☐ Wheezes R ☐ ☐ ☐ L ☐ ☐ ☐ ☐ Diminished ☐ Absent R ☐ ☐ L ☐ ☐ Comments:
Gastrointestinal	☐	☐	**Bowel Sounds** ☐ Hypo ☐ Hyper ☐ Absent **Abdomen** ☐ Firm ☐ Protuberant ☐ Distended ☐ Tender **Bowel Habits** ☐ Frequency ☐ Hemorrhoids ☐ Constipation ☐ Diarrhea ☐ Ostomy ☐ Irregular **Recent Changes** ☐ Bleeding ☐ Incontinent ☐ Color Change ☐ Nausea ☐ Vomiting Comments:
Skin Integumentary	☐	☐	**Problem** ☐ Bruise: ☐ Burn: ☐ Rash: ☐ Cyanotic: **Location** ___ ___ ___ ___ **Problem** ☐ Wound: ☐ Ulcer: ☐ Other: **Location** ___ ___ **Problem** ☐ Cold & Clammy ☐ Diaphoretic ☐ Pale ☐ Jaundice Comments:
Genitourinary Reproductive	☐	☐	**Urinary** ☐ Urgency ☐ Oliguria ☐ Hematuria ☐ Incontinent ☐ Frequency ☐ Hesitancy ☐ Nocturia ☐ Dysuria **Reproductive** ☐ Discharge ☐ Bleeding ☐ Breast Problems ☐ Prostate Problems Comments:
Emotional Mental	☐	☐	☐ Anxious ☐ Uncommunicative ☐ Combative ☐ Upset ☐ Uncooperative ☐ Suicidal Ideations ☐ Withdrawn ☐ Multiple Life Crises Comments:
Pain	☐	☐	Location: ___ Onset: ___ Duration: ___ Intensity (0–10): ___ Quality/Characteristics/Pattern: ___ Comments: ___ Alleviating Factors: ___ Aggravating Factors: ___ Affects on ADL: ___ Relieved by: ___

Plan of Care	Interdisciplinary plan of care/clinical pathway/clinical guidelines ☐ **Reviewed** ☐ **Revised** Discussed with patient/family? ☐ **Yes** ☐ **No**	Referral recommended (yes) requires date and initial of person entering dept. consult/information into Star
Risk for Falls/ Injury	Patient is on falls/injury precautions ☐ **Yes** ☐ **No** If no, proceed with falls/injury reassessment: Altered mobility=2 Altered mental status=2 Fall or near fall=2 Within 24 hrs postop=2 Altered elimination pattern=2 Fails to follow directions=1 **TOTAL SCORE** ☐	High risk for falls/injury (3 or more falls) ___ Initials
Advance Directives	If patient has an advanced directive, is a copy on the chart?	☐ No ☐ Yes Date:___ Initials:___ ☐ N/A
Integument	One or more (√) checks indicates a reevaluation of the plan of care is needed. ☐ Does patient demonstrate a decrease in mobility? ☐ Does patient have any reddened areas on bony prominences? **If (√) checked, refer to the ETN** ☐ Is there a loss of previously intact skin?	☐ No ☐ Yes Date:___ Initials:___
Diabetic Treatment	**If (√) checked, refer to the DTC** ☐ Patient ordered insulin or oral agents in the past 24 hours	☐ No ☐ Yes Date:___ Initials:___
Nutrition	One or more (√) checks, refer to the RD ☐ Change in functional status (i.e., difficulty swallowing, ↓LOC) ☐ New procedure affecting nutrition (i.e., chemotherapy, dialysis) ☐ Altered diet or inadequate nutrition (i.e., TF, TPN, PPN) ☐ Patient on special diet for first time (i.e., ↓ cholesterol, ADA)	☐ No ☐ Yes Date:___ Initials:___
Discharge Planning	One or more (√) checks, refer to the CM ☐ Current discharge plan is not appropriate for patient	☐ No ☐ Yes Date:___ Initials:___
Spiritual Needs	One or more (√) checks, refer to PC ☐ Patient/family needs spiritual or emotional support from hospital chaplain, personal clergy, or religious community	☐ No ☐ Yes Date:___ Initials:___
Functional	One or more (√) checks, refer to OT/SLP/PT ☐ Has there been a surgical procedure or other condition change resulting in change in function? ☐ Change in ADLs ☐ Change in communication ☐ Change in mobility ☐ Change in swallowing	☐ No ☐ Yes Date:___ Initials:___

RN Initials: ___   RN Signature: ___   Date: ___   Time: ___   Unit: ___

Figure 6.2. (continued)

University of Anystate Hospitals

PROGRESS NOTES
PAGE 4 OF 4

PATIENT LABEL

DAILY CARE RECORD

DATE: _____

Activity	7–3	3–11	11–7
Activity Ad Lib			
Bedrest			
Dangle			
Ambulating			
Up in Chair			
Turning Time			
Position: Right Left Back			
Bedside Commode/Bathroom Privileges			
ROM/Leg Exercise			
Incentive Spirometry			
Cough, Deep Breath			
Other:			

Hygiene	7–3	3–11	11–7
Bathtub/Shower/Bed			
Complete/Self/Assist			
Skin Care			
Oral Care/Nasal Care			
Perineal Care			
Other:			

Nutrition	7–3	3–11	11–7
Type of Diet			
Amount Eaten			
HS Snack			
Calorie Count			
Tube Feeding/Supplement			
Other:			

Risk Management	7–3	3–11	11–7
Side Rails (×2 or ×4)			
Call Light in Reach			
Name Band On			
Bed in Low Position			
Fall Precaution Protocol			
Seizure Precautions			
Isolations			
*Self-Injury Precaution			
Other:			

Equipment	7–3	3–11	11–7
Telemetry/Traction			
Ventilator			
IV Pump			
Antiembolism Hose			
O₂ Amount _____ Device _____			
Feeding Pump/Bag Changed			
Suction-Gastric/Thoracic/Oral			
Special Mattress/Bed			
Skin Protectors			
Sequential Compression Device			
Pulse Oximeter			
Other:			

√=Maintained entire shift   *Refer to interdisciplinary progress notes (for equipment that is ordered and recorded in notes).

Maintenance Record

	Site Port	Time Int.

Cap/Δ
Site Care
Site Start/Δ
Size

Primary Caregiver Signatures

7–3	
3–11	
11–7	

Initials	Additional Signatures

Specimen/Tests/Procedures

Specimen	Results
Type	
Blood	
Urine	
Stool/Wound	
X-ray	
Scan	
Diagnostic Test	

Respiratory Care Services

Therapy: □ HHN □ MDI □ CPT □ Other_____
Frequency: _____ Hour _____ ID □ A/C □ WA

7 a.m.	8	9	10	11	12	1	2	3	4	5	6
7 p.m.	8	9	10	11	12	1	2	3	4	5	6

Special Instructions:

Medication & Dose:

Comments:

Site Check: (IV/INT/AV Fistula = q. 8. h.)

Initials = No evidence of redness, swelling, or drainage; rate and fluid checked; and/or presence of bruit and thrill. *Refer to IPN

Site	7–3	3–11	11–7

Sites

SC = Subclavian (R or L)	PC = Portacath
RAV = Right AV Fistula	LAV = Left AV Fistula
H = Hickman	PB = Piggyback
LA = Left Arm	RA = Right Arm
LH = Left Hand	RH = Right Hand
O=	

PROGRESS NOTES
000009 (11/2002)

(EMR), and electronic patient record (EPR) are some of the most common. Currently, the preferred term is **electronic health record** or **EHR**.

Definition of the Electronic Health Record

The American Health Information Management Association (AHIMA) reserves the term *EHR* for record systems that fulfill the Institute of Medicine's vision for computer-based records (Dick et al. 1997). The Institute of Medicine provides health and science policy guidance to all sectors of society.

In its landmark report, *The Computer-Based Patient Record: An Essential Technology for Health Care*, the Institute of Medicine defined the EHR as:

> . . . an electronic patient record that resides in a system specifically designed to support users by providing accessibility to complete and accurate data, alerts, reminders, clinical decision support systems, links to medical knowledge, and other aids. (Dick et al. 1997, 55)

True EHRs are not simply digitized versions of traditional paper records. Rather, they incorporate sophisticated data capture and retrieval technology as well as fully functional decision support systems. In addition, the infrastructure of EHRs automatically protects the security and integrity of clinical documentation and makes it available instantaneously to multiple users.

Many hospitals and other healthcare organizations are currently using computerized health record systems that store information as images rather than as individual data elements. In other words, many existing computer-based records are electronic versions of paper documentation. For example, a record in this type of system might contain a scanned digital image of a patient's history and physical report, but the clinical information contained within the history and physical report is only accessible visually (it cannot be electronically searched). Therefore, this report still functions in the same way that a paper-based record functions, and it has many of the same limitations of paper-based records.

Current computer-based record systems do make patient information more widely accessible, but most lack the decision support capabilities and links to expert medical resources that are characteristic of fully functional EHRs. In today's healthcare environment, few organizations have implemented fully functional EHRs as envisioned by the Institute of Medicine. However, the implementation of electronic imaging technology in mixed-media records stored electronically is probably the first step toward more widespread adoption of true EHRs.

EHR Standards

Health Level Seven (HL7), a healthcare standards development organization, completed the initial work on a functional model for EHRs in late 2003. In early 2004, industry stakeholders, led by the EHR Collaborative, voted to adopt a proposed model. The **EHR Collaborative** is composed of several allied health and trade associations, including AHIMA, which support the universal implementation of EHRs. A new functional model, which lists more than 160 functions recommended for EHRs, was released in 2007 (HL7). AHIMA, along with the other healthcare organizations participating in the EHR Collaborative, has stated that the adoption of a national EHR standard will stimulate the commercial development of more broadly applicable and less costly electronic health record systems.

The **American Society for Testing and Materials (ASTM)** has also developed a standard for electronic health records. This standard, currently titled, Standard Practice for Content and

Structure of the Electronic Health Record (EHR), has been revised several times since its initial release in 1999. The current standard, E1384-07, was revised in October 2007. The standard covers the content and structure of electronic health records and provides guidelines for healthcare organizations planning and implementing new systems.

[handwritten margin note: trying to combine standards]

The vision for a **nationwide network for health data exchange** began more than a decade ago with the Institute of Medicine's report, *The Computer-Based Patient Record* (Dick et al. 1997). In that study, the institute recommended a major, coordinated national effort, with federal funding and strong private-sector advisory support, to accelerate the adoption of computerized medical records. In the years that have followed, consensus has emerged that the nation's medical system must replace its outdated and frequently error-plagued, paper-based approach to information management.

Because moving patient data from paper to electronic methods dramatically increases its potential mobility, discussion has turned to ways that data can be organized and shared to improve care and decrease cost. An early champion was the **National Committee on Vital and Health Statistics (NCVHS)**. In 1997, NCVHS began exploring the concept of a **national health information infrastructure (NHII)**, the framework that would support the appropriate and secure exchange of health information.

[handwritten margin note: dealing with technologies to reduce costs]

The current surge in activity began with President Bush's January 2004 State of the Union Address, which contained a mention of the benefits of computerized health records. This was followed in spring 2004 by an executive order creating the **Office of the National Coordinator for Health Information Technology (ONC)** within the Department of Health and Human Services (HHS). One of the coordinator's duties was to oversee development of an NHII, and within 90 days of its creation, ONC released "The Decade of Health Information Technology," which became better known as the "Strategic Framework" (Thompson and Brailer 2004). Soon after this, NHII disappeared as ONC referenced the **National Health Information Network (NHIN)**. The following year, the title was revised, switching from *national to nationwide*, reflecting an integration of locally managed networks rather than a single, national database.

[handwritten margin note: started RHIO's]

Today, much of the activity in health information technology concerning the private sector comes from within the Department of HHS. The **Agency for Healthcare Research and Quality (AHRQ)** provides funding and information for health information technology projects, including grants to state and regional **health information exchange (HIE)** initiatives. The **National Resource Center for Health Information Technology** provides technical assistance. The Department of HHS plays an active role promoting industry discussion, research, and demonstrations.

The universal adoption of an electronic health records system may still be years off, but the change is inevitable. The primary goals of every health record system are to facilitate the sharing of clinical information and to ensure the quality and safety of patient care. Increasing demands for accurate, secure, and accessible health information will only be fully met through the application of advanced communications technology. The AHIMA Foundation for Research and Education (FORE) funded research on standards for the content of the electronic health record. This study, originally published in *Perspectives on Health Information Management* (2004), is reproduced in appendix F on the accompanying CD.

Format of the Electronic Health Record

The EHR is possible due to the evolution of technology for information capture, storage, and exchange. By design, the EHR addresses many of the limitations in functionality of paper-based health record systems. For example, EHRs are almost always accessible through a network; so the availability problems characteristic of paper-based records do not affect electronic records. EHR advantages that enhance record functionality include the following:

- Indexing and searching databases for more enhanced information retrieval

- Allowing various levels of access and customized views

- Allowing multiple users to access the same information simultaneously

- Performing complex or difficult tasks quickly and accurately

- Permitting ready access to volumes of professional resource information such as practice standards and medical literature

Improved functionality of electronic health records includes the ease with which they can be updated and maintained. Because EHRs can be copied and stored on a variety of electronic media, computer files can be backed up frequently and stored at off-site locations or in secure storage areas within the facility. Thus, they can be more easily protected from damage, loss, and tampering than paper-based records.

However, there are some disadvantages to EHR systems. They can be very expensive to design, implement, and maintain. Like all technological advances, the cost of EHR systems is probably the highest now, when the technology is still relatively new. As national standards are accepted and more customers want the technology, more vendors will begin marketing uniform systems that meet industry standards. Prices should decrease dramatically after the original development costs have been recouped and manufacturing processes have been refined.

EHR systems are expensive to implement because of the extensive training required for health record users. The need to make process changes, redevelop health record policies and procedures, convert existing paper records to electronic formats, and recruit information system support staff also adds to the total cost of implementing a new system.

For healthcare providers and institutions, the implementation of an EHR system can yield significant documentation-capture functionality to support healthcare facility operations and customer care.

Technological Infrastructure for EHRs

Electronic health record systems are very complex. Unlike other digital systems currently used in hospitals to perform relatively narrow functions (such as admitting, administration, or laboratory reporting), EHRs fulfill a number of interrelated communication functions involving virtually every area of the hospital.

Communications technology has evolved quickly over the past fifteen years, and systems developers and health information administrators often find it challenging to keep up with new developments. System administrators also must develop ways to make existing information systems work with new technological devices.

A number of communications technologies support health record systems formats. The most important are databases, database management systems, image processing and storage systems, data capture and retrieval technology, and servers and networks. (See figures 6.3 and 6.4.)

Databases and Database Management Systems

A **database** is an organized collection of data that have been stored electronically for easy access. **Database management systems** make it possible to create, modify, delete, and view the data in a database.

Figure 6.3. Physical and logical data repositories for EHR systems.

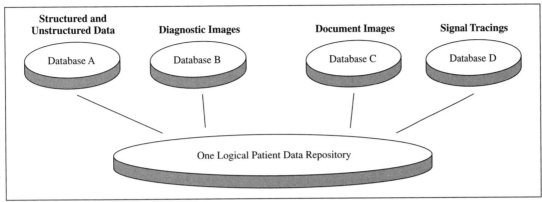

Most health record systems are organized according to one of two database models—the centralized and the distributed—or in a hybrid of the two models. In the centralized system, all of the organization's patient health information and data are stored in a single system. In the distributed model, patient health information and data are distributed in department-based systems or subsystems that are able to exchange information with one another.

The centralized system, using an electronic format, is frequently built around a clinical data repository. A **clinical data repository** is a centralized database that captures, sorts, and processes patient data and then returns them to the user. These functions demand specialized database management capabilities. The most common type of database management system in use today is the relational database, which uses data tables to organize information. New types of database management systems are in development and will probably speed up processing time in the future. (See figure 6.5.)

Figure 6.4. EHR data types and their sources.

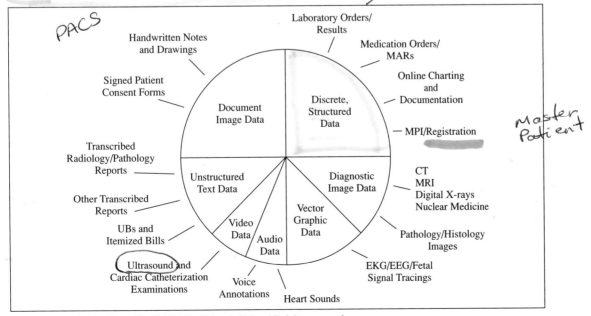

Figure 6.5.   Conceptual model for a health information management system.

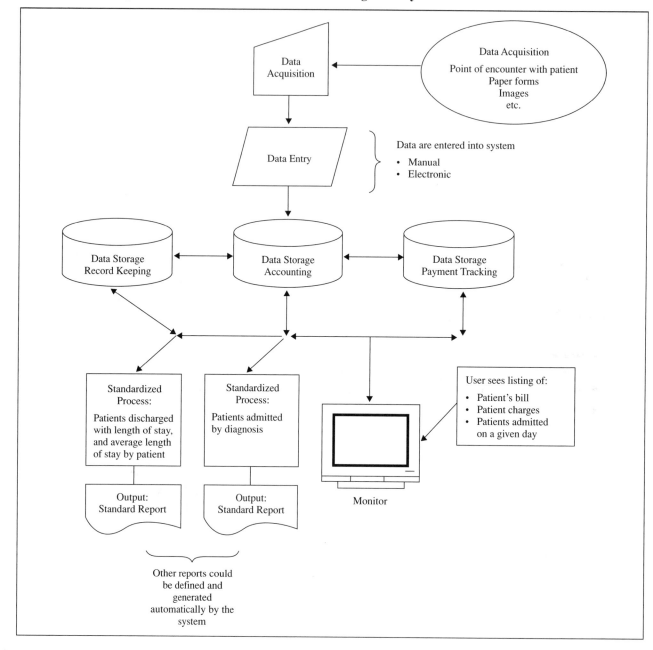

In decentralized systems, health record information is retained in separate departmental computer systems or databases. Data are then exchanged among departmental systems as needed (for example, between the clinical laboratory's system and the obstetrics unit's system).

The decentralized system can work relatively well when all or most of the facility's computers use the same proprietary operating system. However, all of the organization's departments must follow established **messaging standards**, also called interoperability standards or **data exchange standards**, which ensure that all of the organization's data are structured and formatted in the same way (Amatayakul 2007, 242).

Image Processing and Storage Technology

Traditional paper-based health records include few photographs and diagnostic images. With the introduction of clinical imaging devices, it is now possible to combine health record text files with digital diagnostic images (x-rays, CT scans, and so on) as well as digital photographs. With this technology, clinicians at different locations can view the same images at the same time and then compare their diagnostic interpretations.

Many hospitals incorporate documents into their electronic health record systems using image-processing technology. Digital scanners create images of handwritten and printed documents that are then stored in health record databases as electronic files. Using scanned images solves many of the problems associated with traditional paper-based health records. Digital files can be backed up frequently, which helps solve the problem of lost paper and microfilm records. In addition, because digital files are always under the control of a system administrator, access and confidentiality can be protected simultaneously. Digital imaging also makes it possible for more than one clinician to view the same document at the same time from distant locations. However, as noted previously, clinical documentation stored as digital images can only be accessed visually; that is, it cannot be searched electronically.

Data Retrieval Technology

Retrieving specific data elements from a paper record can require a lot of time and effort. Many organizations have attempted to improve retrieval processes by using color-coded file folders, flags, and tabs as well as automated record-tracking systems. Data content required for reporting is often abstracted from the paper chart and entered into a computer system for processing. Although such methods are helpful, they have not completely resolved the problem of inefficient information retrieval. Abstracting data is expensive.

The ultimate goal of every health record keeping system is the fast and secure delivery of accurate and complete health information to authorized recipients when and where they need it. To be effective, data retrieval systems must be based on the needs of the users.

Database systems that use query language applications allow users to perform text searches of electronic health record data. The ability to identify key words and phrases in textual data makes it easier to find and retrieve key pieces of patient information from health records.

The usefulness of text search technology in healthcare applications has been limited by the lack of standardization in medical terminology. Currently, several different medical terms can be used to describe the same condition. For example, angiohemophilia may also be called von Willebrand's disease, von Willebrand's syndrome, constitutional thrombopathy, or vascular hemophilia. As a result, text searches using one of the synonyms for this condition would likely yield only a small portion of the information that is actually available.

To address this problem, healthcare industry groups are working together to develop standardized, controlled medical vocabularies. Of these, the Systematized Nomenclature of Medicine–Clinical Terms® (SNOMED CT®) is the one most likely to be adopted universally.

Data-capture Technology

Creating a workable data-capture process has proved to be one of the biggest challenges in electronic health record system development and implementation. Ideally, the individual responsible for providing each service enters the documentation for the service into the health record database at or near the time the service is performed. Once recorded, the information

227

becomes available immediately to all authorized users who need access. However, many clinicians who graduated from medical school before the widespread use of personal computers are very reluctant to learn how to input data directly into electronic records and instead, use dictation devices. Transcription of dictated reports is still the most common type of data input for health records. Although there are forms of structured data input that clinicians will tolerate, most do not have time to enter data directly into a health record system. The reliability of voice recognition systems is steadily improving, and this technology is expected to become a common clinical documentation tool in the future.

Optical character readers (OCRs) may also play a role in data capture. These devices work like digital scanners and can be used to convert handwritten data into digital data. Additional data-capture tools are being developed for clinical documentation using mobile devices and voice commands. Still in the developmental stage are sophisticated systems that apply natural language processing, which permits narrative text to be converted to discrete data for processing by the computer (Amatayakul 2007, 12).

Healthcare Information System Standards

In the current healthcare environment, there are hundreds of healthcare information system (HIS) vendors but limited standardization of products. The use of proprietary software and technology is widespread. Healthcare professionals, managers, policy makers, regulators, and educators often struggle to locate and share information among incompatible computer information systems.

Unlike other industries, such as banking and air travel, the healthcare industry has been slow to develop and accept information system (IS) standardization. Even in areas where information technology standards exist, noncompliance remains a problem. The slow progress toward industry standardization was a major contributing factor behind the passage of the Health Insurance Portability and Accountability Act (HIPAA) in 1996. (HIPAA regulations are discussed in chapter 2.)

Recent efforts toward the development of healthcare IS standards have gained momentum. Today, the following standards development organizations are working to develop terminology, messaging, and data content standards for healthcare information system:

- Health Level Seven (HL7)
- American Society for Testing and Materials (ASTM)
- The Institute of Electronic and Electrical Engineers (IEEE)
- American College of Radiologists/National Electrical Manufacturers Association (ACR/NEMA)
- International Standards Organization (ISO)
- Systematized Nomenclature of Medicine–Clinical Terms (SNOMED CT)
- National Library of Medicine (NLM)
- Unified Medical Language System (UMLS)
- Certification Commission on Health Information Technology (CCHIT)

For health record systems to function beyond one healthcare facility, several types of HIS standards must be established and followed (LaTour 2007, 180).

- **Structure and content standards** establish and provide clear and uniform definitions of the data elements to be included in EHR systems. They specify the type of data to be collected in each data field, the length of each data field, and the attributes of each data field, all of which are captured in data dictionaries.

- **Functionality standards** define the components that an EHR needs to support the functions for which it is designed. HL7 draft standards for an EHR were developed in 2004 and, at the time of publication, were being tested in the healthcare industry.

- **Technical standards** complement content and structure and **vocabulary standards** are the next step in making interoperability possible. Technical standards provide the rules, often called protocols, for how these data are actually transmitted from one computer system to another.

Standardization of Forms and Views

Documentation for health records is contributed by the clinical team involved in direct and indirect care of a patient. The HIM professional is knowledgeable about the documentation standards of various agencies and accrediting bodies. The HIM professional has access to two tools to guide compliance to these guidelines and influence the quality of record entries: clinical team training and forms design.

Forms management is critical in both electronic data-management systems and traditional paper-based record systems. The standardization of data-capture tools ensures the quality and completeness of health record content in both paper-based and computer-based environments Most acute-care organizations have established forms committees to oversee the development, review, and control of the facilities' data-capturing tools, including all paper forms and on-screen views and interface. The committee should include information users from the following departments (Roberts 2007, 371):

- Health information management

- Medical staff

- Nursing staff

- Purchasing

- Information services

- Performance improvement

- Support and ancillary departments

The forms committee or a representative of the committee usually works directly with commercial vendors to develop health record forms or electronic data-capture systems that fulfill the information needs of the organization. Chapter 5, figure 5.12 provides an example of a physician's order in an electronic format. For comparison, refer to figure 5.11 for an example of a physician's order in a paper-based format.

In an effort to merge paper forms with electronic documentation, healthcare organizations implement document imaging and document management systems. An important function of the forms committee is to develop specific guidelines for forms development and specifications. Guidelines may include paper size and color, page borders, shading, bar code requirements, and page orientation.

The design of on-screen views and data entry interface is one of the most important considerations in developing EHR systems. Electronic systems allow individual users to choose the way data are presented, so designers should understand how clinicians and other users prefer to receive information. For example, physicians generally prefer to find all of the information they need in one place. Therefore, putting as much information as possible on each view meets their needs better than creating less crowded views that require users to scroll down to see the information or to proceed through multiple views.

In both electronic and paper-based health record systems, the most important step in the standardization of forms and views is to establish the information needs of health information users. Every form or view must fulfill its intended purpose by including all of the data required in an appropriate and easy-to-use format.

For example, when the purpose of a form is to provide patient instructions for aftercare, the data elements on the form must provide all of the information the patient will need in language that the patient can understand. Similarly, when the form is meant to be completed by hand, the response areas on the form must allow enough space for handwritten information. When the purpose of a view is to provide clinicians with an update on the patient's condition, the view should contain all of the pertinent information in a format that can be reviewed at a glance. Complete principles of form and interface design are provided in appendix G on the accompanying CD.

Following thoughtful design practices may not always ensure the overall effectiveness of the organization's documentation and data entry tools. Duplication and redundancy can also frustrate users and yield conflicting information. Forms design and management processes should ensure that only one version of each form is available for use at any one time. Processes should also look at the number of different forms in use to determine whether the same information is being collected on multiple forms or views in more than one way.

Standardization of Acronyms, Abbreviations, and Symbols

To avoid ambiguity, facilities should standardize the abbreviations, acronyms, and symbols that are used in health record documentation. Hospital health record policies and medical staff rules should determine which symbols, acronyms, and abbreviations may be used by the clinicians who author health record entries, and the rules should be enforced. As an alternative method, some hospitals develop lists of prohibited acronyms, symbols, and abbreviations rather than approved lists.

In 2003, the Joint Commission published six patient safety goals, one of which requires healthcare organizations to designate the abbreviations that should never be used in health records (Joint Commission 2003). In general, **prohibited abbreviations** are those that have more than one meaning or can easily be misinterpreted in handwritten form, with potentially dangerous results for patients. The Joint Commission now requires hospitals to prohibit the use of the following abbreviations in all handwritten, patient-specific documentation:

- **U** (for unit)
- **IU** or **iu**
- **QD** or **qd**
- **QOD** or **qod**
- **.0** (zero after a decimal point)
- **0.** (zero before a decimal point)
- **MS, MSO4, MgSO4**

Symbols, acronyms, and abbreviations should be limited to those that are the most widely applicable and unambiguous. The list of abbreviations, acronyms, and symbols should include the accepted definition of each entry, and ideally, each abbreviation, acronym, or symbol should have only one meaning. When illustrations, forms, or other complex materials use numerous or unusual abbreviations, the author should provide a legend to explain what the abbreviations mean.

Because of space limitations, symbols, acronyms, and abbreviations are more likely to be used in on-screen, EHR data entry. This can lead to problems in interpretation. To solve this problem, developers should consider creating a feature whereby definitions are made available when users click an abbreviation, symbol, or acronym.

Clinical Support Technology

The AHIMA vision statement "Quality Healthcare Through Quality Information" spotlights the most important function for healthcare records. Imagine a physician attempting to treat a seriously ill patient with no information about the patient's history, past illnesses, or current medications. At best, treatment would be delayed while the physician orders diagnostic tests to learn helpful information. The HIM work of data capture, processing, and storage are all purposed to ensure information is available when needed to provide quality care. Components of the HIS are designed to support this purpose.

Clinical Decision Support Systems

Clinical decision support (CDS) systems help physicians and other clinicians make diagnostic and treatment decisions. A CDS system automatically analyzes health record data and searches for unusual patterns. When a potential problem is identified (for example, a drug interaction), the system issues an alert or a reminder that includes a recommendation for specific corrective action.

The technology that supports these functions of CDS systems may be categorized as rules engines, statistical analyses, search engines, and expert systems that incorporate a variety of analytical tools (Amatayakul 2007, 396).

Links to Secondary Databases

Clinical indexes and registries have been compiled by acute-care hospitals and other healthcare organizations for decades. These secondary databases are a valuable source of information for healthcare policy makers, researchers, and educators. In the past, the information in secondary databases was compiled directly from paper-based health records; so maintaining the databases was labor intensive and expensive.

Today, the availability of clinical information in digital format has made it easier and less expensive to create secondary databases. (For example, information on diagnoses and procedures is routinely collected in the form of ICD-9-CM codes, which are recorded electronically during the coding and billing process.) As a result, the number, size, and complexity of clinical registries, indexes, and other databases have grown rapidly. Database development, however, has not been without its problems. Organizations that manage clinical databases have had to deal with a number of complex issues, including patient confidentiality, health information ownership and control, and data quality and accuracy.

The Hybrid Health Record

Most healthcare entities are in transition from paper-based health records to electronic health records. The speed of this transformation varies from entity to entity based on a variety of internal and external factors. The often-lengthy transition to the electronic health record forces healthcare facilities to manage and maintain a hybrid medical record.

Definition of the Hybrid Health Record

An AHIMA e-HIM Work Group (2003b) used the following to describe the hybrid health record.

A hybrid health record is a system with functional components that:

- Includes both paper and electronic documents
- Uses both manual and electronic processes

Managing health information in this hybrid environment is challenging, particularly given the transition management requirements. Nevertheless, there is some risk to any organization that customer quality of care may be adversely affected if the transition from a paper-based environment to an electronic environment is not effectively managed. See appendix A on the accompanying CD for the AHIMA practice brief, "The Complete Medical Record in a Hybrid EHR Environment" (2003).

Format of the Hybrid Health Record

In essence, the hybrid medical record is a transitional medical record. It is dynamic in nature, and the format and content continuously change as healthcare facilities continue on their journey to a fully electronic health record.

Hybrid records are positive steps toward the EHR, but they also create special challenges. Both manual and computer processes must be supported, policies and procedure are needed for both types of systems, and appropriate safeguards must be in place for privacy and security of both systems. A definition of what constitutes a record in each system must be developed. As the transition occurs, it is also important to regularly update system descriptions, including the location of all care documents, so that patient health information remains readily available to users. The AHIMA e-HIM Work Group (2003) suggested a matrix for this step. See table 6.1 for an example.

As the electronic system develops, different versions of documents may exist, and these also must be monitored and logged for both legal and practice purposes. Additionally, the AHIMA e-HIM Task Force (2003) describes in detail changes in health information processes and procedures that are required as a record transitions from paper to hybrid to fully electronic.

Table 6.1   Hybrid health record legal source legend

Report/Document Types	LHR Media Type (P)aper/(E)lectronic	Source System Application (nonpaper)	Electronic Storage Start Date	Stop Printing Start Date
Organization's Name **HYBRID HEALTH RECORD** **LEGAL SOURCE LEGEND**				
Admission History & Physical	P/E	System 1	1/1/2002	1/1/2003
Attending Admission Notes	P			
Physician Orders	E			
Inpatient Progress Notes	P			
Discharge Summary	E	System 1	1/1/2002	4/1/2002
Inpatient Transfer Note	E	System 1	1/1/2002	
Outpatient Progress Notes	P			
Clinical Laboratory Results— (Preliminary/Interim)	E	System 2	1/1/1999	1/1/1999
Clinical Laboratory Results—(Final)	E	System 2	1/1/1999	1/1/2000
Radiology Reports	E	System 3	7/1/2003	
Care Flow Sheets	E	System 1	6/1/2003	
Medication Records	E	System 1	7/1/2003	
Clinical Consult Reports	E	System 1	1/1/2002	
Preoperative, Preprocedure Notes	P			
Pathology Reports	E	System 2	1/1/1999	1/1/2000
Organ/Tissue Donation or Transplants	P			
Patient Problem List (Summary List)	E	System 1	8/1/2003	
Urgent-Care and Emergency Records	P			
Consents[a]	E	System 4	TBD	
Advance Directive				
Correspondence[a]	E	System 4	TBD	
Preoperative Anesthetic Assessments and Plans	P			
Intraoperative Documentation	P			
Postoperative Documentation	P			
Brief Postoperative Note	P			
Surgical Operative Reports	E	System 1	1/1/2002	

[a]Scanned electronic documents

Source: AHIMA 2003.

Health Record Storage Systems

Paper-based and electronic health records have different storage requirements. As discussed earlier in the chapter, electronic health records are stored digitally in centralized or departmental clinical data repositories. The storage options for paper and mixed-media records include paper-based storage systems, microfilm-based storage systems, and digital image-based storage systems.

Paper-based Storage Systems

No matter what type of identification system a facility uses, most use color coding on health record folders to make storage and retrieval more efficient. Color-coded file folders are available from suppliers, but color-coded labels can also be used to organize records.

Paper-based health record files can be stored in vertical or lateral filing cabinets, open-shelf files, or compressible file systems. Vertical file cabinets are difficult to access and are rarely used to store health records. Lateral file cabinets are easier to access but are used only in low-volume areas of the hospital.

Hospitals usually use open-shelf or compressible files for housing paper-based health records. Open-shelf filing units resemble open bookshelves. Some are always open, and others have recessed doors that can be closed and locked.

Compressible file systems take up less space than fixed storage units. Compressible file systems are similar to open-shelf systems. The difference is that the shelving units are not fixed. In one type of compressible system, the units are mounted on permanent tracks in the floor so that they can be moved. Another type of compressible system is made up of horizontal or vertical carousels. The horizontal, open-shelf carousel contains files that revolve around a central spine or track. The vertical carousel brings all files or records directly to a workstation. Vertical carousel systems are often used to store master patient indexes.

Microfilm-based Storage Systems

Paper-based health records require a huge amount of storage space, but alternative storage options can reduce space needs significantly. Storing images of paper reports and documentation on microfilm is an effective option for inactive or infrequently used health records. Microfilm records are also acceptable as courtroom evidence, because they are difficult to alter (Johns 2007, 348).

The process of microfilming involves making special photomicrographs of the original paper documents. These tiny negative film images are then archived for long-term storage. Anyone who is interested in accessing the stored records must use a special microfilm reader, which magnifies the images.

Image-based Storage Systems

Another solution for health records storage is an **electronic document management system (EDMS)**. Source documents are scanned to create digital images of the original documents. The digital documents can then be stored electronically on optical disks. Some digital scanners can process hundreds or even thousands of documents per day. Access to images stored on optical disks is fast and easy, and scanned information can be made available simultaneously to any number of users. Document scanning is also used to convert stored health record information into images that can be loaded onto new electronic health record systems. See appendix H on the accompanying CD for more information about EDMS.

Health Record Formats Impact on HIM Functions

The format of health records impacts how HIM professionals manage standard departmental functions. For example, managing the health record completion process in a paper-based facility consists of identifying deficiencies by manually reviewing the paper health record. In the hybrid health record environment, adding an electronic process, such as electronic signatures, enables record completion to be accomplished remotely. When a completely electronic health records system is implemented, deficiencies are identified automatically, and health records can be monitored for unsigned reports, unviewed results, and missing reports. Table 6.2 describes HIM functions in paper-based, hybrid, and electronic health record environments.

The transformation of HIM functions is not always easy. The path of change, especially in the hybrid record environment, has many different twists. There is no one right way to do things. The changes are not always efficient, nor are the outcomes perfect—in fact, at times, they may be downright difficult and ugly.

Table 6.2 outlines the transformation that occurs in HIM functions as the format of the health record moves from a paper-based state through the hybrid transformation into the fully electronic health record.

Summary

It is critical to expedite the location of information within health records by adhering to a predetermined, published, standardized format for data entry. With a paper-based record, this is accomplished with well-designed forms that guide the entry of data elements. With an electronic health record, it is accomplished by a well-designed interface and edit prompts that guide data entry. As facilities transition from paper-based health records to electronic health records, hybrid health records require the utilization of features from both formats. By standardizing the format and content of health records, providers can meet requirements for record completion and data quality as well as storing information in a location that facilitates retrieval.

Table 6.2 EHR impact on HIM functions

Function	Paper Health Record	Hybrid Paper-Electronic Health Record	Electronic Health Record
Abstracting data elements	Data is entered manually into computerized system.	Function is streamlined by initiating structured data collection through online forms and data entry templates at the point of care. HIM involvement includes designing and revising documentation forms to meet data collection and regulatory and bylaws requirements.	Function is eliminated with automated data capture. (This excludes free-form documentation such as narrative notes, dictations, and natural language processing.) Qualified HIM staff performs data analysis and administration, verification, and reporting. Documentation templates are developed to conform to state, federal, tribal, and local laws.
Admission and discharge processing and reconciliation	Accounting for records to ensure 100 percent retrieval of cases for filing and coding; function is performed by clerks.	Accounting for paper records to ensure 100 percent retrieval of cases for filing portions of paper record, scanning, and coding; function is performed by clerks or scanning staff.	Accounting for paper records is received from external sources for scanning; function is performed by scanning staff. Online reconciliation of cases for revenue stream; function is performed by coders.
Adoption record change	Minimal	Minimal	Minimal
Analysis (or deficiency analysis)	Assessment for compliance with regulatory and internal medical staff bylaws requirements is performed manually.	Assessment rules and rules to force completion evolve; some analysis work is reduced. Staff can be reallocated, via work queues, to preadmission analysis (such as ensuring that H&P is adequate prior to surgery or MD orders are complete for nursing home or rehabilitation facilities). Physicians receive electronic notification of incomplete items in the health record.	Function is minimal due to automated rules. In the absence of rules, HIM staff checks documents (such as handwritten documents, voice recognition, dictations). Physicians receive electronic notification of incomplete items in the health record.
Assembly of paper record	Manual	Manual for remaining paper documents	Staff is redeployed for document preparation, indexing, imaging, and quality control.
Back up, downtime, and recovery processes	Paper-based charts are used.	Organizations develop "worst-case scenario" plans to address issues such as what to do when EHRs are unavailable. HIM staff directs system disaster efforts (such as printing key documents, maintaining daily backups and paper systems, coordinating data entry, and scanning key data elements after unplanned downtime). Necessary forms revert to paper processes and are readily available. Staff is trained in their use.	Same as hybrid state. The backup system could be a CD with appropriate documents that are accessible from a local drive rather than the network. Downtime processes include use of PDAs or tablet PCs that provide for data uploading after the system is recovered.

Function		
Birth and death certificate preparation	Staff conducts interviews, collects data, types, completes paper forms or electronic submissions, and obtains signatures required by state law.	Clerical staff continues to abstract and collect data for vital records; however, state or county laws may mandate use of an electronic data submission process. Electronic data submission processes may not require validation by providers. Birth facilities may continue to prepare and provide signed paper documents to parents.	Same as hybrid state
Charge description master (CDM) administration	Function moves into the realm of HIM to ensure accurate and timely codes and updates.	HIM staff ensures accurate and timely coding and updates and links codes to online, structured documentation. Staff tests and verifies mapped codes.	HIM staff ensures accuracy of codes and continually performs maintenance updates to link codes to online, structured documentation.

Staff tests and validates mapped codes and application software.

CDM is linked so that there is notification when changes occur. |
| Charge ticket verification | Some HIM departments manually verify all charges on charge ticket against documentation. | HIM staff validates mapped codes—some manually and some online—based on location of the documentation. Super bills can be created by physicians or specialty clinics and are maintained and updated on a regular basis. | Computer-assisted coding requires validation of structured documentation against unmapped codes as well as validation of unstructured documentation against charges. If computerized physician order entry and medication administration records are implemented, this function is completely automated. |
| Coding and documentation training for all providers (physicians, nurse practitioners, physician's assistants) | Provider training for documentation and relationship to coding is rudimentary, generally focusing on specific providers or disciplines where reimbursement is a concern.

Query process for providers for additional documentation of information is typically done on paper. | Same as paper record | Staff positions increase as traditional coding positions decrease. Function is critical to ensure that charge description master and documentation templates correspond to internal and external reporting requirements as well as billing.

HIM staff educates clinicians on changes and develops and maintains templates and charge-capture processes to ensure accuracy of coding and documentation.

Query process for providers requesting additional documentation or information is automated. |
| Coding: CPT | Manual assignment using books or encoders is often done outside the HIM department. | Transition to coder-managed chargemaster eliminates need for manual code assignment. Auditing function is still needed to ensure charges are entered for all documented services rendered. | Coding is automated. Validation of charge capture against documentation is still required. Auditing or coder intervention for ad-hoc documentation is also required. Staff reductions can be expected. |
| Coding: E & M and physicians at teaching hospitals | Manual | Manual | Function changes focus from coding all procedures to validation and comparison of documents with computer-suggested codes. |

Table 6.2 (continued)

Function	Paper Health Record	Hybrid Paper-Electronic Health Record	Electronic Health Record
Coding: ICD-9-CM, ICD-10-CM, and/or ICD-10-PCS	Books or encoders are used; paper documents are the source of information.	Function moves toward automated encoding as online medical record systems support computerized functions.	Computer-assisted coding becomes more of an auditing function to ensure full capture of all codes, especially from free-form sources such as natural language processing. As SNOMED CT is adopted for data reporting and research, providers will be able to document clinical care in the EHR, SNOMED-CT codes will be automatically applied, and mapping tables will be used to identify related codes from other terminology. As rules-based maps develop for multiple-use cases and become increasingly sophisticated, the level of human review at the individual code level diminishes and human roles primarily focus on the development and maintenance (including quality control) of maps for a variety of use cases as well as the development of algorithmic translation and concept representation. Availability of computer-aided coding applications relieves the shortage of expert coders and enables them to perform other critical data management roles in the electronic HIM environment. ICD-10 coding will be important as a global tool.
Data quality, integrity, and reconciliation processes (including EHR and other specialized application work queue management)	Computer reports and statistics are verified against paper records and reports.	HIM staff begins online reconciliation of autogenerated documentation, monitoring EHR inboxes and interface reports (such as files from transcription or laboratory systems) and locating data that fails to transfer and post to the EHR.	Function fully transitions from paper verification to computer-based reconciliation of EHR functions and work queues. Patient-entered data includes the results of self-monitored clinical data (such as daily blood pressure readings), verification of registration data, and scheduling for appointments and tests. Insurance verification is completed automatically during the preregistration process. Patients without coverage are automatically directed to a financial counselor.
Data reporting and interpretation	Ad-hoc and routine reporting	Function transitions to ad-hoc reports and data mining. This shift requires methods for tracking inception of each EHR, as well as revisions to and deletions of either specific online, structured data or the entire EHR.	Data interpretation and data-mining skills are the new focus. Healthcare organizations need staff that understands coded data and classification systems for efficient data mining, accurate reporting, and interpretation as well as development of metadata definitions. Relational database management skills are needed as the healthcare industry moves toward disease management, where the patient is managed across the healthcare continuum and health problems are identified more quickly. Healthcare data is used as the basis for developing treatment protocols and critical pathways for disease management.
Denial management	Manual	Includes both manual and electronic follow-up	Function improves as advancements are made in health plan and benefits validation and claims processing. Additionally, as charge description master software becomes more sophisticated, audits are done virtually. With electronic provision of required documents, turnaround time decreases.

Function	Paper	Hybrid	Electronic
Document and records management	Primary focus is paper health record and some required logs and registers.	As focus moves away from paper medical record management, time shifted to assume organization-wide document management functions, including processes to eliminate shadow medical records, radiographic images, photographs, patient videotapes, business document imaging, image reproduction, retention, storage, access planning, record organization, and data collection.	Same as hybrid record
Document identification	Often manual; a key component of filing paper	Depending on the electronic system implemented, function transforms to bar codes, indexing methods, or optical character recognition. The process must ensure correct posting, including date of service, correct patient, and document type.	Process expands from the hybrid state to all documents in the EHR. Monitoring is necessary to ensure correct posting of electronic documents.
Document preparation, indexing, and scanning	Document repair is performed only as part of record assembly.	Function requires manual document preparation except for COLD-fed records (which come directly and electronically into the EHR). Decisions regarding which documents are scanned translate into policy and procedure.	Generally, this function includes only paper documents received from external sources. It will continue as long as paper documents are part of the EHR. It will decrease as interoperability allows more electronic document exchange to occur.
Documentation improvement training	Minimal except for coding training. This function has increased with programs such as DRG Assurance or through correct E&M coding initiatives.	Same as paper record	Function decreases as structured forms or data fields are designed to capture regulatory and billing needs. HIM staff ensures that rules and structured data fields meet regulatory needs. Automated tools allow online queries of and by providers. Online tools provide training 24 hours a day, seven days a week through real-time feedback.
DRG or documentation auditing program	Manual	Function consists of a combination of manual review of paper records and review of electronic documentation.	Daily concurrent follow-up minimizes as templates and rules are implemented. Initial review is necessary if the primary document is the unstructured H&P. This is performed remotely.
Filing records	Manual	Some manual filing remains through the transition state.	Function is eliminated as move to EHR is completed.
Filing reports concurrent (charting)	Manual	If printed record is maintained, some printing and filing is necessary. However, activity is reduced as documents become available electronically.	Function is eliminated. Staff can be redeployed to prepare documents for scanning, indexing, and other activities in that process.
Filing reports retrospective	Manual	Manual for paper record, but potentially only key documents during transition to fully electronic health record.	New function is resolution of electronic documents and reports that cannot be matched to a record. The frequency of this activity is dependent on system activity and mismatches.
Form and template design	Function includes standardization of data elements, placement (format), and logical flow for data capture.	Function includes screen design, data field definition, and print formats, as well as development of standard online data collection procedures and data dictionary definitions. Processes for requesting and implementing new forms are standardized to optimize use of existing data.	Same as hybrid record. Data dictionary encompasses all medical documentation.
Imaging	Minimal	Function significantly increases during transition to hybrid state and then to a fully electronic health record.	With most documents, online imaging is a function to capture temporary forms and external records only. HIM advisory role develops for imaging acquisitions and implementation for business records. Imaging becomes minimal as external documents become available electronically.

Table 6.2 (continued)

Function	Paper Health Record	Hybrid Paper-Electronic Health Record	Electronic Health Record
Master patient index (MPI) maintenance	Manual or electronic, including card file and online systems; may be limited to HIM applications	Function expands to system-wide database coordination for integrated EHR. For reasons of patient safety, dedicated MPI reconciliation staff is required to maintain up-to-the-minute patient identifiers. Roles expand to person identity management (guarantors) because the number of disparate systems with patient information increases the number of staff dedicated to the function. Number of staff is also influenced by enterprise medical record number needs for integrated health systems. Staff monitors medical record number and corrects source documents with accurate number.	Positive patient identification at the point of registration reduces staff dedicated to this function; however, this depends on the size of immigrant and transient populations. (Population predictions for the next 25 years forecast that immigrant populations will continue to grow; this will prolong MPI challenges, especially in the pediatric population.) Computer algorithmic scripts are implemented that run concurrently and identify duplicate (or possible duplicate) registrations. Photos of patients can be included in the EHR to ensure identification.
Ongoing record review	Manual	Function extends to paper and online records.	Function decreases with use of templates, alerts, and reminders. It is likely based on exception reports for items designated for review using autogenerated reports for review. Focus shifts to follow-up as reporting becomes routine.
Reconciliation of inboxes and other online files	Does not exist	A program capable of concurrently monitoring all systems is developed, and HIM staff performs reconciliation to ensure system files are complete and accurate.	Same as hybrid record
Record completion process	Manual	Electronic signatures are implemented, completion is accomplished remotely.	Rules are in place for automated monitoring of unsigned reports, monitoring of unreviewed results, and missing reports.
Specialized registries (cancer, cardiac, PICU, trauma, Alzheimer's)	Manual or computerized	HIM staff gathers data from EHRs. Rules are implemented identifying cases that require staging (such as cancer) or other specialized documentation. Staff is required to submit paper to state registries until they are capable of electronically accepting data.	HIM staff continues to submit paper abstracts depending on state registry computerization. Staff completes abstracts online and submits electronic data transfer from health facility data repository or warehouse to state system. Data will be coded in SNOMED CT or ICD-10-CM so information can be translated in a global environment.
Release of information for continuity of care	Manual	Manual for caregivers without remote access or without privileges.	Protocols are developed to provide electronic versions of information that can be shared as appropriate. This is made available as a read-only version or placed in a queue with a specific date after which it is no longer accessible.
Release of information, other	Manual	Manual, but process begins for identifying methods that will allow access to both paper and electronic records.	HIM staff continues to assist external sources needing access to PHI through batching individual or groups of records, setting up and monitoring work queues, and tracking disclosures. Depending on state law, organizations may eliminate paper records for legal purposes (such as the courts) and provide a view that is certified as a legal copy using an electronic signature.

Function	Current	Transitional	Future
Release of information to patients	Manual	Function continues to be manual; however, new responsibilities evolve, such as assisting patients with access to their information through secure Web sites or portals.	HIM staff continues to assist patients in accessing records through Web sites as well as on paper for those without computer access. New processes for assisting patients by moving data from the main medical record to the personal health record emerge. Staff continues to assist the court system and other external entities requesting certified copies. Paper copies continue to be generated but are reduced as interoperability progresses and patients are able to access EHRs. Electronic signatures may be developed that signify a view as certified for legal purposes.
Retrieving records	Manual	Record pulling is reduced as scanned or online documents become available, but function is needed for historical files not yet scanned (if there is a decision to scan old files). Physicians are asked to identify information from paper charts that should be scanned to eliminate the need to pull paper charts in the future.	Function is eliminated except for historical files maintained on paper or microform.
Revenue stream management (DNFB, charge entry, provider completion of documentation; organization of follow-up efforts)	Manual	Function includes more online management through computer-generated reports using logic rules.	The revenue cycle is managed completely online.
Security, clinical access by users to the health record	Manual	Function is performed manually and online using role-based context or individual access rights to clinical information. This increases emphasis on auditing access history to ensure adherence to policies.	Routine auditing and monitoring of access history is in place.
Statistics	Manual	Function is performed manually, though some statistics can be produced through automated reporting tools.	Function includes increased use of dashboard and other types of automatically generated statistical reports.
Transcription, natural language processing, direct charting by clinicians	Manual	Addition of processes such as natural language processing to support creation of the EHR begins. HIM role includes training staff, system administration, development of templates, monitoring accuracy, and a new role for transcriptionists as document editors.	There is potential for reduced transcription staff due to use of natural language processing (NLP), direct charting, and point-and-click charting by clinicians. There is potential for increasing the number of typed documents and shifting available transcriptionists to NLP editing or other situations in which structured notes may not be appropriate.

Source: Tegen 2005.

References

AHIMA e-HIM Work Group on Electronic Document Management as a Component of EHR (October 2003).

AHIMA e-HIM Work Group on Health Information in a Hybrid Environment. (October 2003).

AHIMA e-HIM Work Group. 2003b. Practice brief: Speech recognition in the electronic health record. *Journal of American Health Information Management Association* 74(10).

Amatayakul, Margret K. 2007. *Electronic Health Records: A Practical Guide for Professionals and Organizations,* 3rd ed. Chicago: AHIMA.

American Society of Testing Materials (ASTM) Standard E1384-07, 2007. Standard practice for content and structure of the electronic health record (EHR). West Conshohocken, PA: ASTM International. Available online from www.astm.org.

Dick, R., et al. eds. 1997. *The Computer-Based Patient Record: An Essential Technology for Health Care,* revised edition. Washington, D.C.: National Academy Press.

EHR Collaborative. 2004. *EHR Functional Model.* Available online from www.ehrcollaborative.com.

Health Insurance Portability and Accountability Act (HIPAA) of 1996. Public Law 104-191. Available online from www.gpoaccess.gov/cfr/index.html.

Health Level Seven. 2007. EHR Functional model. Available online from www.hl7.org/ehr/downloads/index_2007.asp.

Johns, Merida. 2007. Health information technology functions. Chapter 8 in *Health Information Management Technology: An Applied Approach,* 2nd ed. Edited by Merida Johns. Chicago: AHIMA.

Kohn, Deborah. 2006. Informatics in healthcare. Chapter 3 in *Health Information Management: Concepts, Principles, and Practice,* 2nd ed. Edited by Kathleen LaTour and Shirley Eichenwald-Maki. Chicago: AHIMA.

LaTour, Kathleen M. 2007. Healthcare data sets. Chapter 5 in *Health Information Management Technology: An Applied Approach,* 2nd ed. Edited by Merida Johns. Chicago: AHIMA.

Roberts, Jane. 2007. Health information technology functions. Chapter 8 in *Health Information Management Technology: An Applied Approach,* 2nd ed. Edited by Merida Johns. Chicago: AHIMA.

Tegan, A., et al. 2005. The EHR's impact on HIM functions. *Journal of American Health Information Management Association* 76(5): 56C–H.

Thompson, T. G., and D. J. Brailer. 2004. The decade of health information technology: Delivering consumer-centric and information-rich health care framework for strategic action. Washington, D.C.: National Coordinator for Health Information Technology.

The White House Office of the President. 2004 (April). Transforming Health Care: The President's Health Information Technology Plan. Washington, DC: The White House.

Chapter 7

Best Practices in Health Record Documentation

Diann Brown, MS, RHIA, CHP

Learning Objectives

- Explain the concept and importance of document improvement and identify four guidelines for a successful document improvement program

- Explain the purpose of health record analysis and the differences between quantitative and qualitative analysis

- Discuss the importance of ongoing record review and data quality management

- Define the term "data dictionary," explain its purpose, and describe the steps involved in developing one

- Define the term "authentication" within the context of health records and discuss some of the tools used to achieve it

- Explain the process for correcting errors in paper-based and electronic health records

- Identify four areas of concern when working to prevent fraud in the electronic health record environment

- Discuss the importance of data quality in electronic health records and discuss the ways in which it can be achieved

- Identify and explain three concepts important to developing a litigation response plan for e-discovery

- Define the term "disaster recovery planning" and outline the points a disaster-recovery plan should address

Key Terms

Analysis

Application

Authentication

Biometric identifier

Collection

Data quality management

Deficiency system

Digital signature

Disaster recovery planning

Electronic document management system (EDMS)

Electronic signature

Health data repository

Health record analysis

Hybrid health record

Medical record delinquency rate

Ongoing record review

Physician query process

Qualitative analysis

Quantitative analysis

Unique personal identifier

Warehousing

Introduction

As previously discussed in this book, every healthcare provider is required to document the clinical services performed on behalf of individual patients. How documentation occurs in the healthcare setting changed significantly during the late 1990s. Health information management (HIM) professionals in the healthcare setting have seen their roles evolve from merely keeping health records to the forefront of facilitating how healthcare information is organized and used. HIM professionals play an important role in clinical documentation by providing tools and processes that improve workflow and assist clinical staff in accessing and using information and completing documentation on time. It is vital to the healthcare industry that HIM professionals develop and use best practices as they relate to supporting quality data.

HIM professionals have advanced from managing documentation in a paper-based health record to managing documentation in the electronic health record (EHR). As hospitals transition to an electronic health records system, they find their records in a hybrid state, and HIM professionals play an essential role in implementing systems and processes that permit timely access to clinical data, regardless of how records are documented or stored. Another key role is advocating for quality documentation and data in health records to improve customer care and safety. The American Health Information Management Association (AHIMA) published a practice brief that describes a process for making improvements in health record documentation (Fletcher 1999). The practice brief advocates best practices that support quality and cost-efficient health information documentation requirements. (See figure 7.1.) Several best practices described in this chapter are adopted from AHIMA's practice briefs. AHIMA practice briefs are an excellent way for HIM professionals to stay on top of current best practices in health information management.

Figure 7.1. Recommended best practices in health record documentation.

1. **Consistent and standardized documentation requirements**

   a. Advocate consistent and standardized documentation requirements by working with stakeholders and accrediting and regulatory bodies, including but not limited to the JCAHO, the National Committee for Quality Assurance, the Centers for Medicare and Medicaid Services, the ASTM, and HL7.

   - Eliminate physician attestation requirement.
   - Streamline regulatory activities.
   - Change laws or legislation that requires physician signatures on verbal orders.

2. **Innovative, high-quality, and cost-efficient clinical documentation practices**

   a. Utilize authentication and authorship mechanisms that use available technology.

   b. Reduce record completion time frames. The time from patient discharge to record completion should be as short as possible. Develop policies and practices to facilitate completing records in a timely manner.

   - Collect records of discharged patients quickly.
   - Ensure that incomplete records remain available to physicians for completion. When the record is needed for purposes unrelated to patient care, have the record reviewed in the department.
   - Establish the physician's preferred appointment day and time to complete records and make them available at the appointed time.
   - Develop an equal-access system so that every physician who has deficiencies in the same record can have access to the record.
   - Apply record completions policies uniformly to all physicians without exception.
   - Withhold the paychecks of residents or do not allow them to graduate when they have incomplete records outstanding.
   - Use quality improvement techniques to improve record completion timeliness.
   - Reduce documentation requirements to those required to fulfill accreditation standards, federal regulations, and state laws.
   - Monitor and graphically report improvement efforts.
   - Redesign forms to ensure that they are user-friendly.
   - Decentralize record completion.
   - Work with other hospitals in the system or geographic area to standardize record completion requirements.
   - Analyze records for deficiencies on a concurrent basis.
   - Levy fines, suspend privileges, or otherwise punish physicians who do not complete records in a timely manner.
   - Utilize positive incentive programs for timely record completion.
   - Reduce reliance on paper-based sources of information to reduce or eliminate routine delivery and maintenance requirements.
   - Standardize billing process so that claims are derived exclusively from electronic documentation to reduce or eliminate the need to release paper-based information for reimbursement purposes, claim audits, and record handling.
   - Streamline health record completion guidelines.
   - Minimize the number of unsigned verbal orders.
   - Reduce loose filing backlogs.
   - Allow medical staff to take responsibility for record completion timeliness.

   c. Utilize new and improved technology for documentation.

   - Use speech recognition technology to supplement transcription services.
   - Develop a standardized format for policies and procedures that are accessible electronically.
   - Utilize e-mail to transmit information.
   - Implement telemedical record documentation processes.

Figure 7.1. (continued)

3. **Appropriate measures and monitors to assess health record documentation quality**

a. Develop documentation processes that reflect the organization's uniqueness.

b. Organize an ongoing records review program and monitor its effectiveness using performance improvement techniques.

c. Streamline health record completion guidelines.

d. Educate practitioners and others on the importance of innovative, high-quality, and cost-efficient documentation practices.

e. Recruit a physician to act as a liaison to improve documentation.

4. **Strategic Planning**

a. Develop and implement an electronic health record system.

b. Develop processes to accommodate the emergence of integrated health delivery systems and transition of patient care to nonacute settings.

c. Prepare for the implementation of ICD-10-CM and ICD-10-PCS.

Source: Fletcher 1999.

Documentation Improvement Programs

Documentation improvement programs have proliferated in healthcare facilities around the country. The programs are often precipitated by the need to increase facility revenue. However, this is not the only reason to establish programs to improve the quality of health record documentation. Documentation improvement programs are thought to improve the quality of care through quality documentation.

As prospective payment systems have become the rule (rather than the exception) for reimbursement, lack of a uniform language or guidelines for health record documentation have been revealed. The **physician query process** was instituted as a response to this new problem. It is a communication tool and an educational mechanism that provides a clearer picture of specific resident diagnoses when in question.

"Documentation therapy" is a comprehensive-care plan that combines educational and operational steps to improve physician contributions in the documentation requirements for health records:

> Physicians must be educated that complete documentation helps both the physician and the hospital with regard to compliance and protection from litigation. The key to appropriate documentation lies in physicians' understanding of coding methodology and its clinical interpretation. (Micheletti and Shlala 2006)

Documentation deficiencies can be minimized by thorough evaluation of the patient encounter record. Identifying and correcting problematic documentation can limit reimbursement delays. Gold (2007) states, "a true clinical documentation program must be a medical staff initiative that will eventually result in doctors who make entries into the medical record with words that paint the true picture of their patients so the HIM department can paint the exact same picture in codes."

Documentation improvement is also a core function for HIM professionals as stated by Fletcher (1999):

> In 1998, AHIMA's 1998 House of Delegates approved a resolution titled "Advocating Quality and Cost-efficient Health Information Documentation Requirements." The resolution cited managing and monitoring the quality of documentation in patient medical records as core functions of the health information management profession.

Guidelines for a documentation improvement program include the following:

1. **Consistent and standardized documentation requirements**: Periodic meetings between HIM staff and physicians in each clinical specialty can help improve communication and provide targeted education. HIM managers must develop policies and procedures so that when coders identify documentation deficiencies, the next steps are clearly defined.

2. **Innovative, quality, and cost-efficient clinical documentation practices**: Simplifying documentation can help, also. A list of standardized abbreviations and terms should be available to physicians, and the process for correcting errors in patient documentation entries should be standard. Streamlined forms can significantly improve documentation.

3. **Complete, current, and quality healthcare information**: Promote the development and use of appropriate measures and monitors to assess the quality of health record documentation. Appoint a suitable liaison to assist with physician communication, preferably a physician advisor.

4. **Strategic planning** (Fletcher 1999)

Improving physician documentation requires ongoing education, operational processes that facilitate better communication and monitoring against standards, and periodic reporting of documentation audit results to stakeholders. By implementing effective educational and operational strategies, healthcare facilities will minimize compliance risk, improve financial health, and enhance customer care.

Health Record Analysis and Management

In acute-care hospitals, HIM professionals are responsible for evaluating every health record for completeness. In the paper-based environment, HIM professionals may conduct retrospective reviews after the patient has been discharged because of limited access to the health record while the patient is receiving treatment. However, best practices include implementation of concurrent or ongoing reviews of health record content. Concurrent or ongoing record reviews can assist organizations in meeting accreditation and regulatory requirements because identified documentation issues are addressed in a timely manner. Utilizing clinical staff for ongoing record review at the point of care may be used as a means to educate staff on regulatory documentation requirements and improves the overall quality of health record documentation. Oftentimes, organizations develop health record review policies to define the scope of reviews and to analyze the collection and reporting of data for use within the organization. See figure 7.2 for a sample record review policy.

When HIM professionals perform health record review after discharge, it usually corresponds to **health record analysis**. The purpose of health record analysis is to ensure the quality and completeness of clinical documentation. This process is not an evaluation of the clinical care provided to the patient. However, quality improvement and accreditation organizations depend on health record documentation for evidence that appropriate and effective care is being provided to patients. Furthermore, the quality of clinical documentation significantly impacts the coding and billing processes that lead to reimbursement of provided services.

Traditional health record analysis comprises two separate but related processes: quantitative analysis and qualitative analysis. **Quantitative analysis** consists of a review of the health

after discharge

Figure 7.2.   Sample record review policy.

1.0 PURPOSE

   To establish guidelines for open medical records review process.

2.0 POLICY

   Medical records are reviewed on an ongoing basis at the point of care. The review of medical records is based on hospital-defined indicators that address the presence, timeliness, readability, quality, consistency, clarity, accuracy, completeness, and authentication of data and information within the record.

3.0 SCOPE

   This policy applies to clinical departments/units at ABC Hospital.

4.0 MEDICAL RECORD SAMPLE

   ABC Hospital shall conduct a review of a representative sample of a minimum of six (6) open medical records per clinical/unit area each month.

   The medical record sample population will include inpatient, outpatient, emergency, observation, day-surgery, and clinic patients.

5.0 PROCEDURE

   5.1 Each clinical area will conduct open medical record reviews monthly utilizing the electronic Open Medical Records Review form.

   5.2 Clinical staff will access the Open Medical Records Review form online via the Intranet.

   5.3 Demographic information will be entered and applicable questions related to the medical record being reviewed will be completed.

   5.4 The submit button will be clicked after completion.

   5.5 Health Information Management shall compile reports monthly.

   5.6 The Medical Records Committee will conduct secondary reviews on problem-prone data elements such as prohibited abbreviations, legibility, timeliness of history and physical or operative reports, and other record elements.

6.0 REPORTING DATA

   6.1 The Health Information Management Director shall report summarized data monthly to unit managers and directors. At a minimum, reports will consist of the following:

      6.1.1   Number of charts reviewed by unit

      6.1.2   Monthly unit tally per reviewer

      6.1.3   Percentage summary unit results

      6.1.4   Summary unit results

   6.2 Unit managers/directors shall analyze, conduct follow-up and implement action plans. Action plans will be submitted at least semiannually to the Medical Records Committee.

   6.3 Results are reported to the Medical Records Committee, Accreditation Task Force, and other committees as appropriate.

---

record to determine its completeness and accuracy. **Qualitative analysis** is a review of the health record to ensure that clinical protocols are met and to determine the adequacy of entries documenting the quality of care. Many hospitals are applying a new quality review technique that combines quantitative and qualitative review.

   In hospitals that use traditional, paper-based health record systems, HIM department personnel are responsible for ensuring that health records of discharged, transferred, and deceased patients are received in the HIM department (Coffman-Kadish 2002). (See figure 7.3.) HIM personnel compare records received with discharge lists/logs to ensure all records are accounted for from each unit or department. Depending on the hospital's health record policies, HIM personnel may reassemble the contents of the record in a specific order for storage. However, most hospitals have replaced the reassembly of records with the best practice of maintaining the record in reverse chronological order. The process of assembling the record after discharge

Figure 7.3. **Steps in the flow of paper-based health records after discharge.**

1. Records of discharged patients arrive or are delivered to HIM department.

2. Receipt of records is verified by comparing discharge lists to actual charts received.

3. Folder corresponding to records is pulled.

4. Record is assembled according to prescribed format ensuring that all pages belong to the correct patient and that forms are in correct date order.

5. Deficiencies such as signatures, reports needing completion, and so on are assigned to the responsible provider.

6. Diagnoses and procedures are coded.

7. Record is held for final completion by providers either in incomplete chart area or some other filing area.

8. Charts are rechecked after the providers have done their work to ensure that all have been completed.

9. The complete record is filed in the permanent filing area.

Source: McCain 2006, 188.

is not necessary in facilities that use an electronic document management system (EDMS) or EHR system.

Facilities using an EDMS to organize hybrid health records require a format that facilitates easy retrieval of interfaced and scanned documents. The ideal scanning process would automatically organize documents within the health record through the use of bar codes and tables that are designed to define document location. (See figure 7.4.) The ideal system creates an EHR in which users may set up individual preferences for viewing electronic documentation as information is documented.

Quantitative Analysis   *easily done by computer*

The purpose of quantitative analysis is to assess the completeness and accuracy of patient health records. Quantitative evaluations are based on the regulatory, accrediting, licensing, and reimbursement requirements that apply to the hospital. Therefore, the timing and extent of quantitative health record analysis depend on policies developed by individual organizations. Both paper-based and computer-based records are subject to quantitative review.

Implementing concurrent or point-of-care inpatient record analysis positively impacts patient care and safety when findings are corrected immediately. Technology makes it more efficient to shift from back-end to front-end analysis, which is of greater benefit in many applications in the industry. Another benefit of concurrent review is that content or authentication issues can be addressed before the patient has been discharged, which enhances the timeliness of documentation and quality of the record. In addition, it is an effective way of ensuring that documentation is completed when services are performed.

Deficiencies may be auto-assigned by the EDMS or HIM personnel in the hybrid environment. The EDMS can be configured to present deficiencies in a queue for HIM personnel to review for completeness. HIM personnel assign the deficiency to the appropriate physician for completion. Deficiency types assigned in an EDMS may include missing reports, editing electronic documents, annotating scanned documents, or electronic signatures. After documents are electronically signed, no additional review is required by HIM personnel.

In the EHR, interfacing missing items automatically updates the deficiency from "missing" to "signed." Ideally, electronic systems auto-assign deficiencies based on record completion criteria established by the organization. For example, when the history and physical examination is incomplete and/or not documented in the health record within the established time frame, the system autogenerates a deficiency for the attending physician to complete the required documentation.

Figure 7.4.   Document locations within the electronic health record (EHR) system.

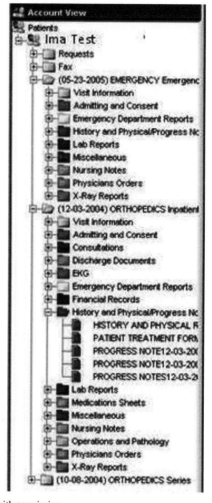

Source: Streamline Health. Reprinted with permission

During record analysis, missing or incomplete information is identified, and the reviewer can attempt to find the missing documentation. If missing documentation cannot be located, HIM personnel can issue deficiency notifications to the appropriate caregivers.

Deficiency systems may be paper-based, computer-based, or electronic. A deficiency system is designed to track and report elements of documentation missing from health records. Paper-based deficiency systems use a checklist to indicate missing reports, signatures, consents, and other documentation. (See figure 7.5 for an example of a paper-based deficiency slip.) Computer-based deficiency systems provide logs for reporting and tracking health record deficiencies. (See figure 7.6 for a sample on-screen view of an electronic deficiency chart.) Deficiencies created in an electronic system are automatically placed in the physician in-box or work queue. The oldest deficiencies are listed first for completion; however, the physician can prioritize deficiencies processing by using the sorting features inherent in the EDMS.

Most HIM personnel periodically remind physicians to complete their patients' records for past admissions. The value of temporarily identifying deficiencies is that it allows the aggregation of information that can be used for performance improvement and credentialing functions. It plays a role in enforcing medical staff bylaws and hospital policies, thus leading to the accreditation measurement of standards compliance through average medical record delin-

Figure 7.5.   Sample paper-based deficiency slip.

Physician/Practitioner's Name: _____
Health Record Number: _____
Patient's Name: _____
Discharge Date: _____
Analyzed by: _____
Date: _____

Signatures Required	Dictation Required	Missing Reports
_____ History	_____ History	_____ History
_____ Physical	_____ Physical	_____ Physical
_____ Consultation	_____ Consultation	_____ Consultation
_____ Operative Report	_____ Operative Report	_____ Operative Report
_____ Discharge Summary	_____ Discharge Summary	_____ Discharge Summary
		_____ Radiology Report
Other	Other	_____ Pathology Report
		_____ Progress Notes
___ _____	___ _____	
___ _____	___ _____	Other
___ _____	___ _____	___ _____
		___ _____
		___ _____

[handwritten: quantitative]

quency rate metrics. Hospitals using an EHR usually achieve single-digit delinquency rates for incomplete records.

Accreditation standards require that hospitals track the number of delinquent medical records. The Joint Commission (2006) requires hospitals to monitor the **medical record delinquency rate** at least quarterly. During the Joint Commission accreditation process, delinquency statistics data are used during accreditation surveys to show past evidence of compliance with record completion standards. The delinquency rate is calculated by dividing the monthly average number of discharges by the monthly average number of delinquent records.

Qualitative Analysis

Qualitative analysis is the systematic review of sample health records to determine whether patient care and record documentation standards are being met. As part of the hospital's quality management program, many organizations implement qualitative analysis at the point of care by clinical or HIM professionals rather than after discharge. The goal of qualitative analysis is to determine the adequacy of the health record as documentation of the quality of care provided to the patient. For example, HIM professionals look for evidence in the record indicating

[handwritten: quality doesn't change whether paper or electronic]

Figure 7.6. Sample on-screen view of an electronic deficiency chart.

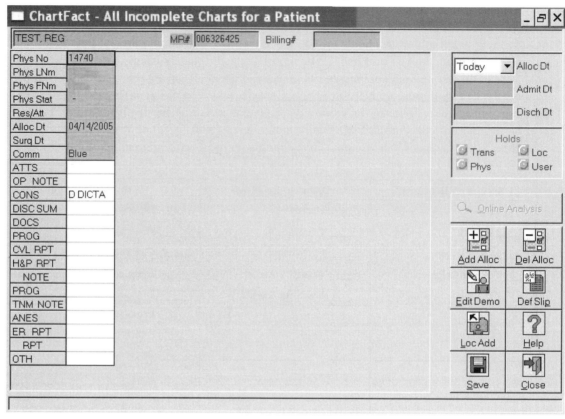

Source: SoftMed Systems, Silver Spring, MD. Reprinted with permission.

that caregivers followed clinical practice guidelines, performed adequate patient assessments, and completed other required tasks.

Hospitals may establish a reporting structure such as a medical records committee or performance improvement manager to receive the results of qualitative analysis. The designated group/person addresses problems identified and implements actions to improve the quality of the health record documentation. Common problems identified during qualitative reviews include the following:

- Inconsistencies in documentation related to the diagnostic information recorded on admissions records, history and physical reports, operative and pathology reports, care plans, and discharge summaries

- Inconsistencies between the patient's pharmacy profile and the medication record

- Inconsistencies in the documentation related to test results, treatment plans, and follow-up instructions

- Ambiguities in documentation resulting from the use of unapproved symbols and abbreviations

- Inconsistencies in nursing documentation related to the patient's pain status compared to physician's orders for analgesics

- Inadequacies in nursing documentation related to interdepartmental transfers that result in time gaps in accounting for patient's location

Ongoing Record Review

Ongoing record review is a continuous health record quality review process. Clinical and/or HIM professionals review the records of current inpatients or outpatients to ensure health records are complete and accurate and that the facility's clinical documentation practices meet relevant accreditation standards, state licensing laws, and federal regulatory requirements. Ongoing record reviews also address quality and patient safety initiatives by improving documentation practices. The Joint Commission (2006) requires review of health records at the point of care. For example, tracking, trending, and reporting data collected about National Patient Safety Goals such as prohibited abbreviations or legibility can produce changes within the organization.

HIM professionals should take the lead to make the review process happen. Providing an automated tool for both clinical and HIM departments for data collection and reporting improves the timely use of data for rapid decision making. Hospitals may purchase vendor software or collaborate with their internal information services (IS) departments to implement electronic data collection tools. The abilities to customize data collection and provide feedback are benefits that allow HIM professionals to easily focus on problem-prone areas, implement action plans, and measure progress. Policies on data collected and reported are vital to the use of data. Policies and procedures should address the functions of the ongoing record review program and include responsibilities of the healthcare staff as well as other clinical disciplines. The result should be to develop a meaningful ongoing record review plan designed to meet the needs of the organization (Lewis and Reinicke 2005).

See figures 7.7 and 7.8 for examples of ongoing records review checklists. Also, see the sample record review policy in figure 7.2. A sample of an electronic ongoing record review is illustrated in figure 7.9.

Data Quality Management

Data quality management is a process that ensures the integrity of data during data collection, application, warehousing, and analysis. In 2006, the AHIMA issued a revised position statement on "Quality Healthcare Data and Information" that calls for the improvement of data quality by developing and implementing standards for data content, data mapping, and documentation within the healthcare industry. AHIMA (2007) advocates for continuous quality improvement strategies that support quality data and information. It is recognized that improving the quality of data, information, and knowledge in the U.S. healthcare system is paramount as the industry transitions from paper to electronic health records. Technology should be designed to support the collection of high-quality data at the point of care, data aggregation, exchange, and retrieval. Everyone involved with documenting or using health information is responsible for its quality. This is a transition from past practices when HIM professionals carried the primary responsibility for record management. According to AHIMA's Data Quality Management Model (2007), there are four key processes for data:

- **Application**: the purpose for which the data are collected
- **Collection**: the processes by which data elements are accumulated
- **Warehousing**: the processes and systems used to store and maintain data and data journals
- **Analysis**: the process of translating data into information utilized for an application

Healthcare quality and safety require that the right information be available at the right time to support patient care and health system management decisions. Gaining consensus on

Figure 7.7.   Open record review checklist: Initial assessments.

Information/Indicator	Record Number	Record Number	Record Number	Record Number	Record Number	Record Number	Record Number
	004303	193847					
1. Nursing unit	11B	12B					
2. Admission date	04/06/200x	04/06/200x					
3. Primary physician	Jones	Smith					
4. Was the history and physical report available within 24 hours of the admission?	**No**	Yes					
5. Does the history and physical report include information of the patient's the past history, examination of heart, lungs, and mental status and other body systems related to the condition for which the patient was admitted?	Yes	Yes					
6. Is the nursing initial assessment complete and free of blanks?	Yes	Yes					
7. Was the nursing initial assessment completed within 24 hours of the admission?	Yes	Yes					
8. Was a functional status screen completed when warranted by the patient's condition?	Yes	Yes					
9. Was a nutritional status screen completed when warranted by the patient's condition?	Yes	Yes					
10. Was the need to plan for discharge or transfer determined?	Yes	Yes					
11. Was the patient's level of pain assessed?	Yes	Yes					
12. Did the patient sign the consent to treatment?	Yes	Yes					
13. Was it determined whether the patient had an advance directive?	**No**	Yes					
Comments							

Actions Needed	Who		When Due
Supply missing report of history and physical.	Dr. Jones		04/08/200x

Figure 7.8. Closed record review checklist: Discharge summary.

Information/Indicator	Record Number 000011	Record Number 000026	Record Number 001000	Record Number 000090	Record Number 000087	Record Number 000560	Record Number 000777
1. Nursing unit	10A	12B	10A	10A	10A	12B	10A
2. Primary physician	Smith	Green	Jones	Smith	Black	White	Jones
3. Discharge date	04/04/200x	04/04/200x	04/04/200x	04/04/200x	04/04/200x	04/04/200x	04/04/200x
4. Was the discharge summary in the record within 30 days of discharge?	Yes	Yes	Yes	Yes	Yes	Yes	Yes
5. Does the discharge summary include the reason for the patient's hospitalization?	Yes	Yes	Yes	Yes	Yes	Yes	Yes
6. Does the discharge summary include documentation of significant findings?	Yes	Yes	Yes	Yes	Yes	Yes	Yes
7. Does the discharge summary include documentation of all of the procedures performed and the other care, treatment, and services provided?	Yes	Yes	Yes	Yes	Yes	Yes	Yes
8. Does the discharge summary include documentation of the patient's condition at discharge?	Yes	Yes	Yes	**No**	Yes	Yes	Yes
9. Does the discharge summary include documentation of the patient aftercare instructions?	Yes	Yes	Yes	Yes	Yes	Yes	Yes
10. Is the discharge summary readable, complete, and free of blanks?	Yes	Yes	Yes	Yes	Yes	Yes	Yes
11. Is the discharge summary free of abbreviations from the prohibited list?	**No**	Yes	Yes	Yes	Yes	Yes	Yes
12. Is the discharge summary signed and dated by the author or otherwise authenticated?	Yes	Yes	Yes	Yes	Yes	Yes	Yes
Comments	Trend						

Actions Needed	Who	When Due
Send Dr. Smith another reminder about the use of prohibited abbreviations from the JCAHO list, specifically SO4.	Tilly	Today
Ask Dr. Smith to add specific information about the patient's condition at discharge.	Dr. Smith	04/10/200x

Figure 7.9.   Sample electronic open medical records review form.

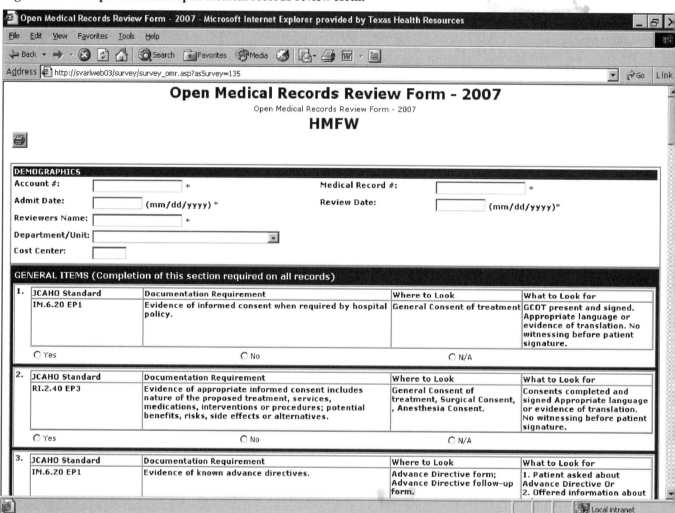

Windows and Internet Explorer are registered trademarks of Microsoft Corporation in the United States and other countries.
Source: Texas Health Resources.

essential data content and documentation standards is a prerequisite for high-quality data in the interconnected healthcare system of the future. Further, continuous quality management of data standards and content is a key component to ensuring that information is useable and actionable (AHIMA 2007).

Developing a Data Dictionary

This section was adapted from AHIMA's e-HIM Work Group on EHR Data Content's Practice Brief, "Guidelines for Developing a Data Dictionary," originally published in the February 2006 issue of the *Journal of American Health Information Management Association*.

Information systems are only as good as their data. Without a mutually agreed-upon set of data elements with clearly defined names and definitions, the validity and reliability of the data contained in a system are suspect at best and must be discounted at worst. The data dictionary and its relationship with the metadata registry are the foundation of an information system and the central building block that supports communication across business processes.

A data dictionary is defined as a descriptive list of names (also called representations or displays), definitions, and attributes of data elements to be collected in an information system or database. The purpose of the data dictionary is to standardize definitions and ensure consistency of use.

Standardizing data enhances interoperability across systems. It also improves data validity and reliability within, across, and outside the enterprise. Communication is improved in clinical treatment, research, and business processes through a common understanding of terms. Standardization provides developers with a common road map to promote consistency across applications.

Lack of a sound data dictionary can cause problems within and across organizations. Organizations may call the same data element by different names, or they may call different data elements by the same name across an enterprise. As a result, an organization may not collect all of the information it needs, or it may be unable to combine or map data across systems because the definitions are not identical. A worse possibility is that an organization may combine data elements it believes to be equivalent and draws incorrect inferences from the invalid data. Multiple users entering data may have different definitions or perceptions of what goes into a data field, thereby confounding the data. For example, are "reason for visit" and "chief complaint" the same or different?

Large complex systems with multiple stakeholders (internal and external) often require use of multiple, differing data sets. Variances among the data sets that are not recognized across the system can affect the information flow as well as the workflow. Maintaining expansive, overlapping data sets costs time and money and affects the organization's ability to provide quality of care. The organization will not be positioned for harmonizing information at the regional or national level.

Guideline Development Process

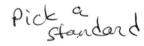

In developing a data dictionary, a healthcare facility may want to consider 11 major industry standard data sets for comparison:

- ASTM International's E1384-02a Practice for Content and Structure of the Electronic Health Record Minimum Essential Data Set

- ASTM International's WK4363 Standard Specification for the Continuity of Care Record (CCR)

- Doctor's Office Quality Information Technology's Data Element Specification v.1.1.2

- Electronic Medical Summary (e-MS)(Canada) Core Data Set

- International Organization for Standardization (ISO)/TS 18308 Health Informatics: Requirements for an Electronic Health Record Architecture

- Joint Commission on Accreditation of Healthcare Organizations Comprehensive Accreditation's Manual for Ambulatory Care: Information Management Standards 6.20, EP1

- Centers for Medicare and Medicaid Services' (CMS) Minimum Data Set, Version 2.0, for Nursing Home Resident Assessment and Care Screening

- National Center for Vital and Health Statistics' Core Health Data Elements

- CMS and the Joint Commission on National Hospital Quality Measures

- AHIMA's Personal Health Record Minimum Common Data Elements

- Health Level Seven's Clinical Document Architecture, release 2

creating a policy [handwritten marginalia]

Design a Plan

Preplanning is imperative. Development, implementation, and continuing maintenance of the data dictionary are topics for preplanning. The development of a data dictionary is part of a larger process. An information model must first be developed to align the workflow with information flow. This includes deciding what data are required, how the data will be used, who will use the data, and how the data will flow internally and externally, including communications with other entities.

This should be a collaborative process, and stakeholders should be encouraged to resist the temptation to collect data simply because they can. In the ideal scenario, data are captured once for use by multiple users. The result of this data mapping is the ability of multiple entities to mine the same data source. Each will know the exact nature of the data element each is accessing. The plan should also include the following:

- The type of media (paper, electronic, spreadsheet, relational database) in which the data dictionary will be developed and maintained. The media choice may depend on the complexity of the enterprise system and the availability of resources.

- Adequate funding and staffing with clearly defined roles and responsibilities for development and ongoing maintenance of the data dictionary. Databases are dynamic and can be affected by new business lines, changes in national standards, and clinical advancements.

- Provisions to ensure that all licensing agreements are in order.

- Ongoing education and training of all staff as appropriate to their use of data elements and their definitions.

Integrate Common Data Elements

Integrate into the data dictionary the common data elements used across an enterprise. One purpose of the data dictionary is to provide consistency and understanding of common data across applications. Preplanning is necessary to accomplish this at an enterprise level. A process must be clearly defined and key stakeholders identified. The process requires collecting data or metadata (data about the data) on each data element found to be common across domains. It is important to define up front what needs to be done before starting the dictionary. This includes defining what metadata will be collected on each element as well as what will not be collected. Examples of metadata include name of element, definition, application in which the data element is found, locator key, ownership, entity relationships, date first entered system, date element terminated from system, and system of origin.

A metadata registry is an authoritative source of reference information about the representation, meaning, and format of data collected and managed by an enterprise. It does not contain the data itself but the information that is necessary to clearly describe, inventory, analyze, and classify data.

Ensure Collaborative Involvement

Ensure collaborative involvement and buy-in of all key stakeholders when defining data requirements for an information system. Stakeholders include data creators, data owners, and data users, both internal and external to the organization. Representation should reflect all geographies (departments, facilities, satellites, corporate representatives, and external entities). Each organization must identify its stakeholders based on its own unique business model, organizational structure, information flow, and reporting requirements. Different stakeholders may have different data element definitions within their local domain. Every attempt should be made to promote collaborative agreement whereby a datum is collected only once even though it may be used by multiple end users.

For example, a large enterprise discovers that it has 40 different representations for data elements with a set of values of "yes" and "no" throughout its data dictionary. These include: Y = yes, N = no; yes, no; 1 = yes, 0 = no; 1 = no, 0 = yes; 1 = yes, 2 = no. These should be standardized as one set of values in the enterprise data dictionary.

Public health and research are examples of external stakeholders. Public health reporting is often forgotten in the data requirements definition phase. As a result, organizations incur extra costs to develop special interfaces and maintain crosswalk tables to meet public health requirements. For example, the Joint Commission, at its discretion, provides crosswalks between its accreditation manuals and CMS Conditions of Participation for specific practice settings, as well as crosswalk documents that describe significant updates or revisions to accreditation manuals.

The collaboration of all data stakeholders (for example, clinical specialties, support services, HIM services, IS services, reimbursement specialists, administrative, legal, and public health agencies) should enhance consensus and understanding of data and their flow across all domains.

Develop an Approval Process

Develop an approval process and documentation trail for all initial data dictionary decisions as well as for ongoing updates and maintenance. It is important to document decisions made about the data dictionary throughout the life of the system. Each subsystem (for example, finance, lab, radiology) should have one authoritative owner responsible for tracking all implemented data dictionary activations, deactivations, relevant dates, events, and decisions.

There must be a maintenance and change control process for adding new values, elements, and enactment dates. The subsystem owner should review and approve any additions to the system and integrate those changes through a collaborative process with other owners into the whole enterprise system. The process should address how a new datum applies in the local setting or domain and across all aspects of the enterprise.

Identify and Retain Details

Identify and retain details of data versions across all applications and databases. Ensure clear mapping instructions for organization-specific definitions. Version control is essential for maintaining data reliability. It is important that the data set version be clearly identified. Differences between versions may be minor or extensive. It is critical that everyone in the enterprise operate on the same version in order to maintain data integrity and continuity. Version control is essential for data dissemination in standard format to satellite or remote facilities. Separate tables may be considered for keeping track of changes such as additions, deletions, and their relative effective dates.

Design Flexibility and Growth Capabilities

The data dictionary should be designed so that it will accommodate architecture changes resulting from clinical or technical advances or regulatory changes. Build expansion capabilities into the fundamental design to accommodate a dynamic system. There should be a plan for future expansion, such as expanding a data field from one element to multiple elements. Expansion must be carefully addressed because of the potential ramifications of concept migration, the change of an idea or concept over time through growth, or change to the system. This becomes problematic when comparing data across time if the meaning of a particular element has changed while its name or representation has not. If a data element is completely revamped, document when that specific data element went into effect and when it was deactivated. If the data element expands into something new, do not migrate the old concept but rather create a new element to move forward. This will affect how the data are stored and retrieved. It may require consultation with vendors where current system limitations exist.

Always strive for concept permanence. Never reuse a concept even if it becomes obsolete. For example, when an ICD code number is retired, never reassign the retired code to a new concept. Always follow the defined coding practices. This becomes particularly important in data comparison. Address architecture flexibility in vendor contracts to allow for system upgrades and room for expansion to accommodate requirements common to provider-specific issues, user groups (multiple sites), or state-based directives.

Design for Expansion

Consider future needs to collapse and expand values to accommodate mapping from a larger to smaller or smaller to larger number of values within a field definition. When setting up the information system, consider how to accommodate multiple systems and how to go from one code system to another. Mapping and transferring guidelines should be clarified between data sets. For example, race or ethnicity is frequently defined with different values. One data set has four items; another has six. The mainframe or core system needs the maximum amount of values. The mapper needs to know the rules to use when collapsing six values into four. Migrating four to six is usually impossible, which creates other issues.

Gender is another core data element that can generate much discussion. Many systems only allow for male and female, while others provide for unknown and other. When an "other" category is an option, there should be a process for monitoring what is captured under that heading. When large numbers begin to appear in the category, there should be a review to determine if a new discrete category is required or if there is misunderstanding in the definition of the core element.

Follow Established Guidelines

ISO/International Electrotechnical Commission (IEC) 11179 guidelines are designed for metadata registry (data dictionary) construction to promote interoperability and automated data sharing. Uniformity of approach in data dictionary development avoids industry fragmentation. In an effort to promote and improve international communications among governments, businesses, and scientific communities, ISO and IEC have developed standards for specification and standardization of data elements. The ISO/IEC 11179 standard consists of the following:

- A framework for the generation and standardization of data elements
- A classification of concepts for the identification of domains
- Basic attributes of data elements
- Rules and guidelines for the formulation of data definitions
- Naming and identification principles for data elements
- Registration of data elements

make sure you can expand

This standard provides excellent, detailed information and examples of how to classify and define data elements. It also includes examples of pitfalls and practices to avoid.

Adopt Recognized Standards

Examine the nationally recognized standards and normalize field definitions across data sets to accommodate multiple end-user needs. It is important to define all data characteristics to be included for each data element for all domains. This includes specifying domain boundaries and identifying linkages across domains. This will require extensive discussion and agreement among all stakeholders. The ideal is the development of a common integrated data and terminology model. Terminologies should be coordinated to eliminate overlaps, redundancies, and inconsistencies. This will eliminate the need for mapping among terminologies.

Beware of Differing Standards

Do not assume that things labeled the same are actually identical or will map one to one. For example, there are several different wound staging protocols. CMS requires one version in the Minimum Data Set Version 2.0 for reimbursement purposes. For clinical care, it requires a different staging protocol that is based on the Agency for Healthcare Research and Quality (AHRQ) Clinical Practice Guideline for Pressure Ulcers. Pain measurement scales are another example of multiple scales for the same concept. Always check with a subject matter expert to ensure valid data.

Use Geographic Standards

Geographic codes and geocoding standards should conform to those established by the National Spatial Data Infrastructure and the Federal Geographic Data Committee, following the guidelines of the Federal Information Processing Standards. Valid street addresses, zip codes, county, state, and country codes are important to information exchange across systems and geopolitical boundaries. Standardization of geographic codes enhances interoperability of systems. Healthcare uses this information for tracking diseases as well as people. Using internationally accepted standards further enhances the interoperability of systems and the exchange of information. The following are recommended resources for geographic codes:

- Federal Information Processing Standards (www.itl.nist.gov/fipspubs)
- Federal Geographic Data Committee (www.fgdc.gov)
- United States Postal Service (www.usps.gov)
- National Spatial Data Infrastructure (www.fgdc.gov/nsdi/nsdi.html)
- International Organization for Standardization (www.iso.org)

Test the System

When the data dictionary is completed, a test plan should be developed to ensure that the system implementation supports the data dictionary. This should include sampling data inputs and outputs for conformance, validity, and reliability, as well as conformance to standards as defined in the data dictionary. This process should also verify interoperability of systems.

Provide Ongoing Education

Train all staff as appropriate to their use of data elements and their definitions.

To ensure consistency of understanding, application, and use of data, it is imperative to provide ongoing education in those definitions. New employee orientation should routinely include exposure to the concepts expressed in the data dictionary.

Ensure Consistency

Assess the extent to which the use of the agreed-upon data elements supply consistency of information sharing and avoid duplication. Ensure simultaneous adoption of new knowledge developed through research and changing terminologies reflective of changes in clinical practice. Specific stakeholders external to most end-user organizations that should be involved in the development and modification of data elements that affect clinical care include all American Board of Medical Specialty recognized specialty societies (for example, American Academy of Pediatrics and the American Academy of Family Physicians). This evaluation and modification process should be ongoing and involve members of the specialty societies at all stages of the process.

The creation and maintenance of the data dictionary is pivotal to the success of an EHR system. Much thought and effort must go into the planning and the maintenance of this foundational information. Collaboration and buy-in by stakeholders across all domains is critical to the success of the EHR implementation. A process for ongoing maintenance and updates as well as version control must be in place. The upfront design must provide room for change, growth, and expansion over time. Organizations should follow established guidelines such as the ISO/IEC 11179 and the geographic code systems where possible to promote interoperability. Normalization of concepts across end users is an ultimate goal, while any variances in business or clinical concepts should be carefully noted. Once the hard work of the build has been completed, the EHR system should be thoroughly tested to ensure it accurately reflects the standards as defined in the data dictionary.

Authentication of Health Record Entries

In the context of health records, **authentication** is the process of providing proof of the authorship of documentation in the health record whether maintained in a paper or electronic format. Federal and state laws govern standards for authentication of health records. Some states have no requirements, while others outline specific procedures for authentication, including acceptable methods and time frames (Welch 2000a). Many state laws apply exclusively to physicians' orders for drugs and services (Dougherty 2001). Additionally, hospitals address authentication requirements for health records in medical staff rules and regulations, which provide minimum authentication requirements for documentation, including how it is authenticated.

Many hospitals produce health records in various formats as the organization transitions to an electronic health record; therefore, HIM professionals should have a good understanding of authentication requirements based on how health records are created. In the paper-based health record, written signatures are usually applied to handwritten documentation as it is created. Often signatures are illegible, and clinicians forget to date and time stamp entries. However, HIM professionals identify missing signatures when reviewing documentation for completeness.

As facilities implement EHRs, their health records become hybrid. A **hybrid health record** is a blend of paper-based and electronic documentation. Therefore, the hybrid health record includes a combination of handwritten and electronic signatures. HIM departments using an **electronic document management system (EDMS)** to manage health records is an example of a hybrid state. An EDMS can be defined as interfaced and paper-based documents scanned into a document imaging system that has workflow functionality. For example, scanned paper-based documents and interfaced, transcribed documents can both be electronically authenticated with an electronic signature. The EDMS can trigger signature deficiencies in interfaced documents, or HIM professionals can assign a signature deficiency to scanned documents. An **electronic signature** is a unique personal identifier that is entered by the author of EHR documentation via electronic means. Benefits of the electronic signature include legibility and automatic dating and time stamping of entries.

Authentication in electronic health record systems is accomplished with electronic or digital signatures. Digital signatures use the same technology as automated credit card authentication systems. A **digital signature** is a digitized version of a handwritten signature. The author of the documentation signs his or her name on a pen pad, and the signature is automatically converted to a digital signature that is affixed to the electronic document (AHIMA e-HIM Task Force 2003a). Electronic authentication executed at the completion of documentation within an application is the best practice because it saves time, and all entries are legible, dated, and time stamped.

not covered by HIPAA

Each individual that has been authorized to document in the electronic health record uses a **unique personal identifier** in the form of a code or password. Some systems may use a combination of a unique logon ID and password as a means to validate the author of the documentation or it may be a **biometric identifier** such as a fingerprint or retinal scans.

Each unique personal identifier must be assigned exclusively to a specific clinician, and a master list of the electronic identifiers must be maintained in a secure environment. Electronic signatures are permitted under Medicare *Conditions of Participation for Hospitals* (2007) regulations and accreditation standards. Some states outline requirements for the use of electronic signatures for authentication. States that do not address this issue may permit the use of electronic signatures with approval from fiscal intermediaries or state authorities. (AHIMA e-HIM Task Force 2003a). Most states have enacted specific laws or regulations addressing electronic signatures, and HIM professionals should be familiar with their own state laws on electronic signatures.

Corrections in Clinical Documentation

When erroneous entries are made in health records, written procedures should have provisions on how corrections are made. Educating clinicians who are authorized to document in the health record on the appropriate way to make corrections will promote consistency and standardization and maintain the integrity of the health record. Errors corrected in the paper-based record may be easier to identify visually than those corrected in electronic documentation systems. The following is the recommended process for correcting errors in paper-based records (Smith 2001):

1. The clinician making the correction should draw a single line in ink through the incorrect entry.

2. The clinician should then print the word error at the top of the entry.

3. The clinician should authenticate the error notation by signing or initialing the notation and noting the date and time. The signature should include the individual's credentials and title. The reason the change is needed should also be noted.

4. The correct information should then be added to the entry as a notation. Late entries should be labeled as such; that is, entries must never be antedated (assigned a date earlier than the current date).

time stamped

Clinicians cannot use the same method of correcting erroneous documentation that has been created and stored electronically. So how does one approach this challenging issue in the electronic health record so the amended documentation can be identified? The practice of correcting transcribed reports has been for the clinician to dictate an addendum to the original report, especially if the report has been signed. However, when the transcribed report is interfaced into an EDMS, the clinician has the ability to edit the original report before applying an electronic signature. After the report is electronically signed, the text-editing feature should not be available for amending documentation. Organizational policy should consider creating an addendum rather than an amendment to a signed document.

A primary concern when making corrections to the electronic health record is the rippling effect of data passing to various data sets, systems, and warehouses in an electronic environment, which magnifies the risk of inaccurate data. When corrections are needed for electronic documentation, data capture methods should include a mechanism for adding corrections to all the data sets to which information has been passed. Following are some best practices for correcting documents in an EHR:

1. Minimize the need for corrections by having documents complete and accurate before electronic authentication occurs.

2. Determine if data was received in the EHR through an interface from another documentation system.

3. Either edit or add an amendment to original documentation and resend it through interface to the EHR.

4. Add amendments to signed documentation by indicating the reason for the amendment.

5. The electronic system should identify authors of documentation and date and time entries.

6. Redistribute corrections to recipients of the original/incorrect documentation.

7. Correct data in all electronic systems to ensure integrity of data collected.

8. Limit the number of persons authorized to make amendments to a signed document.

9. If policy allows editing of signed documents, all versions of the documents must be available for legal purposes.

10. Signed documents in the EHR should never be permanently deleted from the system, but provide a link for accessing the original version of the note or document.

Guidelines for EHR Documentation to Prevent Fraud

This section was adapted from AHIMA's e-HIM Work Group on EHR Data Content's Guidelines for EHR Documentation Practice, "Guidelines for EHR documentation to prevent fraud," originally published in the January 2007 issue of the *Journal of American Health Information Management Association*.

Electronic documentation tools offer exciting, new timesaving and validity-checking features designed to enhance communication for all health record users. They address traditional, well-known requirements for documentation principles, while supporting expansive new HIM capabilities. However, use of these features without appropriate management and guidelines may cause invalid autopopulation of data fields, manufactured documentation to enhance expected reimbursement, and other undesirable outcomes.

There are a number of existing regulations and laws on documentation principles, as well as rapidly accumulating experiences translating core HIM principles into the electronic realm. Existing resources address documentation authorship principles, auditing, and forms development, and new ones are emerging to ensure and preserve documentation integrity in an age of electronic identity theft and changes in the legal evidentiary requirements for electronic business and clinical records.

According to the National Health Care Anti-fraud Association, healthcare fraud is defined as an "intentional deception or misrepresentation that the individual or entity makes knowing that the misrepresentation could result in some unauthorized benefit to the individual, or the entity, or to some other party." EHR users should not expect unintentional deception or misrepresentation to be viewed more gently by payers, evaluators, or litigators. However, one of the many changes HIPAA (2006) legislation rendered is that the standard is now "known or should have known." This shifts burden significantly by including the concept that those submitting claims have a due diligence obligation to proactively identify and prevent fraud, as the burden now is that the deception or misrepresentation need not be known or intentional but should have been known.

There are four areas of concern regarding the EHR environment:

1. **Authorship integrity**: Borrowing record entries from another source or author and representing or displaying past as current documentation and (in some instances) misrepresenting or inflating the nature and intensity of services provided

2. **Auditing integrity**: Inadequate auditing functions that make it impossible to detect when an entry was modified or borrowed from another source and misrepresented as an original entry by an authorized user

3. **Documentation integrity**: Automated insertion of clinical data and visit documentation using templates or similar tools with predetermined documentation components with uncontrolled and uncertain clinical relevance

4. **Patient identification and demographic accuracy**: Automated demographic or registration entries generating erroneous patient identification, leading to patient safety and quality of care issues as well as enabling fraudulent activity involving patient identity theft or providing unjustified care for profit

Authorship Integrity

Authorship is the origin of recorded information that is attributed to a specific individual or entity. (AHIMA 2005a) EHRs must allow more than one party to add additional text to the same entry and retain and display the authorship of each entry. For example, a nurse or alternate user can begin a patient's encounter note, and later, the examining physician can add comments.

[handwritten margin note: add only]

In systems that require a single authorization for visit notes, the entire note may be attributed to the physician, and entries or observations by alternate users may be edited or deleted before final physician authentication despite the alternate users' authentication. Another example includes flowcharts allowing entries by multiple individuals over a period of time and requiring only one signature at the end of the encounter, thus losing the identities of caregivers who posted interim data.

[handwritten margin note: link each entry to one author]

In these situations, it may be impossible to verify the actual provider of care or the amount of work performed by each person providing services. When records are analyzed and clinical codes reported for billing, the claim may reflect the wrong provider and level or type of care. One method of healthcare fraud involves using unlicensed individuals to perform services, while submitting claims under the provider number of a legitimate provider. It is the user's duty to ensure that all documentation authorship is accurately recorded in all approved uses of the documentation tools available.

Auto-authentication or Systematic Authorship Misrepresentation

Progress notes are considered assertions of a person and are authenticated for legal admissibility in a court of law. Auto-authentication methods that do not require an author to review the entry fall short of federal and state authentication requirements and place the organization at legal risk. Some providers choose not to enter their own progress notes electronically and use scribes or assistants to type entries into the system for subsequent authorization. Policies, procedures, and checks and balances must be in place to ensure that the physician or legally responsible individual reviews the health record entries and affixes an authorization compliant with existing law. Since health record documentation drives payment from health plans, inaccurate information may lead to perceived fraudulent activities.

Borrowing Data from Other Sources

Electronic tools make it easier to copy and paste documentation from one record to another or to pull information forward from a previous visit, someone else's records, or other sources, either intentionally or inadvertently. Studies (Embi et al 2004, Hammond et al 2003, Helbig 2004, Weir et al 2003) show that the ability to "copy previous entries and paste into a current entry" lead to a record where a clinician may, upon signing the documentation, unwittingly swear to the accuracy and comprehensiveness of substantial amounts of duplicated or inapplicable information as well as the incorporation of misleading or erroneous documentation. The studies further illustrate that, while helping to improve apparent timeliness and legibility of documentation, additional adverse effects are created by the inability to verify actual authors or to authenticate services provided at any given time. From a billing perspective, defaulting clinical information with previous existing documentation from other patient encounters facilitates billing at a higher level of service than was actually provided.

Because of industry and regulatory payment pressures, physicians may find it necessary to document each component of the history and physical or review of systems during a patient encounter for payment and quality measurement. Time constraints and patient care demands can sometimes make it difficult for clinicians to meet the evaluation and patient management documentation requirements, creating the temptation to copy and paste. Shortcuts developed in the absence of consideration of clinical purpose can result in erroneous records and elevate the potential for fraudulent activity unless clinicians are fully aware of the risk and, therefore, undertake appropriate review. Difficulties resulting from these practices include the following:

- Inaccurate representation of authorship of documentation

- Duplication of inapplicable information (relevant to the original case but not true for current care)

- Incorporation of misleading or erroneous documentation due to loss of context that was available to users in the original source

- Inclusion of entries from documentation created by others without their knowledge or consent

- Inability to accurately determine services and findings specific to a patient's encounter

- Inaccurate automated code generation associated with documentation

Auditing Integrity

If an EHR lacks adequate audit trail functionality, there may be no way to determine if and when corrections or amendments were made to the documentation, by whom, or the nature of the correction or amendment. In addition to the normal unintentional mistakes that occur in documentation, there may be situations where the alteration of records is performed to prevent the discovery of damaging information or to avoid legal action. Without an adequate auditing function always "on" in an EHR system, legitimate changes may not be distinguishable from illegitimate ones, and the latter type may be accepted as fact and may be untraceable. Any changes or deletions made outside of routine record use must be maintained in the EHR system. Any uncertainty as to the integrity of the record creates legal liability for the institution while protecting criminal activity.

automatic

The functionality of the EHR may also determine whether or not an original note or amendment includes the correct date and time. Some systems automatically assign the date that the entry was made, while others allow authorized users to revise the date of entry to the date of the visit or service. It is imperative that any system be able to identify the date the note or amendment originated and the service date that the note or amendment references. Otherwise, the date sequence may be impossible to follow, adversely affecting appropriate patient care and resulting in questionable supporting documentation for reported services. Some EHR systems allow more than one party to add additional text to the same entry; for example, when faculty physicians are required to cosign resident notes. If the EHR does not have functionality to enable both providers to document and sign, it may be impossible to verify the actual provider of care or the amount of work performed by each person providing services. When records are analyzed and clinical codes reported for billing, the claim may reflect the wrong provider or incorrect level or type of care.

never include personal opinions in an EHR

no arguments

know emails all are a permanent part of the record

As stated before, auto-authentication, defined as signing multiple documents at one time without opening the documents, falls short of federal and state authentication requirements and could place the organization at legal risk. Some providers use scribes or assistants to type entries into the system for subsequent authorization. In some situations, the physician or other provider gives his or her access codes to assistants to allow direct entry of the notes. The system recognizes the author as the physician or the other authorized provider of care, instead of the assistant. Checks and balances must be in place to ensure that the physician or other legally responsible individual has reviewed the health record entries and authenticated them compliant with existing law.

Documentation Integrity: Automated Insertion of Clinical Data

Documentation templates are sometimes employed to enter default common findings into health record documents. For example, the automatic generation of common negative findings within a review of systems for each body area or organ system. Template users (often physicians) should document pertinent positive results and delete incorrect auto-generated entries.

The primary reason templates are used is to save time. A physician not fully aware of the consequences of defaulting information in templates may fail to take the time necessary to review all defaulted data for changes and leave incorrect information in the record. This can lead to an inappropriate clinical picture, and the accuracy of the entire documented entry may be questioned. Documentation can be especially suspect when used as the basis for service justification or other payment concerns without evidence of clinical relevance.

EHR systems must allow limited automatic creation of information. In the hands of criminals, autogenerated documentation for health records can enable rapid and plausible claims to both government and private health plans for payment. Clinical coding professionals rely on documentation for code assignments used on health plans. If the documentation is not true, the codes do not accurately reflect the circumstances of the healthcare service even when the codes are completely consistent with the documentation in the record. The "dirty data" resulting from inappropriate use of these tools compromises both good patient care and data-mining capabilities.

Templates often provide clinical information by default and design. When used inappropriately, they may misrepresent a patient's condition and might not reflect changes in a condition. These tools may also include defaults such as "reviewed past, family, and social history" for frequent visits, which is often not indicated or performed each time. Unless the physician or other authorized provider removes the default documentation from the visit note, a higher level of service than is actually provided could be assigned as well as a higher level of service claimed than might be appropriate for the service.

All templates and autogenerated entries, such as laboratory results, have the potential to be problematic. Accordingly, management oversight is necessary. Appropriate care must be taken that the data captured and stored are accurate, complete, and associated with the correct patient record and encounter.

One example of a beneficial feature of EHR systems is the autopopulation of discrete clinical data (such as laboratory results) in the appropriate data fields rather than requiring a physician or other authorized provider to document the results with a progress note. Anecdotal information indicates that data generated as close as possible to the point of care are the most accurate and least likely to be connected with healthcare fraud.

Patient Identification and Demographic Data

Some EHR systems include capabilities for additional efficiency in health service financial management transactions and billing processes. Demographic and insurance data may be defaulted for a patient's encounter. Based on a setting or type of service, the system can automatically assign a registration status or discharge disposition. Audit functions must be implemented to ensure that appropriate and legitimate information results and errors can be tracked for correction and staff training purposes. Health plan or payer policies may include patient-care setting adjustments such as an office, hospital, or outpatient department for physician services. If a registration status is incorrectly assigned, the location of service and technical, professional, or global billing may be inappropriately reimbursed.

Patient identity theft is also an area of vulnerability for healthcare organizations. In the wrong hands, Medicare, Medicaid, and other health plan claims data coupled with the ability to manufacture supporting documentation creates the risk of false claims and criminal activity. Patient safety and quality-of-care issues arise when physician order entry systems fail to provide appropriate safeguards to identify fraud and abuse or business agreements involving data management violate patient privacy or allow unscrupulous providers to provide care that is unnecessary or fails to meet community standards for quality.

Solutions for Success in Fraud Prevention When Using EHR Features

Preventing fraud resulting from deliberate falsification of information requires three primary conditions:

- Organizational desire and commitment to conduct business and provide care in an ethical manner

- Organizations purchasing systems that include functions and capabilities to prevent or discourage fraudulent activity

- Organizations implementing and using policies, procedures, and system functions and capabilities to prevent fraud

Managing Data

A best practice strategy for handling data in the electronic environment necessitates front-end and ongoing monitoring, including point-of-care data quality assessment. The traditional, retrospective auditing and quality-assurance activities traditionally associated with the paper-based health record will continue to be an approach of choice for some data quality checkpoints. However, concurrent data quality checks play a more prominent role to ensure quality of documentation in an electronic environment while retrospective auditing may exist as a parallel set of assessment functions.

To understand how and where data flows throughout the organization, it is important to perform an analysis of current systems and implement organizational policies to optimize standardization toward the assurance of quality. When data are stored or maintained in more than one system, all systems must be cleaned up to prevent bad data from reentering the system. Due to the interconnectivity of many electronic systems, decisions must be made determining which systems should be included in data clean up, how far back to go, and how long it takes to clean up data (AHIMA 2007). See chapter 3 for a discussion of e-Discovery, which expands on data management requirements in relation to the Federal Rules of Civil Procedure (FRCP), which were updated in 2006.

e-Discovery: Developing a Litigation Response Plan

This section was adapted from Kimberly Baldwin-Stried Reich's article "Developing a Litigation Response Plan," originally published in the October 2007 issue of the *Journal of American Health Information Management Association*. This topic is also discussed in chapter 3.

The e-discovery amendments to the FRCP (updated in 2006) and the Uniform Rules Relating to the Discovery of Electronically Stored Information (2007) (approved in August 2007 at the National Conference of Commissioners on Uniform State Laws) are creating new roles and responsibilities for legal counsel and HIM and information technology (IT) professionals. Organizations must begin thinking how they will respond to e-discovery requests for information. The process by which electronic information is produced in response to threatened or impending litigation is changing, and those closely involved with it must be knowledgeable on the requirements for producing information.

Three concepts are important in developing a litigation response plan for e-discovery:

- an organization's duty to preserve documents in the face of threatened or pending litigation,
- the legal hold, and
- the development of an organization's e-discovery response plan.

New Requests, New Responsibilities

In general terms, *discovery* is the formal, pretrial legal process used by parties to a lawsuit to obtain information. Discovery helps ensure that neither party is subjected to surprises at trial. The scope of information that can be obtained through discovery is broad and is not limited to what will be used at trial. Federal courts and most state courts allow a party to discover any information relevant to the claim. Because of the broad nature of this standard, parties often disagree about what information must be exchanged and what is considered "privileged." These disputes are resolved through court rulings on discovery motions.

In e-discovery, the court is alerted early in the litigation, and the district judge, magistrate judge, or special master may take an active role in addressing the handling of discovery of electronically stored information, when it is expected to occur.

While the FRCP amendments apply to civil cases brought before federal (district) courts, it is anticipated that these amendments coupled with the Uniform Rules Relating to the Discovery of Electronically Stored Information will define the standards for discovery and production of electronic information at the state and local court levels.

As a result, it is incumbent upon legal counsel and HIM and IT professionals to evaluate how their roles and responsibilities will change with regard to the discovery and production of electronically stored information.

E-discovery will be most effective when legal counsel has a good understanding of the rules, communicates and negotiates with opposing counsel and the court, and involves HIM and IT professionals in the process.

The Duty to Preserve

The basic principles regarding preservation of relevant electronically stored information are essentially the same as those governing the preservation of relevant paper-based business records. That is, at the moment when litigation is reasonably anticipated (known, threatened, or pending), the normal disposition and processing of information in either format should be suspended.

For example, today some healthcare organizations make a copy of the paper-based record (usually the patient's health record) at the time litigation is known. The original paper-based record is then given to risk management or legal counsel, who secures the record in a locked file. Access to the original paper-based health record is then usually controlled or monitored to prevent unauthorized access or tampering.

The duty to preserve relevant electronically stored information also supersedes an organization's record retention and management policies that would normally result in the destruction of electronically stored information. The basic premise of common law doctrine is to avoid spoliation (intentional destruction, alteration, or concealment) of evidence for use at trial. The courts have inherent powers and rules that govern the imposition of sanctions for spoliation.

The Legal Hold

Once litigation can be reasonably anticipated, an organization should establish a legal (litigation) hold, and reasonable measures should be taken to identify and preserve all information relevant to the claim. A legal hold (also known as a preservation order) may or may not be issued by a court. An organization's key determination in establishing a legal hold is when litigation is "reasonably anticipated." For example, once an individual or organization is served with a complaint, subpoena, subpoena duces tecum, or receives notice of a government investigation, litigation can be reasonably anticipated. A legal hold should then be immediately established and reasonable measures taken to identify and preserve relevant information. The duty to preserve could arise well before an individual or organization is served with any of these documents or notices. Determining when the legal hold should be established is not a rote decision. When faced with potential litigation, the facts of each situation must be carefully weighed.

Organizations and their legal counsel may consider the following general factors prior to establishing a legal hold:

- The potential litigation risk to the organization (type, source, and credibility)

- The potential risk of information loss if a legal hold is not established

- Identification of all individuals identified as potential "record custodians"

- Assessment of the level of knowledge, sources, and location of information within the organization relevant to the potential claim

- Process by which the establishment of the legal hold will be communicated within the organization

- The time frame for reviewing the legal hold and when it can be lifted

The e-Discovery Litigation Response Team

In business, as well as in healthcare, the discovery of electronically stored information is not a simple, inexpensive, or straightforward process. The true costs to search, cull, and retrieve electronic information (including information that is contained in back-up tapes and legacy systems) that may be relevant to a lawsuit could far outweigh the costs of providing photocopies of a patient's health records. Organizations must establish a plan and process to understand the true costs and burdens of producing electronic information.

Effective e-discovery administration requires a team of interdisciplinary professionals serving on a litigation response team. Legal counsel should oversee the e-discovery process and head the team. They will advise senior management and the governing board about any and all impending litigation, and they can define and delineate the measures the organization should take in the identification, preservation, search, retrieval, and production of responsive electronic and other potentially relevant information.

IT and HIM professionals should also be appointed to the team. They are best equipped to advise legal counsel about the forms, formats, methods, status, costs, location, and production burden of potentially responsive information. They also possess knowledge of the technical and administrative processes surrounding the use, management, storage, retention, and destruction of information within the organization.

The time to prepare for e-discovery is now. An e-discovery plan should be prepared well in advance of litigation, and it should be tailored to the needs of the size, scope, and complexity of the organization. By becoming familiar with the FRCP, the Uniform Rules Relating to the Discovery of Electronically Stored Information, and state legislation involving electronic document production, legal counsel and HIM and IT professionals have the unique opportunity to work together to define and shape e-discovery processes for their organizations and states.

Disaster Planning

Another important aspect of health record documentation is planning for how information can be accessed to treat patients during planned or unplanned computer systems down time or during a disaster. Hospitals are required to have backup plans to protect health information from damage and destruction. **Disaster Recovery Planning** is the technological aspect of business continuity planning. HIM professionals assist in designing disaster recovery plans that address how information can be documented in the health record during down time or a disaster.

A well-designed disaster-recovery plan should consider the following:

1. Daily backups and removal of electronic data/information to offsite location for protection

2. Access to information needed to treat patients

3. Backup plan to collect and document health information

4. Protection of computer systems, data, and paper-based records from destruction

5. Protection against unauthorized use and disclosure

6. Safeguards to ensure integrity and confidentiality of information

7. Provision for orderly recovery of information

8. Periodic testing of disaster recovery plans before a disaster occurs

The Hurricane Katrina experience demonstrated that good contingency plans not only should include backing up patient data to other media, but also identified the need to make data accessible as soon as possible. Another lesson learned during Katrina was the importance of thorough planning for health information in disaster preparedness and response (Carol 2006).

Disaster planning must account for manual processes for use during down time even when health information is electronic. HIM professionals play an important part in disaster planning by assuming leadership roles in ensuring health records are safeguarded while the information is accessible.

Disaster recovery best practices include the following:

- Routinely reviewing emergency plans

- Regularly practicing and reviewing contingency plans

- Ensuring employees are knowledgeable and prepared to quickly implement plans

- Ensuring serious dialogue about backup and recovery

- Routinely moving backup data to a remote location

- Routinely testing contingency plans

HIM professionals provide a unique perspective in disaster planning because they understand the workflow of the health record better than any other professional in the organization does, and they can identify strategies for making paper or electronic records available for patient care. HIM should plan how to respond to different levels of disasters and how records will be created or maintained during this process. Additionally, they should plan how to make electronic databases available during a disaster and how quickly information will be recovered.

Figure 7.10. Decision tool.

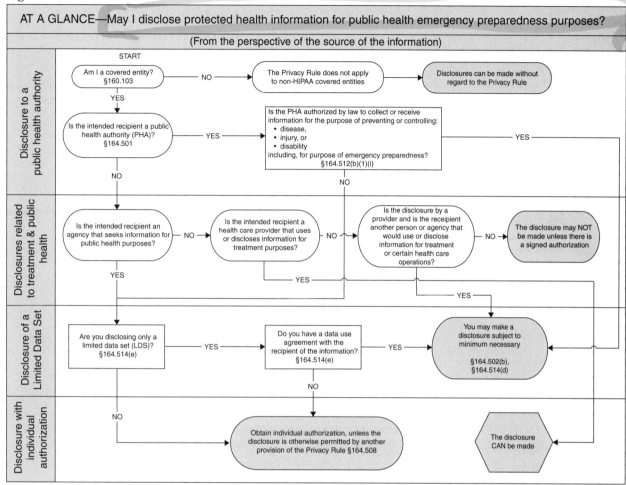

In the aftermath of Hurricane Katrina in 2005, the Veterans Administration initiated the development of the Health Data Repository that will contain real-time copies of local clinical data. The **Health Data Repository** is a database that provides immediate nationwide access to local data in the event of primary system failure or system unavailability. The repository is an effort to improve data accessibility and increase disaster preparedness. See figure 7.10 for a health information release decision tool from the Office for Civil Rights (OCR). This tool focuses on issues relevant to emergency preparedness and does not address other federal, state, or local confidentiality laws that may apply in specific circumstances. Although this tool does not discuss all the Privacy Rule requirements (HIPAA 2003) for the uses and disclosures permitted, it can be used as a guide to develop a contingency plan for releasing protected health information in a disaster.

Summary

HIM professionals' role in healthcare settings has advanced from ensuring compliance with documentation requirements to one of developing and implementing best practices and processes that help support clinical staff to create accurate documentation and complete it in a timely manner. During the process of health record analysis, HIM professionals identify deficiencies in health records that range from authentication to missing documentation. Organizations use data documented in the health record to improve quality of care and patient safety.

Regulatory and accrediting agencies require hospitals to protect health information from damage, loss, and destruction. The importance of protecting health information during a disaster requires effective planning and implementation of disaster recovery and business-continuity plans. Development of a litigation response plan is recommended in light of e-discovery regulations and litigation. HIM professionals play a key role in implementation of disaster planning. HIM professionals provide valuable leadership and knowledge in assisting hospitals with development and implementation of best practices for providing and maintaining quality documentation throughout the healthcare environment, whether in paper or electronic form.

References

AHIMA e-HIM Task Force. 2003a. Practice brief: Implementing electronic signatures. *Journal of American Health Information Management Association* 74(10).

American Health Information Management Association Professional Practice Teams. 2005 (September). Available online from www.ahima.org.

AHIMA e-HIM Work Group on Maintaining the Legal EHR. 2005a. Update: Maintaining a legally sound health record—paper and electronic. *Journal of American Health Information Management Association* 76(10): 64A–L.

AHIMA e-HIM Work Group on EHR Data Content. 2006 (February). Guidelines for developing a data dictionary. *Journal of American Health Information Management Association* 77(2): 64A–D.

AHIMA e-HIM Work Group. 2007 (March). Assessing and improving EHR data quality. *Journal of American Health Information Management Association* 78(3): 69–72.

AHIMA e-HIM Work Group: Guidelines for EHR Documentation Practice. 2007 (January). Guidelines for EHR documentation to prevent fraud. *Journal of American Health Information Management Association* 78(1): 65–68.

American Health Information Management Association. 2007. Position statement: Quality healthcare data and information (revised and adopted October 2006). *Journal of American Health Information Management Association* 78(1): 20.

Carol, Ruth. Lessons from Katrina. 2006. *Journal of American Health Information Management Association* 77(4): 46–50.

Centers for Medicare and Medicaid Services. 2007. *Medicare Conditions of Participation for Hospitals.* Washington, D.C.: CMS.

Coffman-Kadish, Nancy. 2002. Health record analysis. Chapter 5 in *Health Information Management: Principles and Organization for Health Information Services,* 5th ed. Edited by Margaret Skurka. San Francisco: Jossey-Bass.

Dougherty, Michelle. 2001. Practice brief: Verbal/telephone order authentication and time frames. *Journal of American Health Information Management Association* 72(2).

Embi, Peter J., et al. 2004. Impacts of computerized physician documentation in a teaching hospital: Perceptions of faculty and resident physicians. *Journal of American Medical Informatics Association* 11(4): 300–309.

Federal Rules of Civil Procedure, 28USC. 2006. *United States Code.* Available online from http://judiciary.house.gov/media/pdfs/printers/109th/31308.pdf.

Fletcher, Donna. 1999. Practice brief: Best practices in medical record documentation and completion. *Journal of American Health Information Management Association* 70(10): 56A–H.

Gold, Robert S. 2007. What clinical documentation improvement is—and what it's not. *For the Record* 19(6): 8.

Hammond, Kenric W., et al. 2003. Are electronic medical records trustworthy? Observations on copying, pasting and duplication. AMIA Annual Symposium Proceedings: 269–273.

Helbig, Susan. 2004. Copying and pasting in the EHR-S: An HIM perspective. 2004 IFHRO Congress & AHIMA Convention Proceedings. Available online from http://library.ahima.org/xpedio/idcplg?IdcService=GET_HIGHLIGHT_INFO&QueryText=%28Copying+and+Pasting+in+the+EHR%2dS%3a+An+HIM+Perspective%29%3cand%3e%28xPublishSite%3csubstring%3e%60BoK%60%29&SortField=xPubDate&SortOrder=Desc&dDocName=bok3_005520&HighlightType=HtmlHighlight&dWebExtension=hcsp.

Joint Commission on Accreditation of Healthcare Organizations. 2006. *2006 Comprehensive Accreditation Manual for Hospitals; The Official Handbook.* Oakbrook Terrace, IL: Joint Commission.

Lewis, S., and S. Reinicke. 2005 (October). To Review or Not to Review: Finding the Solution for Ongoing Record Review. *Proceedings of the AHIMA 77th National Convention and Exhibit,* San Diego, CA.

McCain, Mary. 2006. Paper-based health records. Chapter 8 in *Health Information Management: Concepts, Principles, and Practice,* 2nd ed. Edited by Kathleen LaTour and Shirley Eichenwald-Maki. Chicago: AHIMA.

Micheletti, J., and T. Shlala. 2006 (February). Documentation Rx: Strategies for improving physician contribution to hospital records. *Journal of American Health Information Management Association* 77(2): 66–68.

National Health Care Anti-fraud Association. What is healthcare fraud? Available online from http://www.nhcaa.org/eweb/DynamicPage.aspx?webcode=anti_fraud_resource_centr&wpscode=ConsumerAndActionInfo.

Office of Civil Rights. n.d. Available online from www.hhs.gov/ocr/hipaa/decisiontool/EmergencyPrepDisclose.pdf.

Reich, Kimberly Baldwin-Stried. 2007. Developing a litigation response plan. *Journal of American Health Information Management Association* 78(9): 76–78, 86.

Roberts, Jane. 2007. Health information technology functions. Chapter 8 in *Health Information Management Technology: An Applied Approach,* 2nd ed. Edited by Merida Johns. Chicago: AHIMA.

Servais, Cheryl. 2008. *The Legal Health Record.* Edited by Neil Olderman and Kelly Trahan. Chicago: AHIMA.

Smith, Cheryl. 2001. Practice brief: Documentation requirements for the acute care inpatient record. *Journal of American Health Information Management Association* 72(3).

Weir, CR, et al. 2003. Direct text entry in electronic progress notes: An evaluation of input errors. *Methods of Information in Medicine* 42(1): 61–67.

Welch, Julie. 1999. Practice brief: Correcting and amending entries in a computerized patient record. *Journal of American Health Information Management Association* 70(8).

Welch, Julie. 2000a. Practice brief: Authentication of health record entries. *Journal of American Health Information Management Association* 71(3).

Welch, Julie. 2000b. Practice brief: Storage media for health information. *Journal of American Health Information Management Association* 71(6).

PART III

Organization and Management of the Health Record

Chapter 8

Accreditation and Regulations

Diann Brown, MS, RHIA, CHP

Learning Objectives

- List and explain the sources of regulations, legal doctrine, and standards that apply to acute-care health records

- Describe the basic hospital licensure process

- List the sources of information on Medicare and Medicaid regulations

- List and explain the documentation standards in the Medicare *Conditions of Participation for Hospitals*

- Explain the concept of deemed status

- Explain the difference between regulatory standards and accreditation standards

- Explain the Joint Commission's accreditation process

- Explain the Joint Commission's sentinel event policy

- Explain the purpose of tracer methodology

- Briefly outline the AOA HFAP accreditation process

- Explain the purpose of establishing uniform data sets

- List and define the five types of health informatics standards

- Describe the status of the HL7 standard on electronic health records

- Describe the purpose of developing health record policies and procedures and explain the difference between a policy and a procedure

Key Terms

Accreditation

Accreditation organizations

American Health Information Community (AHIC)

American Osteopathic Association (AOA)

American Society for Testing and Materials (ASTM)

Board certification

Centers for Medicare and Medicaid Services (CMS)

Code of Federal Regulations (CFR)

Conditions of Participation for Hospitals

Credentialing

Data dictionary

Deemed status

EHR Collaborative

Electronic data interchange (EDI)

Federal Register

Health informatics standards

Health Information Technology Standards Panel (HITSP)

Health Level Seven (HL7)

Health Plan Employer Data and Information Set (HEDIS)

Healthcare Facilities Accreditation Program (HFAP)

Identifier standards

Individual tracer activity

Individual-based system tracer activity

Joint Commission

Licensure

Medical staff bylaws, rules, and regulations

National Committee for Quality Assurance (NCQA)

Periodic Performance Review (PPR)

Policies

Priority focus areas (PFAs)

Priority focus process (PFP)

Procedures

Professional certification organizations

Regulation

RxNorm

Security standards

Sentinel event

Standards

Standards development organizations (SDOs)

Statute

Structure and content standards

Systematized Nomenclature of Medicine–Clinical Terms® (SNOMED CT®)

Tracer methodology

Transaction and messaging standards

Unannounced survey

Vocabulary standards

Introduction

Acute-care hospitals are subject to a number of complex operating requirements. Federal, state, and local branches of government; accreditation organizations; professional medical societies and associations; and national and international standards development organizations establish these operating requirements.

The mandatory rules that apply to hospitals and other healthcare organizations come from several different sources:

- Federal statutes and regulations, which apply throughout the United States

- State statutes and regulations, which apply only within individual states

- County and municipal ordinances and codes, which apply only to local communities

- State and federal judicial decisions, which apply only to the geopolitical areas that fall under the jurisdiction of the court that made the decision

A **statute** is a piece of legislation written and approved by a state or federal legislature and then signed into law by the state's governor or the president. The Health Insurance Portability and Accountability Act (HIPAA) of 1996 is an example of a federal statute. Table 8.1 provides a list of other federal legislation relevant to acute-care records.

A **regulation** is a rule established by an administrative agency of government. The difference between a statute and a regulation is regulations must be followed by any healthcare organization participating in the related program. Administrative agencies are responsible for implementing and managing the programs instituted by state and federal statutes. The **Centers for Medicare and Medicaid Services (CMS)** is an example of an administrative agency. The CMS is the federal agency charged with developing and implementing Medicare and Medicaid regulations, such as the Medicare *Conditions of Participation for Hospitals* (2006).

Acute-care hospitals must meet additional requirements such as the following:

- State licensure requirements

- State health record regulations

- State public health regulations

- State rules on Medicaid qualifications

- County and municipal building safety codes

- HIPAA Privacy and Security Rules

- Legal doctrines of medical liability based on judicial decisions

Table 8.1   Federal laws that affect acute-care documentation

Legislation	Date	Impact on Documentation
False Claims Act	1863	Established federal penalties for cheating the federal government by supplying inferior goods and services
Amendment	1986	Established federal penalties for filing false or fraudulent Medicare and Medicaid claims
Social Security Act	1935	Established the Social Security program
Amendments (Public Law 89-97)	1965	Established the Medicare and Medicaid Programs
Amendment (Public Law 98-21)	1983	Established the prospective payment system for inpatient care
Freedom of Information Act	1966	Established public's right to access information maintained by branches of the federal government
Alcohol Abuse and Alcoholism Prevention, Treatment and Rehabilitation Act	1970	Established patient's right to control the release of information related to his or her treatment for alcoholism
Amendment	2000	Established strict confidentiality requirements for treatment records maintained by facilities that receive federal funding
Drug Abuse Prevention, Treatment and Rehabilitation Act	1970	Established patient's right to control the release of information related to his or her treatment for drug addiction
Amendment	2000	Established strict confidentiality requirements for treatment records maintained by facilities that receive federal funding
Comprehensive Drug Abuse Prevention and Control Act	1970	Established strict federal controls on the dispensing of narcotics, depressants, stimulants, and hallucinogens
Privacy Act	1974	Established requirements for obtaining written consent before disclosure of confidential personal information
Food, Drug and Cosmetics Act, Medical Device Amendments	1976	Established controls on the testing, manufacturing, labeling and distribution of drugs and medical devices,
Utilization Review Act	1977	Established Medicare and Medicaid requirement for continued-stay reviews of acute care services
Tax Equity and Fiscal Responsibility Act	1982	Established efforts to control Medicare spending through the gradual implementation of prospective payment systems
Peer Review Improvement Act	1982	Established Medicare and Medicaid requirements for medical necessity and quality reviews of acute care services
Emergency Treatment and Active Labor Act	1985	Established "antidumping" regulations under the Consolidated Omnibus Reconciliation Act; prohibits hospital emergency departments from transferring medically unstable patients to other facilities because they have no health insurance coverage
Consolidated Omnibus Budget Reconciliation Act	1985	Established reimbursement penalties for providing substandard healthcare services to Medicare and Medicaid patients
Omnibus Budget Reconciliation Act	1986	Established reporting requirements for peer review organizations that identify facilities providing substandard healthcare
Health Care Quality Improvement Act	1986	Established the National Practitioner Data Bank
Omnibus Budget Reconciliation Act	1989	Established the Agency for Health Care Policy and Research
Omnibus Budget Reconciliation Act	1990	Established reporting requirements for peer review organizations that identify practitioners providing substandard healthcare
Americans with Disabilities Act	1990	Established the equal opportunity and physical access rights of people with physical and mental disabilities
Patient Self-Determination Act	1990	Established the rights of patients to refuse medical treatment, make healthcare decisions, and establish advance directives
Safe Medical Devices Act	1993	Established reporting requirements for hospitals that identify potential safety problems with medical equipment and implantable devices
Health Insurance Portability and Accountability Act	1996	Established privacy and security rules to protect the confidentiality and integrity of patient-identifiable information; also established the Healthcare Integrity and Protection Data Bank
Balanced Budget Act	1997	Established Medicare requirement that physicians provide diagnostic information to support orders for services under certain limited circumstances; led to general practice of including diagnostic information on physicians' orders
Benefits Improvement and Protection Act	2000	Established that hospital inpatient PPS should recognize the cost of new medical services and technologies.
Medicare Prescription Drug, Improvement, and Modernization Act	2003	Established standards for an electronic prescription drug program.

Source: Rhodes and Burrington-Brown 2002.

The voluntary rules that apply to acute-care organizations also come from a variety of sources:

- **Accreditation organizations:** professional organizations that set the standards against which healthcare organizations are measured to ensure the quality and safety of their services

- **Professional certification organizations:** private societies and membership organizations that establish professional qualification requirements and clinical practice standards for specific areas of medicine, nursing, and allied health professions

- **Standards development organizations:** private or governmental agencies that develop scientifically based models against which structures, processes, and outcomes can be measured

Although following the recommendations of standards-setting organizations is voluntary, it is generally in the best interest of healthcare organizations and clinical professionals to adopt them as uniform practice. For example, hospitals that have been accredited by the Joint Commission or the **American Osteopathic Association (AOA)** are automatically granted deemed status by the Medicare program.

Similarly, physicians and other clinical professionals who have earned **board certification** through a professional certification organization are generally assumed to be fully qualified to practice in their area of specialty. In addition, the professional practice guidelines developed by a certification organization are generally accepted as the established standard of care for that specialty. A specific procedure performed by a board-certified physician or surgeon according to the practice guidelines established for that procedure, therefore, would be considered to have met the established standard of care.

Hospitals are legally responsible for the quality of nursing and medical care as well as other clinical services provided to inpatients and outpatients in their facilities. When a patient is harmed by an unqualified or negligent clinician in one of the hospital's departments, the hospital as well as the clinician may be held jointly accountable for the patient's injury.

The governing board of every hospital is responsible for establishing policies and procedures to ensure that only qualified clinical practitioners are allowed to provide patient services in the facility. These policies and procedures guide the process of credentialing. **Credentialing** is the process of verifying the educational qualifications, licensure status, and experience levels of healthcare professionals who have applied for the privilege of practicing within a healthcare facility.

Standards development organizations such as the **American Society for Testing and Materials (ASTM)** and **Health Level Seven (HL7)** work with professional and trade associations and governmental agencies to establish uniform operating practices. It is in the interest of hospitals to follow the national standards established by such organizations, especially the standards relevant to data transmission and healthcare informatics. Efficient information sharing is critical to many areas of healthcare operations but especially to reimbursement and performance improvement. The current work being done to establish healthcare informatics standards will be critical to the future implementation and success of electronic health record systems.

Each hospital's location, services, and organizational structure is unique. Therefore, each hospital must design and follow its own operating policies and procedures to ensure that its services and health records fulfill all of the standards and regulations that apply to its situation. In designing health record policies, it is also important to remember that regulatory and accreditation agencies rely heavily on the information documented in health records to determine whether patient-care standards are being met.

State and federal regulations, national accreditation standards, and clinical practice standards are created, updated, and changed frequently. Therefore, health information professionals must make reviewing the sources of regulations and standards a routine part of their responsibilities. Although this chapter cannot describe all of the requirements that acute-care records must fulfill, it will provide general background information as a starting point for health record policy and procedure development. (Tables 8.2 through 8.5 list sources of more specific information on health record regulations and standards.)

Table 8.2   Resources for health record policymaking: State regulations

Resource	Web Site
Manuals covering state regulations on confidentiality and release of information	State and local HIM associations
State health record retention and destruction regulations	Individual state government Web sites and www.alllaw.com
State hospital licensure regulations	State departments of health Web sites and www.astho.org

Source: Rhodes and Burrington-Brown 2002.

Table 8.3   Resources for health record policymaking: Federal regulations

Resource	Federal Agency and Web Site
Health Insurance Portability and Accountability Act, privacy and security standards	U.S. Department of Health and Human Services, http://www.hhs.gov/ocr/hipaa
Patient Self-Determination Act (advance directives)	The Office of the Law Revision Counsel, http://www.fha.org/acrobat/Patient%20Self%20Determination%20Act%201990.pdf
Office of Inspector General, compliance program guidance	Department of Health and Human Services, Office of the Inspector General, http://oig.hhs.gov/authorities/docs/cpghosp.pdf
Privacy Act of 1974	U.S. Department of Justice, www.usdoj.gov/04foia/privstat.htm
Protection of Human Subjects (45 CFR46)	National Archives and Records Administration, *Code of Federal Regulations,* www.access.gpo.gov/nara/cfr/waisdx_01/45cfr46_01.html
Recording and Reporting Occupational Injuries and Illnesses (29 CFR1904)	National Archives and Records Administration, *Code of Federal Regulations,* www.access.gpo.gov/nara/cfr/waisdx_01/29cfr1904_01.html

Source: Rhodes and Burrington-Brown 2002.

Table 8.4 Resources for health record policymaking: Medicare/Medicaid regulations

Resource	Web Site
Centers for Medicare and Medicaid Services, program manuals, memorandums, and transmittals	www.cms.hhs.gov
Medicare *Conditions of Participation for Comprehensive Outpatient Rehabilitation Facilities* (42 CFR488)	www.cms.hhs.gov
Medicare *Conditions of Participation for Drug, Alcohol, and Substance Abuse Treatment Facilities* (42 CFR2)	www.cms.hhs.gov
Medicare *Conditions of Participation for Hospitals* (42 CFR482)	www.cms.hhs.gov
Medicare *Conditions of Participation for Specialized Providers* (42 CFR485) (inpatient rehabilitation facilities)	www.cms.hhs.gov
Medicare acute inpatient prospective payment system (PPS)	http://www.cms.hhs.gov/AcuteInpatientPPS/
Medicare interpretive guidelines	http://www.cms.hhs.gov/home/regsguidance.asp
Medicare inpatient rehabilition facility prospective payment system (PPS)	http://www.cms.hhs.gov/InpatientRehabFacPPS/
Medicare hospital outpatient prospective payment system (PPS)	http://www.cms.hhs.gov/HospitalOutpatientPPS/
Medicare patient's rights	http://www.cms.hhs.gov/Certificationand Complianc/Downloads/PatientsRights.pdf

Source: Rhodes and Burrington-Brown 2002.

State and Local Licensure Requirements

All states require that hospitals and other healthcare facilities undergo licensure. **Licensure** is the mandatory process whereby state governments grant individual facilities permission to operate within a specific geopolitical area and provide a specific range of healthcare services. All fifty states require that physicians, dentists, and nurses undergo an individual licensure process. Additionally, some states license other groups of clinical professionals, such as clinical psychologists and social workers.

State agencies charged with administering hospital licensure programs have a variety of names; the most common is the department of health. Elements of the licensure program are similar in most states. State departments of health are usually charged with performing the following activities (Johns 2007):

- Developing hospital operating standards

- Issuing licenses to hospitals that meet the standards

- Monitoring hospital compliance with the standards

- Sanctioning hospitals that do not comply with the standards

Table 8.5 Resources for health record policymaking: Accreditation standards

Resource	Web Site
American Correctional Association, Agency Manual of Accreditation Policy and Procedure	www.aca.org
American Healthcare Accreditation Commission, Health Network Accreditation Standards	www.urac.org
American Healthcare Accreditation Commission, Healthcare Provider Credentialing Standards	www.urac.org
American Healthcare Accreditation Commission, Healthcare Utilization Management Standards	www.urac.org
American Healthcare Accreditation Commission, Workers' Compensation Utilization Management Standards	www.urac.org
American Osteopathic Association, Accreditation Requirements for Healthcare Facilities	www.osteopathic.org
Commission on Accreditation of Rehabilitation Facilities, Behavioral Health Standards Manual	www.carf.org
Commission on Accreditation of Rehabilitation Facilities, Medical Rehabilitation Standards Manual	www.carf.org
Joint Commission, Comprehensive Accreditation Manual for Ambulatory Care	www.jcrinc.com
Joint Commission, Comprehensive Accreditation Manual for Behavioral Health Care	www.jcrinc.com
Joint Commission, Comprehensive Accreditation Manual for Critical Access Hospitals	www.jcrinc.com
Joint Commission, Comprehensive Accreditation Manual for Home Care	www.jcrinc.com
Joint Commission, Comprehensive Accreditation Manual for Hospitals	www.jcrinc.com
Joint Commission, Comprehensive Accreditation Manual for Integrated Delivery Systems	www.jcrinc.com
Joint Commission, Comprehensive Accreditation Manual for Laboratory and Point-of-Care Testing	www.jcrinc.com
Joint Commission, Comprehensive Accreditation Manual for Long Term Care	www.jcrinc.com
Joint Commission, Comprehensive Accreditation Manual for Office-Based Surgery	www.jcrinc.com
National Commission on Correctional Health Care, Standards for Health Services in Jails	www.ncchc.org
National Commission on Correctional Health Care, Standards for Health Services in Juvenile Detention and Confinement Facilities	www.ncchc.org
National Commission on Correctional Health Care, Standards for Health Services in Prisons	www.ncchc.org
National Commission on Correctional Health Care, Standards for Opioid Treatment Programs in Correctional Settings	www.ncchc.org
National Committee for Quality Assurance, Standards for the Accreditation of Managed Behavioral Healthcare Organizations	www.ncqa.org

Source: Adapted from Rhodes and Burrington-Brown 2002.

In general, state licensure regulations are modeled after the Medicare *Conditions of Participation* (2006) and Joint Commission (2006) accreditation standards. Typical hospital licensure standards address minimum operating requirements in the areas of operational procedures, staffing, and environmental safety. Some states require hospitals to maintain additional licenses for specific services such as laboratory, radiology, renal dialysis, and substance abuse treatment. Most states have separate licensure requirements for pharmacies.

The documentation in health records is an important source of information in licensure surveys. States conduct annual surveys to determine the hospital's continued compliance with licensure standards. Surveys are often unannounced and generally focus on clinical services and the environment of care. In addition, state surveyors conduct reviews in response to specific complaints from consumers. State surveys are also used to validate compliance with Medicaid regulations.

Medicare and Medicaid Administrative Policies and Regulations

In 1965, amendments to the Social Security Act of 1935 established the Medicare and Medicaid programs. Federal healthcare programs were originally administered by the U.S. Department of Health, Education, and Welfare. The Health Care Financing Administration (HCFA) was established in 1977 to coordinate Medicare and Medicaid benefits on the federal level. The agency was renamed in 2001. Today, Medicare and the federal portion of Medicaid are administered by the Centers for Medicare and Medicaid Services (CMS), an agency of the U.S. Department of Health and Human Services. Local Medicaid programs are administered by agencies within individual state governments.

The health records of Medicare beneficiaries are subject to federal Medicare regulations and policies. Likewise, the records of Medicaid beneficiaries must fulfill the requirements of state medical assistance programs. The health records of Medicaid and Medicare patients are subject to other state laws and regulations, national privacy, security, and accreditation standards. Like other third-party payers, state Medicaid agencies and Medicare fiscal intermediaries may request information from patient records to support reimbursement of claims.

Medicaid Participation

The federal Medicaid program helps pay for the healthcare services provided to individuals and families with low incomes and limited financial resources. Medicaid funding is provided through state-run medical assistance programs, which set the requirements for Medicaid eligibility in their geopolitical regions. In order to receive federal funding, state programs must meet specific minimum requirements as established by federal regulations and CMS policies. However, states decide specific service coverage and reimbursement levels.

Medicaid eligibility and services vary significantly among states, and local providers are subject to complex administrative requirements as defined by state regulations. Participation in state Medicaid programs is voluntary for healthcare professionals and organizations. Hospitals that choose to participate must apply to the state agency that administers the Medicaid program in their local area. Hospitals subsequently supply services to Medicaid beneficiaries under contractual arrangements with the state.

Annual surveys are conducted by most states to confirm hospital compliance with Medicaid regulations. The state agency responsible for conducting annual licensure activities is also responsible for ensuring compliance with Medicaid participation requirements.

Medicare Conditions of Participation

The Medicare program provides healthcare coverage for about 40 million retired and/or disabled Americans (CMS 2006). It is the largest single payer for healthcare services in the United States. Although participation in the Medicare program is voluntary, few acute-care facilities would be able to survive economically if they did not provide services to Medicare beneficiaries.

Hospitals supply services to Medicare beneficiaries under contractual arrangements with the U.S. Department of Health and Human Services. To qualify for Medicare participation, hospitals must fulfill the Medicare *Conditions of Participation for Hospitals* (2006). Providers in other specialty areas such as long-term care or ambulatory healthcare services are required to follow the Medicare *Conditions of Participation* that apply specifically to them.

Conditions of Participation for Hospitals

The Medicare *Conditions of Participation for Hospitals* are published under title 42, part 482, of the *Code of Federal Regulations.* The **Code of Federal Regulations** (**CFR**) is updated whenever statutes or regulations are added or changed. Final changes and updates and proposed changes and updates are also published in the **Federal Register,** a daily publication of the U.S. Government Printing Office. Up-to-date information is also available in other print and online resources provided by the Government Printing Office.

HIM professionals are advised to check the *Federal Register* for the most current version of the Medicare *Conditions of Participation for Hospitals*, available online at www.gpoaccess. gov/fr/index.html.

The CMS works directly with accreditation organizations to coordinate the Medicare *Conditions of Participation* with national Accreditation standards. As a result, the Medicare acute-care standards are similar to the acute-care standards published by the Joint Commission and the American Osteopathic Association.

Section 482.24 of the Medicare *Conditions of Participation* (2006) lists the requirements for medical record services in a hospital. According to this section, every "hospital must have a medical record service that has administrative responsibility for medical records. A medical record must be maintained for every individual evaluated or treated in the hospital." This section of the standard comprises three categories: organization and staffing, form and retention of records, and content of records.

The first standard in this section addresses the organization and staffing of the health information (health/medical record) department. Specifically, it requires the organization of medical record services be appropriate to the scope and complexity of the services provided by the hospital. The standard requires staffing of the department must be adequate to ensure the efficient performance of health record functions.

The second standard addresses health record format and retention requirements, specifically as follows:

- The hospital must maintain a health record for every inpatient and outpatient it treats or evaluates.

- Health records must be accurately written, promptly completed, properly filed and retained, and easily accessible.

- The hospital must follow an effective system for authenticating the authorship of health record documentation.

- The hospital must have an effective system for protecting the integrity of health information and maintaining the security of health records.

- Health records must be retained for a minimum of five years.

- The hospital must have a system for coding and indexing the content of health records so information on diagnoses and procedures can be quickly retrieved for evaluations of medical effectiveness.

- The hospital must have an effective system for ensuring the confidentiality of health records.

- The hospital must have a system for releasing confidential health record information to authorized users but preventing unauthorized access.

- Original health records must not be removed from the hospital except in response to federal or state laws, court orders, and subpoenas.

The third standard describes the content requirements for acute-care documentation. The standard requires information in the health record to justify the patient's admission to the hospital as well as continued hospitalization. The standard further stipulates that acute-care documentation must support the patient's diagnosis and describe the patient's progress and response to services, as well as the following:

- All health record entries must be legible and complete.

- All services must be promptly documented and dated by the individual who is responsible for ordering, performing, or evaluating the provided services.

- The author of every entry must be identified by name and discipline, and the author must authenticate the entries by signing his or her full name or initials or by using an electronic verification entry.

- The health record must be completed within thirty days after the patient's discharge, transfer, or death.

- All acute-care records must include the following types of clinical information:

  — Documentation that a physical examination and medical history were performed no more than thirty days before the patient's admission or within twenty-four hours after admission

  — Documentation of the patient's admitting diagnosis or diagnoses

  — Results of any clinical consultations

  — Documentation of clinical evaluations performed by the clinical staff involved in the patient's care

  — Documentation of any complications, hospital-acquired infections, or negative reactions to medications or anesthesia

  — Properly executed informed consent forms for procedures, as required by medical staff rules, state laws, or federal regulations

  — All physicians' orders, nursing notes, treatment reports, medication records, diagnostic results, vital signs logs, and other information gathered in evaluating and monitoring the patient's condition

—A discharge summary that includes the outcome of hospitalization, the disposition of the case, and the provisions for follow-up care

—Documentation of the patient's final diagnosis or diagnoses

Medicare *Conditions of Participation* (2006) Section 482.13 requires hospitals to protect the personal and medical rights of patients. This section of the regulation lists the patient's rights provisions of the Medicare program. It also requires hospitals to provide a notice of rights to patients or their legal representatives, as follows:

1. A notice of the rights of patients must be provided to patients or their legal representatives, and the notice should be furnished in advance of providing or discontinuing services whenever possible.

2. The notice must describe the facility's procedures for receiving and resolving patients' grievances.

3. The patient's rights notice must include the following provisions:

   • The patient's right to participate in the development and implementation of his or her care plan

   • The patient's right to accept or refuse treatment

   • The patient's right to formulate advance directives and expect caregivers to follow those directives

   • The patient's right to have a family member or personal representative as well as his or her personal physician notified promptly of his or her hospital admission

   • The patient's right to personal privacy and safety

   • The patient's right to be free from all forms of abuse and harassment

   • The patient's right to the confidentiality of his or her clinical records

   • The patient's right to access his or her clinical records within a reasonable time frame

   • The patient's right to be free from restraints of any form (physical or chemical) that are not medically necessary and established by a physician's order (specifically, to be free of restraints applied as a means of coercion, discipline, convenience, or retaliation by staff) (42 CFR Section 482.13)

The hospital should ask patients or their representatives to sign acknowledgment forms to document the fact that information about patient's rights was provided.

Several other sections of the Medicare *Conditions of Participation for Hospitals* (2006) also include documentation requirements. These sections can be summarized as follows:

• *Section 482.22, Medical Staff*: The hospital must have a system for documenting the family's (or legal representative's) permission to perform an autopsy on a patient who died while under the hospital's care.

• *Section 482.23, Nursing Services*: (1) A registered nurse must supervise and ensure the documentation, development, and maintenance of a care plan for every patient. (2) All orders for drugs and biologicals must be made in writing and signed by the physician responsible for the patient's care. (3) Telephone and verbal orders must be accepted only by personnel authorized by medical staff rules, consistent with applicable state and federal regulations. (4) Telephone and verbal orders must be signed, dated, and timed by the prescribing practitioner within 48 hours. (5) The hospital must have a procedure in place for reporting transfusion reactions, adverse drug reactions, and medication errors.

- *Section 482.26, Radiology Services:* (1) The radiologist responsible for interpreting diagnostic images must authenticate the reports of his or her findings. (2) The hospital must maintain records of radiology procedures, consultations, and interpretations for at least five years.

- *Section 482.27, Laboratory Services:* The hospital must have a system in place for notifying patients who may have been exposed to infectious diseases through contaminated blood transfusions.

- *Section 482.43, Discharge Planning:* (1) Hospital personnel must complete a discharge evaluation for every patient who is likely to require posthospital services. (2) The discharge evaluation and plan must be completed in time to avoid unnecessary delays in arranging posthospital services. (3) The discharge plan must be documented in the patient's health record.

- *Section 482.51, Surgical Services:* (1) A complete history and physical must be documented in the patient's health record before surgery begins, except in emergencies. (2) A fully executed consent form must be placed in the patient's health record before surgery begins, except in emergencies. (3) The operating room register must be complete and up to date. (4) An operative report that describes surgical techniques, surgical findings, and any tissues removed or altered must be written or dictated and authenticated by the surgeon immediately following surgery.

- *Section 482.52, Anesthesia Services:* (1) A preanesthesia patient evaluation must be performed and documented no more than forty-eight hours before surgery. (2) An intraoperative record must be maintained while the procedure is in progress. (3) For inpatients, a postanesthesia follow-up report must be written within forty-eight hours after surgery. (4) For outpatients, a postanesthesia evaluation must be performed and documented according to medical staff policy.

- *Section 482, Nuclear Medicine Services:* (1) The practitioner approved by the medical staff to interpret the results of diagnostic procedures that use nuclear materials must sign and date the reports of his or her interpretation of the findings. (2) The hospital must maintain records of nuclear medicine procedures, consultations, and interpretations for at least five years.

Table 8.6 shows a sample of a "crosswalk" table illustrating correlations between the Joint Commission and *Conditions of Participation* standards. Be sure to check your sources, which are updated regularly, for the latest information.

Medicare Compliance Surveys

Hospitals accredited through the Joint Commission Hospital Accreditation Program or the AOA's **Healthcare Facilities Accreditation Program (HFAP)** may participate in the Medicare program because the accrediting agency has been granted deemed status by the Medicare program. **Deemed status** means accrediting bodies such as the Joint Commission or AOA can survey facilities for compliance with the Medicare *Conditions of Participation for Hospitals* instead of the government.

Table 8.6 Sample crosswalk between the Joint Commission and *Conditions of Participation* standards

Documentation Requirements	The Joint Commission	Conditions of Participation
The hospital initiates and maintains a medical record for IM.7.1 every individual assessed or treated.	IM.7.1	
A medical record must be maintained for every individual 482.24 evaluated or treated in the hospital.		482.24
Only authorized individuals make entries in medical records. IM.7.1.1	IM.7.1.1	
Every medical record entry is dated, its author identified IM.7.8 and, when necessary, authenticated.	IM.7.8	
Hospitals establish policies and mechanisms to ensure Intent of IM.7.8 that only an author can authenticate his or her own entry. Indications of authentication can include written signatures or initials, rubber stamps, or computer "signatures" (or sequence of keys). The medical staff rules and regulations or policies define what entries, if any, by house staff or non-physicians must be countersigned by supervising physicians.	Intent of IM.7.8	
All entries must be legible and complete and must be 482.24 (c) (1) authenticated and dated promptly by the person (identified by name and discipline) who is responsible for ordering, providing, or evaluating the service furnished.		482.24 (c) (1)
The author of each entry must be identified and must 482.24 (c) (1) (i) authenticate his or her entry.		482.24 (c) (1) (i)
Authentication may include signatures, written initials, 482.24 (c) (1) (ii) or computer entry.		482.24 (c) (1) (ii)
The medical record contains sufficient information to IM.7.2 482.24 (c) identify the patient, support the diagnosis, justify the treatment, document the course and results, and promote continuity of care among healthcare providers.	IM.7.2	482.24 (c)
To facilitate consistency and continuity in patient care, Intent of IM.7 the medical record contains very specific data and through IM.7.2 information, including: • the patient's name, address, date of birth, and the name of any legally authorized representative • the legal status of patients receiving mental health services • emergency care provided to the patient prior to arrival, if any • the record and findings of the patient's assessment • conclusions or impressions drawn from the medical history and physical examination • the diagnosis or diagnostic impression • the reasons for admission or treatment • the goals of treatment and the treatment plan • evidence of known advance directives • evidence of informed consent, when required by hospital policy • diagnostic and therapeutic orders, if any • all diagnostic and therapeutic procedures and test results • all operative and other invasive procedures performed, using acceptable disease and operative terminology that includes etiology, as appropriate • progress notes made by the medical staff and other authorized individuals • all reassessments and any revisions of the treatment plan • clinical observations • the patient's response to care • consultation reports • every medication ordered or prescribed for an inpatient • every medication dispensed to an ambulatory patient or an inpatient on discharge • every dose of medication administered and any adverse drug reaction • all relevant diagnoses established during the course of care • any referrals and communications made to external or internal providers and to community agencies	Intent of IM.7 through IM.7.2	

Table 8.6 (continued)

Documentation Requirements	The Joint Commission	Conditions of Participation
• conclusions at termination of hospitalization • discharge instructions to the patient and family • clinical resumes and discharge summaries, or a final progress note or transfer summary. A concise clinical resume included in the medical record at discharge provides important information to other caregivers and facilitates continuity of care. For patients discharged to ambulatory (outpatient) care, the clinical resume summarizes previous levels of care. The discharge summary contains the following information: • the reason for hospitalization • significant findings • procedures performed and treatment rendered • the patient's condition at discharge • instructions to the patient and family For normal newborns with uncomplicated deliveries, or for patients hospitalized for less than 48 hours with only minor problems, a progress note may substitute for the clinical resume. The medical staff defines what problems and interventions may be considered minor. The progress note may be handwritten. It documents the patient's condition at discharge, discharge instructions, and follow-up care required. When a patient is transferred within the same organization from one level of care to another, and the caregivers change, a transfer summary may be substituted for the clinical resume. A transfer summary briefly describes the patient's condition at time of transfer and the reason for the transfer. When the caregivers remain the same, a progress note may suffice.		
All records must document the following as appropriate: • admitting diagnosis results of all consultative evaluations of the patient 482.24 (c) (2)(iii) • results of all consultative evaluations of the patient 482.24 (c) (2)(iii) and appropriate findings by clinical and other staff involved in the care of the patient • documentation of complications, hospital acquired 482.24 (c) (2)(iv) infections, and unfavorable reactions to drugs and anesthesia • properly executed informed consent forms for 482.24 (c) (2) (v) procedures and treatments specified by the medical staff, or by federal or state law if applicable, to require written patient consent • all practitioner's orders, nursing notes, reports 482.24 (c) (2)(vi) of treatment, medication records, radiology, and laboratory reports, vital signs, and other information necessary to monitor the patient's condition		482.24 (c) (2) (ii) 482.24 (c) (2)(iii) 482.24 (c) (2)(iv) 482.24 (c) (2) (v) 482.24 (c) (2)(iii)
All medical records must document the following as appropriate: • discharge summary with outcome of hospitalization, 482.24 (c) (2)(vii) disposition of case, and provisions for follow-up care • final diagnosis with completion of medical records 482.24 (c) (2) (viii) within 30 days following discharge		482.24 (c) (2) (vii) 482.24 (c) (2) (viii)
A patient admitted for inpatient care has a medical history MS.6.2 and an appropriate physical examination performed by a qualified physician. (Qualified physician: A doctor of medicine or doctor of osteopathy who, by virtue of education, training, and demonstrated competence, is granted clinical privileges by the organization to perform specific diagnostic or therapeutic procedure(s) and who is fully licensed to practice medicine.)	MS.6.2	
Qualified oral and maxillofacial surgeons may perform MS.6.2.1 the medical history and physical examination, if they have such privileges, in order to assess the medical, surgical, and anesthetic risks of the proposed operative and other procedure(s).	MS.6.2.1	

Table 8.6 (continued)

Documentation Requirements	The Joint Commission	Conditions of Participation
Other licensed independent practitioners who are MS.6.2.2 permitted to provide patient care services independently may perform all or part of the medical history and physical examination, if granted such privileges.	MS.6.2.2	
The findings, conclusions, and assessment of risk are MS.6.2.2.1 confirmed or endorsed by a qualified physician prior to major high-risk (as defined by the medical staff) diagnostic or therapeutic interventions.	MS.6.2.2.1	
Dentists are responsible for the part of their patient's MS.6.2.2.2 history and physical examination that relates to dentistry.	MS.6.2.2.2	
Podiatrists are responsible for the part of their patient's MS.6.2.2.3 history and physical examination that relates to podiatry.	MS.6.2.2.3	
The medical staff determines those non-inpatient services MS.6.3 (for example, ambulatory surgery), if any, for which a patient must have a medical history taken and appropriate physical examination performed by a qualified physician who has such privileges. Except as provided in MS.6.2.1 through MS.6.2.2.3.	MS.6.3	
The patient's history and physical examination, nursing PE.1.7.1 assessment, and other screening assessments are completed within 24 hours of admission as an inpatient.	PE.1.7.1	
If a history and physical examination have been performed PE.1.7.1.1 within 30 days before admission, a durable, legible copy of this report may be used in the patient's medical record, provided any changes that may have occurred are recorded in the medical record at the time of admission.	PE.1.7.1.1	
Before surgery, the patient's physical examination and PE.1.8 medical history, any indicated diagnostic tests, and a preoperative diagnosis are completed and recorded in the patient's medical record.	PE.1.8	
There must be a complete history and physical workup 482.51 (b) (1) in the chart of every patient prior to surgery, except in emergencies. If this has been dictated, but not yet recorded in the patient's chart, there must be a statement to the effect and an admission note in the chart by the practitioner who admitted the patient.		482.51 (b) (1)
A physical examination and medical history [are to] be done 482.24 (c) (2) (i) no more than seven days before or 48 hours after an admission for each patient by a doctor of medicine or osteopathy or, for 482.22 (c) (5) patients admitted only for oromaxillofacial surgery, by an oromaxillofacial surgeon who has been granted such privileges by the medical staff in accordance with state law.		482.24 (c) (2) (i) 482.22 (c) (5)
Plans of care are developed and documented in the patient's TX.5.3 medical record before the operative or other procedure is performed.	TX.5.3	
The hospital must ensure that the nursing staff develops 482.23 (b) (4) and keeps current a nursing care plan for each patient.		482.23 (b) (4)
All records must document all practitioners' orders. 482.24 (c) (2) (vi)		482.24 (c) (2) (vi)
All orders for drugs and biologicals must be in writing 482.23 (c) (2) and signed by the practitioner or practitioners responsible for the care of the patient.		482.23 (c) (2)
Verbal orders of authorized individuals are accepted and IM.7.7 transcribed by qualified personnel who are identified by title or category in the medical staff rules and regulations.	IM.7.7	
When telephone or oral orders must be used, they must be: • accepted only by personnel that are authorized to do so 482.23 (c) (2) (i) by the medical staff policies and procedures, consistent with federal and state law • signed or initialed by the prescribing practitioner 482.23 (c) (2) (ii) as soon as possible • used infrequently 482.23 (c) (2) (iii)		482.23 (c) (2) (i) 482.23 (c) (2) (ii) 482.23 (c) (2) (iii)
Signed x-ray reports of all examinations performed 482.26 (d) shall be made part of the patient's hospital record.		482.26 (d)
The radiologist or other practitioner who performs radiology 482.26 (d) (1) services must sign reports of his or her interpretations.		482.26 (d) (1)

Table 8.6 (continued)

Documentation Requirements	The Joint Commission	Conditions of Participation
The medical record thoroughly documents operative or IM.7.3 other procedures and the use of sedation or anesthesia.	IM.7.3	
A preoperative diagnosis is recorded before surgery by IM.7.3.1 the licensed independent practitioner responsible for the patient.	IM.7.3.1	
Operative reports dictated or written immediately after IM.7.3.2 surgery record the name of the primary surgeon and assistants, findings, technical procedures used, specimens removed, and postoperative diagnosis.	IM.7.3.2	
The completed operative report is authenticated by the IM.7.3.2.1 surgeon and filed in the medical record as soon as possible after surgery.	IM.7.3.2.1	
When the operative report is not placed in the medical IM.7.3.2.2 record immediately after surgery, a progress note is entered immediately.	IM.7.3.2.2	
Postoperative documentation records the patient's vital IM.7.3.3 signs and level of consciousness; medications (including intravenous fluids), blood, and blood components; any unusual events or postoperative complications; and management of such events.	IM.7.3.3	
Postoperative documentation records the patient's IM.7.3.4 discharge from the postsedation or postanesthesia care area by the responsible licensed independent practitioner or according to discharge criteria.	IM.7.3.4	
Compliance with discharge criteria is fully documented IM.7.3.4.1 in the patient's medical record.	IM.7.3.4.1	
Postoperative documentation records the name of the IM.7.3.5 licensed independent practitioner responsible for discharge.	IM.7.3.5	
An informed consent for surgery shall be part of the 482.51 (b) (2) patient's chart before surgery is performed. It must be dated, timed, and signed by the patient and the physician informant.		482.51 (b) (2)
An operative report describing the reason for procedure, 482.51 (b) (6) gross findings, operative procedure (techniques), and tissues removed or altered must be written or dictated immediately following surgery and signed by the surgeon.		482.51 (b) (6)
A presedation or preanesthesia assessment is performed for TX.2.1 each patient before beginning moderate or deep sedation and before anesthesia induction.	TX.2.1	
A preanesthesia evaluation is performed within 48 482.52 (b) (1) hours prior to surgery by an individual qualified to administer anesthesia.	482.52 (b) (1)	
An intraoperative anesthesia record is provided. 482.52 (b) (2)		482.52 (b) (2)
With respect to inpatients, a postanesthesia follow-up 482.52 (b) (3) report is written within 48 hours after surgery by the individual who administers the anesthesia.		482.52 (b) (3)
A preanesthesia evaluation is documented by an individual 482.52 (b) qualified to administer anesthesia and is performed within 48 hours prior to the anesthesia event of surgery.		482.52 (b)
The hospital must maintain signed and dated reports of 482.53 (d) nuclear medicine interpretations, consultations, and procedures.		482.53 (d)
The practitioner approved by the medical staff to interpret 482.53 (d) (2) diagnostic procedures must sign and date the interpretation of these tests.		482.53 (d) (2)
When emergency, urgent, or immediate care is provided, IM.7.5 the time and means of arrival are also documented in the medical record.	IM.7.5	
The medical record notes when a patient receiving emergency, IM.7.5.1 urgent, or immediate care left against medical advice.	IM.7.5.1	
The medical record of a patient receiving emergency, urgent, IM.7.5.2 or immediate care notes the conclusions at termination of treatment, including final disposition, condition at discharge, and instructions for follow-up care.	IM.7.5.2	
When authorized by the patient or a legally authorized IM.7.5.3 representative, a copy of the emergency services provided is available to the practitioner or medical organization providing follow-up care.	IM.7.5.3	

Most acute-care hospitals are accredited through a survey process conducted by the Joint Commission or the AOA. Consequently, they are not required to undergo annual Medicare certification surveys. However, CMS policy requires a sample of hospitals with deemed status (approximately 10 percent each year) to undergo a Medicare validation survey soon after the Joint Commission or AOA accreditation survey is completed (Shaw et al. 2007, 315–316).

Medicare/Medicaid certification programs are conducted by state licensure agencies working under contract with the CMS. Hospitals must undergo a Medicare certification survey annually if they do not qualify for deemed status. Such facilities may have chosen not to participate in one of the accreditation programs, or they may have lost their accreditation temporarily because of compliance deficiencies.

The Joint Commission and other accreditation organizations work with the CMS in an attempt to coordinate their accreditation standards with the Medicare *Conditions of Participation.* However, some inconsistencies still exist. For example, the Medicare regulation requires every health record entry to be authenticated, but the Joint Commission standard on maintaining patient-specific information (IM.6.10) establishes a more lenient minimum requirement (Joint Commission 2006, IM-13):

> Medical record entries are dated, the author identified and, when necessary according to law or regulation and hospital policy, they are authenticated.
>
> At a minimum, the following are authenticated by either written signature, electronic signature, or computer key or rubber stamp:
>
> - The history and physical examination
>
> - Operative reports
>
> - Consultations
>
> - Discharge summary

In contrast, section 482.24(c) (1) (i) of the 2006 Medicare *Conditions of Participation for Hospitals* indicates, "the author of each entry [in the medical record] must be identified and must authenticate his or her entry." Section 482.24(c) (1) (ii) of the regulation further defines *authentication* as "signatures, written initials, or computer entry."

As the preceding example shows, the Medicare *Conditions of Participation,* accreditation standards, HIPAA standards, state health record and licensure regulations, and hospital policies often present conflicting guidelines. In such cases, the hospital must develop health record policies based on the strictest regulatory and accreditation requirements that apply. Thus, the hospital can ensure compliance with all regulatory and accreditation agencies (Shaw et al. 2007, 315). See chapter 4 for a discussion of HIPAA impacts on documentation.

Federal Requirements for Special Health Record Protection

The confidentiality of all patient-identifiable health information must be protected, but several types of health-related information are particularly sensitive. The inappropriate disclosure of information related to substance abuse treatment or psychiatric care can have devastating consequences for patients and their families. Information about a patient's human immunodeficiency virus (HIV) status or sexually transmitted illness can lead to discrimination in employment and housing. Concerns related to the release of genetic information and the potential for discrimination based on genetic profiles are a relatively new area of concern. Several federal regulations supplement state laws and voluntary accreditation standards to provide special protection to particularly sensitive health information.

Records of HIV/AIDS Diagnosis and Treatment

The illness caused by HIV (acquired immunodeficiency syndrome or AIDS) has been a worldwide public health concern for more than two decades. In response to the AIDS epidemic in the United States, most state legislatures have enacted laws that require HIV/AIDS reporting. Because individuals infected with HIV often face discrimination in housing, employment, and healthcare services, many state regulations also specifically address confidentiality issues related to HIV testing and AIDS treatment.

HIV Testing

HIV testing has become a common practice. Many individuals at risk for contracting HIV voluntarily choose to be tested. However, individuals may also be compelled by court order to undergo involuntary testing. In addition, many states have enacted statutes that require specific groups of individuals to undergo routine HIV testing, most commonly healthcare workers.

Most HIV testing in the United States is performed on a voluntary basis. Some states have even developed anonymous HIV testing programs to encourage individuals at risk of infection to be tested without identifying themselves by name. In addition, many individuals undergo routine voluntary testing when they donate blood, plasma, semen, and other human tissue to blood and tissue banks. HIV testing has become a routine element in prenatal care, and infants are usually tested shortly after birth when their mothers are known or suspected to be HIV-positive.

Involuntary HIV testing, however, may be required for specific groups of individuals by state statute or for individuals by court order. Where they exist, state regulations mandating HIV testing apply to specific groups whose infection would present the greatest potential threat to public health. Examples of such groups include convicted sex offenders and prison inmates entering or leaving correctional facilities (McWay 2002, 198–199).

Some states require mandatory testing of specific groups of employees while others permit only voluntary employee-testing programs. Other states prohibit mandatory employee testing or allow it only under specific circumstances, that is, when health status affects the employees' ability to perform their jobs safely. Healthcare workers who perform invasive procedures are one example.

Court orders for mandatory HIV testing of individuals differ from state to state. Specific risks may be identified, such as the individual is likely to be infected with HIV and/or that the individual's HIV status presents a serious threat to the health of other individuals.

Discrimination based on disability status is prohibited by law in some states as well as by the federal Americans with Disabilities Act of 1990. Therefore, the collection of information about an employee's HIV status is a serious issue. The federal regulations in this area also apply to applicants for employment. Hospitals and other healthcare facilities must consult legal counsel before establishing policies and procedures related to human resources issues.

Confidentiality Issues Related to HIV/AIDS

In general, most state regulations developed to protect the identity of HIV-positive individuals address confidentiality practices in three areas: consent for testing, general information on testing, and reporting of test results. Individuals must sign a formal informed consent before testing. Most states also require healthcare providers to provide information about HIV testing and AIDS to patients before they perform the test. The provider's method of communicating test results to patients is also covered in many state HIV testing regulations (McWay 2002, 197, 199).

Virtually every state requires providers to report cases of positive HIV results to the state's public health department. Some counties and municipalities may also require reporting. In general, reporting involves the identification of the infected individual. Therefore, the communication of public health reports containing HIV/AIDS information should be accomplished through a confidential medium, specifically, not via telephone, e-mail, or facsimile transmission (Carpenter 1999).

The AHIMA has recommended the following procedures for managing health information related to HIV infection and AIDS (Carpenter 1999):

- HIV employee-screening programs should protect the confidentiality of test results.

- Specific, written informed consent should be obtained from the individual or the individual's legal representative before voluntary testing.

- When state regulations permit the mandatory testing of patients after healthcare workers have been exposed to blood or bodily fluids, the need for testing should be discussed with the patient or his or her legal representative before testing.

- Counseling provided before or after testing should be performed by a qualified healthcare professional.

- The records of HIV-positive patients should not be subject to special handling procedures because special procedures are more likely to draw attention than routine security measures. In states where special handling is required for the records of HIV-positive individuals or HIV test results, the records should be identified with an obscure code or symbol to avoid inadvertent release of HIV-related information.

- Facilities should implement and monitor compliance with clear policies and procedures on the disclosure of health information related to HIV/AIDS. Policies should dictate that HIV/AIDS information must be used only for diagnosis, treatment, and patient care management. Other disclosures, including disclosures for billing and claims purposes, must be allowed only with the patient's written consent and should be limited to the minimum amount needed for the authorized purpose. Authorized disclosures of HIV/AIDS information should include a notice that redisclosure is prohibited except when required by law.

- HIV/AIDS-related information should only be discussed via telephone in emergencies.

- Clinical coding should be based only on the diagnoses verified in patient records and not on the basis of laboratory results alone.

- Information related to the HIV-positive status of healthcare workers, including information on any restrictions to their practice, should be protected according to all applicable state and federal regulations. Such information should only be disclosed to patients upon the advice of legal counsel.

Records Containing Genetic Information

In 2003, the Human Genome Project completed the mapping of the genetic structure of humans. The U.S. Department of Energy (DOE) and the National Institutes of Health (NIH) jointly sponsored the project. The project was one of the largest scientific projects ever undertaken. Its research identified the function of every human gene. This information promises to revolutionize the future of medicine. The DOE promotes scientific and technological innovation, and the NIH supports medical research.

Genetic information can be used to predict an individual's risk of eventually contracting many types of illness, including diabetes, heart disease, cancer, and even mental health disorders such as alcoholism and schizophrenia. For this reason, the potential for using genetic information as the basis of discrimination against individuals cannot be ignored.

Although genetic information is extremely sensitive, it is usually afforded no special protection under state health record regulations. In addition, the results of genetic tests and genetic information based on family history may be referred to in any part of the health record, and so it is difficult to protect such information from inadvertent disclosure.

HIPAA addresses the issue of health insurance discrimination based on genetic information. The act specifically prohibits healthcare insurance plans from basing coverage decisions and premiums on genetic information alone. Several states have enacted similar health insurance and genetic testing regulations, including Missouri, California, Arizona, Maryland, and Wisconsin (McWay 2002, 170).

Federal Patient Safety Legislation

In July 2004, the U.S. Senate passed the Patient Safety and Quality Improvement Act. It was signed into law on July 29 of that year. This legislation creates a confidential and voluntary system for reporting medical errors. The overall goal of the national reporting system is to improve patient safety and reduce the number of medical errors nationwide.

Accreditation Requirements for Acute-Care Hospitals

Acute-care facilities must fulfill the various regulatory requirements of federal, local, and state governments, but most also choose to participate in one or more voluntary accreditation programs. One of the benefits of accreditation is enhancement to the hospital's public reputation for providing high-quality clinical services. In some cases, it also satisfies eligibility requirements for hospitals participating in programs that affect their financial status, such as Medicare and Medicaid. In addition, many state licensure agencies base their licensure requirements for hospitals on Joint Commission standards.

Accreditation is a systematic quality review process that evaluates the healthcare facility's performance against preestablished, written criteria, or **standards**. Healthcare organizations voluntarily seek accreditation from a variety of private, not-for-profit accreditation organizations. Different types of healthcare organizations and services are accredited by different accreditation organizations.

Either the Joint Commission or the AOA's Healthcare Facilities Accreditation Program accredits most acute-care hospitals. Psychiatric and rehabilitation specialty hospitals and hospital departments devoted to psychiatric and rehabilitation services may also be accredited through the Commission on Accreditation of Rehabilitation Facilities. Managed-care programs that provide acute-care services may be accredited through the National Committee for Quality Assurance. Ambulatory-surgery centers and outpatient diagnostic imaging and radiation oncology treatment facilities may be accredited through the Accreditation Association for Ambulatory Health Care.

See Chapters 9 through 12 for information about the Joint Commission regulations pertaining to the ambulatory, long-term care, hospice and home care, and behavioral healthcare settings.

Joint Commission

The **Joint Commission** is a not-for-profit, standards-setting organization whose primary mission is "to continuously improve the safety and quality of care provided to the public through the provision of health care accreditation and related services that support performance improvement in health care organizations." Currently, it accredits more than 15,000 healthcare organizations and programs in the United States. Joint Commission International expands that commitment worldwide by providing consultation, accreditation, publications, and education services to public and private healthcare organizations in more than 60 countries.

The Joint Commission provides evaluation and accreditation services for the following types of healthcare organizations:

- Acute-care hospitals
- Ambulatory-care organizations
- Behavioral healthcare facilities
- Children's hospitals
- Critical-access hospitals
- Group practices
- Home care organizations
- Hospice services
- Independent or freestanding laboratories
- Long-term care (or skilled-nursing) facilities
- Medical equipment services
- Office-based surgery
- Psychiatric hospitals
- Rehabilitation hospitals

In addition, several specialty settings are eligible for Joint Commission certificate programs such as chronic kidney disease, disease-specific care, healthcare staffing services, inpatient diabetes, lung volume reduction surgery, primary stroke centers, transplant centers, and ventricular assist devices.

In 2004, the Joint Commission accreditation process shifted from triennial survey preparation to a continuous improvement philosophy. The new process focuses on systems critical to the safety and quality of patient care, treatment, and services.

Joint Commission Documentation Standards for Hospitals

Organizations seeking Joint Commission accreditation must meet standards in every area of patient care, including clinical documentation and health records. Periodic accreditation surveys test the adequacy of documentation through detailed health record reviews.

The Joint Commission has developed a number of documentation standards that apply to every healthcare setting. These core standards are supplemented by standards that address the additional documentation requirements of specialty settings and specific clinical services. For example, a teaching hospital that hosts medical education programs would be evaluated on its compliance with authentication requirements for documentation created by medical students and unlicensed physicians in addition to other acute-care documentation standards.

Hospitals use the *Comprehensive Accreditation Manual for Hospitals: The Official Handbook* (CAMH) to conduct self-assessments and evaluate staff and facility performance against Joint Commission standards. The CAMH manual is divided into the following three sections: Patient-focused Functions, Organization Functions, and Structures with Functions.

Section I—Patient-focused Functions

1. Ethics, Rights, and Responsibilities

2. Provision of Care, Treatment, and Services

3. Medication Management

4. Surveillance, Prevention, and Control of Infection

Section II—Organization Functions

1. Improving Organization Performance

2. Leadership

3. Management of the Environment

4. Management of Human Resources

5. Management of Information

Section III—Structures with Functions

1. Medical Staff

2. Nursing

The Joint Commission organizes standards into functional chapters. Each functional chapter has an overview that provides background information. Additionally, each chapter includes the following:

- The *standard*, which defines the performance expectations and/or structures or process that must be in place

- The *rationale for the standard*, which provides additional text describing the purpose of the standard

- The *elements of performance* (EPs), which detail specific performance expectations and/or structures or processes that must be in place

Each standard is identified using a numbering system that combines the standard number, rationale, and elements of performance to create a unique label. This simplified numbering scheme improves the process of adding new standards such as the following:

Standard IM.5.10: Knowledge-based information resources are readily available, current, and authoritative.

Rationale for IM.5.10: Hospital practitioners and staff have access to knowledge-based information to do the following:

- Acquire and maintain the knowledge and skills needed to maintain and improve compliance

- Assist with clinical/service and management decision making

- Provide appropriate information and education to patients and families

- Support performance improvement and patient safety activities

- Support the institution's education and research needs

Elements of Performance for IM.5.10:

1. Library services are provided by cooperative or contractual arrangements with other institutions, if not available on site.

2. The hospital provides access to knowledge-based information resources needed by staff in any of the following forms: print, electronic, Internet, or audio.

3. Knowledge-based information resources are available to clinical/service staff, through electronic means, after-hours access to an in-house collection, or other methods.

4. The hospital has a process for providing access to knowledge-based information resources when electronic systems are unavailable.

Scoring each EP determines the hospital's compliance with a standard. The rating scale used to evaluate EPs is as follows:

0 Insufficient compliance

1 Partial compliance

2 Satisfactory compliance

NA Not applicable

Most Joint Commission (2006) standards that directly affect health information management can be located in the "Management of Information" section of the CAMH manual. Management of information standards encompasses six categories: planning, confidentiality and security, information management processes, information-based decision making, knowledge-based information, and patient-specific information. The hospital accreditation manual also has standards relevant to health records and health information listed in other sections of the CAMH manual, such as ethics, rights, and responsibilities; provision of care, treatment, and services; medication management; and medical staff.

Joint Commission Sentinel Event Policy

The Joint Commission reviews healthcare organizational activities in response to sentinel events to support its mission to continuously improve the safety and quality of healthcare provided to the community. The Joint Commission requires accredited hospitals and other healthcare facilities to implement systems for identifying and addressing *sentinel events*. The Joint Commission defines a **sentinel event** as "an unexpected occurrence involving death or serious physical or psychological injury, or the risk thereof. Serious injury specifically includes loss of limb or function" (Joint Commission 2006, SE-1). A sentinel event is not the same as a medical error, because many sentinel events are not the result of errors. Sentinel events signal the need for an immediate investigation and appropriate response.

Hospitals are encouraged to self-report sentinel events to the Joint Commission. Doing so places the facility at an advantage because of the following:

- It enables the hospital to add lessons learned to the Joint Commissions Sentinel Event Database

- It provides opportunity for consultation with the Joint Commission during the development of the root cause analysis and action plan

- It strengthens the hospital's message to the public that it is doing everything possible to prevent the incident from happening again and is committed to reducing the risk of such an event in the future

Examples of reviewable and nonreviewable sentinel events under the Joint Commission's Sentinel Event Policy are listed in figure 8.1.

Joint Commission National Patient Safety Goals

The Joint Commission measures hospital performance against a set of goals designed to complement its longstanding patient safety standards. As the National Patient Safety Goals (NPSG) process undergoes an annual review and update, some goals become standards and are replaced by new, pressing industry quality issues. The purpose of these goals is to promote specific improvements in patient safety.

The HIM role in patient safety is one of direct leadership, and opportunities for providing critical support exist in many areas. Many HIM professionals are directly involved in clinical quality issues and outcomes through quality management programs. Others affect quality through improved medical record documentation, accurate coding, and index integrity (Hjort 2005).

Most patient safety goals focus on system-wide solutions. The 2007 National Patient Safety Goals that affect accredited hospitals include the following:

- **Goal 1**—Improve the accuracy of patient identification

- **Goal 2**—Improve the effectiveness of communication among caregivers

- **Goal 3**—Improve the safety of using medications

- **Goal 7**—Reduce the risk of healthcare-associated infections

- **Goal 8**—Accurately and completely reconcile medications across the continuum of care

- **Goal 9**—Reduce the risk of patient harm resulting from falls

- **Goal 13**—Encourage patients' active involvement in their own care as a patient safety strategy

- **Goal 15**—Identify safety risks inherent in the organization's patient population

Figure 8.1.   Examples of reviewable and nonreviewable sentinel events.

Table 1. Examples of Sentinel Events that are Reviewable and Events that are Not Reviewable Under the Joint Commission's Sentinel Event Policy*

Examples of Sentinel Events that are Reviewable Under The Joint Commission's Sentinel Event Policy

Any patient death, paralysis, coma, or other major permanent loss of function associated with a medication error.

A patient commits suicide within 72 hours of being discharged from a hospital setting that provides staffed around-the-clock care.

Any elopement, that is, unauthorized departure, of a patient from an around-the-clock care setting resulting in a temporally related death (suicide, accidental death, or homicide) or major permanent loss of function.

A hospital operates on the wrong side of the patient's body.

Any intrapartum (related to the birth process) maternal death.

Any perinatal death unrelated to a congenital condition in an infant having a birth weight greater than 2,500 grams.

A patient is abducted from the hospital where he or she receives care, treatment, or services.

Assault, homicide, or other crime resulting in patient death or major permanent loss of function.

A patient fall that results in death or major permanent loss of function as a direct result of the injuries sustained in the fall.

Hemolytic transfusion reaction involving major blood group incompatibilities.

A foreign body, such as a sponge or forceps, that was left in a patient after surgery.

> **Note:** An adverse outcome that is *directly related* to the natural course of the patient's illness or underlying condition, for example, terminal illness present at the time of presentation, is **not** reportable **except** for suicide in, or following elopement from, a 24-hour care setting (*see* above).

Examples of Events that are Not Reviewable Under The Joint Commission's Sentinel Event Policy

Any "near miss."

Full or expected return of limb or bodily function to the same level as prior to the adverse event by discharge or within two weeks of the initial loss of said function.

Any sentinel event that has not affected a recipient of care (patient, client, resident).

Medication errors that do not result in death or major permanent loss of function.

Suicide other than in an around-the-clock care setting or following elopement from such a setting.

A death or loss of function following a discharge "against medical advice (AMA)."

Unsuccessful suicide attempts unless resulting in major permanent loss of function.

Minor degrees of hemolysis not caused by a major blood group incompatibility and with no clinical sequelae.

> **Note:** In the context of its performance improvement activities, an organization may choose to conduct intensive assessment, for example, root cause analysis, for some not reviewable events. Please refer to the "Improving Organization Performance" chapter of this Joint Commission accreditation manual.

* Note: *This list may not apply to all settings.*

Source: Joint Commission 2008.

Joint Commission Survey Process

In 2007, the Joint Commission added "The Accreditation Process" chapter to its CAMH manual. This chapter includes general information about the accreditation process, the application, types of surveys, the Periodic Performance Review, priority focus areas, and clinical/service groups. Policies and procedures in this chapter are relevant to all healthcare organizations interested in Joint Commission accreditation.

The Joint Commission transitioned to an unannounced survey process for hospitals in 2006. This was a significant change from the triennial accreditation and survey process. Joint Commission defines an **unannounced survey** as one in which an accredited organization will receive *no notice*. The change to unannounced surveys has caused hospitals to move toward a continuous ongoing performance improvement process that supports reversing Institute of Medicine (IOM) findings of medical error and death. This redesign of the accreditation process more accurately measures efforts toward quality care delivery and patient safety.

Between 2006 and 2008, hospitals underwent their first unannounced surveys. These occurred in the year in which the facilities were due for triennial survey. On the morning of each survey, a letter of introduction, survey agendas, and the biographies and pictures of the surveyors assigned to conduct the survey were posted to the organization's secure location on the Joint Commission's extranet site. Subsequent unannounced surveys will now occur 18 to 39 months following completion of the first unannounced surveys. However, initial surveys are still announced unless required to be unannounced to meet deemed status requirements.

Periodic Performance Review

A key component in the continuous accreditation process is the **Periodic Performance Review (PPR)**. The PPR helps hospitals incorporate Joint Commission standards as part of routine operations and ongoing quality-improvement efforts. Hospitals have access to the PPR tool continuously throughout the accreditation cycle. Hospitals evaluate compliance with applicable standards, elements of performance, National Patient Safety Goals and Accreditation Participation Requirements. Organizations are required to submit an update to its PPR annually to the Joint Commission. However, hospitals may select different options for compliance. (See figure 8.2.) The annual due dates for the PPR update is at one-year intervals after the hospital's last full survey.

Priority Focus Process

The Joint Commission describes the priority focus process as an important component of the survey process because it guides the surveyor(s) in planning and conducting on-site surveys. The Joint Commission defines the **priority focus process (PFP)** as focusing survey activities on the organization-specific issues that are most relevant to safety and quality of care. Internal and external data about the organization are integrated to identify clinical service groups and priority focus areas for each hospital. The Joint Commission provides the hospital information about its top clinical service groups and priority focus areas on its secure extranet site.

Priority focus areas (PFAs) include processes, systems, and structures that have the most substantial effect on patient-care services. The Joint Commission designates information management as one of fourteen PFAs vital to successful operation in hospitals (Joint Commission 2007, ACC-19).

The Joint Commission uses the tracer methodology for on-site surveys. The **tracer methodology** incorporates the use of the PFP, follows the experience of care through the organization's

Figure 8.2.   Options for Periodic Performance Review.

Option 1

The organization uses the PPR tool to annually affirm that legal counsel advises the organization not to participate in the full PPR. Instead, the organization completes a PPR and Plan of Action and identifies appropriate Measure of Success (MOS).

The organization may use the PPR tool to score compliance and can print and view standards and Elements of Performance (EPs) to conduct its assessment on paper. Entered data are not submitted to the Joint Commission.

The organization affirms that it has completed an assessment of its compliance with applicable EPs and developed Plans of Action and MOS, if needed, but does not submit these data to the Joint Commission.

The organization can submit standards-related issues in the PPR tool for telephone discussion with Joint Commission staff, if desired, and may receive design approval.

Surveyors review any required MOS at full survey.

Option 2

The organization uses the PPR tool to annually attest that, after careful consideration with legal counsel, it has decided not to participate in the full PPR and instead will undergo a limited announced survey. The survey is approximately one-third the length of a full survey, and a fee will be charged. The survey includes tracer methodology and Priority Focus Process output; all standards are subject to review. The surveyor will leave a written report of the findings with the organization.

The organization submits the PPR tool again within 30 days of the survey. The organization creates Plans of Action and applicable MOS for each standard scored not compliant and submits data to the Joint Commission via the PPR tool within 30 days of survey.

The organization may choose to participate in a conference call with the Joint Commission to discuss the Plans of Action and MOS. If a conference call is not requested, the data will be reviewed by Joint Commission staff. Should they determine a conference call is needed, the organization will be contacted to schedule a call.

Joint Commission staff reviews and approves the Plans of Action during the conference call.

Surveyors will review any required MOS during the full survey.

Option 3

The organization uses the PPR tool to annually attest that, after careful consideration with legal counsel, it has decided not to participate in the full PPR and instead will undergo a limited announced survey. The survey is approximately one-third the length of a full survey and a fee will be charged. The survey includes tracer methodology and Priority Focus Process output; all standards are subject to review.

Unlike option 2, however, option 3 stipulates that no written report of findings will be left at the organization. The surveyor delivers an oral report of findings at the closing conference of the on-site survey.

The organization submits the PPR tool again within 30 days of the survey. This submission addresses the choice of a conference call and any topics for discussion with Joint Commission staff.

At the time of the organization's full survey, the surveyors will receive no information relating to the organization's option 3 survey findings.

Source: Joint Commission 2007.

entire healthcare process and allows the surveyor to identify performance issues. Surveyors may perform two different types of tracers: individual tracer activity or individual-based system tracer activity. **Individual tracer activity** permits the evaluation of the care experience of a specific patient while in the hospital. This method analyzes a hospital's system of providing care, treatment, and services used as the framework for assessing standards of compliance. The **individual-based system tracer activity** explores a specific system or process across the organization. The surveyor evaluates the integration of related processes, coordination, and communication among disciplines and departments during the individual-based system tracer. Data use, infection control, and medical management are key components evaluated during the individual-based system tracer activity.

Hospital staff will be involved in the tracer methodology process. The surveyor will ask staff to provide a list of active patients that will include the patient's name, current location, and diagnosis. The surveyor will interview physicians and hospital staff involved in the care of the patient as he or she proceeds through the hospital visiting areas where service was provided.

Joint Commission Accreditation Decision Process

The Joint Commission states the goal of the accreditation decision and reporting approach is to move hospitals away from focusing on achieving high scores to achieving and maintaining safe, high-quality systems of care, treatment, and service. The Joint Commission has six categories in the accreditation decision process, as follows:

1. *Accredited:* The hospital complied with all standards at the time of the on-site survey or has successfully addressed all requirements for improvement in an Evidence of Compliance (ESC) within 45 days following the posting of the Accreditation Survey Findings Report.

2. *Provisional Accreditation:* The hospital failed to demonstrate successful compliance with all requirements for improvement in an ESC within 45 days following the posting of the Accreditation Survey Findings Report.

3. *Conditional Accreditation:* The hospital was not in substantial compliance with applicable standards and must remedy identified problem areas through preparation and submission of ESC and subsequently undergo an on-site, follow-up survey.

4. *Preliminary Denial of Accreditation:* The hospital demonstrated noncompliance with enough standards to warrant a denial of accreditation, but the decision is subject to an appeal process before issuing a final decision.

5. *Denial of Accreditation:* The hospital has been denied accreditation, and all appeals have been exhausted.

6. *Preliminary Accreditation:* The hospital demonstrates compliance with specific standards during the Early Survey Policy.

American Osteopathic Association

The AOA is a professional membership association that represents more than 56,000 osteopathic physicians (DOs) in practice in the United States. The AOA is also the primary certification agency for osteopathic physicians and the accreditation agency for all osteopathic medical colleges and many osteopathic healthcare facilities (AOA 2007).

The practice of osteopathic medicine began at the end of the nineteenth century. Osteopathy is a therapeutic approach to the practice of medicine that uses all the usual forms of medical therapy and diagnosis, including drugs and surgery. However, it places greater emphasis on the influence of the relationship between the organs and the musculoskeletal system than traditional medical science does. Osteopathic physicians recognize and correct structural problems by using manipulation techniques in both diagnostic and therapeutic processes. The manipulation techniques used by osteopathic physicians are similar to the techniques employed by doctors of chiropractic. The difference is that osteopaths attempt to address structural problems within the body through physical manipulation; chiropractors are attempting to address abnormal nerve function. (Unlike osteopaths, however, chiropractors are not considered medical physicians, and their practices are limited to spinal manipulation and other skeletal "adjustments.")

The AOA first initiated its hospital accreditation program in 1945 to ensure the quality of residency training programs for doctors of osteopathy. Today, the association's Healthcare Facilities Accreditation Program (HFAP) accredits a number of healthcare facilities and services, including laboratories, ambulatory-care clinics, ambulatory-surgery centers, behavioral health and substance abuse treatment facilities, physical rehabilitation facilities, acute-care hospitals, and critical-access hospitals.

Healthcare facilities that have been accredited by the AOA earn deemed status from CMS. CMS extended the AOA HFAP deemed status effective through September 25, 2009. Like hospitals accredited by the Joint Commission, AOA-accredited hospitals are not required to undergo yearly Medicare certification surveys; however, as stated previously, a sample of approximately 10 percent of accredited osteopathic hospitals undergo Medicare validation surveys each year (Shaw et al. 2007, 316). State licensure agencies conduct Medicare certification surveys under contracts with CMS. CMS has also granted the AOA accreditation program deeming authority for hospital laboratory services under the Clinical Laboratory Improvements Act (CLIA) of 1988.

Healthcare Facilities Accreditation Program Documentation Standards

The HFAP's acute-care accreditation standards relate closely to the Medicare *Conditions of Participation for Hospitals* (AOA 2007). The AOA's documentation standards are very similar to the Joint Commission standards except in the area of osteopathic medical practice. According to the HFAP's standards, osteopathic physicians are required to perform musculoskeletal examinations in addition to traditional physical examinations shortly before or after a patient's admission to the hospital unless the patient's condition contraindicates such an examination. One standard specifically requires osteopathic physicians to document the results of such examinations in the patient's health record or to document the reason an osteopathic examination was not performed. Failure to meet this standard is one of the most common deficiencies cited during the survey process (AOA 2004a).

Healthcare Facilities Accreditation Program Survey and Accreditation Processes

Similar to the Joint Commission accredited hospitals, hospitals requesting initial accreditation or renewed accreditation from the AOA initiate the process by submitting an application. The HFAP application requests the same types of information that the Joint Commissions application requires. Likewise, the HFAP conducts on-site surveys at accredited hospitals at least once every three years, and accreditation decisions are based on compliance with the HFAP standards and participation requirements (AOA 2004a).

National Committee for Quality Assurance

The **National Committee for Quality Assurance (NCQA)** is a private, not-for-profit organization dedicated to improving healthcare quality by conducting assessments of managed care and other healthcare programs in the United States. The NCQA began accrediting managed-care organizations in 1991. Today, it provides accreditation programs and related services for health maintenance organizations, preferred provider organizations, managed behavioral health programs, and physician organizations. The NCQA's standards focus on patient safety, confidentiality, member satisfaction, and access to services, service quality, and continuous improvement.

Health Informatics Standards

In an increasingly complex healthcare environment, hospitals and other healthcare organizations collect more data and need more information today than a decade ago. Private organizations and government agencies gather data reported to them by healthcare organizations in state and national databases. Reimbursement organizations, quality improvement organizations, clinical researchers, government policy makers, and others plan and manage medical services and healthcare delivery systems based on data from these databases. The universal implementation of electronic health record systems promises to make data collection, sharing, and analysis more efficient, but it also presents its own unique challenges.

One of the biggest obstacles to the widespread implementation of electronic health record (EHR) systems has been the high cost of new and evolving technology. Hospitals have been reluctant to invest large amounts of capital dollars in clinical information technology for two main reasons: the absence of clear financial incentives and the lack of a shared vision of what an EHR should include and how it should perform.

However, due to the development and implementation of the HIPAA law, policy- and lawmakers are increasingly aware of the need to modernize healthcare information management systems. President George W. Bush initially called for the implementation of EHR systems in his January 2004 State of the Union address. Subsequently, in spring 2004, the president announced the creation of a new federal post dedicated to the nationwide implementation of EHR systems within the next ten years. The Office of the National Coordinator of Health Information Technology (ONC) was established within the U.S. Department of Health and Human Services. The charge of the office is to guide the nationwide implementation of information technology in healthcare applications. Specifically, its long-term goals are to inform clinical practice, connect clinicians, personalize patient care, and improve the health of the U.S. population.

The ONC continues to be an active force in the promotion of health information technology issues at the federal level (AHIMA 2008). In October 2007, the National Coordinator of the ONC Robert Kolodner outlined key points in the national health IT plan, including putting an "infrastructure in place to improve the quality and efficiency of healthcare" as well as developing standards for data, technology, and security. He also identified five "pieces of the puzzle" needed to move the healthcare industry, and the nation, to the "tipping point" into a nationwide health IT system.

1. Standards in health IT products

2. Privacy and security policies. These are important both at the federal and state level, Kolodner said. States are beginning to work together, and "We now see a dialogue that has not occurred before to identify issues," he said.

3. National health information network—"to link us together," Kolodner said. He noted that the Department of Health and Human Services (HHS) last week announced awards to nine health information exchanges to form a National Health Information Network (NHIN) collaborative. The intent, he says, is that by next year they will be operational—moving information between each other.

4. Adoption of interoperable health IT

5. Governance—to coordinate all the pieces. Currently governance and oversight have been provided by the American Health Information Community. While this group has "made more progress in three years than has been made in the last two decades," Kolodner said, change is in the wind. Kolodner told the audience that a "next-generation" model of this group is expected to emerge in 2008 to provide continuity of leadership, a sustainable business model, and decisive action.

Health Data Standards

Efforts to standardize healthcare data began in the 1960s, when healthcare facilities first began using computers to process large amounts of clinical data. When regulators and researchers attempted to compare the data from multiple healthcare organizations, it was evident that organizations were not always collecting the same information or labeling the same information the same way. If meaningful data comparisons were to be made possible, facilities needed to start collecting the same data and using the same data definitions.

The first data standardization efforts focused on hospital discharge data. The need to compare discharge data from one hospital to the next led to the development of uniform data sets, lists of recommended or required data elements with uniform definitions. Data sets used most commonly in hospitals today include the Uniform Hospital Discharge Data Set (UHDDS), the Data Elements for Emergency Department Systems (DEEDS), the Essential Medical Data Set (EMEDS), the **Health Plan Employer Data and Information Set (HEDIS)**, and the Uniform Ambulatory Care Data Set (UACDS).

The collection of uniform discharge data sets and the development of clinical databases made up of aggregate discharge data are still vital to healthcare operations and research today. In combination with diagnostic and procedural coded data, discharge data are used in accreditation, reimbursement, clinical research, delivery planning, and quality improvement, as well as many other internal and external processes and programs.

Standardized data sets developed in the 1960s and still in use today were designed for paper-based systems and pre-Medicare healthcare delivery systems. The National Committee on Vital and Health Statistics (NCVHS) led the development of the first uniform data sets, and it is now leading efforts to develop data standards for modern healthcare delivery and computer-based health information systems in the United States. Congress established the NCVHS to advise the HHS on health data, statistics, and national health information policy. The NCVHS serves as an advisory and review body for health data and statistical problems on a national and international basis, conducts studies, and proposes improvement needs for health statistics and information systems. The committee's responsibilities were expanded in 1996 with the advent of HIPAA. Collectively, these new standards are referred to as health informatics standards. **Health informatics standards** are standards that describe uniform methods for collecting, maintaining, and/or transferring healthcare data among computer information systems.

Standards Development Organizations

A number of national and international organizations develop voluntary standards for a variety of industries. Private and governmental organizations that publish standards are often referred to as standards development organizations. **Standards development organizations (SDOs)** design scientifically based models against which structures, processes, and outcomes can be measured. The American National Standards Institute (ANSI) coordinates the development of standards in the United States. The United Nations International Standards Organization (ISO) coordinates international standards development efforts.

Health informatics standards can be classified into five categories. Each of the categories has a specific purpose (Amatayakul 2004, 122–124):

- **Vocabulary standards:** To establish uniform definitions for clinical terms

- **Structure and content standards:** To establish clear descriptions of the data elements to be collected

- **Transaction and messaging standards**: To facilitate **electronic data interchange** (EDI) among independent computer information systems

- **Security standards:** To ensure the integrity of patient-identifiable health information and to protect it from unauthorized disclosure, alteration, and destruction

- **Identifier standards:** To establish methods for assigning unique identifiers to individual patients, healthcare professionals, healthcare provider organizations, and healthcare vendors and suppliers

Many organizations are currently working on the development of health informatics standards. (See the list of SDOs in table 8.7.) For example, HL7 developed a draft functional model of the EHR. This effort was supported by the **EHR Collaborative,** a group of representatives from healthcare-related professional and trade associations dedicated to the development and implementation of uniform EHR systems. Participants included the American Health Information Management Association, the American Hospital Association, and the Health Information Management Systems Society. As discussed in chapter 2, the model stimulated momentum in developing new technology to support interoperability of EHR system.

The HL7 EHR System Functional Model describes how more than 160 EHR functions should operate to "enable consistent expression of system functionality" (HL7 2007). The interoperability model provides standards for characteristics for EHR creation, transmission, and receipt, and also includes profiles for specific healthcare settings. The HL7 standard is an example of a content and structure standard.

To further advance work toward EHR content, AHIMA formed an e-HIM work group to educate members and the industry on the importance of standardizing data content and data definitions within provider organizations and the industry as a driver to quality of care and patient safety. The work group defined a **data dictionary** as a descriptive list of names, definitions, and attributes of data elements to be collected in an information system or database. Guidelines were established to assist in building data dictionaries at the organization level to standardize definitions and ensure consistency of use. Lack of a sound data dictionary can cause problems within and across organizations. Variances among the data sets that are not recognized across the system can affect the information flow as well as the workflow. These guidelines aid in the development of new and existing data content standards, and support national standards harmonization efforts as they relate to data dictionaries (AHIMA 2006). See appendix I on the accompanying CD for AHIMA's guidelines for developing a data dictionary.

The **Health Information Technology Standards Panel (HITSP)**, established by the ONC, is charged with determining which sets of national standards, developed by SDOs, will be used in the United States and for what purpose. The results of this initiative are reviewed by the **American Health Information Community (AHIC)** and HHS to further refine those standards for the healthcare industry. AHIC, a federal advisory body established by the HHS in 2005, comprises nine public and eight federal representatives plus the HHS secretary. AHIC provides input and recommendations to HHS, digitizing health records for interoperability while ensuring privacy and security of those records (Rode 2007).

The ASTM has also developed standards for the content and structure of EHRs. Standard E1384 describes the basic information categories in EHRs and segments the categories into specific data elements.

The **Systematized Nomenclature of Medicine–Clinical Terms (SNOMED CT)** is an example of a vocabulary standard. It was developed jointly by the College of American Pathologists and the National Library of Medicine. SNOMED CT established a common language for capturing, sharing, and aggregating health data across specialties and care settings.

Table 8.7 Health informatics standards development organizations

Organization	Types of Standards	Description
Accredited Standards Committee X12 Data Interchange Standards Association (DISA) 333 John Carlyle Street, Suite 600 Alexandria, VA 22314 Telephone: (703) 548-7005 www.disa.org	Electronic data interchange for billing transactions The committee's particular area of focus has been computer-to-computer communications between healthcare providers and third-party payers	Chartered in 1979 by ANSI, the X12N subcommittee develops and maintains X12 standards, interpretations, and guidelines. X12N is one of the standards for EDI that is specified in the regulations of the Health Insurance Portability and Accountability Act of 1996. Subgroups of X12N include: *WEDI: Workgroup on Electronic Data Exchange* WEDI has been the prime mover in the development of insurance industry standards. In 1995, WEDI became a private standards advocacy group. *HIBCC: Health Industry Business Communications Council*
American College of Radiology— National Electrical Manufacturers Association (ACR-NEMA) American College of Radiology 1891 Preston White Drive Reston, VA 20191 Telephone: (703) 648-8900 www.acr.org National Electrical Manufacturers Association 1300 N. Seventeenth Street, Suite 1847 Rosslyn, VA 22209 Telephone: (703) 841-3200 www.nema.org	Exchange of digitized images	ACR is a professional association, and NEMA is a trade association. They have worked collaboratively to develop the Digital Imaging and Communications in Medicine (DICOM) standard, which promotes a digital image communications format and facilitates development by the American College of Radiology of picture archive and communications systems. DICOM may be used for electronic exchange of X rays, computed tomography (CT), magnetic resonance imaging (MRI), ultrasound, nuclear medicine, and other radiology images. Work is under way to support other diagnostic images.
American Society for Testing and Materials (ASTM) 100 Barr Harbor Drive West Conshohocken, PA 19428 Telephone: (610) 832-9585 www.astm.org	Multiple health informatics standards, including clinical content of patient records, exchange of messages about clinical observations, data security and integrity, healthcare identifiers, data modeling, clinical laboratory systems, Arden syntax (a coding system), and system functionality	Organized in 1898, the ASTM is one of the largest SDOs in the world. It provides a forum for vendors, users, consumers, and others to develop standards for a wide range of materials, products, systems, and services. It is composed of more than 140 subcommittees or working groups identified as E31 and E32. Since 1990, Committee E31 on Healthcare Informatics has developed standards for health information and health information systems. Standard E1384, discussed earlier, is a product of the E31 subcommittee of ASTM.
Health Level Seven (HL7) 3300 Washtenaw Avenue, Suite 227 Ann Arbor, MI 48104 Telephone: (734) 677-7777 www.hl7.org	Electronic interchange of clinical, financial, and administrative information among disparate health information systems	HL7 is an ANSI-accredited SDO. Level 7 refers to the highest level of the Open System Interconnection (OSI) model of the International Standards Organization. The HL7 standard addresses issues that occur within the seventh, or application, layer.
Institute of Electrical and Electronics Engineers (IEEE) 445 Hoes Lane P.O. Box 1331 Piscataway, NJ 08855-1331 Telephone: (732) 981-0060 www.ieee.org	Medical device information and general informatics format	The IEEE's Medical Data Interchange Standard (MEDIX) is a standard set of hospital system interface transactions based on the ISO standards for all seven layers of the OSI model. Another IEEE standard for a medical information bus (MIB) links bedside instruments in critical care with health information systems.
National Council on Prescription Drug Programs (NCPDP) 4201 N. Twenty-fourth Street, Suite 365 Phoenix, AZ 85016 Telephone: (602) 957-9105 www.ncpdp.org	Data interchange and processing standards for pharmacy transactions	The NCPDP has defined standards for transmitting prescription information from pharmacies to payers for prescription management services and for receiving approval and payment information back in near-real time. Other standards address adverse drug reactions and utilization review.

Adapted from Brandt 2000, p. 39.

The SNOMED core terminology includes more than 357,000 healthcare concepts, each with a unique definition. Currently, it is available in English- and Spanish-language versions. Experts expect SNOMED CT to be adopted as a universal vocabulary standard for EHRs. SNOMED CT is available free for downloading as a part of the National Library of Medicine's Unified Medical Language System Metathesaurus (National Library of Medicine 2004).

The National Library of Medicine has also developed a clinical drug nomenclature in consultation with the Food and Drug Administration (FDA), the Department of Veterans Affairs (VA), and HL7. The FDA regulates the safety of food, drugs, medical devices, and cosmetics. The VA provides benefits to military veterans. **RxNorm** provides standard names for clinical drugs and administered dose forms. Like SNOMED CT, the most recent update of RxNorm is available through the National Library of Medicine's Unified Medical Language System Metathesaurus (National Library of Medicine 2004).

The work completed to develop and establish health informatics standards ensures the successful implementation of electronic health record systems. Compliance with such industry standards continues to be voluntary. Hospitals and other healthcare organizations find it beneficial to adopt health informatics standards because efficient information sharing is critical to so many areas of patient care and healthcare operations.

Internal Hospital Policies and Procedures

Every hospital must develop, implement, and enforce policies and procedures to ensure the quality of clinical care and the safety of patients, visitors, and staff. **Policies** are general written guidelines that dictate behavior or direct and constrain decision making within the organization. **Procedures** provide detailed written instructions on how functions and processes are implemented. Procedures should explicitly fulfill the stipulations of general policies.

Hospitals generally model their internal policies and procedures after applicable state and federal regulations, legal guidelines, accreditation standards, clinical practice standards, and voluntary industry standards. However, internal policies must also reflect the facility's own service goals and standards of care.

Policies should use clear language and follow a consistent format. In addition, every policy, procedure, and revision should be dated to ensure effective version control.

Policies and procedures should be reviewed on a regular basis and communicated to employees and the medical staff during initial employee and provider orientation. Employees and caregivers may also be required to review and sign acknowledgments of particularly important policies at regular intervals. Examples might include patient confidentiality and health record access and security policies. Many healthcare organizations post policies and procedures on their internal information networks to make them easy for employees to access.

Policies and procedures may apply across the hospital's departments or pertain specifically to one group of employees or one functional department. Hospital policies and procedures can be grouped into the following general categories:

- Administration, including health information management
- Medical staff
- Nursing services
- Human resources
- Safety
- Environment of care

Health Information Management Policies and Procedures

Health information management (HIM) professionals work with representatives of the hospital's clinical departments to develop health record policies and procedures. Like other hospital policies, health record policies must comply with applicable state and federal regulations, accreditation standards, and clinical standards. Policies and procedures must fulfill the specific legal requirements that apply to the facility. (Figure 8.3 provides an example of an HIM policy. Figure 8.4 lists the policies and procedures commonly maintained by hospital HIM departments.)

Medical Staff Bylaws, Rules, and Regulations

Medical staff bylaws, rules, and regulations govern the conduct of the independent healthcare professionals who provide patient-care services in acute-care facilities. Bylaws are similar to policies in that they describe general guidelines. Rules and regulations, like procedures, describe the specific activities to be performed to carry out the bylaws. The bylaws describe the structure of the medical staff and its membership qualifications, rights, and responsibilities.

Rules and regulations are generally easier to amend and therefore should be used to communicate elements that are likely to change frequently. Medical staff rules and regulations establish the medical staff's specific responsibilities for patient care and health record documentation.

Medical Records Committee

Medical staff bylaws prescribe the duties and functions of the medical records committee. Usually the committee consists of physician members, president or designee, nursing service

Figure 8.3. Sample HIM policy.

Policy on Terminal Controls

Purpose: To prevent unauthorized access to State University data by providing terminal controls

Scope: University terminals

Standard: Proper physical and software control mechanisms shall be in place to control access to and use of devices connected to university computer systems

Guidelines:

1 Hardware terminal locking: In areas that are not physically secured, terminals should be equipped with locking devices to prevent their use during unattended periods. The locks should be installed in addition to programmed restrictions, such as automatic disconnect after a given period of inactivity.

2 Operating system identification of terminals: All terminal activity should be controlled by the operating system, which should be able to identify terminals whether they are hardwired or connected through communications lines. The operating system should inspect log-on requests to determine which application the terminal user desires. The user should identify an existing application and supply a valid user ID and password combination. If the log-on request is valid, the operating system should make a logical connection between the user and the application.

3 Limitation of log-on attempts: Limit system log-on attempts from remote terminal devices. More than three unsuccessful attempts should result in termination of the session, generation of a real-time security violation message to the operator and/or the ISO (and log of said message in an audit file), and purging of the input queue of messages from the terminal.

4 Time-out feature: Ensure that the operating system provides the timing services required to support a secure operational environment. Inactive processes or terminals (in an interactive environment) should be terminated after a predetermined period.

5 Dial-up control: The communications software should ensure a clean end of connection in all cases, especially in the event of abnormal disconnection.

Source: Johns 2007, 868.

Figure 8.4.   Common HIM department policies and procedures.

The following list provides an example of the types of policy and procedures that may be included in a manual for health information services. The titles and content of the policy and procedures may vary by facility or corporation. Some of the policy and procedures are listed more than once for cross-referencing purposes.

Abbreviations
Access to Automated/Computerized Records
Access to Records (Release of Information) by
　　　Resident and by Staff
Admission/Discharge Register
Admission Procedures
　　Facility Procedures–Establishing/Closing the
　　　　Record
　　Preparing the Medical Record
　　Preparing the Master Patient Index Card
　　Readmission–Continued Use of Previous
　　　　Record
　　Readmission–New Record
Amendment of Clinical Records
Audit Schedule
Audit and Monitoring System
　　Audit/Monitoring Schedule
　　Admission/Readmission Audit
　　Concurrent Audit
　　Discharge Audit
　　Specialized Audits (examples)
　　Change in Condition
　　MDS
　　Nursing Assistant Flow Sheet
　　Psychotropic Drug Documentation
　　Pressure Sore
　　Restrictive Device/Restraint
　　Therapy
Certification, Medicare
Chart Removal and Chart Locator Log
Clinical Records, Definition of Records,
　　　and Record Service
General Policies
　　Access to Records
　　Automation of Records (See also
　　　　Computerization)
　　Availability
　　Change in Ownership
　　Completion and Correction of Records
　　Confidentiality
　　Definition of the Legal Record,
　　　　Coding from home
　　Indexes
　　Ownership of Records

Permanent and Capable of Being
　　　Photocopied
Retention
Storage of Records
Subpoena
Unit Record
Willful Falsification/Willful Omission
Closing the Record
Coding and Indexing, Disease Index
Committee Minutes Guidelines
Computerization and Security of Automated
　　　　Data/Records
Confidentiality (See Release of Information)
Consulting Services for Clinical Records and Plan
　　　of Service
Content, Record *(the list provided is not all-*
　　　　inclusive and should be tailored to the
　　　　facility/corporation)
　　General
　　Advanced Directives
　　Transfer Form/Discharge Plan of Care
　　Discharge against Medical Advice
　　Physician Consultant Reports
　　Medicare Certification/Recertification
　　Physician Orders/Telephone Orders
　　Physician Services Guidelines and Progress
　　　　Notes
　　Physician History and Physical Exam
　　Discharge Summary
　　Interdisciplinary Progress Notes
Copying/Release of Records—General
Correcting Clinical Records
Data Collection/Monitoring
Definition of Clinical Records/Health Information
　　　Service
Delinquent Physician Visit
Denial Letters, Medicare
Destruction of Records, Log
Disaster Planning for Health Information
Discharge Procedures
　　Assembly of Discharge Record
　　Chart Order on Discharge

Figure 8.4. (*continued*)

Completing and Filing Master Patient Index Card	Outguides
Discharge Chart Audit	Physician Visit Schedule, Letters, and Monitoring
Notification of Deficiencies	Physician Visits, Delinquent Visit Follow-up
Incomplete Record File	Quality Assurance
Closure of Incomplete Clinical Record	Health Information Participation
Preparation of the Record, Imaging of Records, Quality Review	QA Studies and Reporting
Emergency Disaster Evacuation	Readmission—Continued Use of Previous Record
Establishing/Closing Record	Readmission—New Record
Falsification of Records, Willful	Recertification or Certification (Medicare)
Fax/Facsimile, Faxing	Reconstruction of Lost Record
Filing Order, Discharge (Chart Order)	Refusal of Treatment
Filing Order, In-house (Chart Order)	Release of Information
Filing System	Confidentiality
Filing System, Unit Record	Confidentiality Statement by Staff
Forms Management	Copying/Release of Records—General
Forms, Release of Information	Faxing Medical Information
Forms, Subpoena	Procedure for Release—Sample Letters and Authorizations
Guide to Location of Items in the Health Information Department	Redisclosure of Clinical Information
Guidelines, Committee Minutes	Resident Access to Records
Incomplete Record File	Retrieval of Records (sign-out system)
Indexes	Subpoena
Disease Index and Forms for Indexing	Uses and Disclosures of Protected Health Information, Uses and Disclosures of Deidentified Documentation, Business-Associated Contracts, Audit Trails
Master Patient Index	
Release of Information Index/Log	
In-service Training Minutes/Record	
Job Descriptions	Witnessing Legal Documents
Health Information Coordinator	Requesting Information
Health Unit Coordinator	From Hospitals and Other Healthcare Providers
Other Health Information Staff (if applicable)	Request for Information Form
Late Entries	Retention of Records and Destruction after Retention Period
Lost Record—Reconstruction	Example Statement for Destruction
Master Patient Index	Retention Guidelines
Medicare Documentation	Retrieval of Records
Certification and Recertification	Security of Automated Data/Electronic Medical Records
Medicare Denial Procedure and Letter	General Procedures
Medicare Log	Back-up Procedures
Numbering System	Passwords
Ombudsman, Review/Access to Records	Sign-out Logs
Omission, Willful	Storage of Records
Order of Filing, Discharge	Telephone Orders
Order of Filing, In-house	Thinning
Organizational Chart for Health Information Department	In-house Records
Orientation/Training of Health Information Department	Maintaining Overflow Record
	Unit Record System

Source: Adapted from Amatayakul 2003 and AHIMA n.d.

representative, director of health information services, and others as required to accomplish the duties and responsibilities of the committee at the request of the chairman. Another committee, as defined by medical staff bylaws, can perform the functions of the medical records committee.

Duties of the medical records committee include the following:

- Evaluating medical records using criteria developed and approved by the medical board to assess that records describe the conditions and progress of the patients, the therapies provided, and the results thereof

- Evaluating and making recommendations to the medical board regarding form and format of the medical records

- Monitoring the promptness, adequacy, pertinence, and completeness of medical records

- Referring identified deficiencies to the appropriate department or committee for review

- Reviewing the number of incomplete charts for each practitioner and referring information to the medical board as appropriate

- Preparing reports as requested by the medical board, a division's quality review officer/ committee, or credentials committee for use during the reappointment and renewal of clinical privileges

Summary

Acute-care hospitals are regulated through a complex and constantly changing system of mandatory and voluntary standards promulgated by government agencies, accrediting organizations, professional organizations, and standards development organizations. Regulations vary at the federal, state, and local levels of government, and Medicare and Medicaid have their own *Conditions of Participation* (2006) based on the healthcare setting. Although several accreditation programs are available for modern-day hospitals, the Joint Commission (2006) brings together these disparate regulations and provides a launching point for most healthcare facilities. Efforts at developing standards for electronic health record systems hold promise for the adoption of fully modern documentation practices in the near future.

References

AHIMA e-HIM Work Group on EHR Data Content. 2006 (February). Guidelines for developing a data dictionary. *Journal of American Health Information Management Association* 77(2): 64A–D.

AHIMA. 2008 (January). Healthcare's Future Transformation. *Journal of American Health Information Management Association* 79(1): 56–57.

Amatayakul, Margret K. 2004 . *Electronic Health Records: A Practical Guide for Professionals and Organizations*, 2nd ed. Chicago: AHIMA.

American Osteopathic Association. 2004a. *About the Healthcare Facilities Accreditation Program*. Available at http://do-online.osteotech.org.

American Osteopathic Association. 2007. *Accreditation Requirements for Healthcare Facilities*, 2004–2005. Chicago: AOA.

Brandt, Mary D. 2000. Health informatics standards: *A user's guide. Journal of American Health Information Management Association* 71(4): 39–43.

Bush, George W. Address before a Joint Session of the Congress on the State of the Union, January 20, 2004. *Public Papers of the Presidents of the United States.* Washington, D.C.: Government Printing Office, 2004.

Carpenter, Jennifer. 1999. Practice brief: Managing health information relating to infection with the human immunodeficiency virus. *Journal of American Health Information Management Association* 70(5).

Centers for Medicare and Medicaid Services. 2006 (Dec. 8). Medicare and Medicaid Programs; Hospital conditions of participation: Patients' rights; Final rule. 42 CFR Part 482. *Federal Register* 71(236): 71377–71428. Available online from http://frwebgate6.access.gpo.gov/cgi-bin/waisgate.cgi?WAISdocID=434367226361+6+0+0&WAISaction=retrieve.

Health Level Seven. 2007. HL7 2007 EHR-S Functional Model. Available online from www.hl7.org/ehr/downloads/index_2007.asp.

Hjort, Beth. 2005. Practice brief: The HIM role in patient safety and quality of care. *Journal of American Health Information Management Association* 76(1): 56A–G.

Johns, Merida. 2007. Information security for managerial and clinical support. Chapter 18 in *Health Information Management Technology: An Applied Approach,* 2nd ed. Edited by Merida Johns. Chicago: AHIMA.

Joint Commission on Accreditation of Healthcare Organizations. *2006 (October). Sentinel event policy and procedures.* Available online from www.jointcommission.org/SentinelEvents/PolicyandProcedures/.

Joint Commission on Accreditation of Healthcare Organizations. 2006. 2006 *Comprehensive Accreditation Manual for Hospitals; The Official Handbook.* Oakbrook Terrace, Il.: Joint Commission.

Joint Commission on Accreditation of Healthcare Organizations. 2006. *About the Hospital Survey Process.* Available online from www.jointcommission.org.

Joint Commission. 2007 (January). *Accreditation process: Facts about the Periodic Performance Review.* Available online from www.jointcommission.org/AccreditationPrograms/Hospitals/AccreditationProcess/PPR_QA.htm.

McWay, Dana. 2002. *Legal Aspects of Health Information Management,* 2nd ed. Clifton Park, NY: Delmar Learning.

National Committee for Quality Assurance (NCQA). 2007. NCQA Accreditation Programs. Available online from http://www.ncqa.org/tabid/66/Default.aspx.

National Library of Medicine. 2004. *Unified Medical Language System Metathesaurus.* Available online from www.nlm.nih.gov/research/umls.

Rhodes, H., and J. Burrington-Brown. 2002. Practice brief: Recommended regulations and standards for specific healthcare settings. *Journal of American Health Information Management Association* 73(10).

Rode, Dan. 2007 (April). Connecting the dots: Outlining the organizations involved with EHRs and HIE. *Journal of American Health Information Management Association* 78(4): 18–20.

Shaw, Patricia, et al. 2007. *Quality and Performance Improvement in Healthcare: A Tool for Programmed Learning,* 3rd ed. Chicago: AHIMA.

The White House Office of the President. 2004 (April). Transforming Health Care: The President's Health Information Technology Plan. Washington, DC: The White House.

Chapter 9

Ambulatory Care

Susan Rossiter, RHIA

Learning Objectives

- Define and explain the different terms associated with ambulatory-based services

- Explain the key trends in ambulatory services today

- Evaluate the different accreditation agencies

- Describe the emerging documentation requirements for each type of accreditation

- Compare the differences in acute care and ambulatory care documentation

- Identify the role that state law plays in the ambulatory-care setting

- Describe the challenges of obtaining informed consent in a large multispecialty setting

- Explain the unique difference in the internal policies for a multisite ambulatory health-care organization

- Outline the internal HIM policies that professionals should address to meet current regulation challenges

Key Terms

Accreditation

Accreditation Association for Ambulatory Health Care (AAAHC) *— most commonly used for ambulatory care*

Ambulatory surgical center (ASC)

American Association for Accreditation of Ambulatory Surgery Facilities (AAAASF)

Birthing center

Cancer treatment center

Closing practice policy

Commission on Cancer (CoC)

Community health center

Coordinated school health program

Correctional facility health clinic

Diagnostic imaging center

Elements of Performance (EP)

Failed/missed appointment policy

Family Educational Rights and Privacy Act of 1974 (FERPA)

Hand-off communication

Health maintenance organization (HMO)

Industrial health clinic

Informed consent policy

Managed-care organization

Medication list

Multispecialty group practice

Outstanding record policy

Sentinel event

Shadow chart policy

Specialist

Problem/Summary list

Telephone encounter

Uniform Ambulatory Care Data Set (UACDS)

Urgent-care centers

Urgent Care Association of America (UCAOA)

Introduction

Today, more than half of all healthcare services are performed through an internal or external network of healthcare providers in an ambulatory-care setting with a primary-care physician (PCP) as the gatekeeper of patient care.

Statistics

According to the National Center for Health Statistics in their 2005 report on health in the United States, Americans increased their use of ambulatory services to physician's offices, hospital emergency departments, and outpatient departments by 31 percent over a 10-year period from 1994 through 2004 (NCHS 2005). This was accompanied by a 19 percent increase in utilization per person. PCPs provided approximately 48 percent of these services. Medical specialists provided approximately 18 percent; surgical specialists provided 16 percent, emergency departments provided 10.0 percent, and outpatient departments accounted for 8 percent.

PCPs play a major role in referral and tracking of the patient's use of specialty providers. Each patient forms a personal network that includes the PCP, medical specialists, and other healthcare professionals. The PCP provides a home base from which the patient's care is directed and information about the patient is collected. This is largely due to the frequency of contact that PCPs have with patients and, often, their families. Coordination of care is dependent on the quality of documentation provided by each of the healthcare providers involved in the patient's treatment. Information exchange is critical as medical decisions are based on the documentation and test results provided by each healthcare provider within the patient's personal network.

Ambulatory-Care Settings

Ambulatory services are flourishing. The same research that led to increased understanding of disease processes has also led to changes in the patterns of medical practice and the settings of patient care. The use of advanced technology, such as endoscopes and lasers, has decreased the trauma associated with surgical procedures and shortened the postoperative recovery period. Complex procedures that a decade ago required long hospital stays now are performed routinely in the ambulatory setting. The use of ambulatory services has grown, in part, in response to the public's demand for high-quality, convenient healthcare. Today, patients and physicians alike emphasize the importance of preventive medicine, which is delivered almost entirely within the ambulatory setting. Following is an overview of the various types of ambulatory-care settings and the associated requirements for each.

Ambulatory Surgical Centers

Elective surgical procedures are performed on patients in **ambulatory surgical centers (ASC).** Patients using these facilities are classified as outpatients and typically are released from the surgery center on the same day that the procedure is performed. Surgical procedures are scheduled in advance and usually take from 5 to 90 minutes. Generally, recovery following the procedure requires less than four hours; so patients can leave the same day. There are no emergency services available at ambulatory surgical centers, and patients in whom surgical complications develop are transported to an emergency department at an inpatient facility.

The following is according to the Federated Ambulatory Surgery Association (FASA):

> [In 2005], 70 percent of all surgeries in America are outpatient, and one out of every five of these is performed at an ASC. ASCs throughout the country have outstanding patient safety records while achieving high rates of efficiency and customer satisfaction.

The trend has been continuing . . . According to the Medicare Payment Advisory Commission (MedPAC)'s *Data Book, Healthcare Spending and the Medicare Program* (2007), the number of Medicare-certified ASCs grew at an average annual rate of 7.6 percent from 2000 (3,028) through 2006 (4,707). "The growth rate slowed recently, from 8.9 percent in 2005 to 4.5 percent in 2006. Each year from 2000 through 2006, an average of 351 new Medicare-certified facilities entered the market, while an average of 74 closed or merged with other facilities." MedPAC also reports that "total Medicare payments for ASC services are growing rapidly. Payments increased by 13.3 percent per year, on average, from 2000 through 2006." (MedPAC 2007)

Some of the high volume specialties, listed in order of CMS total annual reimbursement dollars, are gastroenterology, ophthalmology, pain management, and urology (Norwalk 2006).

Ambulatory surgical centers typically seek accreditation from one of three organizations: the Joint Commission, the Accreditation Association for Ambulatory Health Care (AAAHC), or the American Association for Accreditation of Ambulatory Surgery Facilities (AAAASF).

Birthing Centers

Usually staffed by nurse-midwives, **birthing centers** provide delivery services for women who plan to have normal deliveries. A patient must be screened for medical acceptability before she can be scheduled to deliver her child at a birthing center. Some hospitals also offer ambulatory obstetric services for women who are expected to have normal deliveries.

Following are charting guidelines for midwives (Rosenberger 2001):

- Chart a procedure until it is done, but chart it immediately. If your client refuses care, note that along with an explanation.

- Charting requires that a midwife use her skills of observation. We talk about "looking" for symptoms, but we should also be listening, smelling, and touching. As long as a midwife is with a client, she should be continuously observing her, actively watching and listening at every opportunity. We can often learn as much by what is not said as by what is said.

- Charted information may be overt (obvious), covert (hidden), and either objective (measurable by an observer) or subjective (known only to the client). Overt information includes such observations as the client's fundal height or degree of pitting edema. Covert information could include an asymptomatic vaginal infection or the client's hemoglobin count. Objective information includes a client's blood pressure or the fetal heart tones. Subjective information could be the client's report of vaginal itching, burning upon urination, or nausea.

- The ABCs of charting consist of Accuracy, Brevity, and Completeness. You cannot be judgmental ("can't handle pain"). Rather, write "client moaning with each contraction." Avoid vague terms such as "large" ("passed large clot of blood"). Be specific: "passed blood clot approx. 5 cm in diameter." Be sure that abbreviations are proper and commonly used. Be brief; complete sentences are not necessary. Be complete: Review, assess, and explain results of care given.

Cancer Treatment Centers

Cancer treatment centers specialize in providing comprehensive cancer treatment, including radiation and chemotherapy. Many of them also offer patient education and family counseling services.

Established by the American College of Surgeons (ACoS) in 1922, the multidisciplinary **Commission on Cancer (CoC)** sets standards for quality multidisciplinary cancer care. The CoC Approvals Program encourages hospitals, treatment centers, and other facilities to improve their quality of patient care through various cancer-related programs. These programs are concerned with prevention, early diagnosis, pretreatment evaluation, staging, and optimal treatment, as well as rehabilitation, surveillance for recurrent disease, support services, and end-of-life care.

The availability of a full range of medical services along with a multidisciplinary team approach to patient care at approved cancer treatment centers has resulted in approximately 80 percent of all newly diagnosed cancer patients being treated in CoC-approved cancer programs.

Recognizing that cancer is a complex group of diseases, the CoC Cancer Program Standards (CoC 2006) promote consultation among surgeons, medical and radiation oncologists, diagnostic radiologists, pathologists, and other cancer specialists. This multidisciplinary cooperation results in improved patient care.

The following five elements contribute to the success of a Commission-approved cancer program:

- The clinical services provide state-of-the-art pretreatment evaluation, staging, treatment, and clinical follow-up for cancer patients seen at the facility for primary, secondary, tertiary, or quaternary care.

- The cancer committee leads the program through setting goals, monitoring activities, evaluating patient outcomes, and improving care.

- The cancer conferences provide a forum for patient consultation and contribute to physician education.

- The quality improvement program is the mechanism for evaluating and improving patient outcomes.

- The cancer registry and database is the basis for monitoring the quality of care. (CoC 2006)

Records regarding chemotherapy and radiotherapy treatment must be retained for a patient's lifetime. Premature destruction of such documentation may result in a preventable death or inappropriate subsequent treatment.

Community Health Centers

Sometimes called neighborhood health centers, these facilities are usually located in low-income areas. They offer comprehensive, primary healthcare services (both therapeutic and preventive) to patients who otherwise would have limited access to healthcare. **Community health centers** frequently are operated by local and state public health departments, and most of the services are provided by public health nurses. Patients pay for services either on a sliding scale based on income or according to a flat-rate, discounted fee schedule supplemented by public funding.

Correctional Facilities Health Clinics

Ambulatory-care services are provided to prisoners confined to correctional facilities. Inmates are generally given a receiving screening by a trained correctional staff member within hours of being received into a correctional facility. During the screening, health needs are identified, and if necessary, the prisoner is referred to the health clinic. If medical treatment is required, a medical record is created. A copy of the receiving screening should be included in the medical record after it is created.

Neither informed consent nor payment is required to carry out treatment at a **correctional facility health clinic.** This exception is made for treating inmates so a facility will not be held hostage to a manipulative inmate seeking to obstruct healthcare operations.

Medical necessity in correctional facilities is defined by the National Commission on Correctional Health Care (NCCHC) as "a clinical decision by a qualified health practitioner based on clinical judgment in keeping with current community standards of practice to meet a serious health need of the individual in question" (NCCHC 2007). This does not mean that every medical request must be answered in the manner the patient desires, but that each request must be evaluated by the appropriate clinician. Procedures considered elective or experimental and those for cosmetic rather than functional reasons generally are not considered medical necessities. The qualified clinician making this clinical determination should document the decision and steps taken to arrive at it in the medical record of the individual involved.

The NCCHC is the accrediting body for correctional facilities. NCCHC was established in the 1970s to assist correctional facilities in their continued improvement. Accreditation promotes and documents an efficient, well-managed system of healthcare delivery in correctional facilities. The following standards must be met:

- Facility governance and administration

- Maintaining a safe and healthy environment

- Personnel and training

- Healthcare services support

- Inmate care and treatment

- Health promotion and disease prevention

- Special inmate needs and services

- Health records

- Medical-legal issues

Diagnostic Imaging Centers

A freestanding **diagnostic imaging center** provides diagnostic imaging services including MRI (magnetic resonance imaging), CT (computed tomography), and PET (positron emission tomography), as well as ultrasound (ultrasonography), nuclear medicine, picture archival communication systems, digital mammography, and molecular imaging. These technologies enable physicians to diagnose diseases at earlier stages while avoiding more invasive and costly diagnostic procedures.

While it is a significant technological advancement, diagnostic imaging is also the fastest growing physician service in the United States, with an annual 9 percent growth rate that is three times that of other physician services, according to the American College of Radiology (2005). In 1999, the cost of diagnostic imaging was projected to increase 28 percent between 2000 and 2005 to nearly $100 billion annually, according to a Booz Allen Hamilton analysis (2003).

The American College of Radiology (ACR) is the most widely recognized medical imaging accrediting body, with nearly 16,000 accredited facilities in the United States (2007). The accreditation process evaluates a practice's quality assurance activities, personnel, and equipment. When accreditation is conferred, it is an outward sign that a facility is set up to provide quality patient care.

ACR accreditation is an efficient process of both self-assessment by the facility and independent, external expert audit. Using ACR guidelines and technical standards, the accreditation process measures the facility's personnel qualifications, facility policies and procedures; equipment specifications; QA activities; patient safety; and ultimately the quality of patient care.

ACR (2007) accreditation requires that the physicians supervising and interpreting medical imaging meet stringent education and training standards. ACR accreditation also requires that the imaging equipment be surveyed regularly by qualified medical physicists to ensure that it is functioning properly and that the technologists administering the tests are appropriately certified (ACR 2007).

Industrial Health Clinics

Often located in areas that are easily accessible to industrial sites, **industrial health clinics** offer treatment to workers who are affected by work-related injuries and illnesses. Usually, these centers are financed through the employer's workers' compensation insurance plan. Sometimes they also provide preemployment physicals and testing, which are paid for directly by the potential employers. Finally, many industrial health centers collect data on patterns of work-related illness and injury and provide the information to employers on a contract basis.

Health Maintenance Organizations

Health maintenance organizations (HMOs), also called **managed care organizations**, offer a wide range of healthcare services, including acute care and ambulatory care. They provide health coverage to voluntarily enrolled individuals in return for prepayment of a fixed fee, regardless of the services the individual enrollees actually use.

Private Medical Practices

Physicians who provide medical care in office settings may work alone in a solo practice, work in a limited partnership with one or more physicians, or work in a group practice with a number of physicians. Physicians in a group practice share office space, equipment, records, and personnel, and usually employ an office manager. Some group practices provide medical services in a single specialty (for example, internal medicine). A **multispecialty group practice** includes providers who represent a variety of medical specialties. Physician offices are the most common site for the delivery of ambulatory care. Physicians of many specialties deliver ambulatory care. These physicians include **specialists** in family medicine, internal medicine, obstetrics, gynecology, cardiology, gastroenterology, ophthalmology, and dermatology.

Coordinated School Health Programs

According to the Web site for the American Association for School Health, all the strategies, activities, and services that are offered by, in, or in association with schools and designed to promote students' physical, emotional, and social development make up a school's health program.

When a school works with students, their families, and their community to provide these strategies, activities, and services in a coordinated, planned way, the term *coordinated school health program* applies. Ideally, a coordinated school health program includes the following:

- A healthful environment
- Nursing and other health services that students need to stay in school
- Nutritious and appealing school meals
- Opportunities for physical activity that include physical education
- Health education that covers a range of developmentally appropriate topics taught by knowledgeable teachers
- Programs that promote the health of school faculty and staff
- Counseling, psychological, and social services that promote healthy social and emotional development and remove barriers to students' learning

The **Family Educational Rights and Privacy Act** (FERPA) of 1974 was enacted by Congress to protect the privacy of student educational records. Education records maintained by the student's school contain vaccination histories, information about sports physicals, counseling for behavioral problems, and records of visits to the school nurse. Privacy of education records is protected under FERPA. An institution must have written permission from the adult student or the underage student's parent or legal guardian before releasing any information from a student's educational record.

University-based Student Health Services

University student centers provide primary healthcare; disease prevention services; and counseling for personal, academic, and vocational concerns to their students. Promotion of a healthy life style is one of the main goals. FERPA laws and regulations apply to state colleges, universities, and technical schools that receive federal funding.

Urgent-Care Centers

The **Urgent Care Association of America (UCAOA)** estimates that more than 17,000 **urgent-care centers** deliver urgent care in the United States. These centers are designed to evaluate and treat conditions that are not severe enough to require treatment in a hospital emergency department but still require treatment beyond normal physician office hours or before a physician's appointment is available. (UCAOA)

Ambulatory-Care Health Record Content and Formats

Careful documentation is critical in every ambulatory organization no matter the size or scope of patient care. The health record is a compilation of identifying information about the patient and pertinent facts about his or her current health status and medical history. Provided by the healthcare professionals who participate in the patient's care, the information in the health record is used in planning and managing care, evaluating its adequacy and appropriateness, substantiating reimbursement claims, and protecting the legal interests of both the patient and his or her healthcare providers. Moreover, the health record is a tool for communication among the patient's providers along the continuum of care. Finally, it is used for education, research, public health, and organizational activities such as performance improvement, risk management, and strategic planning.

A paper-based health record that incorporates well-designed forms makes data collection easy and guarantees that all of the information needed to fulfill documentation requirements is up to date. Forms and checklists arranged in a logical sequence allow providers to document care completely without having to prepare separate reports.

Effective forms design is critical to the successful implementation of computer-based patient record (CPR) systems. Well-thought-out input screens and data-entry fields make the process of loading information from paper records efficient and reliable. The system for organizing the various sections of the paper record also can be used as a template for determining CPR access categories and assigning responsibility for updating the various types of information in the electronic record.

For documentation in the ambulatory health record to be meaningful, the information must be arranged in a predefined format. This requirement is especially important when multiple providers use the same record. The health record can be arranged according to one of three formats: source-oriented, problem-oriented, or integrated system (see chapter 6).

The advantages and disadvantages of each of these record formats must be weighed against the needs of the providers using the health record. For example, because it was developed to enhance comprehensive patient care, the problem-oriented record system is especially appropriate for HMOs and neighborhood health centers, where a team of professionals offers total patient care. Different practitioners can easily identify existing conditions and current treatments and adjust their own treatment strategies accordingly. In an urgent-care setting, however, an integrated record system may be more suitable owing to the episodic nature of urgent care. Urgent-care patients usually present for treatment of a single acute problem and then return to their PCP for follow-up care. Of course, the record formats also can be combined. The only requirement is that the resulting record contains sufficient information to identify the patient and to support the diagnosis and plan of treatment for each episode of care. Providing discharge instructions to the patient and hand-off information to that patient's other healthcare providers is critical to the patient's continuity of care.

Basic components are required in every record of ambulatory care. These include the following:

- Registration record, which documents demographic data about the patient

- Problem list, which summarizes all of the medical and surgical problems that have long-term clinical significance for the patient's care

- Medication list, which lists pertinent information about the medications the patient is taking

- Patient history questionnaire, which asks the patient for information about current and past medical conditions

- Medical history, which documents the provider's findings on the patient's health status

- Physical examination report, which contains the provider's findings upon examination of the patient

- Immunization and injection records, which chronicle the patient's vaccinations

- Progress notes, which provide a chronological summary of the patient's illness and treatment at each encounter

- Physician orders, which document the physician's instructions to other parties involved in providing the patient's care

The following items are recommended:

- Patient instructions, which document the instructions the provider gave to the patient regarding follow-up care

- Failed/missed appointment form, which documents patient noncompliance with recommendations for follow-up appointments with the provider

- Flow sheets, which can be used to document treatment between patient visits

- Telephone contact records, which document telephone communications between the patient and his or her healthcare providers

Registration Record

The registration record documents the basic demographic data collected before or during the initial patient visit. This information is maintained and updated on subsequent visits, as needed. Because it defines the data elements that ambulatory facilities are required to collect for billing and reporting purposes, the **Uniform Ambulatory Care Data Set (UACDS)** is frequently used as baseline data.

Individual facilities must determine what additional data they need to collect for the purpose of performing various internal activities such as research, utilization management, planning, and marketing. For example, an analysis of basic demographic data might provide answers to questions about the need to hire additional staff or to open facilities in different locations. The goals and objectives of an ambulatory-care facility also play a role in determining what data should be collected. For example, facilities featuring family-centered care may collect basic demographic data on all of the patient's family members. In general, the following data elements are collected and maintained for every patient:

- Surname, first name, and middle name or initial
- Unique identifying number
- Residence address/telephone
- Date of birth
- Gender
- Marital status
- Race or ethnic origin
- Social Security number
- Medicare, Medicaid, or insurance group number
- Insurance company/address/name of subscriber
- Guarantor, if applicable
- Name of insured
- Patient relationship to insured
- Employer
- Occupation
- Business address/telephone
- Name, address/telephone of nearest relative, friend, or guardian or emergency contact
- Any other emergency contact
- Primary-care physician
- Referring physician/address, if applicable

In many clinics, registration (demographic) information is maintained on the clinic's practice management or billing software. Then a copy is printed and placed in the patient's record. This copy may contain only limited data elements. A new registration record may be printed and placed in the patient's record whenever the registration information changes.

For greater efficiency, an identifying number unique to each patient should be assigned. The use of the patient's Social Security number as an identifier is not recommended due to the potential for identity theft and current laws and regulations governing the use of Social Security numbers.

Problem/Summary List

According to the Accreditation Manual for Ambulatory Surgical Centers (Joint Commission 2007), for each patient receiving continuing ambulatory services, a list of known significant diagnoses, conditions, procedures, and drug allergies must be included in the health record by the third visit.

The **problem list** (sometimes called the **summary list**) is a valuable tool in patient care management and should always be visible and easy to read. A single page summarizes all of the major medical and surgical problems that have long-term clinical significance for the patient, including social and psychiatric problems. The dates of onset and resolution are recorded for each problem. The healthcare provider can use the problem list to determine at a glance which problems are active or resolved and can adjust treatment plans accordingly. As a communication tool, the problem list helps specialty physicians make evaluation and treatment decisions about the patients referred to them for care; having this information often eliminates the need to duplicate costly tests. Each provider documents his or her care of the patient on the same list, thereby creating a comprehensive overview of the patient's medical status. For consistency and clarity, facilities should develop guidelines for recording several key elements in the problem list, including problems, dates of onset, active versus inactive status, and resolution dates.

Significant problems include both chronic and acute conditions that affect patient management. For example, both hypercholesterolemia and status post cholecystectomy would be included on the problem list. Although the cholecystectomy occurred in the past, knowledge of this major surgical event could prove valuable in future clinical evaluations. Abnormal signs and symptoms that have the potential to become significant problems also are recorded, but short-term illnesses that were resolved quickly and "ruled-out" conditions are not. Including ruled-out conditions would defeat the list's purpose, which is to provide a quick reference to the patient's confirmed conditions and their management status. The problem list also records allergies, social situations that may have a significant impact on clinical management (for example, the fact that the patient lives alone or has a history of child abuse), and risk factors (smoking, alcohol and drug usage, and personal and family history of conditions such as cancer, diabetes, or heart disease). Every clinician involved in a patient's care should have information on these factors. The National Committee for Quality Assurance (NCQA) requires notation on the use of cigarettes, alcohol, and substances for all patients older than 14 years of age. Frequently, this information is included on the problem list.

Moreover, the date of onset for each problem should be documented. Guidelines should specify which date should be used, that is, the date the patient reported first noting the condition or the date the provider confirmed the condition. Consistency in documentation is important for interpretation and use in evaluation. Each problem should be labeled as active or inactive so that clinicians can determine treatment priorities quickly and develop a treatment plan. Resolved or inactive problems may still be relevant to management of the patient. When its cause is confirmed, the symptom is not erased but, rather, is linked to the new diagnosis. The resolution date is important as an indicator of problems that have been resolved and as a means for monitoring recurrences.

[handwritten margin note: takes into account — time; something that happened in third grade is no longer relevant]

Medication List

The **medication list** is an ongoing record of the medications a patient has received in the past and is taking currently (Joint Commission 2007). This list is required by the Joint Commission, the AAAHC, and the NCQA. Key data elements include:

- Names of medications
- Dosages and amounts dispensed
- Dispensing instructions (with signature)
- Prescription dates and discontinued dates
- Problem numbers for which each medication was prescribed

Organizations may decide to omit medications prescribed for a single, short-term course of therapy, such as an antibiotic prescribed for an infection. In pediatric patients, however, even short-term medications should be included. Many pediatric illnesses (for example, otitis media) are recurrent in nature; so the physician needs a record that shows which medications were effective in past episodes of the illness.

Dates of medication refills often are charted on the medication list. The medication list is an acceptable location for documentation of patient allergies. However, this information should be documented in only one specific location of the chart to ensure its completeness and consistency. The patient's current medications and allergies should be verified during each patient visit, and the chart should be updated appropriately.

When consistent, accurate, and properly updated, the medication list serves multiple purposes, including alerting the physician to drug sensitivities and allergies. When used in conjunction with the problem list, the medication list can help clarify the reason a patient is taking a particular medication (Benson 1988, 197). For those cases in which patients are taking several medications or seeing several practitioners, the medication list helps providers evaluate and adjust the drug regimen appropriately by taking into account potential incompatibilities or interactions.

Patient History Questionnaire

The patient history questionnaire is structured to prompt the patient to provide certain items of information, including the presence or absence of significant conditions that may represent potential medical problems. The responses to specific questions not only provide information but also serve as starting points for the clinician who must gather additional historical data. The patient should be asked to complete a new history questionnaire at periodic intervals (approximately every five years). Placing an updated patient questionnaire in the health record makes it possible to keep a complete, current history in one place and frees providers from having to read through multiple progress notes.

Medical History

A comprehensive medical history should be obtained periodically from the patient or his or her representative. Frequency depends on the patient's age and health status. Often the initial medical history is obtained by questioning patients in detail about their health history. Clinicians may utilize short history forms to supplement and expand the information provided on the patient's general health history questionnaire. Updates to the history often are included in the progress note made during the patient visit (Cofer 1994).

A complete medical history establishes the foundation for comprehensive care by documenting current complaints and symptoms in addition to past medical, personal, and family history. It should include pertinent aspects of basic physiological systems as well. The medical histories obtained by specialists such as gynecologists and gastroenterologists are comprehensive for the particular organ system involved.

Health Information Management (Cofer 1994) suggests including the following information in a complete medical history. Note that the second element, "Present illness," may not be included in a primary-care ambulatory record when the patient presents for preventive care or health maintenance.

- **Chief complaint or reason for visit:** Nature and duration of the symptoms that caused the patient to seek medical attention as stated in the patient's own words

- **Present illness:** Detailed chronological description of the development of the patient's illness, from the appearance of the first symptom to the present situation

- **Past medical history:** A summary of childhood and adult illnesses and conditions, such as infectious diseases, pregnancies, allergies and drug sensitivities, accidents, operations, hospitalizations, and current medications

- **Social or personal history:** Marital status; dietary, sleep, and exercise patterns; use of coffee, tobacco, alcohol, and other drugs; occupation; home environment; daily routine; and so on

- **Family history:** Diseases among relatives in which heredity or contact may play a role, such as allergies, cancer, and infections, psychiatric, metabolic, endocrine, cardiovascular, and renal diseases; health status or cause and age at death for immediate relatives

The medical history is a record of subjective statements made by the patient. The physical examination is a record of the physician's assessment of the patient's current health status. Information on all of the major organ systems should be documented in the physical examination report:

- **Review of systems:** A systemic inventory designed to uncover current or past subjective symptoms

- **Immunization and injection records:** A list of immunizations or injections of medication including the date(s) of administration; information on the manufacturer and lot number, drug, dosage, and route of administration; signature of the person administering the vaccine; and a consent form for the vaccination

Progress Notes

Progress notes present a summary of the patient's status and treatment at each encounter. Progress notes may be structured or narrative, but to be useful to other reviewers of the health record, they must be legible (if paper based) and uniform. The best example of a structured progress note lies in the SOAP format, commonly used with the problem-oriented medical record. In this format, the note itself is divided into four parts, each identified with a letter from the SOAP acronym:

[handwritten margin notes: pertains to reason for visit; completely covered by the UACDS — called the Reason for the Encounter]

- **S**ubjective: Patient's complaints and comments
- **O**bjective: Physical findings and laboratory data
- **A**ssessment: Diagnosis and impression
- **P**lan: Medication, therapy, referral, consultation, and patient education

The SOAP format helps the clinician to structure his or her decision making to match the problems identified on the problem list. The patient's complaints, diagnoses, and treatments can be viewed at a glance. Under "S" (subjective information), the patient's statement of reason for the visit is commonly recorded in quotes. For "O" (objective data), medical facts established during physical examinations and diagnostic workups is recorded. For "A" (assessment), documentation of a diagnosis or status of an identified problem is written. Under "P" (plan), the practitioner records the patient's individualized treatment plan. Every progress note need not contain documentation for every part of the SOAP acronym, but using this format can assist professionals in ensuring their medical documentation is complete.

Physician Orders

Physician orders are the instructions the physician gives to other parties to provide specific medications, services, diagnostic tests, or treatments to a particular patient. Given the nature of ambulatory care, patients frequently have to visit another site for the orders to be carried out; for example, they must go to the pharmacy to have a prescription filled or the laboratory to have blood drawn for testing. Orders for medication are written on prescription forms and presented to the pharmacy. Orders for diagnostic tests are written on requisition or referral forms that the patient may or may not receive. To comply with accreditation standards requiring that information on all studies, tests, and treatments be entered into the patient's health record at each visit, physician orders often are documented in the progress note. The orders must be written legibly and accompanied with the date and the physician's signature. Standing orders, which the medical staff or an individual practitioner has established as routine care for a specific diagnosis or procedure, are commonly given to recovery room staff in ambulatory surgery facilities. Usually, standing orders are preprinted on a single sheet of paper and, like other physician orders, must be signed, dated, and filed in the individual patient's health record.

Patient Instructions

Unlike the hospital setting, where a healthcare team headed by a physician is responsible for all patient care, the ambulatory setting leaves aftercare in the patient's hands. Therefore, it is essential that the patient be given clear, concise instructions. The Joint Commission's *Accreditation Manual for Ambulatory Surgical Centers* (2008) requires that disposition of and recommendations and instructions to the patient are recorded in the health record, including all hand-off provided for continuity of care. The NCQA Standards for Managed Care Organizations (1996) ask for evidence regarding follow-up care, calls, or visits and specified timing of follow-up appointments. Ideally, instructions to the patient should be communicated both verbally and in writing, with a copy of the written instructions filed in the health record. When a group or individual other than the patient has assumed responsibility for the patient's aftercare, the record should indicate that the instructions were given to that group or individual. The healthcare professional should sign the record to indicate that he or she issued the verbal instructions, and the person receiving the instructions should sign the record to verify that understanding. Moreover, patient comments or questions should be documented, along with the clarifications the healthcare professional offered in

[handwritten marginalia: required / includes disposition at discharge]

response. Documentation of patient education during office visits may be accomplished by using forms that prompt the person providing instruction to cover important information.

Missed Appointment Forms

In the ambulatory-care setting, patients assume responsibility for much of their own healthcare. For example, they have their prescriptions filled and take their medications as prescribed, follow a prescribed diet, report to the laboratory to have diagnostic tests performed, or schedule follow-up appointments as their physician advises. By using a simple form or stamp to note when the patient fails to keep such appointments, the practitioner can protect the organization in case of litigation by demonstrating compliance with clinical practice standards and offering evidence of the quality of care provided. It is important that the provider review the reason the patient was scheduled for an office visit and determine whether the patient should be contacted to reschedule. Attempts to contact the patient, and the advice given, should be documented.

Flow sheets can be an effective way to display information about the patient's treatment from episode to episode. Another useful application for flow sheets is to document the healthcare maintenance provided to the patient (such as health maintenance forms). Used in this manner, flow sheets serve to remind providers when tests or exams are due for the patients they serve.

Telephone Encounters

From a risk management perspective as well as a patient-care perspective, it is critical to document any advice (instructions, prescriptions, orders, medication changes, and such) or patient follow-up that is communicated by a **telephone encounter**. Documentation should include the date and time of the call, the caller's name and telephone number, the patient's name and identifying information, reason for the call, the date and time of the response (or attempts to return the call), the response given, and the signature of the person returning the call. Because messages may be relayed among several people, a standard telephone encounter form should be used to document all information regarding phone calls with every patient.

Ambulatory Care Accreditation Standards

The ambulatory care environment is changing rapidly. New technology, prospective payment systems, compliance requirements, an increasing shift in patient volume, competition in the marketplace, and continuous updates in patient quality of care are some of the ongoing pressures. Many regulatory agencies, payers, and managed-care contractors require accreditation for reimbursement, certification, licensure, and participation agreement.

Consumers are concerned about finding the best ways to meet their healthcare needs. When a facility is accredited, it is measured against national standards set by healthcare professionals. An accredited organization complies with standards and continuously makes efforts to improve the care and services it provides. **Accreditation** is defined as recognition by an external entity of achievement of predefined standards of excellence.

- The Joint Commission (2007) defines quality of care as the "degree to which patient-care services increase the probability of desired patient outcomes and reduce the probability of undesired outcomes, given the current state of knowledge."

- The Institute of Medicine defines it as the "degree to which health services for individuals and populations increase the likelihood of desired health outcomes and are consistent with current professional knowledge" (Kohn, Corrigan, and Donaldson 2000, 211).

Advantages of Accreditation

Ambulatory-care organizations derive a number of benefits from being accredited. Recognition from an accrediting association provides the following:

- Enhances community confidence by a visible demonstration of the organization's commitment to improving the quality of patient care and makes a strong statement to the community about the organization's efforts to provide the highest-quality services possible

- Provides a report card or benchmark of quality of the organization's performance standards including performance improvement (PI) concepts

- Assists in performance improvement efforts, enabling the organization to perform a variety of activities to meet its goal of raising the quality of care to the highest possible level

- Assists in the recruitment of professional staff

- Provides an education tool and ongoing educational support

- Assists the organization in meeting certain regulatory agency certification and state licensure requirements

- Assists the organization in meeting the eligibility prerequisites or requirements for insurance reimbursement and expedites payment by insurers and other third parties, ensures participation in managed-care plans, facilitates bidding on contracts, and increases financing capabilities because lenders may require accreditation as a condition of financing

In addition, accreditation enhances the risk management efforts and may improve access to and reduce the cost of liability insurance coverage.

Joint Commission Accreditation Standards

The Joint Commission established the Ambulatory Care Accreditation program in 1975 to encourage quality patient care in all types of freestanding ambulatory-care facilities. These centers may not be owned or operated by a hospital. See figure 9.1 for a list of the types of ambulatory centers that are certified by the Joint Commission.

In 2007, the Joint Commission made available for the first time a separate manual of accreditation standards for ambulatory surgical centers. Until that time, ambulatory care standards were combined into one manual for all ambulatory-care settings. The *Accreditation Manual for Ambulatory Care Organizations* (Joint Commission 2008) provides an in-depth review of required standards for all other freestanding ambulatory-care organizations. Below is a condensed version of the standards pertaining specifically to information management in a freestanding ambulatory surgical center.

- **Information Management Planning**
  IM.1.10: The organization plans and designs information management processes to meet internal and external information needs.

- **Confidentiality and Security**
  IM.2.10: Information privacy and confidentiality are maintained.
  IM.2.20: Information security, including data integrity, is maintained.
  IM.2.30: Continuity of information is maintained.

- **Information Management Processes**

  IM.3.10: The organization has processes in place to effectively manage information, including the capturing, reporting, processing, storing, retrieving, disseminating, and displaying of clinical/service and nonclinical data and information.

- **Information-based Decision Making**

  IM.4.10: The information management system provides information for use in decision making.

- **Knowledge-based Information**

  IM.5.10: Knowledge-based information resources are readily available, current, and authoritative.

- **Patient-specific Information**

  IM.6.10: The organization has a complete and accurate medical record for patients assessed, cared for, treated, or served.

  IM.6.20: Records contain patient-specific information, as appropriate to the services provided.

  IM.6.30: The medical record thoroughly documents operative or other high-risk procedures and the use of moderate or deep sedation or anesthesia. (See also Standards PC.13.40.)

  IM.6.40: For patients receiving continuing ambulatory-care services, the medical record contains a summary list(s) of significant diagnoses, procedures, drug allergies, and medications.

Figure 9.1. Types of freestanding and specialty ambulatory healthcare centers certified by the Joint Commission.

Freestanding Ambulatory Centers	Specialty Care Providers
• Ambulatory surgery centers	• Birthing centers
• Community health centers	• Cardiac catheterization centers
• Group medical practices	• Dental clinics
• Indian health clinics	• Dialysis centers
• Military clinics	• Endoscopy centers
• Mobile services	• Imaging centers
• Multispecialty group practices	• Infusion therapy services
• Occupational health centers	• Laser centers
• Office-based surgery offices	• Lithotripsy services
• Physicians' offices	• MRI centers
• Correctional facilities health centers	• Ophthalmology practices
• Student health services	• Oral and maxillofacial surgery centers
	• Pain management centers
	• Plastic surgery centers
	• Podiatric clinics
	• Radiation/oncology clinics
	• Rehabilitation centers
	• Sleep centers
	• Urgent/emergency care centers
	• Women's health centers

IM.6.50: Designated qualified staff accepts and transcribes verbal or telephone orders from authorized individuals.

IM.6.60: The organization provides access to relevant information from a patient's record as needed for use in patient services. (Joint Commission 2008)

Refer to the most current Joint Commission manual as standards and elements of performance are updated periodically.

Elements of Performance

Elements of Performance (EPs) are the Joint Commission's specific performance expectations and/or structures or processes that must be in place for an organization to provide safe, high-quality care, treatment, and services. Knowledge of EPs pertaining directly to the health record and documentation in the record are critical for the health information management (HIM) professional working in an accredited facility.

The EPs for Standard IM.2.10 states: The organization must have a written policy for addressing the privacy and confidentiality of information that is based on and consistent with law regulation.

This includes compliance with the following federal and state laws and regulations:

- Health Insurance Portability and Accountability Act (HIPAA) *— federal*
- State medical board
- State and local health departments

In addition to having the written policies under Standard IM.2.10, organizations must do the following:

- Implement the policy
- Ensure the policy and any updates have been communicated to all staff members
- Monitor the policy (such as doing an organization-wide HIPAA audit)
- Stay abreast of developments in technology to continually improve privacy and confidentiality
- Preserve the privacy and confidentiality of data and information identified as sensitive
- Inform individuals having identifiable health data and information that is maintained or collected on how their information will be used or disclosed
- Remove personal identifiers to the extent possible for uses and disclosures of health information consistent with maintaining the usefulness of the information
- Protect health information by ensuring that it is used for the purposes identified or as required by law or regulation and not redisclosed without patient permission

outside of TPO must be de-identified — consents

The EPs for Standard IM.2.10 include a requirement to have written policies addressing information security and data integrity consistent with law or regulation.

Sample HIM policies might include the following:

- A policy to allow staff access to the HIM department on a need-to-know basis (for example, HIM staff and physicians)

- A visitor log and policy

- A policy on transporting medical records to and from the clinic

- A chain of custody policy to ensure the medical record is never in the patient's hands without a member of the organization present

Additionally, the same requirement as above concerning implementation and monitoring of any written policy must be implemented.

Developing and implementing controls to safeguard data and information, including the patient record, against loss, destruction, and tampering are included in Standard IM.2.20. Controls to safeguard the data and information include the following:

- Policies indicating when the removal of records is permitted

- Protection against unauthorized intrusion, corruption, or damage

- Minimization of risk of falsification of data and information

- Guidelines for preventing the loss and destruction of records

- Guidelines for destroying copies of records

- Protection of records in a manner that minimizes the possibility of damage from fire and water

- Policies and procedures, including plans for electronic information systems, that address data integrity, authentication, nonrepudiation, encryption as warranted, and auditability as appropriate to the system and types of information (such as patient information and billing information)

The EPs for Standard IM.2.30 include requirements to back up electronic medical record systems. Contingency plans must be available for interruptions of service due to system failures. The plan must be tested periodically as defined by the organization. See figure 9.2 for EPs related to the following:

IM.6.10: Requirements for patient-specific information

IM.6.30: Documentation for operative and high-risk procedures

IM.6.40: Summary list(s) for patients with continuing ambulatory-care needs

IM.6.50: Process for authenticating verbal or telephone orders

The EPs for Standard IM.6.60 require that access to relevant information from a patient is available as needed for use in patient services. To accomplish this, the organization must do the following:

- Have a process for tracking all components of the medical record

- Use a system to assemble required information or make available a summary or information relative to the patient services provided

Utilization of the above comprehensive documentation requirements assists ambulatory healthcare organizations in meeting the goals of improving patient outcomes, improving healthcare documentation, improving patient safety, and improving performance in patient services.

Figure 9.2. Joint Commission elements of performance.

IM.6.10: Requirements for patient-specific information

- Only authorized users make entries in the medical record.

- The organization defines which entries made by nonindependent practitioners require countersigning consistent with law or regulation.

- Standardized formats are used for documenting all services provided to patients.

- Medical record entries are dated, the author identified, and when necessary according to law or regulation, authenticated by written signature, electronic signature, computer key, or rubber stamp. Use of a computer key or rubber stamp requires the author to sign a statement that he or she alone uses the key or stamp.

- The author authenticates the following per above requirements:

  1 History and physical (H & P)

  2 Operative reports

  3 Consultations

  4 Diagnostic and therapeutic procedures

  5 Follow-up or discharge orders

- The medical record contains sufficient information to identify the patient, support the diagnosis/condition, justify the services, document the course and results of services, and promote continuity of care among providers.

- Policy on timely entry of information into the patient's medical record

- Definition of what is a complete record and time frame to complete the record

- Medical records are reviewed on an ongoing basis.

- Review of the record is based on organization-defined indicators that address the presence, timeliness, readability, quality, consistency, clarity, accuracy, completeness, and authentication of data and information contained within the record.

- The retention time of medical record information is determined by the organization based on law or regulation and its use for patient services; legal, research, operational purposes, and educational activities.

- Original medical records are not released unless responding to laws or regulations, court orders, or subpoenas.

- Medical records of patients who have received urgent or immediate services contain 1) time and means of arrival, 2) whether the patient left against medical advice, 3) conclusions at termination of treatment, including final disposition and instructions for follow-up services.

- A copy of the record is available to the practitioner or medical organization providing follow-up care, treatment, and services.

- Documentation and findings of assessments

- Conclusions or impressions drawn from the H & P exam

- Diagnosis, diagnostic impression, or conditions

- Diagnostic and therapeutic orders

- Diagnostic and therapeutic procedures, tests, and results

- Operative and other invasive procedures

- Progress notes made by authorized individuals, including the date, staff person, and service provided

- Reassessments and plan of care revisions

- Consultation reports

- Allergies to food and medications

- Medications ordered or prescribed

- Dosages of medications administered (including the strength, dose, and rate of administration), administration devices used, access site or route, known drug allergies, patient's response to medication, and adverse drug reactions

- Relevant diagnoses/conditions established during the course of services

- Demographic information: patient's name, gender, address, phone number, date of birth, height, weight, phone number of a legally authorized representative, legal status of patient receiving behavioral health services, patient's language and communication needs

---

Figure 9.2. (continued)

- Evidence of known advance directives when indicated, evidence of informed consent, referrals or communications made to external or internal care providers and community agencies

- Treatment summaries and other pertinent documents to promote continuity of care

- Documentation of clinical research interventions that is distinct from entries related to regular patient care

- Records of communication with patient regarding services (such as telephone calls or e-mail)

- Patient-generated information (such as information entered into the record over the Internet or via previsit computer systems)

- When appropriate, summaries of treatment and other documents provided by the organization are forwarded to other care providers.

- Discharge diagnosis

IM.6.30: Documentation for operative and high-risk procedures

- Provisional diagnosis recorded prior to the operative or other high-risk procedure

- Written or dictated reports are recorded immediately after the procedure. The written report must include the name of the licensed independent practitioner and assistants, procedure(s) performed and description of the procedure(s), finding(s), estimated blood loss, specimen(s) removed, and postoperative diagnosis.

- A progress note written immediately after the procedure can take the place of the full report being recorded immediately. However, the full report must be recorded within a specified time frame defined by the organization.

- The completed procedure report is authenticated by the practitioner and made available in the medical record as soon as possible.

- Postoperative documentation records the patient's vital signs and level of consciousness, medications (including intravenous fluids), blood and blood components administered, unusual events or complications (including blood transfusion reactions), and the management of those events.

  - Postoperative documentation records the patient's discharge from the postsedation or postanesthesia care area by the responsible licensed independent practitioner or according to discharge criteria.

  - Use of approved discharge criteria to determine the patient's readiness for discharge is documented in the medical record.

  - Postoperative documentation records the name of the licensed independent practitioner responsible for discharge.

  - For Medicare-certified ambulatory centers, the results of preoperative diagnostic studies before surgery, if performed, must be documented.

IM.6.40: Summary list(s) for patients with continuing ambulatory care needs

- The summary list must be initiated by the third visit and maintained thereafter.

- The summary list must contain known significant medical diagnoses and conditions and operative and invasive procedures.

- Known adverse and allergic drug reactions

- Known long-term medications, including current medications, over-the counter drugs, and herbal preparations

- The summary list must be quickly and easily available for healthcare professionals to access needed information.

IM.6.50: Process for authenticating verbal or telephone orders

- Qualified personnel are identified per law and regulation.

- Verbal or telephone orders are dated and identify the names of the individuals who gave, received, and implemented the orders.

- Authenticated within the specified time frame, if required by law or regulation

- Verification of the complete verbal or telephone order when reporting critical test results by having the person receiving the order record and "read back" the complete order or test result

Source: Joint Commission 2007.

Ambulatory Care and Office-based Surgery National Patient Safety Goals

In 2006, the Joint Commission announced patient safety standards that apply specifically to ambulatory-care facilities. New requirements for **hand-off communication** of patient information between caregivers and improvement in the safety of medication were given special attention.

> **Standard 2E**: Implement a standardized approach to "hand off" communications, including an opportunity to ask and respond to questions.

> **Standard 3D**: Label all medications, medication containers, or other solutions on and off the sterile field in perioperative and other procedural settings. (Joint Commission 2008)

Sentinel Event Policy

The Joint Commission (2008) describes a **sentinel event** as "an unexpected occurrence involving death or serious physical or psychological injury or the risk thereof." Specifically, it includes "loss of limb of function." Sentinel events are immediate in nature. Accreditation standards include having a sentinel event policy that is organization-specific. Examples of a reportable event for an ambulatory-care organization are as follows:

- Operating on the wrong side of the patient's body

- Leaving a sponge or foreign body such as a sponge in a patient after surgery

- Patient fall resulting in death

- Medication errors that cause paralysis, coma, or other permanent loss of function

The Joint Commission's "Improving Organization Performance" indicators are closely tied to management of sentinel events and outcome of service provided.

Accreditation Association for Ambulatory Health Care

The **Accreditation Association for Ambulatory Health Care (AAAHC)** is a nonprofit organization incorporated in 1979. AAAHC states that it is the "leader in developing standards to advance and promote patient safety, quality and value for ambulatory health care through peer-based accreditation processes, education and research" (2008). AAAHC has a fundamental commitment to high-quality healthcare. The association is dedicated to educating providers in quality assurance and accreditation standards and procedures. AAAHC has conducted thousands of accreditation surveys of all types of ambulatory-care organizations, including ambulatory surgical facilities, college and university health centers, single and multispecialty group practices, and health networks. The association currently accredits more than 3,700 organizations nationwide.

AAAHC's Core Standards include the following:

- Rights of Patients

- Governance

- Administration

- Quality of Care Provided

[handwritten margin note: not that different from JACHO]

- Quality Management and Improvement

- Clinical Records and Health Information

- Facilities and Environment

AAAHC requires that the following data be recorded for each patient visit (AAAHC 2008):

- Date, department (if appropriate), provider's name and profession (for example, physical therapist, registered nurse)

- Chief complaint or purpose of visit

- Clinical findings

- Diagnosis or medical impression

- Studies ordered, such as laboratory or radiology

- Therapies administered

- Disposition, recommendations, and instructions given to the patient

- Signature or initials of the practitioner

- When the initials of the practitioner are used, the record also must contain key listing initials and a corresponding full signature

The "Rights of Patients" standard sets the tone and underscores the very essence of the accreditation process, which is to determine that ambulatory-care organizations are positively addressing essential elements not only to ensure the rights of patients, but also to provide the highest level of care possible. Many healthcare groups at the national level sponsor AAAHC. These groups include the following:

funding

- American Academy of Cosmetic Surgery (AACS)

- American Academy of Dental Group Practice (AADGP)

- American Academy of Dermatology (AAD)

- American Academy of Facial Plastic and Reconstructive Surgery (AAFPRS)

- American Academy of Family Physicians (AAFP)

- American Association of Oral and Maxillofacial Surgeons (AAOMS)

- American College Health Association (ACHA)

- American College of Occupational and Environmental Medicine (ACOEM)

- American Society for Dermatologic Surgery (ASDS)

- Association of Freestanding Radiation Oncology Centers (AFROC)

- Federated Ambulatory Surgery Association (FASA)

- Medical Group Management Association (MGMA)

- National Association of Community Health Centers (NACHC)

- Outpatient Ophthalmic Surgery Society (OOSS)

The AAAHC performs assessments of the quality of care provided by health maintenance organizations. More information is available at www.aaahc.org/eweb/StartPage.aspx.

The AAAHC has surveyed managed-care organizations over the years as a part of their regular accreditation activity. In September 1996, AAAHC became the first accreditation organization to conduct a survey of a purely independent physician association (IPA). Based on this experience and its surveys of managed-care organizations, in April 1997, AAAHC adopted special standards for managed-care professional services delivery organizations. These standards focus on system-wide mechanisms for evaluating care providers that function within managed-care systems and for ensuring standards compliance. The standards address such critical issues as communication to patients, grievance resolution, consumer information, appeals procedures, and utilization management. In addition, the AAAHC has undertaken specialized reviews for state agencies in conjunction with state regulatory requirements, which has resulted in extensive involvement in external reviews of managed-care organizations.

American Association for Accreditation of Ambulatory Surgery Facilities

The **American Association for Accreditation of Ambulatory Surgery Facilities, Inc. (AAAASF)** was established in 1980 to develop an accreditation program to standardize and improve the quality of medical and surgical care in ambulatory-surgery facilities while assuring the public of high standards for patient care and safety in an accredited facility. Information on their Web site states, "Today more than 1200 ambulatory-surgery facilities are accredited by AAAASF, the largest not-for-profit accrediting organization in the United States. Many more facilities are in process for accreditation. These numbers have increased dramatically over the last two years. The vast majority of ambulatory-surgery facilities are still unaccredited, operating independent of any peer review and inspection process. A growing number of states and specialty societies, however, are recognizing the need for mandatory accreditation. AAAASF has been and continues to be in the forefront of these legislative efforts" (AAAASF 2007).

California became the first state to mandate accreditation for all outpatient facilities that administer sedation or general anesthesia. AAAASF was instrumental in the development of the California legislation (AB 595) as well as subsequent laws and regulations in Florida, Georgia, New Jersey, Pennsylvania, Texas, and other states.

Mission

It is the mission of the AAAASF to develop and implement standards of excellence that ensure the highest quality of patient care through an accreditation program serving both the medical community and the public interest by establishing a means for measuring medical competence and providing an external source for evaluating patient safety in the ambulatory-surgery setting.

To accomplish this mission, AAAASF has set the following goals:

- To provide the medical community and the public with a means of standardizing and improving the quality of medical and surgical care in the ambulatory environment

- To encourage the highest level of competence for medical and surgical care of patients in the ambulatory setting

- To provide a forum for the discussion of new concepts in ambulatory surgery care and a repository of information that can be disseminated to the public and medical community

- To encourage constant improvement in the quality of care provided to patients in the ambulatory-surgery setting

- To provide a means of measuring medical and surgical competence and ethical conduct by providing an external source for the evaluation of professional credentialing, patient safety, and quality of care

Ethics

The medical staff in an accredited facility with possible ethical violations will be referred to the ethics committee of the society for their specialty. They will be evaluated by the AAAASF Investigative Committee, whose findings could result in probation, suspension, or revocation of the facility's accreditation by AAAASF.

Designed to ensure verifiable quality care with specific requirements, AAAASF standards for ambulatory surgical facilities include the following:

- General environment

- Operating room environment, policy, and procedures

- Recovery room environment, policy, and procedures

- General safety in the facility

- Blood and medications

- Medical records

- Quality assessment/quality improvement

- Personnel

- Governance

- Anesthesia

Accreditation consists of a periodic three-step review that includes a site visit, committee assessment of site visit findings, and successful participation in a peer review/quality assurance program, including mandatory semiannual online reporting to AAAASF.

Regulation and Policy

In some states, regulations covering hospitals differ from those governing ambulatory-care organizations. Independent physician office practices may fall under the guidance of the medical board for physician's offices, not under the regulation for hospitals. The state of Texas is an example. Ambulatory organizations must decide which rule applies to them and coordinate their internal policies accordingly. For example, a large multispecialty group practice in Texas would have guidelines for different copying fees for release of medical records than would hospitals. See figure 9.3 for an example of board rules concerning documentation and maintenance of the medical record. Note that the physician is required to keep a copy of any information obtained from another healthcare provider as part of the medical record. Another notation should be made concerning the fact that HIPAA regulations preempt state law provisions that are "contrary" to a provision or requirement of HIPAA (2003).

Figure 9.3.   Example of board rules on medical records documentation.

TEXAS MEDICAL BOARD
BOARD RULES
Texas Administrative Code, Title 22, Part

§165.1. Medical Records.

(A) Contents of Medical Record. Each licensed physician of the board shall maintain an adequate medical record for each patient that is complete, contemporaneous, and legible. For purposes of this section, an "adequate medical record" should meet the following standards:

(1) The documentation of each patient encounter should include:

(a) reason for the encounter and relevant history, physical examination findings, and prior diagnostic test results;

(b) an assessment, clinical impression, or diagnosis;

(c) plan for care (including discharge plan if appropriate); and

(d) the date and legible identity of the observer.

(2) Past and present diagnoses should be accessible to the treating and/or consulting physician.

(3) The rationale for and results of diagnostic and other ancillary services should be included in the medical record.

(4) The patient's progress, including response to treatment, change in diagnosis, and patient's noncompliance should be documented.

(5) Relevant risk factors should be identified.

(6) The written plan for care should include when appropriate:

(a) treatments and medications (prescriptions and samples) specifying amount, frequency, number of refills, and dosage;

(b) any referrals and consultations;

(c) patient/family education; and

(d) specific instructions for follow up.

(7) Any written consents for treatment or surgery requested from the patient/family by the physician.

(8) Billing codes, including CPT and ICD-9-CM codes, reported on health insurance claim forms or billing statements should be supported by the documentation in the medical record.

(9) Any amendment, supplementation, change, or correction in a medical record not made contemporaneously with the act or observation shall be noted by indicating the time and date of the amendment, supplementation, change, or correction, and clearly indicating that there has been an amendment, supplementation, change, or correction.

(10) Records received from another physician or healthcare provider involved in the care or treatment of the patient shall be maintained as part of the patient's medical records.

(11) The board acknowledges that the nature and amount of physician work and documentation varies by type of services, place of service and the patient's status. Paragraphs (1) - (11) of this subsection may be modified to account for these variable circumstances in providing medical care.

(B) Maintenance of Medical Records.

(1) A licensed physician shall maintain adequate medical records of a patient for a minimum of seven years from the anniversary date of the date of last treatment by the physician.

(2) If a patient was younger than 18 years of age when last treated by the physician, the medical records of the patient shall be maintained by the physician until the patient reaches age 21 or for seven years from the date of last treatment, whichever is longer.

(3) A physician may destroy medical records that relate to any civil, criminal, or administrative proceeding only if the physician knows the proceeding has been finally resolved.

(4) Physicians shall retain medical records for such longer length of time than that imposed herein when mandated by other federal or state statute or regulation.

(5) Physicians may transfer ownership of records to another licensed physician or group of physicians only if the physician provides notice consistent with §165.5 of this chapter and the physician who assumes the records maintains the records consistent with this chapter.

(6) Medical records may be owned by a physician's employer, to include group practices, professional associations, and nonprofit health organizations, provided records are maintained by these entities consistent with this chapter.

Source Note: The provisions of this §165.1 adopted to be effective December 29, 1997, 22 TexReg 12490; amended to be effective September 14, 2003, 28 TexReg 7703; amended to be effective March 4, 2004, 29 TexReg 1946; amended to be effective September 28, 2006, 31 TexReg 8090

Due to the multiple appointment sites inherent in large multisite ambulatory-care organizations, HIM professionals face unique documentation challenges for both new and existing patients. Often, these organizations have a large, campus-type setting where clinics are established in numerous buildings. Very large centers can include as many as 50 different clinical specialties within the same physicians' practice group. At times, a patient may have several visits scheduled at different clinics (such as internal medicine first and then dermatology) on the same day. Without a centralized record tracking system in place, one clinic may think another clinic has completed the required documentation for a patient. Physicians, fearing records may be unavailable when needed, may keep shadow charts of patient information or hold on to the original medical records.

Chart management of underdocumented and overdue records is essential. Usually, multisite facilities have a unit record with a centralized health information management department. As many as 1500 records may be needed for clinic visits on any one day. Location and movement of medical records in these circumstances is challenging, and an electronic record tracking system is vital. Following are some of the different internal HIM policies needed to manage these challenges.

Informed Consent

The **informed consent policy** is a challenge to large multispecialty physicians' practices due to patients' multiple points of entry. One clinic may assume that another clinic has already had a patient sign the informed consent. Options for managing this challenge include the following:

- Having each patient sign a new consent upon each visit
- Establishing a monitoring system that alerts clinics when consent is needed

Patients often respond negatively to the first option due to not wanting to sign a new release each time they visit the facility. The perception is that the organization should know when the consent has been signed. The second choice presents an economic challenge due to the high cost associated with the staff time required for monitoring and auditing for compliance.

Physicians New to Practice

The new to practice policy should outline how physicians coming into a practice handle their medical records from a prior practice. The policy should direct the physician to review information in patient records from his or her previous practice and place copies of those records in new records at the new practice. Often, physicians want to place an original, prior record into the medical record at the new location. When an original record is incorporated into a new medical record in this manner, it becomes a part of the medical record at the new practice and should not be removed, even if the physician decides to leave the new practice.

Missed Appointments

The organization should have a **failed/missed appointment policy** that tracks appointments that are canceled or missed. The policy should state the required documentation of information concerning the missed appointment.

Rapid Response Team

Although it is possible to notify staff of a predicted emergency such as a major storm for which there is warning, emergencies, by nature, rarely give warning. Therefore, the organization should have a team in place to respond in case of an emergency.

Staff may be ranked in tiers, depending on department size, with a core group of first responders who maintain a calling tree or otherwise designated alert system. These are the staff who are able to easily complete all or most key tasks within the department. They should be physically able to climb stairs, handle temperature variances, and be adaptable to unusual situations. Secondary and tertiary responders may be called in as relief staff according to availability.

Staff can be notified using calling trees, pager systems, or public media. However, if there are no utilities, those may not be an option. All staff, but especially rapid responders, should be instructed to report immediately in the case of an emergency. Secondary tiers may follow at intervals suggested by management. Special "crisis-readiness" job descriptions should be written, reviewed, and revised regularly to ensure that everyone knows his or her place on the team and how each person's performance affects others. (Walsh et al. 2009)

Closing Practice

A **closing practice policy** directs an organization to send out letters to patients of physicians who are closing their practice at a facility. Information should include options for the patient to either continue receiving care from another physician at the facility or to receive a copy of their medical record if they decide to transfer to another practice.

[handwritten note in margin: archived w/ state board of health]

Shadow Charts

A **shadow chart policy** should require that all original information and medical reports be kept in the medical record located in the health information management department. Physicians should be discouraged from keeping copies of records or reports in a shadow chart in their offices. Incorporating and reconciling shadow charts from a physician's practice places an economic burden on the healthcare facility and the HIM department.

Outstanding Records

An **outstanding record policy** should detail the time frame in which a medical record can be kept in the clinic or physician's office. The recommended time is no longer than 48 hours.

Chart Delivery

A chart delivery policy should detail the day and time of delivery for records of patients with regularly scheduled appointments. Because regularly scheduled patient appointments are scheduled ahead of time, the HIM department and the clinic can plan for delivery of these records at a time that is convenient for all. Typically, records are delivered the day before the patient's appointment.

Risk Management and Liability

Risk management efforts are designed to minimize the facility's potential risks and, when an incident occurs, its losses. A comprehensive risk management program incorporates the identification, analysis, evaluation, and elimination or reduction of potential liability by addressing the following issues:

- **Liability insurance:** Ambulatory-care facilities must secure adequate liability insurance. Liability for patient or employee injury applies to both physicians and nonphysicians who provide medical care to patients as well as to healthcare facilities with responsibility for supervising the actions of the medical staff.

- **Credentialing and licensure:** Ambulatory-care facilities must obtain state licensure and adopt a method to properly renew and ensure their licensure status. Specific policies and procedures should address credential verification and monitor compliance with continuing education requirements for all licensed and credentialed personnel.

- **Equipment:** Maintenance and quality control policies should be developed to ensure that all equipment is functional, operated properly, and checked on a regular basis and that appropriate parts and supplies are available.

Summary

As more procedures move away from hospitals into freestanding healthcare centers, closing the gap between the demand for patient-care services and the underuse of current information technology will be a vital function for the HIM professional. As the demand for quality and standardization increases, more freestanding facilities see the importance of becoming accredited. Staying in tune with the various accrediting bodies and their requirements is a must for everyone working in the HIM field. Accrediting organizations are raising the bar for patient safety; continuity of care among healthcare providers; and patient-specific information, including detailed medication lists, summary lists of all past and present diagnoses, and hand-off communication of patient information between caregivers. The need for efficient methods of relaying this information in a timely manner is driving the demand for an electronic record that interfaces across the continuum of care.

References

Accreditation Association for Ambulatory Health Care (AAAHC). 2008. *2008 Accreditation Handbook for Ambulatory Health Care.* Skokie, IL: Accreditation Association for Ambulatory Health Care.

American Association for Accreditation of Ambulatory Surgery Facilities. 2007. Mission, history, about accreditation. Available online from www.aaaasf.org.

American Association for School Health (n.d.) Available online from www.ashaweb.org/whatis.html.

American College of Radiology. 2005. ACR chair tells house committee unnecessary and inferior medical imaging lowers quality of care, costs taxpayers. Available online from http://www.acr.org/MainMenuCategories/media_room/FeaturedCategories/PressReleases/Archive/ACRChairTellsHouseCommitteeUnnecessaryandInferiorMedicalImagingLowersQualityofCareCostsTaxpayersDoc.aspx.

American College of Radiology. 2007. Available online from www.acr.org.

American College of Surgeons. 2006. Commission on Cancer, Cancer Program Standards 2004, revised edition. Chicago, IL: American College of Surgeons. Available online from http://www.facs.org/cancer/coc/cocprogramstandards.pdf

Benson, Dale S., et al. 1988. Quality ambulatory care: The role of the diagnostic and medication summary lists. *Quality Review Bulletin*, 197 (June).

Booz Allen Hamilton. (2003). Medical technology cost management strategy. Report prepared for the Blue Cross and Blue Shield Association, Chicago, IL. Available online from http://www.bcbs.com/betterknowledge/cost/Medical_Tech_Drivr_Rept_10.pdf.

Cofer, Jennifer, ed. 1994. *Health Information Management*, 10th ed., revised. Berwyn, Ill.: Physician's Record Company.

Committee for Quality Assurance (NCQA). 2007. MCO Accreditation. Available online from http://www.ncqa.org/tabid/67/Default.aspx. Note that the NCQA Health Plan Accreditation Standards will be available online July 1, 2008, from www.ncqa.org/tabid/499/Default.aspx.

Department of Health and Human Services, Office of Civil Rights. 1996. Health Insurance Portability and Accountability Act (HIPAA) of 1996, Public Law 104-191 45 CFR Part 160 and Subparts A and E of Part 164 December 3, 2002 Revised April 3, 2003. *Federal Register* 61(251): 68697-68698. Available online from www.gpoaccess.gov/cfr/index.html.

Federated Ambulatory Surgery Association. 2005 (April 15). Federated Ambulatory Surgery Association applauds senate finance committee chairman for letter supporting greater access to ASCs for Medicare patients. Alexandria, VA: FASA. Available online from http://www.ascassociation.org/about/press/april15.pdf.

Joint Commission. 2008. *Accreditation Manual for Ambulatory Surgical Centers*. Oakbrook Terrace, IL: Joint Commission.

Joint Commission. 2008. *Sentinel Event*. Available online from http://www.jointcommission.org/SentinelEvents/.

Kohn, L. T., J. M. Corrigan, and M. S. Donaldson, eds. 2000. *To Err Is Human: Building a Safer Health System*. Washington, D.C.: National Academies Press. Available online from www.nap.edu/catalog/9728.html.

Medicare Payment Advisory Commission. 2007. *Data Book: Healthcare Spending and the Medicare Program*. Available online from http://www.medpac.gov/documents/Jun07DataBook_Entire_report.pdf.

National Center for Health Statistics. 2005. Health, United States, 2005. Available online from www.cdc.gov/nchs.

National Commission on Correctional Health Care. 2007. Accreditation. Available online from www.ncchc.org/accred/index.html.

Norwalk, Leslie V. 2006 (Nov. 6). Comments on Proposed Revised Ambulatory Surgical Center Payment System for Implementation January 1, 2008. Alexandria, VA: ASC Association and Ambulatory Surgery Foundation.

Office for Civil Rights. 2006 (June). *HIPAA Privacy Rule*. Department of Health and Human Services. Available online from www.hhs.gov/ocr/hipaa/decisiontool/#intro.

Rosenberger, Lani. 2001. Charting. *Midwifery Today* 33(3).

Texas Administrative Code. Title 22: Examining boards. Available online from http://info.sos.state.tx.us/pls/pub/readtac$ext.ViewTAC?tac_view=2&ti=22.

Walsh, T., B. C. Sher, G. Roselle, S. D. Gamage. 2009. *Medical Records Disaster Planning: A Health Information Manager's Survival Guide*. Chicago: AHIMA.

Chapter 10

Long-Term Acute-Care and Long-Term Care

Ella L. James, MS, RHIT, CPHQ

Learning Objectives

- Understand the definition of long-term acute-care hospitals

- Understand that long-term acute-care hospitals are governed as short-term acute-care hospitals

- Understand the differences between long-term acute-care hospitals and long-term care or skilled-nursing facilities

- Understand the contents of the long-term acute-care hospital and long-term care facility health records

- Understand the health record review process

- Understand medical necessity in long-term care

- Understand the influence of accrediting bodies on long-term acute-care and long-term care facilities' record keeping processes

- Understand the Medicare assessment schedule

- Understand the resident assessment process

Key Terms

Advance directives

American Osteopathic Association (AOA)

Commission on Accreditation of Rehabilitation Facilities (CARF)

Functional independence measures (FIM)

Health record review process

Joint Commission

Long-term acute-care hospital (LTCH)

Medical necessity

Medicare Prospective Payment System (PPS)

Minimum Data Set (MDS 3.0)

Nursing facility (NF)

Physician acknowledgment statement

Physician certification

Physician query form

Principal diagnosis

Problem list

Quality improvement organization (QIO)

Resident Assessment Instrument (RAI)

Resident Assessment Protocols (RAPs)

Skilled-nursing facility (SNF)

State Operations Manual

Introduction

Long-term care encompasses a wide range of nonacute healthcare services that include skilled nursing, rehabilitation, and subacute medical care. Most long-term care is provided in residential environments such as skilled-nursing facilities and assisted-living facilities. The purpose of every long-term care facility is to provide high-quality clinical care and services in the most appropriate healthcare setting. According to the Centers for Medicare and Medicaid Services (CMS), "each resident must receive and the facility must provide the necessary care and services to attain or maintain the highest practicable physical, mental, and psychosocial well-being" (2006c, 136).

This chapter will discuss the documentation needs in another type of long-term care facility, the **long-term acute-care hospital (LTCH)**. These facilities are not to be confused with skilled-nursing facilities (SNFs) and are indeed hospitals that care for patients with acute and chronic diseases. The only differentiation between an LTCH and short-term acute-care hospital is the length of stay. Currently, LTCHs are defined as having a length of stay of 25 days or greater. LTCHs must meet the same *Conditions of Participation* (CoPs) as short-term acute-care hospitals, including the new additions to the CoPs for Medicare that were published on November 27, 2006 (CMS 2006b).

Long-Term Acute-Care Hospital Settings

Medicare defines LTCHs as hospitals that have an average inpatient length of stay greater than 25 days and typically provide extended medical and rehabilitative care for patients who are clinically complex and suffer from multiple acute or chronic conditions. LTCHs that are subject to the requirements of the LTCH prospective payment system (PPS) meet all of the following criteria:

- They are certified under Medicare as short-term acute-care hospitals that have been excluded from the inpatient short-term acute-care hospital prospective payment system (IPPS).

- They meet state licensure requirements for short-term acute-care hospitals under section 1886(d)(B)(iv) of the Social Security Act.

- They are not excluded LTCH units in a facility, although they can be a satellite and/or hospital within a hospital, colocated within another facility. A hospital within a hospital is a hospital located in or on the campus of an acute care or host hospital. The CMS requires an LTCH to have a separate governing body, medical staff, chief medical officer, and chief executive officer. "In addition, the hospital must perform basic functions independently from the host hospital, incur no more than 15 percent of its total inpatient operating costs for items and services supplied by the hospital in which it is located, and have an inpatient load of which at least 75 percent of patients are admitted from sources other than the host hospital" (CMS 2007).

- They are identified by the last four digits of the Medicare provider number, which ranges between 2000 and 2299.

- They must have a provider agreement with Medicare in order to receive Medicare payment (CMS 2007).

- They are required to have physician acknowledgment statements signed and dated from the attending physician at the initial time of credentialing for admitting privileges just as is required for short-term acute-care hospitals. The **physician acknowledgment statement** notifies physicians that Medicare payment to the facility is partly based on the patient's principal and secondary diagnoses, as well as the major procedures performed, and that falsification of records can lead to fines, imprisonment, or civil penalty under federal laws (HHS 1999b).

- They must have an agreement with a **quality improvement organization (QIO)** for review to include the following:
  — The medical necessity, reasonableness, and appropriateness of hospital admissions and discharges

  — Inpatient hospital care for which outlier payments are sought

  — Validity of the hospital's diagnostic and procedural information

  — Completeness, adequacy, and quality of the services furnished in the hospital

  — Medical or other practices with respect to beneficiaries or billing for services furnished to the beneficiaries

The Medicare reimbursement for LTCHs is under a PPS based on the Medicare diagnosis-related groups (DRG) system used by short-term acute-care hospitals and referred to as LTC-DRGs. The same short-term acute-care DRGs are used, but "have been weighted to reflect the resources required to treat the medically complex patients treated at LTCHs." (Elements of LTCH PPS are available online from www.cms.hhs.gov). Each LTC-DRG includes an established Average Length of Stay (ALOS) for a patient assigned to the LTC-DRG. LTC-DRGs are paid according to the federal payment rate, including adjustments. Other reimbursement methods would be exactly as an acute-care setting.

Since the patient population in an LTCH is considered acute care, many of the same documentation requirements that apply to a short-term acute-care facility apply to the LTCH setting. There may be differences based on state requirements for hospitals. For example, many freestanding LTCHs do not have an emergency department, maternity ward, or surgery suites on-site, however, some states may require the LTCH to have an emergency department available. Regardless, the functions of the LTCH health record are exactly as those for a short-term acute-care setting.

LTCH settings provide long-term acute-care and rehabilitative services for the chronically, critically ill patient. Documentation of these intensive rehabilitation services may set the LTCH apart from the short-term acute-care setting as a multidisciplinary approach to care is typical. Services such as lab, radiology, and laundry may be provided in-house or as purchased services depending on the LTCH setting. LTCH may be freestanding or satellite facilities (hospitals within hospitals). Regardless of the type of arrangement, the LTCH must have a separate board of directors established.

LTCH Health Record Content

The organization and management of the LTCH health records would be consistent with those used in a short-term acute-care facility. The policies that govern the uniformity and content of the health record must be developed and maintained as they are in the short-term acute-care setting. Refer to chapter 6 for details about the format of health records.

A typical LTCH health record may contain the information and forms listed in figure 10.1. In an electronic environment, rather than forms, these elements will be required data fields. Each facility determines how each data point on each form will be captured and stored to create the final electronic health record.

Many of these forms have been described earlier in this book, and their function and purpose is the same in the long-term acute-care hospitals or long-term care facilities.

Face Sheet

The face sheet is usually the first page of a patient's health record. It contains the demographic data and insurance information for the patient. In an electronic format, the data captured on the face sheet may be captured in several screens but displayed in a logical manner to those who need to use the information. For instance, clinical staff caring for the patient should be able to quickly identify the patient by name, health record number, and account number, as well as locate emer-

Figure 10.1.   Content of the LCTH health record.

1. Face sheet	12. Specialty reports
2. Physician query form	13. Flow sheets
3. History, physical, and referral information	14. Graphical data
4. Admission data	15. Care plans
5. Physician orders	16. Education
6. Progress notes	17. Functional independence measure (FIM)
7. Problem lists	18. Procedure records
8. Consultation records	19. Miscellaneous data
9. Reevaluations and assessments	20. Medication administration records
10. Advance directives	21. Discharge documentation
11. Laboratory reports	

gency contacts for the patient; whereas the billing office needs the patient name, account number, and insurance information. While electronic health record systems may display information differently, all the information gathered for the health record is available onscreen on a need-to-know basis (James 2007). See chapter 3 for additional information about admissions forms.

Physician Query Form

The **physician query form** is used to help clarify principal and secondary diagnoses. A physician query form is used if conflicting, ambiguous, or incomplete information about significant conditions or procedures is in the health record. This should be kept to a minimum in any healthcare setting. It should be guided by AHIMA's *Standards of Ethical Coding* (2000) and official guidelines. Medical staff in conjunction with coding professionals should develop the specific clinical criteria for a valid query.

History, Physical, and Referral Information

The history and physical must be completed and placed in the health record within 24 hours of a patient's admission to the LTCH. The format of the history and physical is characteristic of a short-term acute-care hospital examination. Documentation of allergies and the allergic symptoms should be contained in the history and physical and throughout the health record as determined by facility policy.

It is essential for physicians to understand the ICD-9-CM principal diagnosis selection guidelines and Uniform Hospital Discharge Data Set (UHDDS) definitions. See chapter 5 for additional information.

Principle Diagnosis

One of the most difficult documentation issues facing the long-term care environment including the LTCH is the determination of the **principal diagnosis** or the actual reason for admission to the long-term care setting. Typically the history and physical documentation regurgitates everything that occurred in the short-term acute-care setting and tends to accentuate the acute phases of illness that have already been studied. Recent ICD-9-CM Official Guidelines for Coding and Reporting (2005) discuss the importance of the determination of the appropriate diagnoses to be reported in any setting. The official guidelines are updated regularly.

The admission history and physical should provide not only the history of the patient's illness but also the specific reason the patient is being admitted to the long-term care setting. The reason for admission should be clear and should reflect why the patient is coming into the long-term care facility. The plan of care or *impression* should discuss what specific treatments and services will be provided for the patient's stay. It should focus on the activities of care and provide clear rationale for the admission and continued stay in the long-term care setting. As stated previously, without this documentation, the assignment of the proper diagnostic code is very difficult. This is a key aspect of documentation in the LTCH as well as other long-term care environments.

In many instances, the reason for admission into the LTCH is an acute condition such as respiratory failure, complications of surgeries or devices, infections (including septicemia and pneumonias), wounds, osteomyelitis, congestive heart failure, cancer, or many other conditions of disease. Whatever the reason for the admission to the LTCH, it should be clearly documented when the patient is admitted into the facility. Many times, the *after study* in the definition of the principal diagnosis has already been completed in the acute-care setting, and therefore, it should be easier to determine the actual reason for the admission into the LTCH.

Admission Data

Admission data typically contains information such as the immunization record, nursing admission assessments, initial therapy assessments, interdisciplinary evaluation, central line data sheets, initial pain assessment, case management assessments, nutritional screening, initial nutritional assessment, safety assessment, social services intake, general consent, and a preadmission report of contact. The preadmission report of contact helps determine if the patient is being placed in the most appropriate healthcare setting.

Physician Orders

Physician orders contain medication orders, parenteral nutrition orders, do-not-resuscitate orders, admission protocols, or orders that trigger the physician to include other orders such as diet, ventilator setting, required tests and labs, medical precautions, activities, treatment orders, and consults, as appropriate. These orders include all orders from physicians, physiatrists, or consultants.

Progress Notes

Progress notes may be written by physicians with each discipline having its own progress note section, or the progress notes may all be contained in the progress note section and be interdisciplinary in nature. If they are interdisciplinary, each discipline notes their entry as nursing, physical therapy, MD as appropriate. See figure 5.22 (p. 135) for a sample progress note. Progress notes as discussed earlier in the text capture clinical data about the patient.

Problem Lists

Problem lists may be utilized in an LTCH to better track the extensive issues that face the chronically/critically ill patient. A **problem list** captures relevant past and current problems of each patient. It provides a mechanism to organize each of the patient's medical or physical issues. The problems are listed numerically, with the date each problem was identified and the date the problem resolved. In some LTCHs, it may be nursing driven or physician driven. The list is patient specific and includes the patient and problems. It may also contain the attending physician, principal diagnosis, allergies and adverse drug reactions, and symptoms of allergic/drug reactions. Not all facilities utilize problem lists.

Consultation Records

Consultation records include all consultations by surgeons, cardiologists, podiatrists, urologists, and other physicians, as well as dental records. These documents are similar to those discussed in the short-term acute-care hospitals.

Reevaluations and Assessments

Reevaluations and assessments include notes from neurological, nursing, therapies, pastoral care, and social services, which support the care, treatments, and functional changes that occur over the longer length of stay in the LTCH setting.

Advance Directives

Advance directives are required in the LTCH setting. The types of advance directives vary by state but typically include living wills, healthcare surrogate designation or durable power of attorney for healthcare (also called a *healthcare power of attorney*), and anatomical donation.

The healthcare surrogate names another person as the patient's representative to make medical decisions in the event that the patient becomes mentally or physically unable to make his or her own healthcare decisions or communicate his or her intentions. An anatomical donation indicates the resident's wish to donate all or part of his or her body at death. It is used to indicate whether organs and tissue are to be donated to those in need or whether the resident's whole body is donated for research or education (James 2007).

Through the use of advance directives, residents are able to authorize another person to make those decisions for them should they became incapacitated. The same types of advance directives are utilized in the long-term care environment that are seen in the short-term acute care of LTCH settings.

Another type of advance directive is the advance beneficiary notice (ABN). This is used when a provider suspects that a service may be denied by Medicare because it is deemed unnecessary. Patients must be notified prior to treatment. (See figure 10.2.)

A do-not-resuscitate (DNR) order is a physician's order documenting a patient's (or surrogate's) desire for no resuscitation attempts. A DNR order results from a desire expressed in an advance directive. (See chapter 11 for more information, and see also figure 11.12.)

Laboratory Reports

Laboratory reports may become extensive in the LTCH due to a patient's length of stay. These reports are sometimes divided between chemistry, hematology, urinalysis, and microbiology. Facility policy will determine how these reports are permanently filed in the patient's health record or how they are interfaced and housed in an electronic health record. In an electronic data management system (EDMS), if an interface cannot be developed, documents may be filed as paper or scanned into the patient's health record for easier access. An interface is the ability for electronic systems to communicate with each other using languages and codes between two or more applications. For example, the laboratory system used may not be a component of the EHR system and may have been purchased separately from the EHR software. In this case an interface between the EHR and the laboratory system would be required to integrate lab data and the EHR.

Specialty Reports

Radiology reports, cardiac reports, swallow results, sleep studies, pulmonary function tests, pulse oximetry, sleep oximetry, arterial blood gas, and other specialty reports may be completed during the patient's stay in the LTCH to further diagnose health issues related to the patient's condition. Facility policy will clarify how these reports are filed or stored in the patient's health record. In the electronic health record environment, interfaces may be required to view the specialty reports online.

Flow Sheets

Flow sheets are used in the LTCH setting to capture valuable clinical data. These may include interdisciplinary flow sheets or discipline specific data such as nursing flow sheets and therapy flow sheets. Other flow sheets that may be found in an LTCH health record could include those used to capture abnormal involuntary movement, antipsychotic medication, bladder training, blood glucose monitoring, hemodialysis records, critical care or code sheets, heparin injections, intake and output, monthly nursing summaries, observation sheets for one-on-one care, respiratory therapy ventilation reports, respiratory treatments, and seizure records.

Figure 10.2. Advance beneficiary notice (ABN).

Patient's Name:	Medicare # (HICN):

ADVANCE BENEFICIARY NOTICE (ABN)

NOTE: You need to make a choice about receiving these health care items or services.

We expect that Medicare will not pay for the item(s) or service(s) that are described below. Medicare does not pay for all of your health care costs. Medicare only pays for covered items and services when Medicare rules are met. The fact that Medicare may not pay for a particular item or service does not mean that you should not receive it. There may be a good reason your doctor recommended it. Right now, in your case, **Medicare probably will not pay for –**

Items or Services:

Because:

The purpose of this form is to help you make an informed choice about whether or not you want to receive these items or services, knowing that you might have to pay for them yourself. Before you make a decision about your options, you should **read this entire notice carefully.**

x Ask us to explain, if you don't understand why Medicare probably won't pay.

x Ask us how much these items or services will cost you (**Estimated Cost: $**_____), in case you have to pay for them yourself or through other insurance.

PLEASE CHOOSE **ONE** OPTION. CHECK **ONE** BOX. **SIGN & DATE** YOUR CHOICE.

Option 1. YES.   **I want to receive these items or services.**

I understand that Medicare will not decide whether to pay unless I receive these items or services. Please submit my claim to Medicare. I understand that you may bill me for items or services and that I may have to pay the bill while Medicare is making its decision. If Medicare does pay, you will refund to me any payments I made to you that are due to me. If Medicare denies payment, I agree to be personally and fully responsible for payment. That is, I will pay personally, either out of pocket or through any other insurance that I have. I understand I can appeal Medicare's decision.

Option 2. NO.   **I have decided not to receive these items or services.**

I will not receive these items or services. I understand that you will not be able to submit a claim to Medicare and that I will not be able to appeal your opinion that Medicare won't pay.

Date   **Signature of patient or person acting on patient's behalf**

NOTE: Your health information will be kept confidential. Any information that we collect about you on this form will be kept confidential in our offices. If a claim is submitted to Medicare, your health information on this form may be shared with Medicare. Your health information which Medicare sees will be kept confidential by Medicare.

OMB Approval No. 0938-0566   Form No. CMS-R-131-G   (June 2002)

Graphical Data

Graphical data typically includes blood sugar monitoring and vital signs sheets. (See figure 5.20, p. 132.) LTCH pediatric patients' records may also include growth charts. Graphical data are important because they provide a picture of data points over a grid, demonstrating increases and decreases in clinical data such as the blood sugars or blood pressure while growth chart graphs demonstrate the child's development against a norm. In an electronic environment, these data points can be displayed in list or graphical format.

Care Plans

Care plans are required documentation in an LTCH. (See figure 5.17, p. 125.) Some LTCHs may use critical paths (or clinical pathways) for specific patients. Nursing care plans begin upon admission and must be kept current throughout a patient's stay in the LTCH. Care plans are governed by the federal *Conditions of Participation for Hospitals* and may also be governed by state regulations.

The care plan is a snapshot of a patient's status and includes everything from social issues to disease processes. The critical paths and clinical pathways are focused on a specific disease process or pathway. For example, if the patient has pneumonia, the clinical pathway spells out the steps to take for the patient. *for that diagnosis*

A care plan dictates the nursing care that will be provided to a patient. It provides the details that the nurse will apply to manage and treat problems identified by nursing assessment and not just the admitting diagnosis. There are various care plans developed for each problem for which the patient is treated. Plans are developed based on the patient's individual needs, strengths, limitations, and goals as outlined in the Joint Commission standards. The care plans typically include the following:

- Patient name

- Date of initiation

- Assessed problem—usually one problem per sheet in the paper-based record or one screen in the electronic health record

- Subjective and objective data about the problem

- Nursing diagnoses

- Expected outcomes or goals of care and treatment, and the date the expected outcomes or goals will be reached

- Interventions and the time frame for the interventions, expected date of resolution of the problem, and responsible clinical staff

- Final evaluation on the goal date to determine if the goals were met

If goals are met, the care plan is discontinued. If goals are not met, the care plan is reevaluated, revised appropriately, and reinstituted. As new problems arise, new care plans are created to assist the nursing staff in resolving each identified problem.

Depending on the electronic environment, care plan development may flow from assessments to help reduce duplicate documentation. Once problems have been identified at the time of the assessment, the software system may have the capability to open the care planning session. This process eliminates the need to reenter the problem and allows the interventions to be assigned more fluidly.

Education

Education is provided to all LTCH patients. This should include all areas of education mandated by federal and state laws and regulations and those recommended by accreditation standards. Family meetings or family conferences may also be evident in an LTCH setting.

Functional Independence Measures

Functional independence measures (FIM) are completed in some LTCH settings because the focus of care is on extensive rehabilitation of the patient. FIM scores can also be used as outcome measures by LTCHs.

The State University of New York at Buffalo, along with providers and advocate groups, developed FIM in the early 1980s through a grant from the Department of Education. FIM was developed to measure outcomes of patients with various disabilities (HHS n.d.).

There are 18 items measured by FIM. For each item, the level of independence is scored on a scale of 1 to 7, with 1 being the most dependent and 7 being the most independent. Total scores range between 18 and 126. See table 10.1.

used on submission

Procedure Records

Procedure records are used in the LTCH setting and must meet all Joint Commission standards for operative and invasive procedures. While many LTCHs do not have operative suites, many do perform operative services such as central line placement, chest tubes, gastrostomy tubes, tracheostomy tubes, and other services. Blood transfusions are also performed in the LTCH setting. Facility policy dictates which procedures performed require an informed consent. All Joint Commission standards for informed consent apply to the LTCH setting as well if the facility is accredited.

Miscellaneous Data

Miscellaneous data also exists in the LTCH setting and may include some of the following data: authorizations, patient transfer records, preadmission forms, ambulance transportation forms, and interagency transfer forms (which may include specific state requirements). Many of these forms or documents may be generated by the referring facility or service agencies. In an electronic environment, many of these documents may require scanning to include them in the electronic health record.

Medication Administration Records

Due to the extended length of stay in an LTCH setting and multiple medications that the patient is prescribed, medication administration records may be voluminous.

Discharge Documentation

Discharge documentation is required in the LTCH setting and includes the discharge summaries, discharge instructions, discharge medication listings, discharge nursing summary, home activity and exercise plans, skilled-nursing facility placement forms, nursing home applications, and organ tissue donation, death certificate, and autopsy reports if applicable. The LTCH discharge summary is similar to the short-term acute-care hospital discharge summary requiring the same data fields. There may be state-specific criteria for the discharge summary, so it is important to include any state-specific data elements as well.

Table 10.1   Functional independence measures (FIM)

FIM™ Instrument

L E V E L S	7 Complete Independence (timely, safely) 6 Modified Independence (device)	**NO HELPER**
	Modified Dependence 5 Supervision (subject = 100%) *Spotter* 4 Minimal Assistance (subject = 75%+) 3 Moderate Assistance (subject = 50%+) **Complete Dependence** 2 Maximal Assistance (subject =25%+) 1 Total Assistance (subject = less than 25%)	**HELPER**

	ADMISSION	DISCHARGE	FOLLOW-UP
Self-Care A. Eating B. Grooming C. Bathing D. Dressing - Upper Body E. Dressing - Lower Body F. Toileting			
Sphincter Control G. Bladder Management H. Bowel Management			
Transfers I. Bed, Chair, Wheelchair J. Toilet K. Tub, Shower			
Locomotion L. Walk/Wheelchair M. Stairs	W Walk C Wheelchair B Both	W Walk C Wheelchair B Both	W Walk C Wheelchair B Both
Motor Subtotal Score			
Communication *language* N. Comprehension O. Expression	A Auditory V Visual B Both A Auditory V Visual B Both	A Auditory V Visual B Both A Auditory V Visual B Both	A Auditory V Visual B Both A Auditory V Visual B Both
Social Cognition P. Social Interaction Q. Problem Solving R. Memory			
Cognitive Subtotal Score			
TOTAL FIM™ SCORE			

NOTE: Leave no blanks. Enter 1 if patient is not testable due to risk.

LTCH Accreditation Standards and Regulations

Accreditation and regulatory requirements for the LTCH setting are the same as those used in the short-term acute-care setting. An LTCH is regulated by the same federal and accrediting standards used within the short-term acute-care facility, while state requirements may differ from state to state. The audit process mirrors the short-term acute-care hospital process. An LTCH may also seek accreditation from the following:

- **Joint Commission**: Standards are the same in the long-term acute-care hospital as they are in the short-term acute-care hospital (see chapter 8)

- **American Osteopathic Association (AOA)**: Accreditation process for the long-term acute-care hospital is similar to a short-term acute-care facility (see chapter 8 for AOA accreditation standards)

- **Commission on Accreditation of Rehabilitation Facilities (CARF)**: Nonprofit organization establishing standards for rehabilitation services *— very difficult to get, standards are very high*

As with any healthcare setting, a separate health record is maintained for each patient admitted to the LTCH. The content must meet federal and accrediting body standards for short-term acute-care hospitals. The LTCH may have different state requirements for health record content. In the state of Connecticut, for example, there are different requirements for the completion of the health record in an LTCH as opposed to a short-term acute-care hospital. An LTCH health record in Connecticut must be completed within fourteens days of discharge, while the short-term acute-care hospital has a 30-day completion requirement. It is very important to check with individual state requirements for health record content.

LTCH facilities must adopt and enforce medical staff bylaws and rules and regulations that govern medical staff responsibilities as outlined in the Medicare *Conditions of Participation* (2006b). These are also similar to the short-term acute-care hospitals medical staff bylaws.

LTCH Policies and Procedures

Health information policies and procedures will encompass typical HIM practices excluding policies on services that are not covered in the LTCH such as birth or tumor registries. See chapter 4 for more information about registries.

Health record review activity is completed in the LTCH setting and is defined by facility policy. Open records are the focus of audits that examine clinical pertinence and health record completion. It is important to include discharge documentation monitoring in the **health record review process** to ensure that requirements and standards for discharge documentation are met as well. Health records are typically examined at the point of care by various clinical and HIM staff. Facility policy will drive how data are gathered and disseminated. Figure 10.3 shows a sample audit tool for open and closed records. Such tools are used by HIM staff to examine the discharge records and ensure compliance with documentation standards for discharge summaries.

LTCH facilities may have several indicators that are deemed pertinent to their patient population and licensure or accreditation requirements. If the LTCH is accredited by the Joint Commission, the facility must report ORYX indicators. (ORYX supports the integration of outcomes data and other performance measurement data into the accreditation process.) These indicators will differ between LTCHs as deemed appropriate by each facility's policy. If the LTCH is

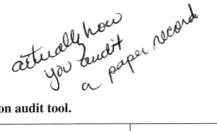
actually how you audit a paper record

Figure 10.3. Documentation audit tool.

Patient Name:				
MR#/VOL#:				
INDICATOR	**YES**	**NO**	**N/A**	**Comment**
History & Physical (H&P)				
H&P completed and on record within 24 hours of admission				
Diagnosis/impression recorded on H&P				
Reason for admission is documented				
Treatment plan documented in the H&P				
Family history				
Social history				
Allergies are addressed				
Review of systems				
Reflection of comprehensive physical exam				
Temperature				
Pulse				
Respiration				
Blood pressure				
Handwritten H&Ps are legible.				
Discharge Summary	**YES**	**NO**	**N/A**	**Comment**
Dictated within 14 days of patient discharge				
Final/discharge diagnoses and all other pertinent diagnoses relevant to the hospitalization				
Procedures performed				
Condition of patient at time of discharge/transfer to acute facility				
Disposition/conclusions				
Instructions to patient or family after discharge regarding discharge medications and follow-up care				
Reason for hospitalization				
Significant findings				
Physician orders are dated/timed when written.				
Indication included for use of antibiotics, antipsychotics, PRN meds.				
INDICATOR	**YES**	**NO**	**N/A**	**Comment**
Orders IM				
TO/VO include time/date of receipt (Nursing)				
Number of TO/VO monitored				
DATED				
TIMED				
SIGNED				
Discharge order present.				
Physician orders are legible.				

electronically can be done automatically rather than having to walk over and look it up.

Figure 10.3.   (continued)

Progress Notes	YES	NO	N/A	Comment
Notes are objective; include observations/results of therapy/plan of action.				
Physician notes are dated/timed when written.				
If death, a final progress note is present.				
Physician progress notes are legible.				
Other	**YES**	**NO**	**N/A**	**Comment**
Allergies are present.				
Prohibited abbreviations are not used when writing orders.				
INDICATOR Clinician	**YES**	**NO**	**N/A**	**Comment**
Assessments				
Nutrition screening done within 2 working days of admission (admission or evaluations/assessment sections, progress note on COU, RCU, and PD)				
Initial pain assessment is completed.				
Initial nursing assessment within 24 hours of admission (on new admissions only)				
Physical status by nursing (monthly summary, progress notes)				
Psychological status (H&P, SW intake, psych consult, chaplain admission section as well)				
Social status (check H&P, SW intake)				
When warranted by patient need, nutritional status is assessed (nursing monthly summary, dietician progress notes, preadmission note).				
When warranted by patient need, functional status is assessed. Done for each RHB patient—chronic as needed (H&P/consults evaluations).				
Clinical progress notes are timed and dated (RN, RT, OT, PT, SLP, Other).				
Need for discharge planning is assessed (case management notes/SW intake).				
Monitoring of medication effect on patient includes assessment based on collective observations, including patient's own perception of effect. (Check progress notes/MARs as necessary.)				
Clinical observations, including the results of therapy, are documented.				
Goals of treatment and treatment plans are documented.				
Care planning considers patient-specific needs, age-specific needs, severity level of condition, impairment, or disability.				
Patient's learning needs, abilities, preferences, readiness to learn are assessed.				
Assessment includes consideration of cultural values, religious beliefs.				
Barriers to learning are incorporated into care plans.				
Spiritual and cultural assessment is completed for the dying patient.				

Figure 10.3.   (continued)

INDICATOR	YES	NO	N/A	Comment
Reassessment				
Reassessment includes patient response to care.				
A significant change in the patient's condition results in reassessment.				
Have staff members integrated information from various assessments of the patient to identify and assign priorities to care needs?				
In reassessments, were care decisions based on the identified patient needs and care priorities?				
Education	YES	NO	N/A	Comment
Educational processes consider the physical, cognitive, cultural, social, and economic characteristics of the patient.				
The educational process is coordinated among appropriate staff or disciplines.				
Patient education is based on assessed needs, abilities, preferences, and readiness to learn, as appropriate.				
When appropriate, the patient/family is educated about safe and effective use of medications. Patient/family is preparing for self-administration of meds.				
When appropriate, the patient/family is educated about nutrition interventions, modified diets, or oral health, when applicable.				
When appropriate, the patient is educated about safe and effective use of medical equipment or supplies.				
When appropriate, the patient is educated about pain and effective pain management.				
When appropriate, the patient is educated about habilitation and rehab techniques.				
When appropriate, the patient is educated about available community resources.				
When appropriate, the patient is educated regarding self-care activities.				
Education is done timely (quarterly entry on patient). Family education sheet, LTC units only, excluding NB				
Patient/family education completed prior to discharge.				
When appropriate, academic education is provided to children and adolescents.				
INDICATOR	YES	NO	N/A	Comment
General Items				
Discharge summaries are completed—PT.				
Discharge summaries are completed—OT.				
Discharge summaries are completed—Other.				
Existence of advance directives NOT APPLICABLE ON PATIENT'S 17 OR YOUNGER				
All diagnostic and therapeutic procedures and test results such as pathology and clinical laboratory exams are in the record.				
Face sheet is present in the record.				
All entries are signed.				
All entries are dated.				
General consent is signed and in the record.				

Figure 10.3.   (continued)

Pediatric Care: As appropriate, the assessment of infants, children, and adolescents includes:	YES	NO	N/A	Comment
The assessment of infants, children, and adolescents includes a length/height (on nutritional evaluation—yearly) q 3 months, 0–2 yrs old, and q 6 months > 2 yrs old.				
Head circumference is documented on admission and then every year for patients 0–2 yrs old. It is done more often if deemed medically necessary. (Check growth charts, admission history database, and H&Ps.)				
Emotional, cognitive, communication, educational, social, and daily activity needs				
Developmental age				
Weight				
Immunization status				
Consideration of the patient's education needs and daily activity				
Family/guardian expectations for and involvement in the assessment, initial treatment, and continuing care of the patient are documented.				

accredited by CARF, it will focus on rehabilitation outcomes, again as appropriate to the facility's determination. For these outcome measures, the incorporation of FIM scores may be used.

Outcomes measures differ among LTCH settings because although LTCHs care for chronically, critically ill patients, LTCHs across the nation manage care for different patient population types. While one LTCH may care for a large volume of ventilator patients, another LTCH may care for cancer patients, wound patients, or even those patients requiring psychiatric care. It is difficult to benchmark outcomes measures across the industry because LTCH patient populations differ greatly in geographic regions. LTCHs are unevenly distributed across the United States, and most are in the Northeast, South, and West. As of 2003, Louisiana had 35 LTCHs, the most of any state, and 16 of these were established in and after 2001 (Kaplan and White 2004). Figure 10.4 shows the location of LTCHs in 2003.

Skilled Nursing and Nursing Facilities

An LTCH is a hospital and not a skilled-nursing facility (SNF) or nursing facility (NF). This section provides details about these special types of long-term care (LTC) facilities.

Skilled-nursing care is care provided to a patient that requires a skill level of a qualified individual, such as a registered nurse. Nursing care is provided when an individual's needs do not require the specific skill set of SNF providers. For example, a nursing facility may help a resident with dressing and/or going to the bathroom, whereas a patient in an SNF has a tube feed administered by a nurse. The difference between a skilled-nursing facility and a nursing facility relates to level of skilled care individuals require.

According to the CMS (2006c, 5), a **skilled-nursing facility** is as follows:

> . . . an institution (or a distinct part of an institution) [that] is primarily engaged in providing skilled-nursing care and related services for residents who require medical or nursing care, or rehabilitation services for the rehabilitation of injured, disabled, or sick persons, and is not primarily for the care and treatment of mental diseases; has in effect a transfer agreement . . . with one or more hospitals . . . ; and meets the requirements for a SNF. . . .

[handwritten margin note: Can be known as a Nursing home]

Figure 10.4.   Location of long-term care hospitals.

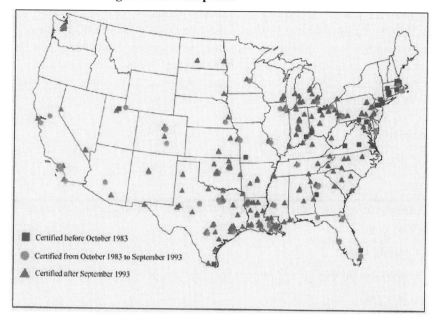

- LTCHs are unevenly distributed across the United States, as shown on this map. On this map, the red triangles represent the LTCHs that opened since 1993 and demonstrate the recent rapid growth of these facilities. LTCHs are concentrated in some areas. For example, there are 35 LTCHs in Louisiana; 16 of these were established in and after 2001, and more are opening. There are press reports that HealthSouth™ is opening a LTCH nursing home in Louisiana.

- The necessity of LTCHs can be questioned if they are present in some areas and not in others. Also, where are patients who need long-term care treated if no LTCHs are located in their areas?

A **nursing facility** is (CMS 2006c, 6) as follows:

. . . an institution (or a distinct part of an institution) [that] is primarily engaged in providing skilled-nursing care and related services for residents who require medical or nursing care, rehabilitation services for the rehabilitation of injured, disabled, or sick persons, or on a regular basis, health-related care and services to individuals who because of their mental or physical condition require care and services (above the level of room and board) which can be made available to them only through institutional facilities, and is not primarily for the care and treatment of mental diseases; has in effect a transfer agreement . . . with one or more hospitals . . . and meets the requirements for a NF . . .

SNF Health Record Content

The functions of the SNF health records are the same as those in the acute-care hospital settings. They function as the documentation and communication tools to facilitate the patient care delivery and legal recording of care and treatment provided to the individuals served. In the SNF setting, health records documentation is a key link to state and federal quality reporting through the required use of the Minimum Data Set. (See "Minimum Data Set," later in this chapter for more information.)

Admission paper work contains a number of documents needed to be completed before a resident can be admitted to a long-term care facility. Requirements depend on the regulations of the state in which the facility operates. In addition to the documentation of preadmission and admission assessments, some or all of the forms, records, consents, or data fields in the electronic health record may be created and maintained in the resident's health record. As in the acute-care setting, a face sheet is typically the first page of a patient's health record.

A completed admission application is usually kept in the admitting office. If it is electronic, it may only be accessible to those who need access to the file. Admission applications may be scanned into the electronic health record because they required the resident's or surrogate's signatures for the following:

- Consent to treat

- Consent to photograph (per facility policy)

- Physician certification for Medicare

- Interagency transfer form (from the referring facility, and this may be a state requirement)

- Acknowledgments

- Mental illness and mental retardation form (state specific)

- Face sheet for the health record

- Acknowledgment of the Notice of Privacy Practices

- Resident bill of rights (depending on facility policy)

- Admission agreement (depending on facility policy)

Several different types of consent and authorization forms are used in long-term care organizations. Consents provide a means for residents to convey to healthcare providers their implied or expressed permission to administer care or treatment or other medical procedures. Authorizations, however, document the resident's formal, written permission to use or disclose his or her protected health information for purposes other than treatment, payment, or healthcare operations. In the electronic environment, these types of documents may have to be scanned into the resident's health record. Advance directives, as described above, also are included.

Admission Assessments

Federal, state, and accreditation organizations drive the assessment and documentation process in long-term care. In an effort to capture the supporting documentation of the Resident Assessment Instrument (RAI), which includes the Minimum Data Set (MDS), a federally mandated resident assessment must be done for every resident in a nursing home. Facilities have developed several types of assessments. These assessments establish mechanisms for gathering appropriate and necessary information about each resident.

State-specific guidelines may require specific areas to be included in the admission assessment. Admission assessment requirements differ by state but may include initial assessments of resident health status and function. The initial assessment form should contain areas to identify, determine functional status, and include health problems that the resident may have.

The assessment process is an ongoing evaluation of the resident's needs, functional abilities, and requirements, and is used to identify and provide appropriate interventions and services. The entire assessment process is fundamental to the care-planning requirements of federal, state, and accrediting bodies.

The physician history and physical must be completed as specified by state regulations. The Joint Commission sets requirements for completion of the history and physical or medical assessment as within 24 hours before admission or within 72 hours after admission (Joint Commission 2007, PC.2.120). A history and physical that is received from the attending physician or licensed independent practitioner and completed within 30 days prior to admission may be used as long as it summarizes the patient's condition and care prior to admission and describes the resident's current physical/psychosocial status (Joint Commission 2007, PC.2.120).

While there are no federal time frame requirements for completing the admission nursing assessments, states may have their own regulations and accreditation bodies. In 2007, the Joint Commission stipulated that "the organization initiates nursing assessments within 24 hours of admission. . . . At minimum, the organization completes assessments within five calendar days after admission for all disciplines pertinent to the reason for admission or as required by law and regulation" (Joint Commission 2007, PC.2.120).

Initial nursing assessments must be completed as established by law or facility policy, but no later than fourteen days after admission. In addition, several Joint Commission requirements address the assessment of each resident. The organization must have a process for assessing and reassessing residents, and reassessments must be conducted at regular intervals. These assessments must be overseen by a registered nurse. Initial assessments also must specifically address the status, needs, and potential of each resident and include information on his or her medical, physical, functional, psychosocial, and nutritional status (see figure 10.5).

Figure 10.5.   Relevant past medical history and medical status.

- Diagnoses
- Medications
- Allergies
- Treatments
- Results of diagnostic or laboratory studies
- Prognosis
- Limitations
- Precautions
- Neuropsychiatric status: Mental, affective, cognitive, sleeping patterns or memory, recall ability, decision-making ability, and behavior
- Communication status: Hearing, speech, language, voice, and modes of expression
- Rehabilitation status: Previous and current functional status, ADLs, mobility, balance, strength, bowel and bladder function, sensory capacity and impairments, vision, ability to swallow, orientation, and rehabilitation potential
- Psychosocial status: Level of functioning, cultural and ethnic factors, current emotional status, social skills, family circumstances, family relationships, current living situation, relevant past history, past roles, and response to current status
- Spiritual status: Spiritual orientation; including the dying individual's self-esteem
- Physical status: Musculoskeletal, cardiorespiratory, gastrointestinal, integumentary, and foot care
- Level of activity: Use of free time; personal preferences, preadmission hobbies, interests, and lifestyle; past and current activities; and ability to participate
- Nutritional and hydration status: Potential nutritional risk and deficiencies; cultural, religious, or ethnic food preferences; special dietary requirements; and nutrient-intake routines
- Dental status and oral health: Condition of the oral cavity, teeth, and tooth-supporting structures; natural teeth or dentures; functioning with or without natural teeth or dentures
- Level of pain: Origin, location, severity, alleviating and exacerbating factors, and current treatment and response to treatment
- Response to stress caused by present situation, illness, and treatment
- Educational needs: Needs, preferences, abilities, and readiness to learn to include family members

Source: James 2007.

Resident Assessment Instrument (RAI)

The **Resident Assessment Instrument (RAI)** is used to complete comprehensive assessments and collect information for the Minimum Data Set for long-term care (MDS 3.0). Every long-term care facility must complete a comprehensive assessment of every resident's needs by using the RAI specified by the state in which the facility operates. The content of RAIs is ultimately determined by each state and may differ from state to state. The RAI consists of a standard Minimum Data Set (MDS), Resident Assessment Protocols (RAPs), and utilization guidelines. The RAI's purpose is to standardize the collection of patient data and determine assessment protocols in the long-term care environment. This assessment process uses version 3.0 of the Minimum Data Set for long-term care (CMS 2007).

The MDS is a primary document in the resident's health record. The RAI is used to evaluate new residents of long-term care facilities within fourteen days of admission, but the interdisciplinary team must take steps to complete further assessments and reassessments to enhance the MDS data gathering process. Evaluations are conducted every quarter, every year, and whenever there is a significant change in the resident's status.

The completion schedule for residents who are eligible for Medicare benefits is slightly different than the schedule for other residents. Medicare's schedule is shown in table 10.2. Note the "assessment type" is the time frame for which an assessment is completed, while the "assessment window" is how long a facility has to complete the assessment.

Minimum Data Set

Minimum Data Set for long-term care (MDS 3.0) is a resident assessment instrument required by long-term care facilities that are certified to participate in the Medicare and Medicaid programs. The MDS is the first component of the RAI. It is used to gather information about specific health status factors and include information about specific risk factors in the resident's care. This comprehensive MDS is used to plan the ongoing care and treatment of the resident in the long-term care facility. It must be printed and placed in the resident's paper record and also sent electronically to the state for reporting.

The three components of the RAI are the MDS, the Resident Assesment Protocols, and the utilization guidelines, which provide a comprehensive tool for the assessment of each resident.

Resident Assessment Protocols

Resident Assessment Protocols (RAPs) "are problem-oriented frameworks for additional assessment based on problem identification items (triggered conditions). They form a critical

Table 10.2   Medicare assessment schedule

Assessment Type		Assessment Window	
Maximum Days		Payment Days	
5-day	Days 1–8[a]	14	1–14
14-day	Days 11–14	16	15–30
30-day	Days 21–29	30	31–60
60-day	Days 50–59	30	61–90
90-day	Days 80–89	10	91–100

[a]When a patient expires or transfers to another facility before the five-day assessment is complete, the facility must still prepare a Minimum Data Set (Transmittal 372).
Source: James 2007.

link to decisions about care planning. The RAPs guidelines provide guidance on how to synthesize assessment information within a comprehensive assessment. The triggers target conditions for additional assessment and review, as warranted by MDS item responses. The RAPs guidelines help facility staff evaluate 'triggered' conditions" (CMS 2007).

The RAPs include the principal components of a long-term care resident's care plan. They are used to further define the resident's care-planning needs and treatment. Moreover, they are used in conjunction with the MDS to ensure that the resident's assessment is comprehensive and the care-planning process is complete. Currently, long-term care facilities are required to use the RAI version 2.0. CMS recently released Minimum Data Set MDS 3.0 (CMS 2006a).

During the RAI process, several assessments should be considered to support the MDS documentation and may include the following:

- Physician history and physical exam
- Nursing assessment
- Wound and skin assessment
- Fall assessment
- Bowel and bladder assessment
- Pain assessment
- Basic mental/cognitive examination
- Restraint assessment (only if applicable)
- Minimum Data Set assessment
- Nutritional assessment
- Therapy assessments, as required
- Therapeutic recreation assessment
- Pastoral care assessment

3. Utilization guidelines

Continued Assessments and Reassessments

Documentation gathered through the resident assessment process provides a clear and accurate representation of the resident's health status. The documentation in the health record supports the resident's care plan and treatment program. Assessments are an ongoing evaluation of the resident's health status, needs, and conditions. Reassessments are required at regular intervals throughout the resident's stay to support continuing treatment and services and the MDS assessments for Medicare. The reassessment process determines areas of improvement and decline in the long-term care resident.

Preadmission Screening Assessment and Annual Resident Review

The Preadmission Screening Assessment and Annual Resident Review (PASARR) is both a federal- and state-mandated requirement that provides a mechanism for screening mental illness and mental retardation (MI/MR). The PASARR for MI/MR is required under the Omnibus Budget Reconciliation Act of 1987 (OBRA). It is completed preadmission and annually (National Long-term Care Ombudsman Resource Center 2001).

all assessments so back to FIM score assessment

369

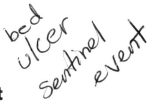
bed ulcer
Sentinel event

Skin Assessment

A skin assessment is conducted as part of the admission assessment process to determine whether the resident is at risk for skin conditions such as pressure ulcers. The assessment helps detect areas of concern such as location and size of decubitus ulcers, bruises, skin lesions, skin tears, and other skin conditions. *then create a care plan if there are problem areas*

Fall Assessments

Fall assessments should be completed to determine residents who are at risk for falling. Federal regulations require that "each resident receives adequate supervision and assistance devices to prevent accidents" (CMS 2006c, PP-229).

Bowel and Bladder Assessment

The bowel and bladder assessment is used to evaluate the resident for any bowel and bladder issues, and it provides valuable data on any existing bowel and bladder problems such as incontinence; frequency of incontinence; and bowel patterns such as constipation, diarrhea, or impaction.

Restraint Assessment

The restraint assessment should be utilized to ensure that facility practice is according to regulation. The facility must always seek the least-restrictive device when implementing a restraint. The facility should strive to be restraint free, but in specific circumstances to maintain or improve the resident's medical condition, a least-restrictive restraining device may be required. "The intent of this requirement is for each person to attain and maintain his/her highest practicable well-being in an environment that prohibits the use of restraints for discipline or convenience and limits restraint use to circumstances in which the resident has medical symptoms that warrant the use of restraints" (CMS 2006c, PP-55).

Psychotropic Medication Assessment

The psychotropic medication assessment is used to evaluate those residents who are taking antipsychotic medications. It helps to determine whether the dosage of the medication can be reduced as appropriate to clinical indications. "Residents who have not used antipsychotic drugs are not given these drugs unless antipsychotic drug therapy is necessary to treat a specific condition as diagnosed and documented in the clinical record" (CMS 2006c, PP-240).

Behavioral and Mood Problems Assessment

Behavioral and mood problems assessment is used to ensure that "A resident who displays mental or psychosocial adjustment difficulty, receives appropriate treatment and services to correct the assessed problem" (CMS 2006c, PP-221). These assessments can address resident wandering, verbal abuse, physical abuse, inappropriate or disruptive behavior, and resistance to care. The assessment should include the number, frequency, intensity, and the ability to alter the behavioral symptoms. See chapter 12 for additional information about behavioral care documentation.

Self-Administration Assessment

A self-administration assessment demonstrates whether the resident is indeed capable of self-administering his or her own medications. "An individual resident may self-administer drugs if the interdisciplinary team...has determined that this practice is safe" (CMS 2006c, PP-39).

Nutritional Assessments

Nutritional assessments are used to guarantee that all residents have adequate nutritional status and to identify any nutritional problems. "The facility must ensure that a resident maintains acceptable parameters of nutrition status, such as body weight and protein levels, unless the resident's clinical condition demonstrates that this is not possible" (CMS 2006c, PP-230).

Activities, Recreation, and Leisure Assessment

The activities, recreation, and leisure assessment evaluates the resident to determine an appropriate program that incorporates the resident's needs, preferences, and abilities and reflects the resident's requirements for recreational activities. "The facility must provide for an ongoing program of activities designed to meet . . . the interests and the physical, mental, and psychosocial well-being of each resident" (CMS 2006c, PP-28).

Social Service Assessment

A social service assessment supports the need to "provide medically related social services to attain or maintain the highest practicable physical, mental, and psychosocial well-being of each resident" (CMS 2006c, PP-102). This assessment should help the resident to adjust to the new environment. The initial assessment is completed at the time of admission with continuing updates during care planning.

Restorative/Rehabilitative Nursing Assessment

A restorative/rehabilitative nursing assessment ensures that "a resident who enters the facility without a limited range of motion does not experience reduction in range of motion unless the resident's clinical condition demonstrates that a reduction in range of motion is unavoidable; and [that] a resident with limited range of motion receives appropriate treatment and services to increase range of motion and/or to prevent further decrease in range of motion" (CMS 2006c, PP-219–220). These assessments are a mechanism to help the resident achieve his or her highest functional level.

The Care Plan

The care plan is the "comprehensive care plan for each resident that includes measurable objectives and timetables to meet a resident's medical, nursing, and mental and psychosocial needs that are identified in the comprehensive assessment" (CMS 2006c, 127). Although state and accrediting bodies may have specific requirements for the care plan criteria, the care plan must be completed and updated as the resident's care and treatment needs change over time.

The care plan is "the 'living and breathing' document that drives the resident's ultimate attainment and achievement of the highest practicable physical, mental, and psychosocial well-being." The care plan "is the basis for all care and treatment modalities the resident requires. It directs the interdisciplinary team to the care and treatment needed for each resident. Moreover, it is the primary source for ongoing documentation of the resident's care, condition, and needs." The resident-specific care plan considers the resident's needs, desires, preferences, and abilities to achieve the highest physical and emotional functioning and well-being. Each care plan is individualized and can easily identify the resident's problems and needs (James 2007).

SNF Accreditation Standards and Regulations

A major change for long-term care occurred in 1987 when President Ronald Reagan approved a revision to Medicare and Medicaid that requires LTC providers to provide services so each resident can "attain and maintain [the] highest practicable physical, mental, and psychosocial well-being" (National Long-Term Care Ombudsman Resource Center 2001).

Long-term care facilities are subject to several intricate operating requirements. These include both voluntary and mandatory requirements, which can include the following:

- Federal statues and regulations

- State licensure

- State health record regulations

- State public health codes

- State regulations for Medicaid qualifications

- County and municipal building safety codes

- Federal health information privacy and security standards

- Joint Commission standards—voluntary requirements

It is imperative that long-term care facilities consult all of these areas to ensure compliance with all regulations and standards.

Medical Necessity and Medicare Documentation

The federal government requires accurate, timely, and complete health record documentation of the skilled nursing and therapeutic services provided to Medicare beneficiaries. The resident's health record must substantiate the clinical indications and **medical necessity** for Medicare Part A coverage as well as the skilled services required and the resident's continued need for coverage. Documentation that supports skilled services are medically reasonable and necessary is required for all charges submitted on the UB-04 (CMS 2002).

Medicare's *Conditions of Participation* require that physician's orders describing the resident's immediate care requirements be provided to the facility at the time of admission. A physician's certification of the resident's need for long-term care services also is required at any time the resident is eligible for Medicare benefits. In addition, Medicare regulations stipulate that a health record must be established for every resident at the time of admission.

Each Medicare resident must have a Medicare Part A certification and recertification executed and signed by the physician who knows the resident's care and treatment requirements. Certification/recertification includes the reasons for Medicare coverage and the skilled services that will be provided. Certification is mandated upon admission; recertifications are mandated for as long as the resident continues to receive Medicare Part A benefits. The recertification is also required when a resident returns to a long-term care facility after a temporary acute-care hospital stay as long as the resident still qualifies for Medicare coverage.

[handwritten margin note: reimbursed per day based on utilization guidelines (time spent with patient and how much care)]

[handwritten margin note: Length of stay is what matters in reimbursement for LTC]

Physician Certification

Staff and attending physicians must periodically certify the need for long-term care services within an SNF. **Physician certification** is required upon admission or as soon as possible thereafter. The first recertification is required no later than the fourteenth day of the patient's stay, and additional recertifications are required every 30 days (CMS 2007, 6).

Standards Governing Assessments

Documentation of the assessments conducted in the long-term care setting is driven by federal and state regulations and accreditation standards. **Medicare prospective payment system (PPS)** requirements also affect clinical documentation efforts. Depending on state requirements, the admission process may start when potential residents are placed on the facility's waiting list. The waiting list may be a state-specific requirement. All states, however, require that residents of long-term care facilities remain under the care of a physician throughout their stay. This is demonstrated through the documentation process of the long-term care health record.

The Joint Commission states that the long-term care facility should admit and treat only those residents whose "identified care, treatment, and services needs it can meet" (Joint Commission 2007, PC.1.10, PC 3). Additionally, information about each potential patient is used "to match an individual's need with the appropriate setting, care level, and intervention" (Joint Commission 2007, GL 3).

CARF examines "service design and delivery that focus on the needs of the persons served" and determines whether "accomplishment of predicted outcomes" was achieved among other valuable quality components of rehabilitation or assisted-living facilities. CARF standards focus on the goals and activities of the resident and the outcomes of care (CARF n.d.). Thus, CARF standards look at the needs of the resident, proper placement, and the outcomes of care.

Documentation of Physician Services

According to CMS, "a physician must personally approve in writing a recommendation that an individual be admitted to a facility. Each resident must remain under the care of a physician" (2006c, PP-368). The facility also must demonstrate that a physician oversees the medical care of each resident at all times. This is done through physician documentation. The documentation of the physician validates that the medical oversight or supervision of care for long-term care residents has occurred. The interdisciplinary team and care-planning process must involve the physician. In the long-term care environment, the physician is not required to visit the resident every day but, rather, as the resident's needs dictate. However, the physician must be informed of the resident's status changes or identified medical problems to ensure that proper care is provided in a timely manner (James 2007). The exact time frames for physician visits are defined in the CMS **State Operations Manual** as follows (2006c):

1. The residents must be seen by a physician at least once every 30 days for the first 90 days after admission, and at least once every 60 thereafter.

2. A physician visit is considered timely if it occurs not later than 10 days after the date the visit was required." (2006c, 371)

Physician documentation includes but may not be limited to the following (James 2007):

- Certification or recertification for Medicare services
- History and physical at admission and annually (if required by state laws or accrediting bodies)
- Medication and treatment orders
- Progress notes
- Consultations
- Discharge summary (if required by state law)
- Discharge order as per state requirements

Progress Notes

An admission progress note is completed when the resident is admitted to the long-term care facility. This "admission note should be entered into the resident's health record that includes the date and time of admission, how the resident arrived at the facility (for example, by ambulance), the reason for the admission, and the resident's current condition and health status. State regulations include specific requirements for admission documentation, time frame for completion, and other specified requirements" (James 2007). Often times these notes are very short and succinct, but in reality these notes should reflect and support the reason for admission to the long-term care setting.

Additional progress notes are entered as determined by federal, state, and accrediting body regulations and standards. Each time the resident is seen by a physician, a progress note should be entered.

Physician Orders

The physician's order must include the frequency, duration, and scope of treatment and be dated and signed. These orders are written when changes, additions, or deletions are required in care and treatment of the resident. They include, but are not limited to, medications (pharmacy orders), treatments such as dressing changes, services such as therapies, ancillary tests such as laboratory blood draws and cultures or radiology studies, and diet orders (James 2007).

Physician Consultations

Consultations may be required when the resident's health status dictates that a specialist examine identified problems encountered in the care and treatment of the resident. Such specialists may include podiatrists, cardiologists, pulmonologists, or surgeons. Consultations are usually kept for easy access in a separate section in the resident's health record. In an electronic environment, consultants who make visits to the resident in the facility require access to the electronic health record to complete the consult documentation. If the resident is sent outside the facility for the consultation, the consult may need to be scanned into the health record so that staff has easy access to the information. Consultations in a long-term care facility contain the same data elements as both the short-term acute-care and long-term acute-care hospital.

Other Documentation

Other documentation includes monthly summaries, education records, activities of daily living, therapy, flow sheets, laboratory and special reports, medication administration records, discharge documentation, accident and incident reports, and organization/management.

Monthly Summary

A monthly summary may be completed in the long-term care setting to help summarize the care given to the resident over time. There are no federal requirements for a summary note; however, state laws may be more specific. The monthly summary is a mechanism to capture concise monthly updates reflecting gains and declines of the resident's condition and health status. The monthly summary should correlate with the resident's care-planning process and further support the MDS assessments.

Education Records

Education of the resident should be documented as provided and completed by the time of discharge. The documentation should be an interdisciplinary team effort. Based on Joint Commission documentation requirements, the resident is assessed for needs, abilities, preferences, and readiness to learn, as appropriate, and the education plan considers the physical, cognitive, cultural, social, and economic characteristics of the resident. The education documentation should include the following (James 2007):

Available community resources

Habilitation and rehabilitation techniques

Nutrition interventions, modified diets, or oral health, when applicable

Pain and effective pain management

Safe and effective use of medical equipment or supplies

Safe and effective use of medications

Self-administration of medications

Self-care activities

Activities of Daily Living

Activities of daily living (ADL) should be documented. Although there is no federal requirement for documentation of ADLs, they are part of the MDS, and many LTC facilities capture this information as supporting documentation. The resident's ADLs indicate the resident's functional status. The documentation of ADLs supports the MDS assessments. Functional ability can be divided into the following categories:

- Bed mobility
- Transfer
- Walking
- Locomotion

- Dressing
- Eating
- Toilet use
- Personal hygiene
- Bathing

Therapy

Rehabilitative therapy comprises those services provided by the licensed therapist staff. These individuals are allied health professionals in physical therapy, occupational therapy, speech-language therapy, and respiratory therapy. Rehabilitative therapy should not be confused with nursing restorative care. The federal government sets stringent standards for nursing homes "to attain or maintain the resident's highest practicable physical, mental, and psychosocial well-being" (CMS 2006c, PP-127). Rehabilitative therapy provides another mechanism to ensure that residents do achieve the best quality outcomes of care. Rehabilitative therapy services documentation include the assessments, daily flow sheet charting, diagnostic evaluation, education, management, and treatments.

Flow Sheets

Flow sheets are used in various ways in the long-term care setting and are used by all clinical staff to capture the health and functional status and responses to treatment. "The common purpose of all of these flow sheets is to document that required services were delivered to the facility's residents and to provide a means of communication among healthcare workers" (James 2007). In the long-term care setting flow sheets are usually discipline-specific rather than interdisciplinary.

Laboratory and Special Reports

Laboratory reports contain information gathered from many kinds of laboratory and diagnostic test results. These reports help establish the correct diagnosis and treatment plan for each resident and they further help to assess changes in residents' health conditions and status.

Special reports include the results of imaging and pathology testing, among other procedures. Imaging may include a full range of radiological service diagnostic test results, including the more common x-ray, EKG, Holter monitor, MRI, CT scan, and respiratory therapy reports (such as pulmonary function testing and pulse oximetry results). X-ray reports are the most common test result found in the resident's health record (James 2007).

Medication Administration Records

Medication administration records (MARs) are tools used to capture the delivery of each drug to the resident. The MAR identifies medications a resident is scheduled to take, how often they should be administered, and at what dose they are to be administered (James 2007).

Discharge Documentation

Federal regulations require that the reason or need for the transfer or discharge be documented in the resident's health record. In addition, each resident must be notified in writing of the reasons for the transfer or discharge and the facility bed-hold policy. Discharge documentation refers to those records that must be completed at the time the resident is transferred to another facility or discharged from the facility. These documents include the following:

- Medication education and drug discharge documentation
- Clinical discharge summaries for all disciplines treating the resident
- Comprehensive assessment (MDS)
- Discharge plan of care
- Discharge instructions to the resident or resident's family as appropriate
- Transfer forms or interagency transfer forms
- Physician discharge summary

Risk Management and Liability

In chapter 3, the liability issues associated with short-term acute-care were discussed. Identical liability issues exist in the long-term acute-care and long-term care settings. These types of facilities also look at risk management concerns, incident reporting, and medical staff credentialing and privileging and rely on the health record documentation to support these areas. While long-term care may have more issues with the longer stays and accidents or injuries within the facility, the liability factors discussed under short-term acute-care apply in these care settings.

Accidents or incidents may occasionally occur in the long-term care setting. When they do, they must be reported in an accident or incident report. Additionally, the facts of the event must be documented in the resident's health record. The actual accident or incident report does not get filed into the resident's health record. Facility policy must outline how the facts of the occurrence should be documented: ". . . documentation does not indicate that an incident report has been filed, nor does it refer to the report in the documentation. However, the resident's health record must reflect the facts of the injury and how it was received" (James 2007).

The same standards for documentation and management of the acute-care setting apply in the long-term care setting. The resident's health record is the principal communication instrument for planning, coordinating, and managing the resident's care. It is the legal business record of the facility. Moreover, it is the facility's defense against malpractice claims.

Summary

Long-term care includes not only skilled and nonskilled-nursing facilities, but also long-term acute-care hospitals. Long-term care processes include governance, accreditation, and documentation guidelines, and mirror short-term acute-care hospital processes, although many long-term care facilities do not have emergency services, surgical suites, or maternity care. While the terms are used interchangeably throughout the industry, this chapter details the differences between skilled-nursing facilities (SNFs), nursing facilities (NFs), and long-term acute-care facilities (LTCHs).

The clinical documentation for long-term care encompasses a broad range of information, assessments, and medical services. Much of the information captured is similar to that for the short-term acute-care hospitals. The LTCH Medicare Prospective Payment System uses short-term acute-care hospital diagnosis-related groups (DRGs), but mandates the use of LTCH DRGs. While these DRGs are the same as those used in short-term acute-care, the LTCH DRGs have different weights and length of stays attached to them. The importance of the principal diagnosis is detailed.

The Resident Assessment Instrument, Minimum Data Set, and Resident Assessment Protocols assist in assessing the resident's condition and health status and in defining the resident's care-planning needs and treatment. The documentation in the long-term care health record provides a summary showing compliance with regulations and standards determined by federal, state, and accrediting bodies. Additionally the health record provides proof of services for reimbursement from Medicare, Medicaid, and/or third-party payers.

References

AHIMA Coding Policy and Strategy Committee. 2000. AHIMA's *Standards of Ethical Coding*. Chicago: AHIMA.

Centers for Medicare and Medicaid Services. 2002. *Long-term Care Hospital PPS Training Guide*. Available online from http://www.cms.hhs.gov/LongTermCareHospitalPPS/03_ltch_train.asp.

Centers for Medicare and Medicaid Services. 2006a. *MDS 3.0 for nursing homes*. Available online from www.cms.hhs.gov/NursingHomeQualityInits/25_NHQIMDS30.asp# .

Centers for Medicare and Medicaid Services. 2006b (Nov. 27). Conditions of participation for hospitals: Final rule. 42 CFR Part 482. *Federal Register* 71(227): 68672 –68695. Available online from http://a257.g.akamaitech.net/7/257/2422/01jan20061800/edocket.access.gpo.gov/2006/pdf/E6-19957.pdf.

Centers for Medicare and Medicaid Services. 2006c. Appendix PP—Guidance to surveyors for long-term care facilities, Revision 22. In *State Operations Manual*. Available online from www.cms.hhs.gov/manuals/Downloads/som107ap_pp_guidelines_ltcf.pdf.

Centers for Medicare and Medicaid Services. 2007. (Oct. 1). Prospective payment systems for inpatient hospital services. 42 CFR Part 412.22 *Federal Register*. Available online from http://a257.g.akamaitech.net/7/257/2422/16nov20071500/edocket.access.gpo.gov/cfr_2007/octqtr/pdf/42cfr412.22.pdf.

Centers for Medicare and Medicaid Services. 2007. *CMS's RAI Version 2.0 Manual: Medicare SNF PPS*. Available online from www.cms.hhs.gov/NursingHomeQualityInits/20_NHQIMDS20.asp#TopOfPage.

Commission on Accreditation of Rehabilitation Facilities. n.d. Available online from www.carf.org.

Department of Health and Human Services. n.d. *The FIM*. Available online from www.os.dhhs.gov/healthit/documents/chiinitiative/DFCPAForms.pdf.

Department of Health and Human Services. 1999a (Oct. 1). Medical review requirements: Physician acknowledgement; Final rule. 42 CFR 412.46. *Federal Register* 60(170): 45847. Available online from www.access.gpo.gov/nara/cfr/waisidx_99/42cfr412_99.html.

Department of Health and Human Services. 1999b (Oct. 1). Conditions of participation: Nursing services; Final rule. 42 CFR 482.23 . *Federal Register* 3(Parts 430 to End): 351-352. Available online from www.access.gpo.gov/nara/cfr/waisidx_99/42cfr482_99.html.

Department of Health and Human Services. 2005. The ICD-9-CM Official Guidelines for Coding and Reporting. Available online from www.cdc.gov/nchs/data/icd9/icdguide.pdf.

James, Ella. 2007. *Documentation and Reimbursement for Long-term Care,* 2nd ed. Chicago: AHIMA.

Joint Commission. 2007. *Comprehensive Accreditation Manual for Long-Term Care*. Oakbrook Terrace, IL: Joint Commission.

Kaplan, S., and C. White. 2004. *Annual research meeting report: Long-term care hospitals' role in Medicare post acute*. Available online from www.medpac.gov.

MedPac. 2004 (June). Defining long-term care hospitals. Chapter 5 in *Report to the Congress: New Approaches in Medicare*. Available online from www.medpac.gov/publications%5Ccongressional_reports%5CJune04_ch5.pdf.

National Long-Term Care Ombudsman Resource Center. 2001. Federal Nursing Home Reform Act from the Omnibus Budget Reconciliation Act of 1987. Available online from www.ltcombudsman.org/ombpub-lic/49_346_1023.cfm.

U.S. Social Security Administration. 1982. Payment to hospitals for inpatient hospital services Sec. 1886. [42 U.S.C. 1395ww] (d)(II)(B)(iv). *United States Code.* Available online from http://www.ssa.gov/OP_Home/ssact/title18/1886.htm.

Chapter 11

Home Care and Hospice

Margaret J. White, MS, NHA, RHIA, CPHQ

Learning Objectives

- To identify the key components of the home care and hospice health record database

- To develop an understanding of Medicare Home Care and Hospice Benefits

- To introduce the Medicare Home Care survey process

- To discuss the documentation challenges for the prospective payment system and OASIS

- To provide the quantitative record review guidelines

- To introduce the Home Care and Hospice legal issues

- To define Outcomes Management and Quality Requirements of Home Care and Hospice

- To reinforce the importance of confidentiality of Performance Improvement activities and OASIS

Key Words

Advance directive

Analysis

Application

Civilian Health and Medical Program of the Uniformed Services (CHAMPUS)

Collection

Community Health Accreditation Program (CHAP)

Comprehensive assessment

Descriptive outcome

Do-not-resuscitate (DNR) order

Home Assessment Validation and Entry (HAVEN)

Home care

Home health

Home health agency (HHA)

Home health resource group (HHRG)

Medicare-certified

National Association for Home Care & Hospice (NAHC)

OASIS

Omnibus Budget Reconciliation Act of 1987 (OBRA)

Outcome and Assessment Information Set (OASIS)

Outcomes

ORYX®

Patient outcome measures

Patient's rights

Patient Self-Determination Act (1990)

Performance improvement (PI)

Performance measurement

Plans of care

Prospective payment system (PPS)

Regional Home Health Intermediary (RHHI)

Request for anticipated payment (RAP)

RHHI Outcomes and Assessment Information Set Verification (ROVER) protocol

Risk-adjusted outcome

Tax Equity and Fiscal Responsibility Act of 1982 (TEFRA)

Warehousing

Introduction

Home care in the United States is a diverse and dynamic service industry. Within this industry, home health agencies, home care, personal-care providers, and hospices have come to be known collectively as home care organizations. More than 20,000 providers deliver home care services to some eight million individuals who require services because of acute illness, long-term health conditions, permanent disability, or terminal illness. It should be noted that the term *home care* is often interchanged with ***home health*** and should be regarded as one and the same. Annual expenditures for home health were estimated to be $38.3 billion in 2003. The growth of the agencies themselves has also been dramatic. The 1880s saw the establishment of the first home care agencies. By 1963, the number of agencies totaled nearly 1,100. Today that number exceeds 20,000 (NAHC 2004).

According to the **National Association for Home Care & Hospice (NAHC)** data (2004), **Medicare-certified** home health agencies grew more than threefold, from 1,753 to 5,983 in the time period of 1967 through 1985. However, in the 1980s, the number of Medicare-certified home care agencies leveled off to approximately 5,900 as a result of increasing Medicare paperwork and unreliable payment policies. Both of these problems led to a 1987 lawsuit brought against the Centers for Medicare and Medicaid Services (CMS) by a coalition of U.S. congressional members, consumer groups, and NAHC. After the successful conclusion of the lawsuit, Medicare's annual home care benefit increased significantly and the number of agencies rose to more than 10,000. Yet, once again, the number of Medicare-certified agencies has declined to 7,265 since 2003. NAHC believes the 31.5% decline in agencies since 1997 is the direct result of changes in Medicare home health reimbursement enacted as part of the Balanced Budget Act of 1997 (NAHC 2008).

Medicare added hospice benefits in October 1983, 10 years after the first hospice was established in the United States. The number of Medicare-certified hospices has grown from 31 in January 1984 to 3,078 as of December 2007. Home care and hospice growth occurred in a changing healthcare environment—a more competitive, managed-care environment. This environment challenges providers to develop information management systems that encourage documentation of standardized, high-quality, and accessible data and information to support patient and family care, quality improvement efforts, strategic planning, and other essential activities (NAHC 2004).

Background

Various key factors have driven the need for improved health information management in home care and hospice organizations.

Compliance with Federal Regulations

The CMS, through its Home Health Initiative, developed a quality-monitoring system that makes highly specific data collection and information management demands on home care providers. The Balanced Budget Act of 1997 (BBA) and the **Omnibus Budget Reconciliation Act of 1987 (OBRA)** mandated the implementation of a new prospective payment system for skilled-nursing facilities, home healthcare agencies, outpatient rehabilitation services, and other outpatient services provided to Medicare beneficiaries. The **prospective payment system (PPS)** became effective on October 1, 2000. The PPS changed Medicare and Medicaid home care reimbursement from a cost-based system to a system of fixed-fee reimbursement based on a patient-need classification system. The BBA bundled all services covered and paid for on a reasonable cost basis under the Medicare home health benefit, including medical supplies, into the prospective payment.

Standard Core Assessment Tool

One of several challenges in revising the home health *Conditions of Participation* was the development of a standard core assessment tool. The management tool is designed to be used by providers and eventually by government agencies and healthcare consumers to compare patient indicators and outcomes across providers. CMS made outcome-based quality management reports available to providers in early 2000.

Conditions of Participation and Joint Commission Standards

CMS revised *Conditions of Participation* and the Joint Commission revised its standards to focus on outcomes of care and to eliminate unnecessary procedural requirements. The

[handwritten: quality assessment tool- OASIS CMS]

[handwritten margin note, left side: Must be homebound if receiving Medicare or Medicaid]

[handwritten margin note: Quiz]

challenge for revising *Conditions of Participation* and the standards was to standardize assessments and develop data collection methods useful as management tools for providers. In addition, the revisions were meant to enable government agencies, accreditation and licensure, surveyors, and healthcare consumers to compare indicators and outcomes across home health organizations.

Standardized Definitions for Data Elements

In 1993, the National Association for Home Care's board of directors charged the information resources and quality assurance committee with the task of developing standardized definitions for home care and hospice data elements through a consensus conference process. The board recognized that a uniform minimum data set was a necessary first step toward achieving standardized, comparable home care and hospice data. The consensus conference was held in December 1993. In 1997, the information resources and quality assurance committee added the **Outcome and Assessment Information Set (OASIS)** to the uniform minimum data sets (UDS). OASIS is a group of data elements that represent core items in a comprehensive assessment for an adult home care patient. The data elements form the basis of patient outcome measurements used for outcome-based quality improvement. *[handwritten: evaluation tool measures patient outcomes]*

Uniform Minimum Data Sets

A uniform minimum data set is a minimum set of informational items that have uniform definitions and predefined categories. Uniform minimum data sets are designed to meet the essential information needs of multiple users in the healthcare system. The framework adopted to guide development of the data set for home care and hospice services was based on the U.S. Department of Health and Human Services' concept of a UDS. The UDS is intended to meet the common data needs of multiple users, and so it will not necessarily meet the total data needs of any one organization, nor does it limit additional data collection by an organization to meet its specific information needs. The UDS addresses data documentation and collection at the organizational level and at the individual patient level. This data set is being used for data collection efforts conducted by the NAHC. Other entities involved in home care and hospice are encouraged to use these definitions when constructing surveys and questionnaires (NAHC 2004).

Compliance with Accreditation Standards

Organizations that choose to be accredited by the Joint Commission must meet its management of information (IM) standards (Joint Commission 2007). Home care and hospice organizations may also decide to participate in the Community Health Accreditation Program (CHAP), whose core standards are related to information management, clinical records, and management information systems.

Framework for Providers

Through the Management of Information Standards in the Joint Commission's 2007 *Comprehensive Accreditation Manual for Home Care* (CAMHC), a series of required processes provide a framework for home care and hospice providers to more effectively and productively manage their information. The 2007 standards are functionally based, and IM is viewed as a function integral to the provision of care and services. Joint Commission IM standards describe the effective and continuous improvement of information management in healthcare organizations. The organization's leaders are responsible for achieving, maintaining, and improving an organization-wide approach to information management and ensuring the education and training of staff in managing and using information.

The Managed-Care Environment

To vie for managed-care contracts and to survive in the current competitive healthcare environment, home care and hospice providers need data and information to document the quality, outcomes, and costs of services provided. Providers who can demonstrate that their services and outcomes are superior (through comparisons with norms or comparative data) have a competitive edge.

Increasingly Complex Organizations

As healthcare organizations become more diverse, the need for available organization- and patient-level process and outcome data and information grows. Reliable, standardized systems for data documentation are essential, as are efficient methods for sharing data and information among providers within an organization.

Government Influences

The state and federal governments need home care and hospice information to examine such issues as access to healthcare services and the quality, outcome, utilization, and costs of services provided. Having such information is especially vital when reformed systems are introduced.

This trend is evidenced by two initiatives to capture outcome data: the Joint Commission's ORYX and CMS's OASIS. Both data sets are functioning as benchmarks of **performance improvement (PI)** within and among organizations. However, the raw data that each data set gathers must be collected in such a way that data quality is ensured. To do so, organizations must invest in quality technology and quality staff. Attaining quality comes under the practice of data quality management (DQM). DQM functions involve continuous improvement for data quality throughout an organization and include four key processes for data (AHIMA 2006):

- **Application:** The purpose for which data are collected
- **Collection:** The processes by which data elements are accumulated
- **Warehousing:** Processes and systems used to archive data and data journals
- **Analysis:** The process of translating data into information utilized for an application

Home Health and Hospice Record Content

The information provided upon referral is essential when determining whether a patient is suitable for admission to home care or hospice. Organizations develop admission criteria for determining the appropriateness of a patient's admission. These criteria depend on the types of care and services provided and on the care philosophies of the organizations, as well as Medicare coverage guidelines. In hospices, typical criteria include a terminal prognosis, the inappropriateness of curative treatment, a patient's desire for palliative treatment, a physician's order and, depending on hospice philosophy, the availability of a willing and able caregiver. Four general categories govern admission criteria (Haddad 1987):

1. Medical stability (with the exclusion of hospice patients)

2. Desire for home care (or hospice)

3. The suitability of the home environment

4. Financial resources

The Office of Inspector General (OIG) started monitoring all Medicare beneficiary access to **home health agencies (HHAs)** in 1999. In 1999, the OIG concluded that there appeared to be no widespread problem with placing Medicare hospital patients with HHAs. The 2007 OIG work plan continued to monitor home health outliers, enhanced payments for home health therapy, cyclical noncompliance, accuracy of data on the Home Health Compare Web site, and accuracy of coding claims for Medicare Home Health Resource groups and home health rehabilitation therapy services. Many HHAs use select OASIS questions to prescreen potential referrals. The OIG work plan increases the importance of documenting referrals not admitted.

The health record database originates with intake/referral data, and these data form the basis for initial care planning. Intake personnel commonly receive referral data via telephone or facsimile. Some organizations have nurses working in hospitals to assist in discharge planning and admitting patients to home or hospice care. Accurate referral data are a result of such early collaborative efforts, which are vitally important for continuity of care, especially in cases where patients are receiving clinical respiratory or pharmaceutical/infusion therapy.

At times, the information received via telephone from referral sources such as hospitals or physicians is not complete. The ideal method for providing patient referral information is to transmit it electronically. This will become more common as home care and hospice organizations develop links with managed-care organizations or healthcare networks. Faxing is also an efficient and preferred method of sending data from healthcare facilities, because the resulting data are more accurate and complete.

The intake or clinical record documentation must specify a start-of-care date. According to the Medicare CoP 484.55, the initial assessment visit must be held within either 48 hours of referral or 48 hours of the patient's return home or on the physician-specified start-of-care date. In the absence of a physician-specified start-of-care date, the initial assessment visit is conducted within 48 hours of the referral. When the physician specifies a start-of-care date, this supersedes the 48-hour time frame. The intake or clinical record documentation must specify a start-of-care date.

Recommendations for the content of referral and intake data in home care and hospice are listed in figure 11.1.

Documentation of a patient's physical limitations (such as blindness) is also desirable so that any problems with delivery of services can be anticipated.

Within 10 days, written transfer information, including transfer discharge summaries and other pertinent portions of the clinical record, should be received from the transferring facility (CMS 2005a).

Home Care and Hospice Assessment Information

Although the initial assessment may begin in the hospital or long-term care facility from which the patient is referred, it more commonly begins on the first home care visit or admission to hospice. The type, content, and comprehensiveness of the assessment should correspond to the types of care and services to be provided. It is essential to include the suitability of a home environment in the assessment, as well as any safety measures that are needed, especially relating to the placement of durable medical equipment (DME) and the provision of infusion therapy. It is also essential to assess the ability of a patient and family to use the equipment provided. In

Figure 11.1. Home care and hospice documentation requirements.

A. Documentation requirements for professional home care services

  1. Admission/referral/general information should include the following:

    a. Patient-identifying data and social information

    b. Name, address, and telephone number of next of kin or significant other

    c. Emergency contact

    d. Referral source

    e. Attending physician identification

    f. Reimbursement information

  2. Initial clinical information should be received from the attending physician, referral source, and/or patient or family, and documented prior to the first home visit. This includes the following:

    a. Admitting diagnosis(es), principal and other

    b. Surgical procedures related to home care admission

    c. Significant history and presenting problems, including the patient's social and emotional status, activity limitations, and limitations to healthcare access

    d. Allergies

    e. Initial medication and treatment orders including type and frequency of services to be provided and the supplies and equipment needed, in the form of verbal orders until signed orders are received

    f. Any dietary restrictions

    g. Patient's living arrangements

    h. Availability of able and willing caregiver

    i. Other agencies involved in care

B. Documentation requirements for hospice patient services

  1. Admission/referral/general information should include the following:

    a. Patient-identifying data and social information

    b. Name, address, and telephone number of next of kin or significant other

    c. Primary-care person's name, when applicable

    d. Referral source

    e. Physician identification

    f. Referral information

    g. Any other information that standards/regulations require

  2. Initial clinical information should be received from the attending physician (directly or through approved personnel) and documented prior to admission. This includes the following:

    a. Admitting diagnosis(es), principal and other

    b. Prognosis

    c. Current medical findings, including present physical, social, and emotional status of the patient

    d. Allergies

    e. Pain status

    f. Initial medical and treatment orders, including medications

    g. Input in establishing, and concurrence with, tentative treatment plan

    h. Any dietary restrictions

    i. History and physical examination

    j. For Medicare hospice patients, physician certification of a life expectancy of one year or less

    k. Any other information that standards/regulations require

C. Nonmedical services *Durable medical equipment*

  1. The following information should be received regarding homemaking services or durable medical equipment (DME) with no professional services provided.

    a. Client-identifying information, including client's name, address, and telephone number

    b. Demographic and social information, including sex, birth date, race, ethnicity, marital status, and usual living arrangement

    c. Emergency contact

addition, an assessment should include the availability of an able and willing caregiver, living arrangements, and family composition. This information, together with an assessment of activity and functional limitations, helps to determine the extent of required support. Nonhospice home care also uses this information to begin to plan for home care discharge.

Home Care and OASIS

Before comprehensive assessment and OASIS data collection can occur, the HHA must inform Medicare and Medicaid patients about OASIS and explain their rights with respect to the collection and reporting of the data. (Note: OASIS data collection is not required for non-Medicare or non-Medicaid patients.) These rights include the following:

- The right to be informed that OASIS information will be collected and for what purpose

- The right to have the information kept confidential and secure

- The right to be informed that OASIS information will not be disclosed except for legitimate purposes allowed by the Privacy Act

- The right to refuse to answer a specific question

- The right to see, review, and request changes on their assessment

A standard notice to patients that explains these rights in plain language was published in the *Federal Register* on June 18, 1999, and is available in English and Spanish on the OASIS Web site. HHAs must present and explain this required notice to beneficiaries before their initial OASIS assessment (CMS 2006).

When professional home care services are provided, the assessment becomes more comprehensive, documenting the presence as well as the absence of problems. The OIG work plan in years past included a determination on how assessment information helps to establish the case-mix adjustment used in determining the level of Medicare payment to an HHA for a particular patient.

Medicare CoP 484.55 requires a **comprehensive assessment** of patients. Each patient must receive, and an HHA must provide, a patient-specific, comprehensive assessment that accurately reflects the patient's current health status and includes information that may be used to demonstrate the patient's progress toward achievement of desired outcomes. The comprehensive assessment must identify the patient's continuing need for home care and meet the patient's medical, nursing, rehabilitative, social, and discharge planning needs. For Medicare beneficiaries, the HHA must verify the patient's eligibility for the Medicare home health benefit, including homebound status, both at the time of the initial assessment visit and at the time of the comprehensive assessment. The comprehensive assessment must also incorporate the use of the current version of OASIS items, using the language and groupings as specified by the secretary. The comprehensive assessment includes the collection of OASIS data items by a qualified clinician, such as a registered nurse, physical therapist, occupational therapist, or speech language pathologist.

For Medicare patients, there are additional requirements. Agencies are expected to conduct an assessment that accurately reflects the patient's current health status and includes information to establish and monitor a plan of care. The plan of care must be reviewed and updated at least every 60 days or as often as the severity of the patient's condition requires. The requirement to conduct a drug regimen review applies to all patients serviced by the HHA.

Federal regulations require a comprehensive assessment, with OASIS data items integrated, for all patients who receive skilled services except for those patients who are younger than age 18, receiving maternity services, receiving only housekeeping or chore services, or receiving only personal care services. This includes Medicare, Medicaid, managed care, and private pay patients accepted by the HHA. It also includes Medicaid patients receiving services under a waiver program. Although comprehensive assessments are required for all patients, the OASIS is not required for non-Medicare and non-Medicaid patients.

Subsequent updates on the comprehensive assessments must be conducted at certain intervals after admission. These updates must include specific data items in the current OASIS data set. OASIS data items are not meant to be the only items included in an agency's assessment process. They are standardized health assessment items that must be incorporated into an agency's own comprehensive assessment tool. For therapy-only cases, the comprehensive assessment should incorporate OASIS data items with other assessment data that the HHA currently collects for therapy patients, as opposed to simply adding them at the beginning or end (CMS 2006).

Hospice and Assessment

For hospice care, a patient and family assessment is performed. This involves a psychosocial assessment of patient and family needs, including adaptive and coping abilities. A spiritual assessment is also performed. This may be included on a psychosocial assessment form or on a separate assessment form. As is made evident in the context of the preceding discussion, the assessment of needed bereavement support begins on hospice admission.

When a hospice patient is experiencing pain, a pain assessment is performed to document the effectiveness of pain medication. Pain is considered the fifth vital sign according to the Joint Commission (1995) and should be assessed whether the patient has a history of pain or not. As discussed earlier, the content of assessment forms for particular categories of patients may conform to information items indicated by a critical path, with opportunity for individualization. A large number of home care and hospice organizations record pain assessment information electronically via hand-held devices or portable computers.

Figure 11.2 lists the recommendations for the content of initial assessment information for home care and hospice patients.

Home Health Plans of Care

In this section, the term *plans of care* refers to the Medicare-required home health plans of care that are documented on CMS form 485. Although the form is no longer required, the information contained within the form is required. Agencies may choose to use form 485 to meet the required documentation (CMS 2003). (See figure 11.3.) Plans of care may also be referred to as physician's orders. A description of care plans follows.

Based on the problems and needs identified during assessment and documented on the problem list, care plans are comprehensive and include documentation of care or services to be provided by all disciplines, independent contractors, organizations, and volunteers. The Joint Commission requires that an organization design the process, including required documentation, for care planning, review, and when necessary, revision. A policy for care plan review and revision must exist (Joint Commission 2007). Care plans include goals and objectives, as well as indicating the person/discipline responsible for implementing the plan(s), frequency of services to be provided, and the medications prescribed. Hospice care plans are interdisciplinary. Record documentation reflects the participation of patients, physicians, and pharmacists in care planning (Joint Commission 2007).

Figure 11.2.   Content of initial assessment information for professional home care and hospice patient services.

A. Content of initial assessment information for professional home care services

   1. The health record documents including the following initial nursing assessment information:

      a. Diagnoses and problems

      b. Past medical history and present illness

      c. Review of systems

      d. Present medications and treatment

      e. Activities of daily living and functional limitations

      f. Patient-care requirements, including equipment and supplies needed

      g. Dietary and nutritional information

      h. Suitability of the patient's residence and safety measures required to protect the client from injury

      i. Composition of household and relevant information regarding the family and caregiver

   2. When skilled nursing is required, the home care nursing staff obtains the initial nursing assessment on the first day of admission; when skilled-nursing care is ordered later during admission, the assessment is obtained at the first skilled-care visit. Be aware that some states require a nursing assessment even when skilled-nursing care is not provided. The record should also include documentation of the initial clinical evaluations of other disciplines or services that may have been involved in care of the patient (for example, physical therapy, occupational therapy, and pharmacy). The start of care begins at the first billable visit according to PPS regulations.

   3. Relevant x-ray, pathology, laboratory, or other test findings are documented.

B. Content of initial assessment information for hospice patient services

   1. The hospice record including the following relevant information:

      a. Diagnoses

      b. Past medical history

      c. Review of systems

      d. Present treatment

      e. Activities of daily living

      f. Functional limitations

      g. Patient-care requirements

      h. Dietary or nutritional information

      i. Pain assessment

      j. Psychosocial assessment

      k. Spiritual assessment

      l. Safety measures required to protect the patient from injury

      m. Equipment needed in the home

      n. Suitability of the patient and family residence

      o. Relevant information regarding the primary caregiver

   2. The appropriate hospice clinical staff obtains the initial assessment on the first day of admission or on the first home visit. The record should also include documentation of the initial clinical evaluations of other disciplines involved in the care of the patient (for example, physical therapy, occupational therapy, and pharmacy).

   3. Relevant x-ray, pathology, laboratory, or other test findings are documented.

   4. A problem list, based on the initial assessment, is documented.

C. Nonmedical services

   1. When nonmedical services, such as homemaker/chore services or DME are administered with no professional service provision, assessment information is much more limited than in the preceding cases. Referencing Joint Commission (2007) requirements is recommended in these instances.

Figure 11.3. Home health certification and plan of care (CMS form 485).

Department of Health and Human Services
Centers for Medicare & Medicaid Services

Form Approved
OMB No. 0938-0357

HOME HEALTH CERTIFICATION AND PLAN OF CARE

1. Patient's HI Claim No.	2. Start Of Care Date	3. Certification Period		4. Medical Record No.	5. Provider No.
		From:	To:		

6. Patient's Name and Address

7. Provider's Name, Address and Telephone Number

8. Date of Birth	9. Sex ☐ M ☐ F	10. Medications: Dose/Frequency/Route (N)ew (C)hanged

11. ICD-9-CM	Principal Diagnosis	Date

12. ICD-9-CM	Surgical Procedure	Date

13. ICD-9-CM	Other Pertinent Diagnoses	Date

14. DME and Supplies

15. Safety Measures:

16. Nutritional Req.

17. Allergies:

18.A. Functional Limitations

1 ☐ Amputation	5 ☐ Paralysis	9 ☐ Legally Blind
2 ☐ Bowel/Bladder (Incontinence)	6 ☐ Endurance	A ☐ Dyspnea With Minimal Exertion
3 ☐ Contracture	7 ☐ Ambulation	B ☐ Other (Specify)
4 ☐ Hearing	8 ☐ Speech	

18.B. Activities Permitted

1 ☐ Complete Bedrest	6 ☐ Partial Weight Bearing	A ☐ Wheelchair
2 ☐ Bedrest BRP	7 ☐ Independent At Home	B ☐ Walker
3 ☐ Up As Tolerated	8 ☐ Crutches	C ☐ No Restrictions
4 ☐ Transfer Bed/Chair	9 ☐ Cane	D ☐ Other (Specify)
5 ☐ Exercises Prescribed		

19. Mental Status:

| 1 ☐ Oriented | 3 ☐ Forgetful | 5 ☐ Disoriented | 7 ☐ Agitated |
| 2 ☐ Comatose | 4 ☐ Depressed | 6 ☐ Lethargic | 8 ☐ Other |

20. Prognosis: 1 ☐ Poor   2 ☐ Guarded   3 ☐ Fair   4 ☐ Good   5 ☐ Excellent

21. Orders for Discipline and Treatments (Specify Amount/Frequency/Duration)

22. Goals/Rehabilitation Potential/Discharge Plans

23. Nurse's Signature and Date of Verbal SOC Where Applicable:	25. Date HHA Received Signed POT

24. Physician's Name and Address	26. I certify/recertify that this patient is confined to his/her home and needs intermittent skilled nursing care, physical therapy and/or speech therapy or continues to need occupational therapy. The patient is under my care, and I have authorized the services on this plan of care and will periodically review the plan.
27. Attending Physician's Signature and Date Signed	28. Anyone who misrepresents, falsifies, or conceals essential information required for payment of Federal funds may be subject to fine, imprisonment, or civil penalty under applicable Federal laws.

Form CMS-485 (C-3) (02-94) (Formerly HCFA-485) (Print Aligned)

Source: CMS 1994.

For home care reimbursement purposes, CMS form 485 is used to document the physician's plan-of-care orders. The physician uses CMS form 485 to certify the patient's need for home health service. Most home health agencies have computer-based applications to assist them in completing CMS form 485 and in tracking the need for recertification, which is required every 60 days. Hospice certifications are required after the first 90 days, the second 90 days, and 60 days thereafter.

When a Medicare-certified hospice contracts with an inpatient facility, the inpatient care must be based on the interdisciplinary care plan of the hospice. The hospice maintains control of the care, and this must be made evident in the health record. Policies, procedures, and contracts define the relevant information to be shared among providers, so gaps in care are prevented, and the hospice record documents all services provided. Procedures should provide for written and oral communication among hospice team members and inpatient care providers throughout the inpatient care episode.

Standardized care plans and protocols are available for specific service provision and for medical and nursing diagnoses. Any standardized care plans that are used must be individualized for each patient and caregiver. When critical paths are used, standardized or structured care plans may also be used for documentation.

Regardless of an organization's Medicare certification status, a care plan conforms to the physician's plan-of-care orders. The care plan is based on the nursing initial assessment, as well as the initial assessments of other disciplines involved in the care of the patient. An interdisciplinary care plan is recommended, but separate discipline care plans may be documented when they are filed together in the health record.

Figure 11.4 lists the content of interdisciplinary care plans for professional home care and for hospice patients.

Physician's Orders and Plans of Care

As indicated by the type of care service provided, the health record includes legible, complete, signed, and dated physician's diagnoses and therapeutic orders. The person authorized to accept the orders must record, date, and sign all verbal or telephone orders, and the attending physician must countersign and date the orders within the time period specified in organization policy and required by state regulations. When pharmaceutical care is provided, the pharmacist reviews prescriptions and verbal orders before dispensing medication.

CMS views the initial percentage payment as a **request for anticipated payment (RAP)** rather than a Medicare claim for home health PPS purposes. The first percentage payment under home health PPS does not require a physician-signed plan of care before submission. The RAP for the episode may be submitted based on verbal orders. To request anticipated payment for the initial percentage based on a physician's verbal orders, a copy of the plan of care with all physician's verbal orders—in writing with the date of receipt by the registered nurse or qualified therapist responsible for furnishing or supervising the ordered services—must be completed and immediately sent to the physician for signature. The RAP may be submitted when the HHA has a signed referral prescribing the physician's detailed orders for services and the patient's condition. Signed orders must be obtained as soon as possible and before the claim for services is submitted for the final percentage payment of each episode. The claim for the final percentage payment requires a signed plan of care prior to billing.

The RAP will be canceled and recovered unless the claim for the episode is submitted within 60 days from the end of the episode or the issuance of the anticipated payment. This split-percentage payment approach helps alleviate cash flow concerns but increases the need for timely signed orders.

Clinical and Progress Notes

For this discussion, the term *clinical note* refers to a note documenting care services provided, and *progress note* refers to a summary note. A progress note may be documented upon any transfer between hospice care levels, on discharge, or when physicians or others need a summary of recent services provided.

Figure 11.4. Content of interdisciplinary care plans for professional home care services and for hospice patients.

A. Content of interdisciplinary care plan for professional home care services

  1. The care plan documents the following information:

    a. Identified patient problems

    b. Expected outcomes, long- and short-term goals

    c. Plans and interventions, including medications prescribed and required medical equipment to be provided to meet the identified goals

    d. Discipline responsible for carrying out plans and achieving goals

    e. Dates when expected outcomes are met

    f. Signature of the nurse or care coordinator for the patient

  2. Verbal orders should be appropriately documented and signed by the attending physician within the required time and prior to billing; care plan should be updated when an additional discipline enters the care of the patient or when change occurs in care management.

  3. The care plan should undergo interdisciplinary review, even when separate discipline care plans may be documented. The service providers and, whenever possible, the attending physician, should perform this review. When care services are provided through contractual agreement, persons who provide these services should also participate in care plan review.

  4. Care plan reviews should be individualized to each patient and occur at least every 60 days. Reviews should be documented in case conference minutes or elsewhere in the health record. Care plan changes should also be documented.

  5. The record should clearly reflect coordination of care planning between all disciplines, paraprofessionals, organizations, and other care providers, as well as between the organization, the attending physician, and the patient.

B. Content of interdisciplinary care plan for hospice patient services

  1. It is recommended that, within one week of admission, an interdisciplinary care plan be developed for the patient and family. This plan should conform to physician's orders and be based on clinical information in the initial database and problem list. The care plan documents the following information:

    a. Identified patient and family problems and needs

    b. Identified goals that are realistic, achievable, and measurable

    c. Care and services to be provided to meet identified goals, including medications prescribed and required medical equipment

    d. The signature of the attending physician and team coordinator for the patient and family

  2. Verbal orders should be appropriately documented and signed by the attending physician; care plan should be updated when an additional discipline enters the care of the patient and family or when change occurs in care management.

  3. The planned frequency of interdisciplinary care plan review should be documented. Although each care plan is individualized to the patient, reviews should occur no less than every two weeks after admission. Care plan changes should be documented, and when appropriate, there must be documentation of new orders signed by the attending physician.

  4. Record documentation should include the findings and conclusions of team case conferences.

  5. Continuing discussions among the attending physician and members of the interdisciplinary team should be documented.

C. Nonmedical services

  1. When nonmedical services are provided, the health record should contain documentation of the services performed. Refer to Joint Commission (2007) standards for additional guidance.

Clinical Notes and Visit Documentation

Clinical and visit notes are designed to give a clear, comprehensive picture of the patient's clinical status, the care being provided, and the patient's response to that care. Policies, procedures, and forms can ensure that documentation is entered efficiently into the record and that such important aspects of care as supervision of care and patient and family education are documented. Documentation incorporates conversations with physicians, pharmacists, relatives, and others who have an impact on patient care.

When nonmedical services are being provided and there is no professional service provision, a checklist may be used to document the services provided.

When professional services are provided, visits by licensed certified staff are documented in a signed and dated clinical progress note or flow sheet entry, which includes the following information:

- A description of the patient's physical and psychosocial signs and symptoms or changes in signs and symptoms

- Any treatment, service, or medication rendered and the patient's reaction

- Any changes in the patient's condition or the patient's and family's psychosocial status

- Any patient and family instruction given, as well as patient and family demonstration or verbalization of knowledge of instructions given

- Plans for future visits

When flow sheets are used to document interventions or progress toward care goals, clinical notes are then used to record supplemental information such as assessment of findings, interventions and plans, telephone conversations, and nursing supervisory visits every 14 days. When flow sheet documentation uses a coding system, a legend should appear on the form.

The comprehensive assessment must include a review of all medications the patient is currently using in order to identify any potential adverse effects and drug and food reactions, including ineffective drug therapy, significant side effects, significant drug and food interactions, duplicate drug therapy, and noncompliance with drug therapy. This requirement applies to all patients being serviced by the HHA, regardless of whether OASIS-specific requirements apply.

When authorized home care or hospice staff administers medications, the action is documented in the health record, as well as any beneficial effects and presumed adverse drug reactions. When pharmaceutical and infusion therapy services are provided, patients are continually monitored for medication effectiveness and actual or potential medication-related problems. This is a collaborative process involving the pharmacist, and documentation will show evidence of this collaboration. The health record provides evidence that conclusions and findings of medication monitoring are communicated to all healthcare professionals involved in the patient's care (Joint Commission 2007). When pharmaceutical services are provided, pharmacy records are filed with health records (Joint Commission 2007). The American Society of Health-System Pharmacists (2003) has developed educational materials on the health record and the pharmacist's record documentation.

Home Health Aide Documentation

Agencies must provide enough home health aide services to meet the needs of the patient. Home health aides who are employees of the home care or hospice, as well as aides used by the agency hospice under an arrangement or contract, must meet the personnel qualifications specified by the *Conditions of Participation*. Home health aides are selected on the basis of such factors as a sympathetic attitude toward the care of the sick; ability to read, write, and carry out directions; and maturity and ability to deal effectively with the demands of the job. They are closely supervised to ensure their competence in providing care. A registered nurse provides written patient-care instructions and monitors the services provided by the home health aide. This nurse also visits the patient's residence at least once every two weeks if aide services are provided, in order to assess aide services and relationships and determine whether goals are being met. The on-site visit need not be made while the aide is furnishing services. Home health aide services should be adequately documented in the health record, including nursing orders for the home health aide and an assignment sheet, flow sheet, and narrative notations documenting services rendered. The nurse or therapist should also include documentation of coordination with the aide and continuing supervision of the aide's services. It is recommended that home health aides record the services they provide in a checklist format. Aides should document short narrative notes only when reporting unusual occurrences (for example, changes in the condition of the patient or phone calls) or when state regulations require it.

Dietary and Nutritional Information

Health record documentation should reflect, as appropriate, the patient's nutrient intake, dietary instructions to the patient and family, and demonstration or verbalization from the patient and family of dietary instructions given. A diet history and nutritional evaluation by a dietician should be completed when appropriate as defined in organization policy.

Progress Notes and the Discharge Transfer Record

Upon a patient's discharge or death, a summary is documented. This report includes the following information:

- Admission and discharge dates and type of discharge

- Care and support provided by each discipline

- Status of goal attained upon discharge or death

- When discharged alive, the status of the patient and the reason for discharge

- Discharge diagnoses or problems

- Any unmet needs and referrals for continuing care

- For hospice settings, time (if known) and place of death, as well as plans for bereavement follow-up

Home care or hospice organizations may also include other outcome monitoring information on their discharge summaries. OASIS data are collected and completed by the qualified clinician when a patient transfers to an inpatient facility with or without discharge, discharge to community, or death at home. Agencies may take up to seven calendar days after the date of completion of the comprehensive assessment to enter (encode) the OASIS data into their computers using **Home Assessment Validation and Entry (HAVEN)** software or a similar application. The day the clinician completes the assessment is day zero for purposes of calculating the seven-day window. Encoding of all OASIS data items must be complete, or locked, in order to accurately compute the information (Health Insurance Prospective Payment System [HIPPS] code set) necessary for billing Medicare patients under the prospective payment system.

When hospice patients are transferred between home and inpatient care, a transfer note is created. The documentation summarizes the patient's status, care, and support being provided, as well as the reason for transfer.

For Medicare-certified home health agencies, a discharge summary that includes a patient's medical and health status at discharge must be made available to the patient's attending physician, and physicians must be informed of this availability. The discharge summary may be incorporated into the routine summary reports already furnished by the physician (CMS 2005a).

Notations should be appropriately labeled and should provide an overall, comprehensive view of the patient's total progress and current summary report including social, emotional, and behavioral adjustments relative to the diagnosis, treatment, rehabilitation potential, and anticipated outcomes toward recovery or further debilitation. Medicare regulations do not dictate the frequency with which progress notes must be written.

The Medicare Hospice Benefit

It is essential that health information managers working in hospice know what makes a patient eligible for the Medicare hospice benefit and how to document provision of care. Most hospice reimbursement hinges on meeting those requirements. Medicare coverage for hospice care began with enactment of section 122 of public law 97–248, the **Tax Equity and Fiscal Responsibility Act of 1982 (TEFRA)**. The *Code of Federal Regulations* (Medicare CoP 484.55) defines the Medicare hospice benefit and documentation requirements. Interpretive guidelines provide additional guidance on required documentation. Throughout this section, definitions and requirements have been abstracted from these sources. Patients must elect hospice care from a Medicare-certified hospice to be eligible for Medicare reimbursement. When patients elect hospice care, they waive their rights to Medicare reimbursement for treatment of their principal (terminal) diagnosis and related conditions outside of care provided by the designated hospice, by another hospice provided under arrangements made by the designated hospice, or by the individual's attending physician when that physician is not an employee of the designated hospice or receiving compensation from the hospice for those services. An individual can revoke the Medicare hospice benefit and then reelect the benefit after revocation. An individual can also elect to change the designated hospice program. Election, revocation, and reelection of the Medicare hospice benefit—as well as change of the designated hospice—must be documented in the health record, and that documentation should clearly show that the patient or the patient's legal representative was well-informed. Patients can elect the hospice benefit at any time. The periods consist of the following:

[handwritten margin note: must be terminally ill. Life expectancy of less than 6 months]

1. The initial 90-day period

2. The subsequent 90-day period

3. The subsequent extension of an unlimited number of 60-day periods when the patient is certified terminally ill with a six-month prognosis if the disease runs its normal course

To be eligible for the hospice benefit, a patient must have a physician-certified terminal illness. A written certification must be obtained for each of the four periods in the preceding list, and the certification must indicate a life expectancy of six months or less if the terminal illness runs its normal course. The health record should contain evidence of this certification.

Medicare hospice fiscal intermediaries are beginning to conduct focused medical reviews of hospice claims. One area these intermediaries are questioning concerns the validity of the terminal certification of some patients. Some cases of long lengths of stay and patients with chronic diagnoses have led to this questioning.

To prevent denials, coding personnel are advised to use the most specific diagnosis codes and to ensure that the terminal diagnosis is always listed as the principal diagnosis. All complications of chronic conditions should be documented and coded as appropriate. In addition, health record documentation on admission and throughout a hospice episode must support a patient's terminal status. When a claim is selected for medical review, it is recommended that copies of all health record documentation, including the admission assessment, be submitted to a fiscal intermediary for review (Hospice Association of America 2005).

The Hospice Association of America (HAA), in conjunction with CMS and the National Hospice Organization, has developed guidelines on screening hospice patients who have illnesses other than cancer for admissions and recertifications. Guidelines address determining a patient's prognosis, what to look for, and what to document (HAA 2005).

Provision of Care under the Medicare Hospice Benefit and Documentation

Medicare has defined four general hospice care levels and has assigned different reimbursement rates to each:

1. Routine home care

2. Continuous home care

3. Inpatient respite care

4. General inpatient care

A hospice must maintain management control of a patient's care, regardless of the treatment setting, and the health record must contain evidence of this control. According to Medicare regulations, hospices that cannot provide inpatient care directly must contract with an inpatient care provider.

Hospice regulations require an interdisciplinary group to plan and provide or supervise the care and services provided to patients and families. This group includes at least the following hospice employees:

*   A doctor of medicine or osteopathy

*   A registered nurse

*   A social worker

*   A pastoral counselor or another type of counselor

The care plan becomes the basis for team decision making and can be considered the map for team interventions.

Medicare requires that volunteers be used in administrative or direct patient care roles. In many hospices, volunteers provide services and support to the patient, family, or significant other. Volunteers are considered members of the interdisciplinary team.

Following is a summary of the advice included in this chapter regarding documentation and the Medicare hospice benefit:

*   The health record must contain evidence that the interdisciplinary team plans and manages a patient's care across all settings of care.

- The health record must contain evidence that hospice interdisciplinary care continues when a patient is admitted for inpatient hospice care.

- Health record documentation must justify the level of hospice care the patient is receiving. When the status of a patient changes, requiring continuous home care or inpatient care, clinical notes must document this change, and the care plan must be revised to indicate any new problems or changes in plans.

Volunteer Documentation

Volunteers are defined in 42 CFR 418.3 as hospice employees who facilitate compliance with the hospice core services requirement. The hospice uses volunteers, in defined roles, under the supervision of a designated hospice employee. The hospice must provide appropriate volunteer training consistent with the specific tasks that volunteers perform. The interdisciplinary group conducts an assessment of the patient's and caregiver's need for a volunteer. Volunteers must be used in administrative or direct patient care roles. Agencies must document the roles assigned to that hospice's volunteers. Hospices use volunteers to supplement the care being provided by the paid staff who work directly with patients and their family members, both in the patients' homes and the inpatient setting. Hospices must document the cost savings of volunteers, which must include the identification of necessary positions occupied by volunteers, work time spent by volunteers, and estimates of the dollar costs that the hospice would have incurred if paid employees occupied the positions. Hospices must document a continual level of volunteer activity and expansion of care and services achieved through the use of volunteers, including the types of services and the time worked (CMS 2005a).

In hospice settings, volunteers write notes after each visit and include them in the hospice record using separate volunteer documentation forms. The volunteer coordinator or nurse team coordinator reviews the volunteer's notes and initials them before they are filed. Volunteer's notes include the following information:

- New issues, special concerns, or significant changes observed in the patient or family since last contact

- The volunteer's response and interventions to changes/concerns at this contact

- The volunteer's plan for next contact

- The request for special consultation/contact from other staff when needed

Bereavement Documentation

Bereavement counseling services are often provided to the family and caregivers after a patient's death. Counseling is provided on the basis of an assessment of the family's and caregiver's needs, the presence of any risk factors associated with the patient's death, and the ability of the family and caregivers to cope with grief. The supervisor of bereavement services may be the interdisciplinary group social worker or other professional with documented evidence of training and experience in dealing with grief. Documentation for bereavement counseling does not necessarily have to be contained in the clinical record, but it must be maintained by the hospice in an organized, easily retrievable manner for a specified time period.

The hospice record includes an initial and follow-up bereavement assessment of the family and significant others that documents the physical and emotional status of the family and significant others. It is recommended that the initial bereavement assessment be completed at the team meeting following the patient's death. The bereavement follow-up assessment is completed within four weeks of the patient's death. Subsequent bereavement assessments are completed as deemed necessary by the hospice bereavement staff and as stated in hospice policy. Notes are written after each bereavement visit. These notes document the general emotional and physical status of the family and significant other at that visit, any counseling that was performed or follow-up action taken, and any changes in plans. On discharge from bereavement follow-up, a summary is written. This summary includes appropriate information regarding services provided to the family and significant other and the status of the family and significant other during the last bereavement contact.

Justification of Hospice Skilled Care Levels

Employees in Medicare-certified hospices must be conscientious when documenting a patient's need for inpatient and continuous home care and the actual provision of services. To be considered continuous by Medicare, home care must be provided for at least 12 hours in one 24-hour period (for example, 12 a.m. to 11:59 p.m.), and care must be predominantly skilled-nursing care. Continuous care is initiated during periods of crisis (such as severe pain, hemorrhaging, and imminent death) or when active palliation or management of acute medical symptoms is needed. Record documentation must describe the crisis and include the date and time it occurred. In conjunction with this, the patient's care plan is revised to reflect the changes in the problems and care provision. During continuous care, an extensive nursing note is written at least hourly, and it is signed with the date and time, as are all record notations during this period. When inpatient care is required, a medical crisis such as "symptoms out of control" is documented. On admission and continuously throughout the inpatient care period, documentation reflects the patient's need for acute care. As with continuous care, the interdisciplinary care plan is modified to reflect new or exacerbated problems, as well as changes in care provision. The hospice furnishes a copy of the patient's plan of care to the inpatient provider and specifies the inpatient services to be furnished.

Short-term inpatient care may be provided in a Medicare hospice inpatient unit. The Medicare conditions for each of these providers of service apply to all patients regardless of payment source, unless a specific exception is provided in the regulations. Services provided in an inpatient setting must conform to the hospice patient's written plan of care and must be reasonable and necessary for the palliation of symptoms or the management of the terminal illness. General inpatient care may be required to adjust and monitor the patient's pain control or manage acute or chronic symptoms that cannot be managed in another setting. Inpatient admission may also be furnished to provide respite for the patient's family or other persons caring for the individual at home. Respite care is the only type of inpatient care that may be furnished in a nursing facility. The hospice is accountable for all hospice services provided under arrangement at nursing facilities. The hospice furnishes the inpatient provider a copy of the patient's plan of care and specifies the inpatient services to be furnished. The hospice health record includes a record of all inpatient services and events and a copy of the discharge summary (CMS 2005a).

The Medicare Home Care Benefit

Successful health information managers working in home health often refer to the Medicare *Benefit Policy Manual*, chapter 7 "Home Health Services" (CMS 2005a). Referencing the policy manual is key to understanding how the Medicare home care benefit drives documentation requirements for patient care, home health certification, CMS form 485, Medicare home care surveys, and the prospective payment system. The following sections describe some of those requirements.

Home Health Prospective Payment System

Medicare reimburses all home health agencies (HHAs) under a prospective payment system (PPS). PPS is designed to promote efficiency and help prevent waste and abuse within the home health payment system.

Between 1990 and 1997, home healthcare expenditures grew from 2.9 percent to nearly 9 percent of all Medicare payments. The earlier cost-based system was creating growth in home health spending, due in large part to the lack of incentives to efficiently provide care. Previously, HHAs had been paid based on the costs of providing care, which was only subject to a per visit limit. Thus, the more visits HHAs provided and the greater the cost increases, the greater the payments to those HHAs. The old system encouraged abuse, as evidenced by the increase in per-beneficiary visits, which more than doubled from 36 in 1990 to 80 in 1997. The General Accounting Office reported in 2002 that Medicare payments to home health agencies were considerably higher than payments for full home healthcare episodes (on average, about 35 percent higher than the estimated cost of home healthcare when figures were compared for the first six months of 2001) (GAO 2002). In 2005, according to CMS Health Care Information System (HCIS) data, the average number of beneficiary visits was 31 with an average payment per patient of $4050.00.

The interim payment system, which was mandated by the Balanced Budget Act of 1997 and replaced three years later with the PPS, was based on the lowest of reasonable costs, an aggregate cost limit per visit, or an aggregate cost limit per beneficiary. Such limits removed incentives to provide unnecessary visits in order to increase payment.

Under the PPS, HHAs are now paid a predetermined base payment that may vary per each 60-day episode of care depending on the patient's severity of illness and home health needs. As identified through completion of the OASIS documentation, the services that are reimbursed include home health aide visits, skilled-nursing visits, supplies, medical social services, and therapy. Key points of the PPS include the items listed in figure 11.5.

The Medicare Home Care Benefit and Documentation of Eligibility

Medicare certification of Part A home care providers includes the home health agency. Because Medicare Part B providers (such as DME, pharmacy, and others) are considered vendors, they are not certified. The Home Health Agency Manual defines the Medicare home care benefit and documentation in relation to such. Interpretive guidelines provide additional directions concerning required documentation. Throughout this section, definitions and requirements have been abstracted from these sources (all other sources are referenced).

To be eligible for Medicare-reimbursed home healthcare, a Medicare beneficiary must meet the following conditions:

- The beneficiary is confined to home.

- The beneficiary is under the care of a physician, who establishes and approves the plan of care for the individual.

- The beneficiary needs intermittent, skilled-nursing care, physical therapy, speech therapy services, or continuing occupational therapy.

Figure 11.5. Key points of home health agency (HHA) prospective payment system (PPS) reimbursement.

- Medicare will reimburse HHAs for each 60-day episode of care as long as the patient remains eligible and the services are medically necessary.
- Beneficiaries who have greater home healthcare needs will warrant higher payment rates to their HHAs.
- National payment rates ranging from $1,100 to $5,900 for each 60-day episode of service will be used. Payment is determined by the intensity of care provided. Data documented from patient assessments (which is already a requirement for all Medicare-participating HHAs) will be used to support payment rates. Payment rates are also adjusted by area wage differences.
- In cases where the patient's care results in unusually high home healthcare costs, outlier payments will be made for a portion of the amount of costs beyond the set threshold.
- In order to streamline the approval process and ensure adequate payment when an HHA accepts a new Medicare patient, the Centers for Medicare and Medicaid Services (CMS) will pay up front 60 percent of the initial episode reimbursement. The HHA will receive the remaining 40 percent of payment at the end of that initial episode of care. Episodes of care that follow will be paid based on equally divided payments between the beginning and end of those care episodes.
- Patients who have a significant change in their condition during an episode of care will have an adjustment made to their payment rate.
- HHAs will get a partial episode payment according to PPS regulations when a patient chooses to transfer or to discharge from and return to the same agency that warrants a new clock for payment. This is considered a "beneficiary elected transfer." When a new 60-day episode begins, the original 60-day payment is proportionally adjusted to reflect the time the beneficiary remained under the agency's care before the intervening event. (CMS 2005a)
- HHAs and suppliers will be paid separately for durable medical equipment if it is medically necessary.
- CMS will perform extensive reviews to assess errors or trends within this new payment system as well as to ensure that the quality of patient care is maintained.

Home Confinement (Homebound Status)

Patients should be essentially homebound. This does not mean that the patient must be bed-ridden, but leaving home must present considerable difficulty and be infrequent and of short duration unless for medical reasons. The reason(s) for homebound status and the fact that the patient is homebound must be recorded on CMS form 485 or facsimile, on the comprehensive assessment, and periodically in the clinical notes. Documentation regarding homebound status should be descriptive. Why is a patient homebound? What happens when a patient walks too far? When the patient visits the doctor, what type of assistance is provided? Nursing and therapy documentation should be congruent, not conflicting. OASIS items MO350–MO380 and Life System Profile items MO640–MO820 should also support the patient's homebound status. According to CMS regulations, driving does not necessarily render a patient nonhomebound (CMS 2005a).

Home Health under the Care of a Physician

The beneficiary's physician is responsible for signing the home health certification CMS form 485 upon the initiation of any plan of care. Upon the completion of every 60-day episode during which the patient received continuous home healthcare from the same home health agency, the beneficiary's physician is responsible for home health recertification. The home health prospective payment system should not have changed the plan of care. It remains the beneficiary's physician's responsibility to develop a plan of care based on his or her intimate knowledge of the medical condition of the home health patient. The plan of care developed in consultation with the agency staff covers all pertinent diagnoses, mental status, types of services and equipment required, frequency of visits, prognosis, rehabilitation potential, functional limitations, activities permitted, nutritional requirements, medications and treatments, safety measures to protect against injury, instructions for timely discharge or referral, and any other appropriate items.

The patient's physician approves the patient's plan of care and certifies the need for home health services by signing a home health certification and plan of care, CMS form 485 (figure 11.3, p. 391). CMS now allows for physician review, care plan oversight, and certification update reimbursement. Upon the completion of every 60-day episode if the patient continues to receive continuous home healthcare from the same home health agency, the beneficiary's physician is responsible for recertification of the plan of care.

Skilled Services Requirement for Benefit Eligibility

The patient must require skilled services. The three required skilled services include intermittent skilled-nursing care, physical therapy, and speech therapy. Patients receiving one of these three services are also eligible to receive medical social services and occupational therapy; the occupational therapy may be continued if required after other skilled services have been discontinued.

The skilled care being provided must be reasonable and necessary. A fiscal intermediary's decisions must be based on the individual patient's health status and medical need as reflected in his or her plan of care and health record. Although intermediaries have edit screens to detect questionable claims, the information from these screens cannot be the only reason for denying coverage, and documentation must also be reviewed.

According to CMS, reimbursable skilled-nursing care consists of services that are reasonable and necessary to the treatment of illness or services that must be performed by or under the direct supervision of a licensed nurse if the safety of the patient is to be ensured and the desired result achieved. General categories of reimbursable skilled services include the following:

- Observation and assessment when significant changes in the patient's condition could occur that would require the skills or evaluation of a skilled nurse and that may result in changes in the client's plan of treatment or in possible institutionalization

- Teaching and training activities that require nursing skills or knowledge

- Performance of skilled procedures such as the insertion and sterile irrigation of catheter, intravenous and intramuscular injections, and wound care

- Management and evaluation of the care plan

The Medicare *Benefit Policy Manual*, chapter 7, "Home Health Services," includes additional discussion regarding coverage for skilled care services, as well as for other reimbursable services (CMS 2005a). Documentation throughout the record must continually confirm the need for and provision of skilled services.

When a patient begins receiving one of the skilled services described in the preceding material, he or she qualifies for other reimbursable services. These other services include medical social services provided to patients under direction of a physician, part-time or intermittent home health aide services, medical supplies (other than drugs or biologicals), and DME available from the agency. Recent changes to Medicare home care regulations allow medical social services of a brief duration to be provided to families of patients.

Intermittent or Part-Time Home Care Benefits

For coverage of home care benefits, skilled nursing and aide services must be provided on an intermittent or part-time basis. Medicare *Benefit Policy Manual* (2005a) defines the terms intermittent and part-time in detail.

Home Health Certification and Plan of Care

Home Health Certification and Plan of Care, CMS form 485, is designed to meet regulatory requirements for the physician's plan of care; although as previously stated is not a mandated form. It documents a physician's certification and recertification that a patient needs home health services and meets the Medicare requirements for receipt of home health services. Medicare *Benefit Policy Manual*, chapter 7, offers detailed instructions on how to provide this information (CMS 2005a). The agency must document this before the final claim for each episode can be submitted to the Medicare fiscal intermediary. The patient's physician must review, update, and recertify the plan of care at least every 60 days.

Medicare Home Care Surveys

Medicare home care surveyors use medical, nursing, and rehabilitative care indicators to determine the quality of a patient's care and the scope of the home health agency services provided to the client. These surveyors use the CMS Home Health Functional Assessment to document data from home care record reviews and patient visits. During a standard Medicare survey, an agency's admission volume determines the number of records to be reviewed, and surveyors review a stratified sample of clinical records.

Based on record review, employee interviews, and home visits to patients, Medicare surveyors make their conclusions about the areas listed in figure 11.6.

Medicare guideline CoP 484.20(a) instructs surveyors on presurvey and on-site survey activity related to OASIS data collection. Before the survey, surveyors check with the state OASIS education or automation coordinator and review OASIS data management reports to determine whether encoding is completed within seven days after completing the OASIS data set. On-site, surveyors check to see if the HHA is transmitting its own data or has an arrangement with an outside entity acting on behalf of the HHA to electronically submit OASIS data to the state agency. If so, surveyors confirm that a written contract exists that describes the

Figure 11.6. Information documented by Medicare surveyors from home care record reviews and patient visits.

Partial or extended Medicare surveys can focus on the following standards:

CoP 484.10 Patient's rights

CoP 484.11 Release of patient-identifiable OASIS information

CoP 484.12 Compliance with federal, state, and local laws; disclosure and ownership information; and accepted professional standards and principles

CoP 484.14(g) Coordination of services

CoP 484.18 Acceptance of patients, plans of care, and medical supervision

CoP 484.36 Home health aide services

CoP 484.48 Clinical records

CoP 484.14 Organization, services, and administration

CoP 484.16 Group of professional personnel

CoP 484.30 Skilled-nursing services

CoP 484.32 Therapy services

CoP 484.34 Medical social services

CoP 484.38 Qualification to furnish outpatient physical therapy or speech therapy

arrangement the HHA has with the outside entity to enter and transmit OASIS data on behalf of the HHA. Surveyors determine the process for encoding and locking OASIS data being readied for transmission to the state. When questions are raised through interview or record review, surveyors review the HHA's policies regarding encoding time frames. New HHAs seeking initial certification must apply for appropriate state and federal HHA identification and passwords and be able to demonstrate compliance with collecting, completing, encoding, and reporting OASIS data for all applicable patients in an electronic format that meets CMS specifications prior to the initial survey (CMS 2006).

Home Care Medicare Reimbursement Documentation Guidelines

Whether federally or privately funded, insurance programs employ specific guidelines to determine patient eligibility for home care benefits. When a home care organization accepts a client for care, it also assumes the responsibility for documenting that the client meets the eligibility guidelines at the time of admission and throughout the period of time that the client receives care. Failure to do so can lead to additional costs for the agency should claims be denied.

Medicare is the largest single payer for home care services. Other public funding sources for home care include Medicaid, the Older Americans Act, Title XX social services block grants, the Veterans' Administration, and **Civilian Health and Medical Program of the Uniformed Services (CHAMPUS)**. Private insurance accounts for only a small portion of home care payments. Slightly more than one-fifth of home care services is financed through out-of-pocket payments. Clearly, it serves the best interests of home care organizations to be familiar with the requirements of the various third-party payers and design documentation systems that not only facilitate the provision of high-quality care but also ensure documentation of specific information required for reimbursement.

Initial Agency Contact Documentation

Documentation of the initial agency contact must establish that the client is eligible for services that are reimbursed by the third-party payer and that the professional caregiver has rendered a necessary service during the contact. Many third-party payers will only reimburse for conditions of an acute nature. The assessment must give a clear picture of the patient's status before the onset of the acute illness, report the date of onset of the acute illness, and describe the patient's limitations that resulted from the illness and make it necessary for home care services to be provided.

Physician Plan of Care

Third-party payers require that professional services be provided under a plan of care that a physician has established. The plan of care, which documents physician's orders, should reflect an accurate diagnosis and list treatments and services to be provided. In addition, the plan of care should indicate the frequency and duration expected for each treatment modality. Subsequent documentation should note that services have been provided within the bounds of the plan of care and any subsequent physician's orders. The third-party payer has no obligation to reimburse for services that are provided that have not been specifically ordered or were provided more frequently or for a longer duration than ordered. It is important to note that the services provided must be appropriate to the patient's diagnosis(es). For example, when physical therapy services are ordered, the patient's diagnosis(es) must reflect that the client has a problem that requires the services of a physical therapist.

Homebound status must be established during the initial visit. The Medicare Home Health Agency Manual states that, by definition, homebound status is retained when the patient can leave home only with some difficulty for medical appointments or for occasional other purposes. Continuing documentation substantiates this homebound status.

First Visit Criteria

It is also important for the professional caregiver to document any care given during the initial visit to the client. Most third-party payers will not reimburse a visit made for assessment purposes alone. If the nurse assesses a healing wound during an initial assessment and then changes the dressing, the assessment and change of dressing must be documented. Documentation language is important. The third-party payer wants to see that the client is receiving the care that the skilled professional is trained to give; so record documentation must demonstrate that the care has been provided. Need-based charting is a must. Each entry must stand alone in its ability to demonstrate that a problem or need existed, that it was within the realm of reimbursable services, that intervention was taken by a skilled professional, and that the effects of the intervention taken were assessed. Instead of simply saying that a leg wound was dressed, nurses must describe the wound, the amount and type of drainage, any odor, and the diameter and depth. Documentation must specifically indicate what kind of wound dressing was used, the client's response to the procedure, the client's understanding of his or her role in the care of the wound, and the plan for future visits.

Because of the need for detailed, specific documentation, it has become increasingly important that the format of the record expedite documentation of these factors. However, some third-party reviewers have not been receptive to forms that use a checklist format to facilitate documentation on flow sheets. The professional caregiver must be acutely aware of how entries in the record are documented. Simple remarks such as "walks with walker" may signify to the reviewer that the patient is no longer homebound when the caregiver may have meant that the patient requires the use of a walker to ambulate from the bed to the living room or that the patient continues to be unable to ambulate without the assistance of a walker. Specific statements about the extent to which the client is able to ambulate are also important in documenting homebound status: for example, the caregiver could state that the patient is unable to ambulate more than 10 feet without stopping to rest.

Premature Judgments and Ambiguity

Care should be taken to avoid making premature judgments about the client's condition. For example, if the nurse on the second visit finds that the client's blood pressure is within normal limits, a statement such as "blood pressure stable on medication" could indicate to the reviewer that the client no longer requires nurse visits. The nurse would be better advised to record that the client's blood pressure is responding to diet and medication intervention and then go on to describe what continuing needs for nursing care are present. On the next visit, documentation could reflect that the client is continuing to respond to diet and medication intervention. As a general rule, it will be easier to convince a reviewer to acknowledge that a problem continues to be present when the caregiver focuses on what else needs to occur in order for the client to be ready for discharge, rather than on progress made to date.

Ambiguity can also cause denial of a benefits claim, because the reviewer does not have enough information to substantiate that skilled care was given. For instance, if the nurse were seeing a newly diagnosed diabetic patient and wanted to indicate that diet was assessed and instructions were given on specific food exchanges during the visit, documentation should specifically reflect these details rather than simply stating that the diet was reviewed and food exchanges discussed. Most third-party payers will not reimburse for reviews and discussions; however, they will pay for assessments and instructions.

At the time of discharge, the record should include the skilled services that were rendered on the final day of care. If the client no longer needed assistance to ambulate, then a question could arise as to whether the client continued to be homebound and in need of home health-care. It could be argued that such details are trivial and foolish. However, claims have been denied because documentation lacked details.

The burden of proof lies with the home care organization. Although an organization has the right to appeal a claim denial, such appeals are costly in terms of delays in receiving reimbursement and in the staff time required to complete the paperwork involved. Potential denials are best avoided by following the rules and providing details up front. Denials should be categorized and reported by reason so that corrective action may be taken. Medicare regional home health intermediaries can provide quarterly cumulative denial data. Audit and billing activities should be set up accordingly.

Timeliness of Documentation

A final point about charting for reimbursement is that documentation must be timely, or payment may be jeopardized. An organization can better accomplish this task by following two steps. First, the organization must be aware of paperwork submission deadlines for services payment; then the organization must share this information with the staff who submits claims for reimbursement.

Documentation Challenges for PPS and OASIS

Many home health providers are overwhelmed by the burden of documentation for the PPS and OASIS. For patients to whom OASIS applies, Medicare CoP 484.55 requires that the comprehensive assessment must be completed in a timely manner, consistent with the patient's immediate needs, but no later than five calendar days after the start of care. Item M0090 on the OASIS data set reflects the final date the qualified clinician completed the actual patient assessment. This is usually the date of the last home visit made to complete the comprehensive assessment but may reflect a date subsequent to the on-site visit when the qualified clinician needs to follow up with the patient's family or physician in order to complete an OASIS clinical data item. The agency has 30 additional days from the date that the patient assessment is completed to encode, enter, edit, check, lock, and export the data for future submission to the state survey agency.

Every month, agencies must electronically report all OASIS data collected on all applicable patients in a format that meets CMS electronic data and editing specifications. OASIS data on non-Medicare and non-Medicaid patients receiving skilled services must be reported once the masking requirement is effective. Agency software must mask non-Medicare and non-Medicaid OASIS data so that the patient-identifiable information remains anonymous, except to the reporting HHA. At that time, HHAs using software developed by private vendors must use software that appropriately masks non-Medicare and non-Medicaid records for all assessments in a similar manner to the functionality provided by the HAVEN software.

Medicare CoP 484.20 requires OASIS data collection by a qualified clinician as part of the comprehensive assessment at start of care, resumption of care, follow-up, transfer to inpatient facility with or without discharge, significant change in clinical condition, discharge to community, and death at home. Encoding of OASIS data items must be complete and locked in order to accurately compute the information (HIPPS code) necessary for billing Medicare patients under the PPS (CMS 2006).

As the experiences of home care and hospice providers make evident, the paperwork burden is not abating; although, the OASIS is not required for hospice patients. The need for accountability and the health record data and information continue to increase. Considering this, home care and hospice organizations are addressing the paperwork burden by implementing more efficient documentation systems. However, the process for reducing the time needed for documentation is complex and time consuming. Computerizing the record alone is no panacea for reducing the documentation burden. Gains in productivity can arise from computerization or even a new manual system when organizations plan carefully through an assessment of needed data, revised processes, staff education, and monitoring of the effectiveness of the new system. Regardless of whether an organization's health record is manual or computerized, efficiency can be gained through well-designed forms and data-entry screens that are logically sequenced and discourage redundant data entry.

Communication and Timeliness of Documentation

To offer well-coordinated care, an individual care provider needs ready access to information on the care and services that all disciplines and organizations provide to patients. In addition, providers need information on patients' response to care, and any changes in care plans and goals.

The possibility of inadequate transmission of treatment-related information among home care staff and between home care programs and other organizations providing patient care is a negligence risk. This risk is equally high for hospice programs, perhaps more so when hospices contract for inpatient or skilled-nursing facility services. Maintaining timely communication can be challenging, because physicians, the actual care setting, and many individual care providers are physically distant from the home care or hospice organization. The health record serves as one vehicle for communication. Other communication vehicles include computer terminals, telephones, and facsimile machines. In addition to serving as a vehicle for communication, the health record contains evidence of continuing communication. A good standard of practice obligates the home care and hospice program to provide information to patients and their families.

Timely health record documentation affects communication and the coordination of care. An organization's policies address the time requirements for incorporating OASIS, encounter information, and signed orders into the health record. Healthcare practitioners should record their findings at the point of care or within 24 hours of an encounter to adequately support patient care. State laws frequently define timeliness, especially in relation to signatures on physician's orders. Failure to obtain signed orders in accordance with policies and state laws puts an organization at a liability risk and raises red flags for payers and surveyors. Additionally, Medicare and some third-party payers cannot be billed unless signed orders are present.

Home care and hospice organizations must go to great lengths to promptly incorporate documentation and signed orders into paper-based health records, and it may be difficult to meet state requirements for timely documentation. Computer-based record systems can make it possible for care providers to document at the point of care on hand-held or portable computers brought to the patient's home and to transmit current patient information to the organization's centralized computer through modems in the individual caregiver's home. Such computer systems are becoming increasingly common in the home care and hospice settings. Computer networks to physician offices are also needed, so that information can be efficiently shared and orders can be signed electronically. This application is currently far less common.

Consistent and Complete Documentation

A litmus test for an accurate and up-to-date health record is whether an alternative care provider can review the record on any given day and obtain a clear, consistent picture of the patient's status, care plans and goals, and the care and services recently provided. Although passing this litmus test takes some effort, the alternative could be incomplete and inconsistent documentation that might lead to serious problems involving care, legal, reimbursement, licensure, and accreditation issues. Timely documentation and reference-based, up-to-date documentation policies, procedures, and practices promote completeness and consistency in documentation. In addition, ongoing record reviews that monitor record completeness and consistency can target problem areas needing improvement.

Because home care and hospice programs have come under increased scrutiny during investigations for Medicare fraud, incomplete or inconsistent documentation poses particular legal concerns (Harrison and Cole 2005). Section 1128B of the U.S. Social Security Act prohibits obtaining money from the federal government to which one is not entitled, by submitting inaccurate information, by over-utilizing services, or by falsifying the information provided. Billing for services not provided may be alleged under this prohibition when documentation does not agree with claims that have been submitted. For example, documentation may not be present for services provided, or documentation of a patient's status may not be consistent. Complete, consistent documentation that includes dates of service provided and signatures of providers goes a long way toward avoiding (and when necessary, defending against) fraudulent claim allegations. Complete records also protect an organization from unsubstantiated lawsuits and judgments.

Development of Documentation Policies and Procedures

Specific and clear documentation policies and procedures result in health records that reflect evidence of care and service provision in keeping with community standards. Policies and procedures guide the practice and documentation of a home care or hospice organization. When based on community standards and reimbursement regulations, policies and procedures also define what disciplines can and cannot do and give directions on how to perform a particular responsibility, including documentation. For example, a policy and procedure would delineate who notifies a physician of a change in a patient's condition, when this notification is necessary, and how this notification should be conveyed and documented.

A discipline's professional practice standards reflect community standards. Such standards define a discipline's scope and practice. Professional practice standards are developed and published by such professional organizations as the American Nurses Association (ANA), National Association of Social Workers, American Occupational Therapy Association, American Physical Therapy Association, and the American Speech and Hearing Association. The ANA has standards for home health nursing practice. States have practice acts or statutes that define professional practice for nurses and other disciplines. CHAP and Joint Commission (2007) standards, as well as federal and state regulations, also reflect community standards. These standards and regulations may be referenced in a court of law even when an organization has chosen not to be accredited or Medicare certified. Joint Commission standards (2007) require numerous documentation policies and procedures.

Up-to-date, standard operating procedures that are monitored for compliance help to ensure high-quality, consistent care and legally protect the individual provider and the organization. Policies and procedures that are consistently reviewed and updated to reflect changes in community standards, laws, organizational structure, and technology are an organization's key to risk management (Harrison and Cole 2005).

Quantitative Record Review Guidelines

Quantitative record review should be conducted at regular intervals. Routine quantitative record review of all hospice and home care records ensures that the required documentation is present, accurate, consistent, and timely.

The quantitative record review described in this section differs from the qualitative home care clinical record review that Medicare requires. Clinical record review may focus on completeness, but it also examines quality and utilization of services. Requirements call for it to be completed only quarterly on a sample of health records.

Trained staff or health information management professionals, known as registered health information technicians (RHITs) and registered health information administrators (RHIAs), often perform quantitative record review. Health records should be reviewed on admission, on discharge, and on a regular basis every 30 to 60 days. Monitoring processes should ensure timely documentation of the services provided and the timely signature of physician's plans of care and orders. Policies and procedures should address the process of record review, as well as administrative mechanisms for ensuring staff compliance in completing records.

The fact that the Medicare PPS is reimbursed on the basis of the home health resource group is not a reason to skip the review of Medicare documentation. The OIG's compliance program guidance addresses the importance of accurate documentation of care reflected in charges. The reason for this is that annual updating and calculation of norms for the PPS are driven by actual charges. As with compliance, tracking actual charges makes good business sense; it helps the organization measure its efficiency in resource utilization. For compliance purposes, all documentation that serves as the basis for the generation of a bill for patient care should be reviewed. This type of review is different from the type of review that occurs for coding purposes. Documentation monitoring, performed concurrently, ensures that the documentation reflects the full extent of the care provided. At a minimum, the following types of documentation should be monitored concurrently:

- Documentation generating charges (especially higher dollar amounts like infusion care)

- Documentation for any physician charges

- Documentation for ancillary service billing

The HIM department should manage documentation monitoring. However, it is important to involve expert clinical staff when necessary. This not only validates the process, but also involves more of the organization's staff in the compliance process. Clinical staff expertise may be needed for some parts of the review or for the clinical record review process required by Medicare *Conditions of Participation* (Krouth 2000).

Part of Joint Commission's assessment of an ongoing record review process will be determining whether problems were identified and corrected. For this reason, it is important to demonstrate that action was taken. Copies of minutes are good pieces of evidence. In addition, agencies should review about 5 percent of their discharges. For example, if an agency discharges 1,000 patients each quarter, the ongoing record review should include 50 records each quarter, or about 17 records per month (Ongoing 2000).

Hospice Inpatient Record Review

All hospice inpatient records should be reviewed shortly after admission to and on discharge from inpatient care. In cases where patients are inpatients for extended time periods, the records should also be reviewed every 30 to 60 days. Shortly after the admission of the patient, the health record is reviewed for the information listed in figure 11.7.

On discharge of the patient and on an ongoing basis, the health record should be reviewed for the information listed in figure 11.8.

Figure 11.7. Information reviewed after hospice admission.

• Dates and signatures on all documents	• Advance directives
• Patient's name on all documents	• Do-not-resuscitate (DNR) and other applicable "do not" orders
• Correct filing of all documents	• Required assessments
• Referral information	• Current physical examination
• Patient and family identification data	• Interdisciplinary care plan
• Properly completed consent forms	• Copies of documents from transferring facility
• Patient's rights documentation	• Other documents as required by an individual hospice

Figure 11.8. Information reviewed upon hospital discharge.

• Date and signature on all documents	• Team case conference documentation
• Patient's name on all documents	• Clinical/progress notes
• Correct filing of all documents	• A discharge summary to include discharge diagnosis and the applicable bereavement assessments
• Updated care plans	

Home Care Record Review

Clinical record review is a concurrent process at home health organizations. Records are reviewed for completeness, timeliness, and accuracy at admission, as visits are made, and at discharge. In addition, home health organizations must have a tracking process to ensure the prompt return of physician's plans of care and orders.

Admission Review

Shortly after a patient's admission to home care or hospice, the health record should be reviewed for the information listed in figure 11.9.

Figure 11.9. Information reviewed upon home care admission.

• Dates and signatures on all documents	• Copies of advance directives, when applicable
• Patient's name on all documents	• Required comprehensive initial assessments
• Correct filing of all documents	• Signed physician plan of care and physician orders
• Referral information	• Care plan for each discipline providing service and/or for each type of service being provided (interdisciplinary for hospice)
• Patient identification data	
• Properly completed consent forms and service agreements	
• Documentation of provision of patient's rights and advance directive information	• Copies of documents from transferring agencies
	• Other documents as required by an individual organization

Discharge and Ongoing Review

On discharge and on an ongoing basis (every 30 to 60 days), the home care health record should be reviewed for the information listed in figure 11.10.

Figure 11.10   Information reviewed upon home care discharge and ongoing review.

- Date and signature on all documents
- Patient's name on all documents
- Correct filing of all documents
- Team case conference documentation (interdisciplinary for hospice and interdisciplinary preferred for other providers)
- Updated and signed plans of care and orders by attending physician
- Updated care plans for all disciplines providing service and for each type of service being provided (interdisciplinary for hospice)
- Clinical progress notes, home health aide notations, or volunteer documentation for each visit made
- Home health aide supervisory visits by a nurse or therapist
- Evidence of review of volunteer notes
- Discharge summary documenting care and support provided by each discipline, whether goals were met, discharge type, discharge medical and health status and reason for discharge when patient is discharged alive, unmet needs and plans for follow-up care, discharge diagnoses and problems, admission and discharge dates; and, for hospice, applicable bereavement assessments

Visit Documentation Review

To ensure that records are complete, many home care and hospice providers monitor visit documentation. The HIM professional or trained staff can accomplish visit reviews by documenting visits against visit itineraries or schedules. To ease the review process, individual providers can attach or consolidate clinical notes to their itineraries and provide this documentation to review personnel for verification before filing. Alternatively, review personnel can be presented with itineraries and schedules to check against handwritten or typed notes before filing. When the notes are computer-based, the review personnel can compare itineraries and schedules against the computer-based documentation. A computer-based system also makes it possible to routinely check schedules against clinical progress note documentation. Visit documentation review should be included in routine processes, so that the review does not delay the filing of clinical progress notes.

Physician's Documentation Review

Home care organizations can rely on the mail or fax to obtain required signatures from physicians on plans of care and orders. It is recommended that a system be put in place to monitor the timeliness of signatures and to follow up when signatures are late. When problems persist even with a monitoring system, the entire process should be reviewed to determine how to better achieve timeliness. Although the organization has little control over the behavior of physicians, it does have the power to reduce its own time lags. A monitoring system should address the points detailed in figure 11.11.

Home Care and Hospice Legal Issues

In home care and hospice, patient's rights, advance directives, do not resuscitate orders, and issues related to the withholding of life-sustaining treatment are at the fore of pertinent legal issues. To avoid pitfalls, organizations should review written policies, procedures, and organization-specific documentation requirements carefully for redundancy.

Patient's Rights

Home health organizations have a responsibility to inform patients of their rights with respect to care provided. Patients whose data will be collected and used by the federal government

Figure 11.11.   Physician's documentation review monitoring guidelines.

• Physician's offices should be notified about any items not returned within a specific time period. • Staff must confirm that the orders were sent to the correct physician at the correct office before resending orders for signature. • Establishing trends in delinquent orders by physician groups will allow the organization to determine whether some referral relationships continually put the agency at financial or compliance risk. • Agency managers should know how many claims are on hold due to unsigned orders.	• The following methods can be used to monitor return of plans and orders from physicians. — Copies of mailed or faxed documents should be kept in a tickler file by order date. Upon return of the signed order, the tickler file copy can be pulled and appropriately destroyed. A specified time frame should be established to review and resend orders. — A manual or computer-based log of unsigned documents should be maintained, in which attempts to retrieve signed orders are logged. A review of report details will help identify delinquent signatures. — Home health order-generating software that includes documentation tracking modules can be employed. Some software systems even allow document tracking through bar codes and bar code readers.

must receive a notice of their privacy rights. The health record provides evidence that patients are fully informed consumers, actively involved in their care. The protection and promotion of patient and family rights and responsibilities in home care and hospice programs is addressed by CHAP and Joint Commission (2007) standards, as well as by Medicare home care and hospice Conditions of Participation.

The **Omnibus Budget Reconciliation Act of 1987 (OBRA)** requires organizations receiving Medicare and Medicaid funds to document that home care and hospice patients are informed of their rights and that they agree to their care plans. To inform them of their rights, patients are provided with a bill of rights. This form can be used as is or modified to reflect state licensure requirements, any new accreditation standards, and/or reference to hospice instead of home care.

Medicare regulation CoP 484.10 confirms a **patient's right** to be informed and to participate in planning care and treatment, and the right to be informed, in advance, about the care to be furnished, any financial liability, and of any changes in the care plan. The patient is also to be informed of any changes and any financial liability for care rendered. The HHA must advise the patient in advance of the disciplines that will furnish care and the proposed frequency of visits. The HHA must advise the patient in advance of any change in the plan of care before the change is made. The patient has the right to participate in the planning of care. The HHA must advise the patient in advance of the right to participate in planning the care or treatment and in planning changes in the care or treatment (CMS 2005a).

The OASIS database is subject to the requirements of the federal Privacy Act of 1974 (5 USC § 552a). The privacy act allows the disclosure of information from a system of records without an individual's consent if the information is to be used for a purpose that is compatible with the purposes for which the information was collected. However, under patient's rights regulations, the HHA must provide the patient with a written notice of the collection of OASIS information in advance of furnishing care to the patient.

Determining care includes the right of a patient to refuse treatment, which the U.S. Supreme Court supported in *Cruzan vs. Director of the Missouri Department of Health* (1990). In the Cruzan decision, the court affirmed both the right of a patient to refuse medical treatment and the status of artificial tube feeding as medical treatment. The decision affirmed a patient's right to refuse both life-sustaining treatment and life-saving treatment (Brent 2005).

Patient Self-Determination Act of 1990

In 1990, OBRA's **Patient Self-Determination Act** was enacted. It requires home care and hospice organizations receiving Medicare and Medicaid funds to inform patients of their rights under state law to make advance decisions concerning medical care by activating advance directives. **Advance directives** are instruments patients can use to clarify treatment choices in the event that they are no longer capable of doing so. State laws recognize different types of advance directives. Two common types are living wills and durable powers of attorney. A home care and hospice organization's written policies and procedures on advance directives should reflect required documentation, including the following (Brent 2005):

- A discussion with the patient regarding the presence of advance directives
- Provision of written information to the patient on state laws and the organization's advance directive policies
- Medical orders to carry out the patient's wishes
- The physical presence in the record of the advance directive itself

When an existing advance directive is not filed in the health record, documentation explains the reason why, such as patient refusal.

Do-Not-Resuscitate Orders

A **do-not-resuscitate (DNR)** order is a physician's order documenting a patient's (or a substitute decision maker's) desire for no resuscitation attempts. (See figure 11.12.) Although a DNR order results from a desire expressed in an advance directive, it does not replace the need for that directive. In hospice care cases, routine-care-only orders (or consent for care that indicates routine care only) do not substitute for a specific DNR order. Prior to writing a DNR order, a discussion should take place between the attending physician and other team members, the patient, and the next of kin or significant other. The health record contains documentation of the content and outcome of this discussion, and the record must also be clearly flagged to indicate the presence of a DNR order. This is especially important in the hospice inpatient setting. If the DNR form is missing, there is a risk of resuscitating a person in error.

In relation to other life-sustaining measures, "do not" orders in home care and in hospice are necessary. "Do not" orders include such orders as "do not hospitalize" and "do not treat." These orders should also be documented and flagged, as appropriate. When hospices document routine-care-only orders to cover "do not" orders, policy must clearly reflect the meaning of the routine-care-only orders, and their meaning should be conveyed to the patient and/or family.

Hospices as well as other healthcare providers need to develop mission statements reflecting their care philosophies. These mission statements must be shared with patients and their families or significant others. The sharing of an organization's care philosophies should be documented, especially in relation to DNR orders, "do not" orders, and philosophies regarding other life-sustaining measures. Joint Commission standards and Medicare home care and hospice regulations require that patients and their families be informed of healthcare providers' care philosophies.

Written policies and procedures on DNR orders, "do not" orders, and the withholding or withdrawing of other life-sustaining treatment should specify the documentation required and reflect an organization's care philosophies, review of legal requirements, and input from legal counsel. State laws vary significantly regarding DNR orders and the withholding or discontinuance of other life-sustaining treatment. Organizations should be cognizant of their state laws, as well as the legal climate surrounding them.

Figure 11.12.   Sample do-not-resuscitate (DNR) order.

DO-NOT-RESUSCITATE • DNR • DO-NOT-RESUSCITATE • DNR • DO-NOT-RESUSCITATE • DNR

Illinois Department of Public Health

(Page 1 of 2)

UNIFORM DO-NOT-RESUSCITATE (DNR) ADVANCE DIRECTIVE

Patient Directive

I, _____, born on _____, hereby direct the following in the event of:
(print full name)   (birth date)

1. **FULL CARDIOPULMONARY ARREST (When both breathing and heartbeat stop):**

   ☒ **Do Not Attempt Cardiopulmonary Resuscitation (CPR)**
   (Measures to promote patient comfort and dignity will be provided.)

2. **PRE-ARREST EMERGENCY (When breathing is labored or stopped, and heart is still beating):**

   SELECT ONE

   ❑ **Do Attempt Cardiopulmonary Resuscitation (CPR) -OR-**

   ❑ **Do Not Attempt Cardiopulmonary Resuscitation (CPR)**
   (Measures to promote patient comfort and dignity will be provided.)

   Other Instructions _____

   _____

Patient Directive Authorization and Consent to DNR Order (Required to be a valid DNR Order)

   I understand and authorize the above Patient Directive, and consent to a physician DNR Order implementing this Patient Directive.

_____   _____   _____
Printed name of individual   Signature of individual   Date

-OR-

_____   _____   _____
Printed name of (circle appropriate title):   Signature of legal representative   Date
legal guardian
OR agent under health care power of attorney
OR healthcare surrogate decision maker

Witness to Consent (Required to have two witnesses to be a valid DNR Order)

   I am 18 years of age or older and have witnessed the giving of consent by the above person.

_____   _____   _____
Printed name of witness   Signature of witness   Date

_____   _____   _____
Printed name of witness   Signature of witness   Date

Physician Signature (Required to be a valid DNR Order)

   I hereby execute this DNR Order on _____.
                              Today's date

_____   _____   _____
Signature of attending physician   Printed Name of attending physician   Physician's telephone number

◆ *Send this form or a copy of both sides with the individual upon transfer or discharge.* ◆

DNR • DO-NOT-RESUSCITATE • DNR • DO-NOT-RESUSCITATE • DNR • DO-NOT-RESUSCITATE

Figure 11.12. **(continued)**

(Page 2 of 2)

Illinois Department of Public Health
UNIFORM DO-NOT-RESUSCITATE (DNR) ADVANCE DIRECTIVE

Patient's name _____

Summarize medical condition:

When This Form Should Be Reviewed

This DNR order, in effect until revoked, should be reviewed periodically, particularly if –

- The patient/resident is transferred from one care setting or care level to another, or
- There is a substantial change in patient/resident health status, or
- The patient/resident treatment preferences change.

How to Complete the Form Review

1. Review the other side of this form.
2. Complete the following section.
   If this form is to be voided, write "VOID" in large letters on the other side of the form.
   After voiding the form, a new form may be completed.

Date	**Reviewer**	**Location of review**	**Outcome of Review**
			❑ No change
			❑ FORM VOIDED; new form completed
			❑ FORM VOIDED; **no** new form completed

Date	**Reviewer**	**Location of review**	**Outcome of Review**
			❑ No change
			❑ FORM VOIDED; new form completed
			❑ FORM VOIDED; **no** new form completed

Date	**Reviewer**	**Location of review**	**Outcome of Review**
			❑ No change
			❑ FORM VOIDED; new form completed
			❑ FORM VOIDED; **no** new form completed

Advance Directives

I also have the following advance directives: **Contact person** (name and phone number)

❑ Health Care Power of Attorney   _____

❑ Living Will   _____

❑ Mental Health Treatment
Preference Declaration   _____

◆ *Send this form or a copy of both sides with the individual upon transfer or discharge.* ◆

Printed by Authority of the State of Illinois • P.O.335136   100M   5/05

Source: Illinois Department of Public Health 2005.

Home Health Initiative and Home Care Outcome Monitoring

In 1994, CMS began the Medicare home health initiative to identify opportunities for improvement in the Medicare Home Health Benefit. Among the primary recommendations, CMS was advised to develop home health *Conditions of Participation* that include a core standard assessment data set and patient-centered, outcome-oriented performance expectations that stimulate continuous quality improvement in healthcare. OASIS has become part of the same information system that was designed to collect and report beneficiary-specific outcomes and provider performance across a multitude of delivery sites (CMS 2006).

On the basis of comments received, minor modifications were made to the Outcome and Assessment Information Set (OASIS-A2). CMS published the Outcome and Assessment Information Set (OASIS-B1) in June 1998. **OASIS** is a group of data elements that represent core items of a comprehensive assessment for an adult home care patient. In addition, OASIS forms the basis for measuring patient outcomes for purposes of outcome-based quality improvement (OBQI). OASIS serves as a key component in fostering and monitoring improved home healthcare outcomes in the partnership between Medicare and the home care industry. It is also an integral part of the revised *Conditions of Participation* for Medicare-certified home health agencies. Outcome measures are the crux of OBQI, which is a systematic approach HHAs can implement and follow to continuously improve the quality of care they provide. OASIS data significantly improve each state's ability to identify areas of potential quality concerns. See the CMS OASIS data sets Web page for further information: www.cms.hhs.gov/HomeHealthQualityInits/12_HHQIOASISDataSet.asp#TopOfPage.

Most data items in the OASIS were derived in the context of a national research program to develop a system of outcome measures for home care. Outcome-based quality improvement and OASIS evolved over a ten-year developmental period. The core items were refined through several iterations of clinical and empirical research. Other items were later added by a group of home care experts to augment the outcome data set with selected items deemed essential for patient assessment. The goal was not to produce a comprehensive assessment instrument, but to provide a set of items necessary for measuring patient outcomes and essential for assessment, which home health agencies could augment as needed. OASIS items are used in outcome monitoring, clinical assessment, care planning, and other internal agency-level applications.

OASIS encompasses sociodemographic, environmental, support system, health status, and functional status attributes of adult (nonmaternity) patients. In addition, selected attributes of health service utilization, such as therapy utilization, are included. These different attributes should be part of a comprehensive patient assessment (CMS 2006).

Currently, there are 41 Home Health Quality Initiative (2006) measures. Of these, 30 are risk-adjusted quality measures and 11 are descriptive quality measures.

Patient Outcome Measures

Patient outcome measures are calculated on a completed episode of care that begins with admission to a home health agency (or a resumption of care following an inpatient facility stay) and ends with discharge or transfer to inpatient facility. This is different than a Home Health Prospective Payment episode of 60 days. A patient **outcome** is defined as a change (lack of change) in a patient's condition during an episode of care.

The outcomes are divided into the following two groups:

- **Risk-adjusted outcome** rates are adjusted to compensate for differences in the patient population served by different home health agencies, including differences between states.

- **Descriptive outcome** rates are not adjusted. Observed (actual) outcomes are aggregated across all eligible patients served by home health agencies in each state and further aggregated to obtain national observed rates. These observed rates are what appear in the report.

See figure 11.13 for details of the outcome measures.

Figure 11.13. Patient outcome measures.

Risk-adjusted Outcomes	Descriptive Outcomes
Improvement in grooming	Stabilization in management of oral medications
Stabilization in grooming	Improvement in speech and language
Improvement in upper body dressing	Stabilization in speech and language
Improvement in lower body dressing	Improvement in pain interfering with activity
Improvement in bathing	Improvement in number of surgical wounds
Stabilization in bathing	Improvement in status of surgical wounds
Improvement in toileting	Improvement in cognitive functioning
Improvement in transferring	Stabilization in cognitive functioning
Stabilization in transferring	Improvement in anxiety level
Improvement in ambulation/locomotion	Stabilization in anxiety level
Improvement in eating	Improvement in behavior problem frequency
Improvement in light meal preparation	
Stabilization in light meal preparation	
Improvement in laundry	
Stabilization in laundry	
Improvement in housekeeping	
Stabilization in housekeeping	
Improvement in shopping	
Stabilization in shopping	
Improvement in phone use	
Stabilization in phone use	
Improvement in management of oral medications	
Improvement in dyspnea	
Improvement in urinary tract infection	
Improvement in urinary incontinence	
Improvement in bowel incontinence	
Improvement in confusion frequency	
Discharged to community	
Acute-care hospitalization	
Any emergent care provided	

Source: CMS 2006.

Quality Requirements

Home care and hospice programs that seek accreditation through the **Community Health Accreditation Program (CHAP)** or the Joint Commission (2007) or elect to seek Medicare (2006) certification must meet the performance improvement requirements of these groups. Organizations in states with licensing regulations that require quality management must also meet state requirements.

Community Health Accreditation Program Improved Performance Standards

CHAP standards emphasize the need for healthcare organizations to establish an organizational structure that supports a consumer-oriented philosophy and consistently provides for high-quality services and products. CHAP standards also stress the need for organizations to possess adequate resources and a strong potential for long-term viability. The organization's focus on quality must be reflected in its strategic plans, staff orientation and development programs, and quality commitment (CHAP 2005).

CHAP standards require planned efforts to ensure continuous quality improvement. In addition, the organization must develop quality improvement measures and monitoring processes for the following factors (CHAP 2005):

- Client outcome data

- Client satisfaction assessment

- Clinical record reviews

- Peer reviews

- Program evaluations

The standards address the required content of the quality improvement plan and specifics regarding expectations for monitoring. The standards also require that organizations document evidence illustrating how the organization used quality improvement results in service planning and problem resolution. Evidence should also show that the organization's quality improvement efforts resulted in actual improvements (CHAP 2005).

Joint Commission Performance Improvement Standards

Joint Commission standards are statements of the performance expectations that, when followed, lead to positive outcomes. Performance expectations for each function are addressed in the *Comprehensive Accreditation Manual for Home Care* (Joint Commission 2007). Joint Commission standards on improving organizational performance provide a framework for improving the functions addressed in the manual. The framework for PI emphasizes quality and focuses on the common causes of problems and processes. Although the Joint Commission's standards do not require continuous quality improvement (CQI) per se, they do require a process in which planning, design, measurement, assessment, and improvement focus on and lead to PI. A brief discussion of the requirements for each of these components follows. The standards themselves should be referenced for specifics.

Planning Standards

Standards require evidence of a planned, systematic, and organization-wide approach to PI (Joint Commission 2007). Planning must address the processes for conducting PI and ensure that multiple services and staff are involved in planning efforts. Collaboration among disciplines and services should be evident in PI efforts, and contracted services should be included in planned PI activities (Joint Commission 2007).

Design Standards

Design standards address the concept of building quality in at the front end of the process, and thus they focus on the design of new processes. Design standards require that the design of new processes take into consideration the following factors:

- The organization's mission, vision, and plans

- Needs and expectations of patients, staff, and others

- Up-to-date sources of information related to designing processes, such as practice guidelines or parameters

- Performance of the processes and their outcomes in other organizations, such as information from reference databases

Measurement of Performance

Performance measurement is considered to be at the heart of all PI activities. Through evaluation of measurement data, home care and hospice organizations address the need for improved processes. Joint Commission (2007) requires certain measurements to be conducted systematically for the following factors:

- Processes and outcomes

- Performance of processes pertaining to the functions addressed in the accreditation manual

- Quality control activities in at least the following areas, where applicable:

    — Clinical laboratory services

    — Equipment provided to patients

    — Equipment used in providing care

    — Pharmacy equipment and preparations

Data for measurement can be collected to focus on issues chosen as priorities for improvement and to judge the stability of a particular process or the predictability of a particular outcome (also known as a *continuous measurement*). Performance measurement of the functions addressed in the accreditation manual must be continual and focus on processes that meet the following characteristics (Joint Commission 2007):

- Affects a large percentage of patients

- Places patients at serious risk when not performed well, or when performed when not indicated, or when not performed when indicated

- Has/have been or are likely to be problem prone

Assessment of Measurement Data

Joint Commission requires organizations to have a systematic process in place for assessment of measurement data. This assessment should incorporate the use of statistical quality control techniques. The assessment should also incorporate internal and external comparisons of organization process and outcome data over time. External comparisons include comparison to sources such as practice guidelines, data from other organizations, and reference databases. Home care and hospice organizations are advised to obtain Joint Commission input on the expected level of compliance regarding required comparisons.

Joint Commission standards require that intensive assessment be performed when undesired variation in performance occurs. This variation may be represented by an important single event (the Joint Commission uses the term *sentinel event*), such as a blood transfusion reaction, or by a significant variation from either the standards or comparative performances of other organizations. In addition, organizations may choose to perform intensive review to further improve performance. The Joint Commission requires intensive assessment when any of the following sentinel events occur: confirmed transfusion reactions, significant adverse drug reactions, or significant errors related to medication use. When systematic data assessment reveals that an individual's performance presents an opportunity for improvement, the person responsible for patient services ensures that steps for assessing and improving competence are followed (Joint Commission 2007).

Performance Improvement Process

The last component of Joint Commission's improving organizational performance standards concerns the PI process itself. Standards require the PI process to be systematic and standardized throughout the organization. Because every opportunity for improvement cannot be addressed, the standards require organizations to establish criteria for determining organization improvement priorities. The standards specify considerations that the criteria should address. They also specify operational issues that must be considered when designing or improving an activity, as well as the planning, measurement, and assessment that must occur before an improved process is fully implemented (Joint Commission 2007).

Medicare Conditions of Participation for Home Care

The Omnibus Budget Reconciliation Act of 1987 (OBRA) had a major impact on the delivery of home healthcare services. The revised *Conditions of Participation* focused on the health and safety of patients and emphasized patient's rights and the competency of home health aides. Initially published in the *Federal Register* in 1989, the *Conditions of Participation* were revised in 1990, 1991, and 1995. In 1999, CMS added a new condition on comprehensive assessment and the Outcome and Assessment Information Set (OASIS). In 2000, CMS revised some conditions as part of the final rule for the PPS. The interpretive guidelines define the conditions and provide surveyors with direction for the survey process. The guidelines were originally published in the State Operations Manual in 1991 and revised in 1993, 1997, 2000, and 2007. The reader is advised to refer to the most current Medicare *Conditions of Participation* in place.

The Home Health Initiative

The revised *Conditions of Participation for Home Health Agencies* (HHAs) include requirements for an internal quality improvement system based on OASIS data. These outcome measures are both global and focused on specific patient groups. Monitoring clinical progress and financial exposure by episode under the PPS is a challenge requiring effective, time-efficient reviews week after week.

OASIS is intended to support home care assessment and outcome monitoring. OASIS gave **Regional Home Health Intermediary (RHHI)** auditors a new audit tool. The **RHHI Outcomes and Assessment Information Set Verification (ROVER) protocol** is an automated accuracy software application used to assist in the medical review of home health claims submitted by HHAs that are paid under the HHA PPS. According to CMS Medicare Claims Processing Manual, ROVER uses health records to verify that the information contained on an HHA-completed OASIS reflects the condition of the patient and the services actually delivered during a particular episode in time. The program guides medical review staff through a review of information in the clinical record. The reviewer can document whether the case-mix OASIS items have been validated by the information contained in the record. The end results are twofold: a recommended **home health resource group (HHRG)** classification based on the input data and a reporting database containing information from the reviews. Therefore, the information gained by the use of ROVER applies not only to data verification but also to intermediary data analysis and provider education (CMS 2006).

how they assess info from OASIS

Case-Mix and Adverse Event Reports for Outcome-based Quality Management

CMS recommends a two-stage outcome-based quality improvement process. The first stage includes outcome analysis; collecting needed OASIS data; processing, editing, and transmitting data; and reviewing risk-adjusted outcome reports. The second stage, outcome enhancement, involves targeting outcomes for enhancement, evaluating the care for targeted outcomes, and developing a plan of action to change care.

CMS prescribes the following quality management process:

1. Review each report
2. Prioritize adverse event outcomes
3. Conduct review of care
4. Identify problematic care
5. Develop plan to change care
6. Implement the plan
7. Monitor the plan
8. Determine whether change made a difference

CMS requires
1 — Quality Improvement
2 — Use Resource group and assess these 8 areas
3 — ORYX — accrediting review

Agencies should prioritize adverse events and outcomes with the highest incidence and then investigate those most clinically relevant to their organization. After reviewing comparison charts and listing the clinical actions expected to prevent adverse events, HHAs can design chart audit tools. By using record review findings, HHAs can refine subsequent investigations and identify both appropriate and problematic care.

CMS warns HHAs against assuming that change will happen. Instead, HHAs should develop improvement plans to change the care that is provided. As part of a plan, the HHA states the care delivery expectations, implements the plan, and then monitors the care provided. CMS also encourages HHAs to incorporate monitoring plans into other record activities and determine what positions should receive monitoring results. Only then can HHAs expect incremental changes.

State Survey Agencies

State survey agencies will periodically review case-mix and adverse event reports. Reports may also be used during the survey process under the CoP 484.52 agency and program evaluation, policy and administrative review, and clinical record review.

The *Conditions of Participation* for Medicare-certified HHAs requires an annual evaluation of the agency's overall program and a quarterly clinical record review. Patient care services are identified as one component of the agency's total program that must be included in this evaluation. The use of the case-mix and adverse event outcome reports to review and improve patient care delivery is congruent with these program evaluation components. It is also anticipated that state survey agencies will incorporate the adverse event outcome reports into the off-site presurvey preparation and actual on-site survey.

Written Policies

Home health regulations require agencies to have written policies requiring an annual evaluation of the agency's overall program. The evaluation assesses the extent to which the agency's program is appropriate, adequate, effective, and efficient. Results of the evaluation are reported to and acted upon by those responsible for the operation of the agency and are maintained separately as administrative records. As part of the evaluation process, the policies and administrative practices of the agency are reviewed to determine the extent to which they promote patient care that is appropriate, adequate, effective, and efficient. Mechanisms are established in writing for the collection of pertinent data to assist in evaluation (CoP 484.52a). On a quarterly basis, appropriate health professionals who represent the scope of the program review a sample of both active and closed clinical records to determine whether established policies are followed in furnishing services directly or under arrangement. There is a continuing review of clinical records for each 60-day period that a patient receives home health services to determine adequacy of the plan of care and appropriateness of continuation of care (CoP 484.52b).

The agency is expected to have policies and administrative practices in place to promote patient care that is appropriate, adequate, effective, and efficient. Further, it is noted that mechanisms are established in writing for the collection of pertinent data to assist in evaluation. The investigation of adverse event outcomes provides evidence of the agency's review of potential problems in care provision. When problems in care provision are discovered, the development and implementation of the improvement plan demonstrates the agency's goals of overcoming or minimizing existing problems. The use of a chart audit tool for the adverse event outcome investigation provides evidence of the collection of pertinent data to assist in evaluating patient care. Utilizing the adverse event outcome investigation partially addresses this standard. Agency policies and procedures must address how reports are incorporated into the program evaluation.

Quarterly Record Review

Quarterly record review is required to determine whether established HHA policies are being followed in the provision of care. Two aspects of the adverse event outcome report investigation address this standard. It is expected that the chart audit tool used to investigate the adverse event outcomes will incorporate any relevant HHA policies for care provision. Similarly, the monitoring of clinician compliance with new or revised care practices should incorporate relevant HHA policies. When the investigation process is conducted in a phased manner, the adverse events can be investigated and monitored on a quarterly basis. In this way, the associated record review is incorporated into an HHA's current quality monitoring requirements. The investigation of adverse event outcomes becomes part of the HHA's overall quality monitoring program. Although these reports represent many HHAs' first exposure to the use of outcomes for quality improvement activities, the utility of the reports for the HHA's overall quality monitoring program is clear. The benefit to patients is also evident as agencies focus on continuously improving the quality of care they provide.

Adverse Event Outcome Reports

Both state survey agencies and HHAs have access to the adverse event outcome reports. State survey agencies review available reports prior to going on-site as part of their presurvey preparation. The reports help surveyors identify areas of focus during the on-site survey. Surveyors expect HHAs to use the information in the reports to improve patient outcomes. Surveyors assess the HHA's use of the reports for quality monitoring, including how the HHA addresses systemic issues that may be present, in an effort to reduce the incidence of similar adverse events in the future. For example, surveyors may review the specific patient situations included in the adverse event outcome reports to determine whether any events might have been prevented. Another focus of the surveyor's review may be to determine whether any of the adverse event outcomes was due to noncompliance with the *Conditions of Participation* on the part of the HHA. HHAs are strongly encouraged to take advantage of the information presented in their reports for their ongoing quality-monitoring program (CMS 2006).

Medicare Conditions of Participation for Hospices

Medicare CoP reads as follows (CMS 2006):

> A hospice must conduct an ongoing, comprehensive, integrated, self-assessment of the quality and appropriateness of care provided, including inpatient care, home care and care provided under arrangements. The findings are used by the hospice to correct identified problems and to revise hospice policies if necessary. Those responsible for the quality assurance program must
>
> - implement and report on activities and mechanisms for monitoring the quality of patient care,
>
> - identify and resolve problems, and
>
> - make suggestions for improving care. (CMS 2006)

Surveyors examine structures and processes contributing to the quality of hospice services. The principal survey focus is the outcome of the hospice's practices in implementing hospice requirements and the effect of the hospice's services on the patients. Home visits must be made to a sample of Medicare and Medicaid hospice patients if the surveyor determines that home visits are necessary to confirm the hospice is in compliance with all conditions and standards. The hospice self-assessment should include all provided services and the patients' and caregivers' responses to those services. It should also include those services that may have been provided but were omitted. Special attention should be given to the ability of the hospice to deal with symptom management, pain control, stress management, continuity of care, and inpatient care. Suggestions for improving care and any problems identified in providing hospice care should receive the appropriate consideration from the hospice management or governing body (CMS 2006).

Interpretive guidelines contained in the CMS *State Operations Manual* (2006) indicate that a hospice must establish a system to evaluate the care and services provided as well as services that might appropriately have been provided but were not. The governing body should support the quality assurance program, and it should encompass critiques by the patients' families, monitoring of staff performance, and an annual program evaluation of the hospice's total operation. There should be annual studies of at least the following areas:

- Symptom management
- Stress management
- Continuity of care
- Inpatient care

A representative of the governing body must be involved in the annual program evaluation, as should representatives from the various disciplines and representatives from home care inpatient services. Throughout the process, a reporting mechanism to the governing body is required (CMS 2006).

The Joint Commission's Performance Measurement Data

The Joint Commission surveyors assess how home care organizations have integrated and used ORYX performance measurement data in their performance improvement activities. During the PI interview, surveyors ask organization leaders what process was used to select performance measures, how ORYX data have been integrated into internal PI activities, and what results emerged from these activities. ORYX initiatives are designed so that expectations should increase over time. The initial phase of the ORYX initiative offers accredited healthcare organizations significant flexibility by allowing them to select the performance measurement system and individual measures that best serve their strategic measurement goals. More than 15,000 performance measures from nearly 300 performance measurement systems have already been cataloged in the Joint Commission's database as part of this initiative.

The next phase of the ORYX initiative includes the identification of specific core performance measures and the opportunity for listed systems to embed some, or all, of these measures in their own systems. Core measures are grouped into measure sets. In time, measure sets may include clinical performance, client perception of care, health status, and administrative or financial measures. The initial core measures focus primarily on clinical performance. The identification and use of core measures allow comparisons of processes and outcomes of patient care among healthcare organizations across the country, regardless of which performance measurement system the organization is using. The Joint Commission is gradually transitioning core measure sets into ORYX requirements (Joint Commission 2007).

The ORYX Initiative

ORYX is the name of Joint Commission's initiative to integrate performance measures into the accreditation process. The Joint Commission introduced its ORYX initiative in 1997. The ORYX initiative requires organizations to collect quarterly performance measurement data and submit the information via their selected vendors to Joint Commission. ORYX integrates outcomes and other performance measurement data into the accreditation process. The goal is to provide a continuous, data-driven accreditation process that focuses on the actual results of care (performance measurement) and is more comprehensive and valuable to all stakeholders. The Joint Commission strives for its primary mission of improving of the quality of care provided to the public through the provision of healthcare accreditation and related services that support PI in healthcare organizations. The ORYX initiative is the critical link between accreditation and the outcomes of patient care, allowing Joint Commission to review data trends and patterns and to work with organizations as they use data to improve patient care. ORYX performance measures supplement and help guide the standards-based survey process by providing more targeted bases for the regular accreditation survey, continuously monitoring actual performance, and guiding and stimulating continuous improvement in healthcare organizations.

Home health organizations with an average annual census of 120 patients or more, accredited prior to January 1, 2001, were required to select and participate in a performance measurement system. The organizations chose six clinical or perception-of-care measures by December 31, 2000, and began data collection on January 1, 2001. They selected measures most relevant to their patient populations and strategic measurement objectives. The resulting data were reported by the performance measurement system to the Joint Commission by July 31, 2001.

Selecting or participating in a performance measurement system was optional for home health organizations with an average annual census of less than 120 patients or organizations undergoing their initial survey in 2001. However, these organizations chose six measures that were most relevant to their patient populations and strategic measurement objectives. They selected measures from existing performance measures. Sources included listed performance measurement systems, the professional literature, internally developed measures, and measures from professional associations. Measure selections were reported to the Joint Commission on a standardized reporting form.

Surveyors assessed organizations' use of selected measures in their PI activities during the on-site survey process. Organizations were expected to demonstrate, for each measure, the ability to collect data reliably, conduct credible analyses of the data, and initiate appropriate system and process improvements.

Summary

It is important for the HIM practitioner to understand the key components of the home care and hospice health record database and the regulatory environment under which home care agencies and hospices operate. Although many of the health record database components will be familiar to practitioners from other healthcare settings, there are specific components that are unique to each home care and hospice organization. The Centers for Medicare and Medicaid Services has identified core components that present many documentation challenges related to the Medicare home care prospective payment system, the OASIS, and the provision of care under the Medicare hospice benefit, all of which clinicians in home care and hospice settings strive to meet while caring for their patients.

It is vital that the health information management practitioner understands the importance of continually reviewing the documentation to confirm that health records meet all applicable home care and hospice regulations and standards. Additionally, it is critical that the health information management practitioner assists his or her agency in understanding the outcomes management and quality initiatives under way by CMS and other accrediting organizations. The health information management practitioner must recognize the ever-changing regulatory environment and keep abreast of the changes and challenges faced by home care and hospice agencies.

References

American Health Information Management Association. 2007. Position statement: Quality healthcare data and information (revised and adopted October 2006). *Journal of American Health Information Management Association* 78(1): 20.

Brent, Nancy J. 2005. Protecting the AIDS patient's right to make treatment decisions. *Home Healthcare Nurse* 12(2): 10–11.

Centers for Medicare and Medicaid Services. 1994. CMS form 485 (C-3) (02-94). OMB No. 0938-0357.

Centers for Medicare and Medicaid Services. 1999 (Jan. 25). Reporting outcome and assessment information set (OASIS) data; Final rule. 42 CFR Part 484. *Federal Register* 64(15): 3748–3763. Available online from www.cms. hhs.gov/OASIS/Downloads/reporting.pdf.

Centers for Medicare and Medicaid Services. 2000 (July 3). Medicare program; prospective payment system for home health agencies; Final Rule. 42 CFR Parts 409, 410, 411, 413, 424, and 484. *Federal Register* 65(128): 41127–41214.

Centers for Medicare and Medicaid Services. 2003 (June 20). CMS Medicare Manual System, Pub. 100-8 Program Integrity, Transmittal 42. Available online from www.cms.hhs.gov/Transmittals/Downloads/R42PI.pdf.

Centers for Medicare and Medicaid Services. 2005a (Aug. 12). Home health services. Chapter 7 in *Medicare Benefit Policy Manual, Rev. 37*. Available online from www.cms.hhs.gov/manuals/Downloads/bp102c07.pdf.

Centers for Medicare and Medicaid Services. 2006 (Aug. 18). Home health agency billing. Chapter 10 in *Medicare Claims Processing Manual, Rev. 1036*. Available online from www.cms.hhs.gov/manuals/downloads/clm104c10.pdf.

Centers for Medicare and Medicaid Services. 2006 (Aug. 23). Home Health Quality Initiatives. Available online from www.cms.hhs.gov/HomeHealthQualityInits/10_HHQIQualityMeasures.asp#TopOfPage.

Centers for Medicare and Medicaid Services. 2006 (Nov. 9). *OASIS User Manual*. Available online from www.cms.hhs.gov/HomeHealthQualityInits/14_HHQIOASISUserManual.asp#TopOfPage.

Centers for Medicare and Medicaid Services. 2006. Chapter 2 in *State Operations Manual*. Available online from www.cms.hhs.gov/Manuals/IOM/list.asp.

Centers for Medicare and Medicaid Services. 2006b (Dec. 8). Conditions of participation: Patients' rights; Final rule. 42 CFR Subchapter G, Part 482. Section 482.13. *Federal Register* 71(236): 71377. Available online from www.cms.hhs.gov/InpatientRehabFacPPS/04_IRFPAI.asp.

Community Health Accreditation Program. 1997. *Standards of Excellence for Home Care Organizations*. New York: National League for Health Care and Community Health Accreditation Program.

Cruzan v. Director, Missouri Department of Health, 497 U.S. 261 (1990).

General Accounting Office. 2002 (May). Report to congressional committees: Medicare home health care; payments to home health agencies are considerably higher than costs. GAO-02-663. Available online from www.gao.gov/new.items/d02663.pdf.

Haddad, A. M. 1987. *High Tech Home Care: A Practical Guide*. New York: Aspen Publishers.

Harrison, B. A., and D. Cole. 2005. Managing risk to minimize liability. *Caring* 13(5): 26–30.

Hospice Association of America. 2005. Region IV hospices face new claims review edit and new policy regarding limitation of liability. *Hospice Forum* 9(13): 1–2.

Illinois Department of Public Health. 2005 (May). Uniform do-not-resuscitate (DNR) advance directive. Available online from www.idph.state.il.us/public/books/dnrform04b.pdf.

Joint Commission on Accreditation of Healthcare Organizations. 1995. *Understanding the Patient's Perspective: A Tool for Improving Performance*. Oakbrook Terrace, IL: Joint Commission.

Joint Commission. 2007. *Comprehensive Accreditation Manual for Home Care* (CAMHC). Oakbrook Terrace, IL: Joint Commission.

Joint Commission. 2007. *Facts About ORYX for Home Care Organizations.* Available online from www.jointcommission.org/AccreditationPrograms/HomeCare/ORYX/.

Krouth, Mary. 2000. Monitoring content and quality of documentation. *HIM Connection* 2000 2(43): 2–4.

National Association for Home Care & Hospice. 2008. Basic Statistics about Home Care. Washington, D.C.: National Association for Home Care & Hospice. Available online from www.nahc.org/facts/hospicefx07.pdf.

Office of Inspector General. 2007. Work plan, 2007. Available online from www.oig.hhs.gov/publications/docs/workplan/2007/Work%20Plan%202007.pdf.

Omnibus Budget Reconciliation Act of 1987 (OBRA). 1987. Public Law 100-203, (101 Stat. 1330), SEC. 4001. [2 U.S.C. 902 note]. *United States Code.* Available online from http://www.ssa.gov/OP_Home/comp2/F100-203.html.

Ongoing record review: One hospital's pathway to success. 2000 (November). *Medical Records Briefing* 15(11): 1–3.

Patient Self-Determination Act. 1990. Public Law 9621, (1395aa. 1395cc. 1395dd. and 1395hh) and sec. 602 (k) of Pub. L. 962), [42 U.S.C. 1302.1395x. 1395ww note]. *United States Code.* Available online from http://www.fha.org/acrobat/Patient%20Self%20Determination%20Act%201990.pdf.

U.S. Department of Justice. (1974, 2004). Federal privacy act; Final Rule. 5 U.S.C. § 552a *United States Code.* Available online from www.usdoj.gov/oip/04_7_1.html.

Chapter 12

Behavioral Healthcare

Kathleen M. Munn, RHIA

Learning Objectives

- List and explain the sources of regulations and standards that apply to behavioral healthcare records

- Describe the variety of settings for behavioral healthcare services

- List and describe the documentation issues unique to behavioral healthcare settings

- Describe the content of the behavioral health record

- Define and describe psychotherapy notes and their special protection under HIPAA privacy regulations

- List and describe the many outside forces affecting behavioral healthcare

Key Terms

Conservatorship

Day treatment

Early Childhood Intervention (ECI)

Employee Assistance Programs (EAPs)

Family Educational Rights and Privacy Act of 1974 (FERPA)

Health Insurance Portability and Accountability Act of 1996 (HIPAA)

Healthcare reengineering

Inpatient facilities

Integrated delivery system (IDS)

Managed behavioral healthcare organizations (MBHOs)

Managed care organization (MCO)

Mental Health America (MHA)

National Council for Community Behavioral Healthcare (NCCBH)

Outcomes assessment

Outpatient facilities

Partial stay

Personal health information (PHI)

Residential facility

Substance Abuse and Mental Health Services Administration (SAMHSA)

Introduction

It is estimated that one in five Americans, roughly 22 percent, will suffer from a diagnosable mental illness in any given year (NIMH 2001). These conditions, which encompass a wide variety of cognitive, emotional, and behavioral illnesses, along with mental retardation, developmental disabilities, and substance abuse, are classified in the *Diagnostic and Statistical Manual of Mental Disorders, fourth edition (Text Revision* 2000*)*, or DSM-IV-TR®. DSM-IV is the classification system utilized in the United States to diagnose and classify mental illness.

Behavioral health has unique documentation challenges. Clients may be at high risk for suicidal or homicidal behavior. Often they are committed to a behavioral healthcare facility involuntarily or are required to receive treatment against their wishes. Clients who voice suicidal thoughts or exhibit suicidal behaviors present organization staff with significant challenges in terms of care and safety. Consequently, staff must have an organized system for documenting and addressing such behavior (Youngberg 1998, 328–339).

Behavioral healthcare poses unique challenges to patient rights. Even though clients may be at high risk for suicidal or homicidal behavior as a result of mental illness, they have the right to refuse psychiatric treatment. Clients are often committed involuntarily to a psychiatric institution, and the institution must define the fine line between safeguarding the client's rights and protecting the interest of society. Clients who complain of suicidal thoughts or display overtly suicidal behaviors, yet persist in refusing care, present healthcare providers with significant care and safety challenges. Complete and timely documentation of these situations is critical.

The Recipients of Behavioral Healthcare Services

According to the surgeon general, it is estimated that more than 54 million Americans are currently diagnosed with a mental health disorder. Mental illness is prevalent in all races, ages, and social settings and affects almost every family in the United States (USPHS 1999).

Today's healthcare system offers a number of mental health or "behavioral" healthcare services to individuals living with these conditions. The terms *mental health* and *behavioral health* may be used interchangeably throughout this chapter as both are frequently used in treatment settings around the country.

The individuals who seek these services are commonly referred to as *clients*, although they may also be referred to as *patients*, *consumers*, or *recipients*. These terms are used interchangeably throughout this chapter as well.

Behavioral healthcare services may be initiated through court-ordered treatment. The need for treatment in the forensic population (jails, prisons) continues to grow, and the provision of behavioral healthcare services is increasing to forensic populations as funding for these special-needs clients increases.

Organization and Operation

Behavioral healthcare facilities may be private, standalone entities or affiliated with an area hospital or larger healthcare organization. In addition, some behavioral organizations are part of a chain, with a main corporate office and facilities in a specific region or throughout the nation. Many organizations today are owned, operated, and funded by the individual states or counties.

In most states, healthcare plans such as Medicaid or those run by individual counties are responsible for providing funding for individuals with behavioral healthcare problems. If an individual has private insurance that covers behavioral healthcare services, the state or local government may be responsible for paying the difference.

Settings

Today's behavioral healthcare environment allows for an individualized approach to treatment and providing treatment in the least restrictive setting possible. Treatment is specifically prescribed after a diagnosis has been established, and careful consideration is given to the individual's social, medical, and financial circumstances and service needs. It may be provided by a psychiatrist, a psychologist, or a variety of rehabilitative or social work specialists. In many settings, a combination of these individuals is used.

Care typically is prescribed through a treatment or service plan developed by the provider or provider team in response to the individual's needs. In today's environment, the client and his or her family, if available, are often encouraged to actively participate in development of the treatment or service plan.

Additionally, there are unique areas in behavioral healthcare that need to be addressed in an organization's medical staff rules and regulations including the use of seclusion and restraint, psychotropic medication, and other treatments (such as suicide watch, which may be forced on a patient due to self-imposed danger or threat to others). Documentation for these issues is discussed later in this chapter.

Although terminology, licensure, documentation, and staffing requirements may vary from state to state, there are three basics types of behavioral healthcare settings: inpatient, residential, and outpatient. Other special settings include community mental health entities, employee-assistance programs, and schools and universities.

Inpatient Facilities

Inpatient facilities provide patients with around-the-clock care. Of the 5.4 million people who sought mental health treatment in 1990, less than 7 percent required hospitalization. More than half of those who needed inpatient-care had schizophrenia, one of the most severe forms of mental illness (MHA 2007).

Inpatient facilities may be a dedicated portion of a hospital or may stand alone. In some circumstances, clients are in need of partial-stay services or partial hospitalization. Such services are provided to individuals who fall between the need for inpatient and outpatient services and would benefit from a short stay at an inpatient mental health facility or hospital. Figure 12.1 lists some of the elements to review regarding medical necessity for inpatient behavioral facility hospitalization (Martins and Nicholson 2008).

Partial Stay or Day Treatment

Partial stay or **day treatment** programs provide individuals with mental health treatment that is more intense than the services provided on an outpatient basis. Most payers (including

Figure 12.1.   Elements to review for inpatient behavioral facility hospitalization.

- Any evidence of self-injurious behavior?
- Any evidence of threatening behavior?
- Any evidence of disorganized behavior?
- Any evidence of disordered thinking?
- Description of mood and affect.
- Is patient compliant with treatment plan?
- Is patient eating? How much?
- Is patient sleeping adequately? How many hours?
- Is patient attending to ADLs appropriately?
- Is patient compliant with medication? Medication education provided?
- Use of PRNs and response
- Documentation of severity of symptoms whether they have increased or decreased, or different symptoms emerged.
- Does patient require 24-hour professional observation?
- Passes: Documentation of why passes are needed and response to pass
- Groups: Attendance and participation level
- Patient's ability and willingness to participate in discharge planning?
- Is family/significant other participating in patient's treatment?
- If patient has substance misuse or abuse issues, is the patient willing to address this in treatment?

Source: Martins and Nicholson 2008, 241.

Medicare) cover this service when determined medically appropriate by the physician (CMS 2003).

Day treatment/day care/partial hospitalization services include the following:

- Social and recreation activities for individuals who require general supervision during the day

- Psychosocial programs for social interaction

- Family counseling services directed toward a family member's problem in relation to the patient's condition

- Vocational training for employment opportunities, work skills, or work settings

Residential Facilities

Often referred to as *group homes* or *foster homes*, **residential facilities** are staffed by behavioral health professionals who provide supervision and training to the residents in an alternative to the inpatient setting. Clients of such facilities are often encouraged to achieve independence in daily functions with little assistance from the provider. The residence provides a somewhat stable environment that helps many individuals with mental illness to assimilate into the "real world."

Outpatient Facilities

Outpatient facilities provide clients with access to a stable treatment provider on an outpatient basis. Such care may occur in a formal office setting or in the comfort of the individual's home or residence. In some circumstances, outpatient services are provided in homeless shelters in an effort to reach the estimated hundreds of thousands of homeless individuals in America who suffer from mental illness (CMHS 1992).

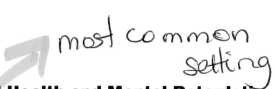
most common setting

Community Mental Health and Mental Retardation Centers

The **National Council for Community Behavioral Healthcare (NCCBH)** lists the following principles for recording information regarding their consumers. Documentation from mental health and mental retardation (MHMR) centers should do the following (NCCBH 2007):

- Reflect the consumer's strengths, competencies, problems, and needs

- Reflect the recognition of family strengths and individuality of family caregivers and others in the consumer's support network

- Use respectful and nonjudgmental language regarding consumers and their support network

- Be treated as a mechanism for enhancing communication

EAPs

Employers also are acknowledging the need for mental health services for their employees by providing access to **employee assistance programs (EAPs)**. These outpatient programs are designed to provide employees immediate access to psychological counseling on a limited basis and may be provided on-site or through local providers.

Schools and Universities

Schools and universities commonly provide outpatient mental health assistance to their students through formal clinics, guidance therapy, or direct collaboration with area community-based providers. Moreover, schools often provide crisis therapy or counseling to students exposed to significant trauma due to violence in the school or community or following major devastating events such as terrorist events or natural disasters. Such therapy or counseling services are commonly provided by local mental health providers.

very, very confidential

Incidents of violence in schools spurred the Bush Administration to reconsider whether state and federal laws properly address "the fundamental interests of privacy and individual freedom, safety, and security," and how these laws assist those with mental health needs in getting appropriate care (Report to the President 2007, 3). A 2007 Report to the President includes several recommendations for state and federal actions including the following:

- Developing guidance that clarifies how information can be shared legally under the **Health Insurance Portability and Accountability Act of 1996 (HIPAA)** and the **Family Educational Rights and Privacy Act of 1974 (FERPA)**, and disseminating it to the mental health, education, and law enforcement communities

- Ensuring that emergency management state and local communities have clear guidance on the sharing of information as it relates to educational records and FERPA (20 USC § 1232g; 34 CFR Part 99)

- Coordinating best practices in disseminating information about threat assessments for colleges and universities

above and beyond HIPAA

only patient can consent to authorization

The report also discusses coordinating state and federal firearms laws. "Only 23 states currently provide any information to the National Instant Criminal Background Check System (NICS) on persons disqualified from possessing firearms under federal law for reasons related

strictest documentation guidelines

to mental health, and many of those that do provide information provide very few records" (Report to the President 2007, 14).

Documentation Issues to Consider in Behavioral Healthcare

Behavioral healthcare requires documentation for many types of treatment that may not regularly occur in other settings. These include such issues as seclusion and restraints, suicide watch, minors seeking services, conservatorship, and psychotherapy sessions.

Seclusion and Restraints

duty to warn

must be monitored inside or just outside the room

least restrictive

must document why harm themselves or others

within 24 hrs must have face to face – how to avoid in the future

As mentioned in chapter 5, in most states, only licensed physicians are allowed to issue orders for the use of seclusion or restraints. In some states, however, psychologists, physician's assistants, and certified nurse-practitioners are also allowed to write orders under limited conditions. In all cases, health record documentation must support the medical necessity of the services and materials ordered. See figures 12.2, 12.3, and 12.4 for sample forms related to the use of seclusion and restraints. The form used in the behavioral healthcare setting is similar to that used in other healthcare settings.

Orders for physical or pharmaceutical restraint or seclusion must comply with Medicare regulations, state laws, and accreditation standards. In general, orders for restraint or seclusion should be issued only when the procedures are necessary to protect the patient or others from harm. Regulations and standards require specific time limits and continuous observation to prevent injuries to the patient, such as suffocation. Accreditation standards for psychiatric facilities provide guidelines that are more specific.

Suicide Watch

sitters – just sit in the room and monitor the patient

Patient observation, such as one-to-one staffing or 15-minute checks, should be documented in a patient's medical record. (See figure 12.5 for a sample form.) Studies have found that in some facilities up to 13 percent of psychiatric inpatients require constant observation. Despite observation and monitoring, however, about 75 percent of patients admitted with suicidal thoughts who committed suicide in the hospital denied these thoughts during their last communication with hospital staff (Grant 2007). The cost of constant observation can be significant for a behavioral healthcare facility—as much as 20 percent of the total nursing budget (Grant 2007).

According to the American Psychiatric Association (2003):

> The most frequent lawsuits, settlements, and verdicts against psychiatrists are for patients' suicides. . . . If a malpractice claim is brought against the psychiatrist, documentation of suicide risk assessments assists the court in evaluating the many clinical complexities and ambiguities that exist in the treatment and management of patients at suicide risk.
>
> The failure to document suicide risk assessments and interventions may give the court reason to conclude they were not done. . . . Thus, it is crucial for the suicide risk assessment to be documented in the medical record.

Minors Seeking Services

Indiana does

Some states permit minors to admit themselves into mental health treatment facilities without parental consent; they also permit minors to authorize disclosure of **personal health**

parents don't have access to information

Figure 12.2. Restraint order in paper format.

Anytown Community Hospital

RESTRAINT ORDER

PATIENT LABEL

Patient Behavior/Criteria Present:
- ☐ Climbing out of bed
- ☐ Pulling at dressings, lines, or tubes
- ☐ Attempting to remove dressings, lines, or tubes
- ☐ Unable to follow directions with results that may injure self or others
- ☐ Standing up from chair
- ☐ Other: _____

Patient Behavior Related To:
- ☐ Confusion
- ☐ Delirium
- ☐ Marked agitation
- ☐ Sedation/analgesia
- ☐ Impaired attention and/or concentration
- ☐ Impaired learning ability
- ☐ Other: _____

Type and Number of Restraints:
- ☐ ×1 ☐ ×2 Soft wrist restraint
- ☐ ×1 ☐ ×2 Soft ankle restraint
- ☐ ×1 ☐ ×2 Soft mitten restraint
- ☐ ×4 Leather restraint
- ☐ Vest restraint
- ☐ Chair restraint
- ☐ Other: _____

Time Limitation:
- ☐ Continuous usage
- ☐ At night only
- ☐ When up in chair
- ☐ When family/visitors not at bedside
- ☐ Other: _____

within 24 hrs there must be a face to face interaction if restraints were used

---

Renewal Order Only
- ☐ Patient examined by physician.
- ☐ Alternatives to use of restraints reviewed by physician/staff.
- ☐ Patient continues to demonstrate behavior leading to use of restraints, as indicated above.

_____
Physician Signature   Date/Time

Telephone/Verbal Order:
Dr. _____/
_____,RN _____
                              Date/Time

RESTRAINT ORDER
000011 (11/2002)

Figure 12.3.   Restraint or seclusion assessment.

PRECIPITATING EVENT: Behaviors leading to restraint or seclusion: _____ _____ _____ _____ _____ _____	Nursing Staff Prompts: _(Check all when completed)_ ☐ 1:1 initiated by Charge Nurse ☐ MD evaluation within one (1) hour ☐ Clothing search complete ☐ Denial of Rights Form complete ☐ Order obtained every 4 hours ☐ Add to Treatment Plan _(CRU only)_

Clinical interventions used prior to restraint or seclusion: _(check all that apply)_

☐   **Medication Intervention**   ☐   **De-escalation**   ☐   **Voluntary Time Out**

☐ **Threat Reduction** _(for fear)_
   ☐   Mirror person as far as eye contact
   ☐   Give reassurance of safety
   ☐   No touching without permission
   ☐   Stand with arms at side, palms facing forward
   ☐   Calm, confident vocal tone
   ☐   Slow gestures
   ☐   Use rule of five _(no more than 5 words-each word 5 letters or less)_

☐ **Control** _(for frustration)_
   ☐   Maintain eye contact
   ☐   Assess origin/cause of frustration
   ☐   Stand with palms facing down
   ☐   Speak in confident manner
   ☐   Moderate tone of voice
   ☐   Use rule of five

☐ **Detachment** _(for manipulation)_
   ☐   No direct eye contact
   ☐   Speak in firm voice
   ☐   Turn at an angled position
   ☐   Use rule of five
   ☐   Act in a disengaged manner

☐ **Consequation** _(for intimidation)_
   ☐   Use rule of five
   ☐   Confident posture
   ☐   Maintain direct eye contact
   ☐   Don't threaten or argue
   ☐   Identify consequences

Patient's response to above interventions: _____
_____

(circle one below)

Less restrictive interventions have been attempted unsuccessfully and **seclusion/restraint/ambulatory restraint** is necessary to prevent the following: ☐ Harm to self   ☐ Harm to others

The patient was given the following explanation of reason for seclusion or restraint:_____
_____

Patient grants permission to notify family of seclusion or restraint   ☐Yes (if yes, document in Progress Notes)
                                                                          ☐ No

☐ Signed consent for involvement of interested party obtained

(If yes, name of person contacted): _____

Release criteria: ☐ Contracts for safety   ☐ Reduced agitation/impulsively
                       ☐ No longer danger to self and/or others

Explain: _____

RN Signature:_____   **Date:**_____   **Time:**_____

County of San Diego
Health and Human Services Agency
Mental Health Services
San Diego County Psychiatric Hospital
RESTRAINT OR SECLUSION ASSESSMENT
HHSA:MHS-225 (11/02)

Patient Identification

436

Figure 12.4. Restraint or seclusion flow sheet.

TITLE:	RESTRAINT or SECLUSION FLOW SHEET
FORM NUMBER:	HHSA: MHS-226
WHEN	For use of Restraint or Seclusion procedures and ambulatory restraints.
ON WHOM	All patients in seclusion, restraints or ambulatory restraints.
COMPLETED BY	The flow sheet will be completed by RNs, and LVNs, PTs and/or MHAs.
MODE OF COMPLETION	Handwritten
FORMAT	Restraint or seclusion flow sheet is a preprinted form to include patient's identification, date, shift, time initiated, and initiator RN signature.

The type of Restraint or Seclusion initiated will be checked.

A new form will be used when the first form is completed or when a new date starts.

Signatures and initials of those staff using the form will be placed in the respective boxes.

- **"Describe Patient Behaviors" Section:**
  - RNs shall document when a patient is placed into seclusion, restraint, or ambulatory restraints and when these measures are renewed, reduced, or discontinued.
  - Additional pertinent information shall be documented here at least once every hour.
  - Code numbers from the top of the page shall be used, when applicable.
  - Additional information may be added to the progress notes.
- **"Every 15 minutes" Section:**
  - May be completed by RNs, LVNs, PTs or MHAs
  - Add time and initials (end of row)
  - Check blanks corresponding to each section
  - Add code numbers in "brief behavior description" column
- **"Every 2 hours" Section:**
  - May be completed by RNs, LVNs, PTs or MHAs
  - Add time and initials (end of row)
  - Check and complete blanks corresponding to each section
- **"Debriefing" Section:**
  - **Shall be completed by an RN**
  - **Add reason for "no" and additional comments as indicated**
  - **If there are no additional comments, write N/A in the blanks provided.**

EXCEPTIONS	None.

06/02

Figure 12.4. (*continued*)]

Date: _____	Shift: _____	Time Initiated: _____	_____

Initiator RN Signature   *Date*

Check One:	☐ Seclusion	☐ Restraint	☐ Ambulatory Restraints

CODES		Document/check each area every **15 MINUTES** or more frequently as needed.	Document/check each area every **TWO (2) HOURS** or more frequently as needed.

1. Beating on door/wall	6. Standing still
2. Yelling/screaming	7. Walking/pacing
3. Crying/cursing	8. Thrashing/spitting
4. Laughing/singing	9. Quiet
5. Mumbling	10. Disrobing/sexually inappropriate

11. Other:_____

(RNs, LVNs, PTs, MHAs)

Initials	Signatures

Table columns (read vertically):
- Time
- Continual visual & auditory observation
- Patient is breathing without difficulty **CIRCULATION CHECKS**
- Restraints intact, extremities assessed
- Brief behavior description **(USE CODES)**
- Offer of foods/fluids
- Offer bathroom/ bedpan
- Range of Motion (10 minutes)
- Pulse & B/P Temperature & Respiration Rate

Initials

Time	*Describe Patient Behaviors* **(document once every hour)**	*RN Initials*								

Debriefing within 24 hours after episode ☐ Yes ☐ No If no, give reason_____

Comments:_____

_____

County of San Diego
Health and Human Services Agency
Mental Health Services
San Diego County Psychiatric Hospital

RESTRAINT OR SECLUSION FLOW SHEET

Patient Identification

HHSA:MHS-226 (06/02)

Figure 12.5. **Inpatient assessment of suicide risk (pre- and postdiscontinuation of suicide precaution).**

Assessment Factor	Low Risk (1 Point)	Moderate Risk (2 Points)	High Risk (3 Points)
Suicidal ideation	No current suicidal thoughts	Intermittent or fleeting suicidal thoughts	Constant suicidal thoughts
Suicide plan	No plan	Has plan without access to planned method	Has carefully thought out plan with actual or potential access to method
Lethality of plan/incident	Low lethality of plan/ incident (such as superficial scratching)	Moderate lethality (such as hidden sharps or contraband items)	High lethality of plan/ incident (such as hanging, suffocation attempt)
No Harm Contract	Reliably signs No Harm Contract	Signs No Harm Contract but is ambivalent	Unwilling or unable to sign No Harm Contract
Behavioral symptoms: • Anxiety • Hopelessness • Helplessness • Anger/rage • Guilt/shame • Impulsivity • Isolation	None to two symptoms present	Three to four symptoms present	Five to seven symptoms present
Support systems	Several friends, coworkers and relatives available	Few or only one friend	None available
Comments:		Total Score:	
		RN Signature:	
		Date & Time:	
Scoring Directions: 1. Assess each assessment factor. 2. Circle one descriptor for each assessment that best describes the patient. 3. Assign appropriate points (1, 2, or 3) to each factor. 4. Add the points for each assessment factor to arrive at a total score.			
Scoring Key: 6–10 points = Low risk (Zero [0] precautions) 11–14 points = Moderate risk (Alert—continue assessment for another shift) 15 points or above = High risk (Notify physician)		**Patient Label**	

information (PHI). Likewise, according to 42 CFR 2, Subpart B, 2.14, if state law permits minors to seek admission for services in a substance-abuse program without parental consent, unless the minor lacks the capacity to make rational choice, only the minor can authorize disclosure of his or her PHI, including the disclosure of information to parents.

Psychotherapy Sessions

A patient's behavioral healthcare record must indicate that the client has a psychiatric illness or demonstrates emotional or behavioral symptoms sufficient to intervene with normal functioning. In addition, it must include the time spent in psychotherapy encounters and show that cognitive skills such as behavioral modification, insight and supportive interactions, and discussion of reality were applied to produce therapeutic change. For interactive psychotherapy, the medical record also must indicate that the client does not have the ability to interact through normal verbal communication means (for instance, art therapy or family therapy).

The special confidentiality protections afforded psychotherapy notes under HIPAA (2003) require programs to handle them cautiously. For this reason, organizations must be clear in their understanding of HIPAA's definition of what constitutes psychotherapy notes.

Psychotherapy notes are also referred to as *process notes*. They capture the therapist's impressions of the client obtained from conversations during private counseling sessions or group, joint, or family counseling sessions. The notes contain details considered inappropriate for inclusion in the medical record and are used by the provider for future sessions. Psychotherapy notes exclude medication, prescription, and monitoring information; counseling session start and stop times; the modalities and frequencies of treatment furnished; results of clinical tests; and any summary of diagnosis, functional status, treatment plan, symptoms, prognosis, and progress to date.

To qualify as psychotherapy notes, the notes must contain extended direct quotations from both client and therapist. In addition, they must include repeated and systematic references to interpretive insights to the client's intrapsychic dynamics as discussed in the therapy sessions. Finally, the documentation in the notes must weave together the client's unresolved past conflicts or issues with current difficulties. Notes that do not meet these criteria are much better identified as counseling progress notes, which are meant to be useful to the entire treatment team as well as the client.

This distinction is important because psychotherapy notes may not be released unless specifically identified on an authorization form and only with the author's permission.

However, not all therapy documentation requires special handling. Some therapy documentation may be released with a valid authorization. Such documentation includes the following:

- Records of the prescription and monitoring of medication

- Counseling session start and stop times

- Modalities and frequency of treatment

- Results of clinical tests

- Any summary of the client's diagnoses, functional status, treatment plan, symptoms, prognosis, and progress to date

In psychiatric settings, clinical observations are typically documented in progress notes. The requirements are similar to that for the acute-care record in that they create a chronological report of the patient's condition and response to treatment during his or her course of treatment, coordination of services provided, and chronological records of vital signs.

Conservatorship

When a person is unable to provide for personal needs such as food, shelter, or clothing as the result of a mental disorder, and thereby is gravely disabled and unwilling or incapable of accepting voluntary treatment, he or she may be recommended for **conservatorship** placement—that is, placed under the care of an appointed guardian. Mental health conservatorship requirements may vary from state to state. Acceptable conservatorship documents are created by attorneys and the courts in each state and may differ in format. Conservatorship documents become part of the medical record.

Behavioral Health Record Content

The acute psychiatric healthcare record contains a number of assessments and reports pertaining to the patient's treatment.

Psychiatric Assessment

This assessment identifies the client's physical, cognitive, behavioral, emotional and social status. It also identifies facilitating factors and possible barriers that prevent the patient from reaching his or her goals beyond the presenting problems. (See figure 12.6 for items to be included in the psychiatric assessment.)

Medical and Psychiatric History

A complete history documents the client's current complaints and symptoms and lists his or her past medical, personal, and family history.

Physical Examination Report

The physical examination report represents the attending physician's assessment of the patient's current health status. This report should document information on all of the patient's major organ systems.

Mental Status Exam

The mental status exam is as crucial to psychiatry as the physical exam is to other areas of medicine. Adolf Meyer developed the mental status exam in 1918. He believed that it was important to ask the same questions of every patient so that certain standards could be achieved. The exam describes various mental functions, including appearance, speech, thought process, behavior, affect, orientation, memory, mood, motor skills, intellect, judgment, and insight.

Diagnostic and Therapeutic Orders

Physician's orders are the instructions the physician gives to the other healthcare professionals who actually perform diagnostic tests and treatments, administer medications, and provide

Figure 12.6. Components of the psychiatric assessment.

Component
Physical factors, including disabilities
Cognitive disorders
Behavioral disorders
Emotional disorders
Mental disorders
Communicative disorders
Social and environmental factors, including social status
Substance abuse, dependence, and other addictive behaviors
Developmental disabilities
Vision and hearing impairments and disabilities
Symptoms that may be associated with a disease, condition, or treatment

specific services to a patient. These orders must be written legibly and include the date and the physician's signature.

Standing orders are orders the medical staff or an individual physician has established as routine care for a specific diagnosis or procedure. Standing orders are commonly used in hospitals, ambulatory-surgery facilities, and long-term care facilities. Usually standing orders are preprinted on a single sheet of paper. Like other physician's orders, they must be signed, dated, and filed in the patient's medical record.

Physicians may communicate orders verbally or via the telephone when the healthcare organization's policies and procedures or medical staff rules allow. State law and medical staff rules specify which practitioners are allowed to accept and execute verbal and telephone orders. How the orders are to be authenticated and the time period allowed for authentication should also be specified.

Restraint and Seclusion Orders

Specific documentation guidelines and procedures to follow with regard to the use of restraint and seclusion procedures vary by state. However, the guidelines to follow in these matters are those outlined in the Joint Commission manual that is updated annually.

Refer to the "Seclusion and Restraints" section in this chapter for additional discussion regarding seclusion and restraints.

Consultation Reports

Consultation reports document clinical opinions requested from physicians outside the case by the patient's primary or attending physician. They are based on the consulting physicians' examination of the client and a review of his or her health record.

Diagnostic and Therapeutic Procedure Reports

The results of all diagnostic and therapeutic procedures are permanently filed in the patient's medical record. Diagnostic procedures include laboratory tests performed on blood, urine, and other samples from the patient.

Mandated Reporting

Many states mandate that certain types of reports be completed and forwarded to the appropriate authorities. Examples of mandated reports include, but are not limited to:

- Abuse reports (domestic, child, and elder abuse)
- Tuberculosis
- Human immunodeficiency virus (HIV)
- Sexually transmitted diseases
- Legal/police reports, including recommendation to revoke a driver's license
- Duty-to-warn report: Mental health professionals have a duty to warn reasonably identifiable victims when there are known serious threats of violence against them. Most states title these reports differently (for example, in California, the Tarasoff Report) (*Tarasoff v. Regents of the University of California* 1976).

- Firearms prohibition: According to California statutory law (CCR 2004), mental health organizations are required to submit reports to the state to prevent clients from owning, possessing, receiving, or purchasing firearms for a period of five years from the date of admission to a mental health organization. This prohibition applies to all persons taken into custody as a danger to themselves or others. Other states may have similar regulations.

Treatment/Care Plans

Treatment or care plans are developed based on the patient's needs as identified via the assessments. Plans must specify the patient's goals and objectives as well as the actions or interventions needed to meet them and time frames in which to accomplish them. Patients are to be involved in the formulation of their plans and asked for input. They also are asked to agree to the planned course of treatment, care, or services. Each state defines the person in that state who may act as a case manager. Case managers prepare assessments and care plans, which then are included in the client's health record.

Care plans are updated when clinically appropriate and when required by organizational policy, state guidelines, and clinical path protocols.

Treatment/care plans may be documented via the following:

- Handwritten notes
- Electronic records
- Standards of practice
- Decision algorithms
- Care paths or maps
- Individualized preprinted plans of care

Outpatient Crisis Plan

Because of the nature of mental illness, clients often develop crisis plans with their therapists. A crisis plan might be viewed in the same way that an advance directive is viewed for individuals in an acute-care setting. It is the client's direction on what to do and who to contact should he or she become mentally incapable of communicating his or her wishes. The crisis plan does not supersede an advance directive but, rather, complements it.

Psychotherapy Notes

Psychotherapy notes contain details considered inappropriate for inclusion in the medical record and are used by the provider for future sessions. Psychotherapy notes do not include medication, prescription, and monitoring information; counseling session start and stop times; the modalities and frequencies of treatment furnished; results of clinical tests; or any summary of diagnosis, functional status, treatment plan, symptoms, prognosis, or progress to date.

Organizations must be clear in their understanding of HIPAA's (2003) definition of what constitutes psychotherapy notes.

Refer to the "Psychotherapy Sessions" section in this chapter for a detailed discussion of psychotherapy notes.

Progress Notes

In psychiatric settings, clinical observations are typically documented in progress notes. The purpose of documenting the clinical observations of physicians, nurses, and other caregivers is to create a chronological report of the patient's condition and response to treatment during his or her course of treatment.

The rules and regulations of the healthcare organization specify which healthcare providers are allowed to enter progress notes into the health record. Typically, these individuals include the patient's attending physician, any consulting physicians who have medical staff privileges, house medical staff, nurses, nutritionists, social workers, and clinical therapists. Depending on the record format used by the hospital, each discipline maintains a separate section of the health record or all provider observations are combined in the same chronological or integrated health record.

Progress notes serve to justify further treatment in the facility. In addition, they document the appropriateness and coordination of the services provided. For Medicare purposes, each note must be able to stand alone and justify medical necessity.

Nurses keep chronological records of the patient's vital signs (blood pressure, heart rate, respiration rate, and temperature) throughout his or her hospital stay. Moreover, it has increasingly become the practice to take vital signs routinely at outpatient care programs. Nurses often keep separate logs showing what medications were ordered and when they were administered.

Documentation of Medication Administration

Healthcare providers are required to obtain written consents and authorizations before providing treatment or disclosing confidential patient information. In addition, acknowledgments may be sought from the patient confirming that he or she has received specific information from the healthcare facility.

Consent to Treatment

Many healthcare facilities obtain consent to treatment from patients or their legal representatives before providing care or services except in emergency situations. The consent to treatment documents the patient's permission to receive routine services, diagnostic procedures, and medical care (Abdelhak et al 2007, 104). The need to obtain the patient's consent before medical and surgical procedures is based on the legal concept of battery, which is the unlawful touching of a person without his or her implied or expressed consent.

Individual states may have laws or regulations that define the content of authorizations. When such laws or regulations exist, the treatment program should consult the HIPAA (2003) Privacy Rule to determine how to apply the state requirements.

Implied consent is assumed when a patient voluntarily submits to treatment. The rationale behind implied consent is that one can reasonably assume that the patient understands the nature of the treatment or would not submit to it. Expressed consent is a consent that is either spoken or written. Although courts recognize both verbal and written consent, verbal consent is more difficult to prove.

It is primarily the physician's responsibility to ensure that the patient understands the nature of the procedure, as well as alternative treatments, and its risks, complications, and benefits before it is performed. Medical staff rules or healthcare provider policies usually list the types of services and procedures that require written consent from the patient. Generally, procedures involving the use of anesthetics, the administration of experimental drugs, the sur-

[handwritten margin note: Sometimes not voluntary]

gical manipulation of organs and tissues, and significant risk of complications require written consent. In addition, some states have passed laws that require written consent forms for certain types of testing procedures (for example, HIV testing).

Advance Directives

An advance directive is a written document that names the patient's choice of legal representative for healthcare purposes. The person designated by the patient then is empowered to make healthcare decisions on behalf of the patient in the event the patient is no longer capable of expressing his or her preferences. Living wills and durable powers of attorney for healthcare are two examples of advance directives.

Certifications for Holds, Restraints, or Seclusion

When a patient is found by his or her treating psychiatrist or psychologist to be a danger to others or him- or herself or to be gravely disabled as defined by state law, the patient may be held against his or her will for various periods of time, depending on state statute. In some states, the patient can request a judicial review. Patients also may petition the treating physician regarding capacity to consent or refuse antipsychotic medication.

Documentation of Conservatorship

As noted earlier, behavioral health patients may require documentation of conservatorship. This may be recommended when a person is unable to provide for him- or herself. Conservatorship documents become part of the medical record.

Refer to the "Conservatorship" section in this chapter for further discussion of conservatorship.

Discharge Summaries and Client Instructions

The discharge summary is a concise account of the patient's illness, course of treatment, response to treatment, and condition at the time of discharge from the service. The functions of the discharge summary include the following:

- Ensuring the continuity of future care by providing information to the patient's attending physician, referring physician, and any consulting physicians

- Providing information to support the activities of the medical staff review committee

- Providing concise information that can be used to answer information requests from authorized individuals or entities

The discharge summary must be signed by the attending physician. However, there are some exceptions to this rule. For example, some states allow nurses to sign discharge summaries in chemical dependency programs.

The discharge summary also includes instructions for the patient's follow-up care. It is vital that the client or his or her caregiver be given clear, concise instructions. Ideally, those instructions are communicated both verbally and in writing. The healthcare professional who provides them should sign the health record to indicate that verbal instructions have been issued. In addition, the person receiving the instructions should sign to verify that he or she understands them. A copy of the written instructions is then filed in the health record.

When someone other than the patient assumes responsibility for the patient's aftercare, the record should indicate that the instructions were given to the party responsible. Documentation of patient education may be accomplished through forms that prompt the person providing instruction to cover important information.

Despite the best efforts of hospital caregivers and physicians, some patients die while hospitalized. In such cases, the attending physician should add a summary statement to the patient's health record documenting the circumstances surrounding the patient's death. The statement can take the form of a final progress note or a separate report. It should indicate the reason for the client's admission, his or her diagnosis and course in the hospital, and a description of the events that led to his or her death.

Information Pertaining to Emergency Care

The delivery of emergency care services occurs primarily in hospital-based emergency departments and freestanding psychiatric hospitals. However, it also occurs "in the field" with various outreach programs that include psychiatric emergency response teams working in conjunction with the police or emergency medical services. Emergency care documentation is limited to information about the patient's presenting problem and the diagnostic and therapeutic services provided during the episode of care. The services provided in emergency situations focus on diagnosing the problem and stabilizing the patient. Unlike physical illness in which minor injuries and illnesses may require no further medical treatment, psychiatric emergency patients must be referred to ambulatory-care providers for follow-up care. Seriously ill patients are admitted to a hospital for ongoing acute psychiatric care treatment. At times, it is necessary to do this even against the patient's will. In this scenario, the client is determined to be incompetent to provide for his or her own care.

In emergency care records, it is extremely important to document the instructions given to the patient as well as the patient's presenting complaint, evaluation, and assessment. Thorough documentation is needed to justify reimbursement, to protect the organization or the patient in future legal proceedings, and to ensure continuity of care.

The following information must be entered into the patient's health record for each emergency care visit:

- Patient's identification (or the reason it could not be obtained)

- Time and means of the patient's arrival at the organization

- Pertinent history of the illness or injury and physical findings, including the patient's vital signs

- Emergency care given to the patient prior to arrival

- Diagnostic and therapeutic orders

- Clinical observations, including the results of treatment

- Reports of procedures, tests, and results

- Diagnostic impression

- Conclusion at the termination of evaluation/treatment, including final disposition, the patient's condition on discharge or transfer, and any instructions given to the patient, the patient's representative, or another healthcare facility for follow-up care

- Documentation of cases where patients left the hospital or emergency department against medical advice

Behavioral Health Accreditation, Regulation, Industry, and Advocacy

Numerous forces in the healthcare environment have an impact on behavioral healthcare and documentation. These forces come from several sources, including accrediting bodies, governmental regulations and recommendations, and changes in the healthcare industry.

Accrediting Bodies

For behavioral healthcare organizations, there are five widely accepted accrediting bodies: Joint Commission, Commission on Accreditation of Rehabilitation Facilities (CARF), American Osteopathic Association (AOA), National Committee for Quality Assurance (NCQA), and Council on Accreditation (COA). These entities issue accreditation and documentation standards that behavioral healthcare organizations may use as benchmarks.

The Joint Commission

The Joint Commission bases its accreditation outcome on the ability of the healthcare organization to demonstrate compliance with specific performance standards. The Joint Commission began accrediting behavioral healthcare facilities in 1971. The accreditation process includes an on-site survey by an interdisciplinary survey team that evaluates ongoing compliance with the performance standards specific to the healthcare setting (Joint Commission 2003).

The Joint Commission has specific documentation requirements for behavioral healthcare. Joint Commission Standard IM.6.10 requires that behavioral healthcare facilities maintain complete and accurate medical records for patients assessed, cared for, treated, or served. Medical records must be reviewed on an ongoing basis at the point of care. See figure 12.7 for a sample record review (audit) form. This review form details the Joint Commission's documentation requirements for behavioral healthcare organizations.

Behavioral healthcare services currently accredited include mental health, addiction services, and child welfare and developmentally disabled care in a variety of treatment settings. Depending on the type of state licensure and the funding source, some behavioral healthcare organizations continue to be surveyed under the hospital standards instead of the behavioral health standards.

As in other healthcare settings, Joint Commission accreditation includes an intensive on-site survey process at least once every three years.

Commission on Accreditation of Rehabilitation Facilities

The Commission on Accreditation of Rehabilitation Facilities (CARF) is similar to the Joint Commission in that it is a not-for-profit organization devoted to ensuring continuous quality improvement in healthcare; however, CARF specifically accredits organizations for quality excellence in rehabilitative and human services. Like the Joint Commission, CARF has developed performance standards that must be met in order for a healthcare organization to pass the survey process (CARF 2004).

CARF has specific behavioral health standards and surveys a variety of behavioral health settings, including mental healthcare, substance-abuse care, and other addiction programs. The CARF General Program Standards, Section 2G for behavioral healthcare documentation, state that the individual records communicate information in a manner that is organized, clear,

Figure 12.7. Behavioral healthcare ongoing record review form.

	Reviewer Signature					Date					
Date:											
Unit:											
REVIEW QUESTIONS	Enter review date in boxes below										
	Yes							No: Corrected			N/A
General Information											
Patient identification data on all pages											
All consents completed and signed as required											
Compliance with prohibited abbreviations											
Documentation of "Read back" for telephone order/critical values (within time frame)											
Times and means of patient arrival											
Documentation if "Left against medical advice"											
Conclusions at termination of treatment, including final disposition, condition, and instructions for follow-up care, treatment, and services (at D/C)											
Initial Screenings & Assessment											
Nursing assessment/documentation complete (no blanks)											
Is there documentation in the computer that the patient was asked about advance directives?											
Is a copy of the advance directive present on the record?											
Is there documentation of the pain scale used to assess the patient's pain?											
Is pain reassessed and pain med effectiveness documented?											
Evidence/documentation that the following screenings/ assessments were performed at point of entry and upon admission according to practice:											
a. Current medication list for reconciliation											
b. Nutritional screening for diet, meals											
c. Universal screening for abuse											
d. Immunizations											
e. Spiritual/educational and cultural needs											
f. Discharge needs											
g. Hx of violence											
h. Fall risk score											
i. Drug/alcohol/tobacco use											

Figure 12.7. (*continued*)

Interdisciplinary care plan:	Yes								No: Corrected		N/A
Is present											
All required elements complete—strength/weakness											
All required signatures present including patient's											
Reassessment											
Are reassessments documented every shift and when a change occurs in the patient condition?											
Is there documentation of the patient's response to all interventions including response to medications?											
Documentation of Care											
Is the care plan revised in response to changes in patient condition or in response to changes in the assessments of other disciplines involved in the care?											
Is there documentation of multidisciplinary discharge planning?											
Is there documentation of discharge instructions/education to patient and/or family?											
Documentation of all elements on graphics present											
Thorough and complete documentation when seclusion/ restraint interventions are utilized											
Physician Care											
Documentation of diagnosis, condition, or indication for—use for each medication ordered											
H&P within 24 hours or documentation of ongoing attempts in progress notes											
Evidence of clinical interpretation of test reports											
Patient and Family Education											
Is there evidence in the record that the education process considers the physical, cognitive, cultural, social, and economic characteristics of the patient?											
Is there evidence that the patient's education is based on the assessed needs, abilities, preferences, and readiness to learn?											
Is there documentation of teaching delivered by appropriate staff or between disciplines?											
Is there documentation that the patient/family has been offered education as appropriate on:											
a. Safe and effective use of medications											
b. Nutrition interventions: modified diet/oral health											
c. Available community resources											
d. Self-care activities/smoking cessation											
e. Discharge instructions											

complete, current, and legible. All documents that require signatures must have original or electronic signatures.

An individual's record must include the following:

- The date of admission

- Information about the individual's personal representative, conservator, guardian, or representative payee, if any of these have been appointed, including the name, address, and telephone number

- Information about the person to contact in the event of an emergency, including the name, address, and telephone number

- The name of the person currently coordinating the services of the person served

- The location of any other records

- Information about the individual's primary-care physician, including the name, address, and telephone number, when available

- Healthcare reimbursement information, if applicable

- The person's:

  — Health history

  — Current medications

  — Preadmission screening, when conducted

  — Documentation of orientation

  — Assessments (See figures 12.8 and 12.9 for sample psychiatric assessment forms.)

  — Individual plan, including reviews

  — Transition plan, when applicable

The discharge summary must include the following elements:

- Date of admission and date of discharge

- Identification of the presenting condition

- Description of the extent to which established goals and objectives were achieved

- Description of the services provided

- The reasons for discharge

- The status of the person served at discharge

- A list of recommendations for services or supports

See figure 5.14 (p. 116) for a sample discharge form.

Other items to include are correspondence pertinent to the person served, authorization for release of information, and documentation of internal or external referrals.

Entries to the records of the persons served follow the organization's policy that specifies time frames for entries. If duplicate information or reports from the main record of a person served exist, or if working files are maintained, such materials are not substituted for the main record, are considered secondary documents, with the main record of the person served

Figure 12.8.   *General* Psychiatric assessment.

This is a psychiatric assessment billed as an MMD provided on site for _____ minutes.

PRESENTING PROBLEM:

    IDENTIFYING DATA/CHIEF COMPLAINT:

    HISTORY OF PRESENT ILLNESS:

CURRENT NEEDS:

    PAST PSYCHIATRIC HISTORY:

DRUG/ALCOHOL HISTORY:

    MEDICAL HISTORY:

    SOCIAL HISTORY:

    CULTURAL & RELIGIOUS ISSUES:

    INSURANCE STATUS:

    VITAL SIGNS:
      Blood pressure: _____ Temperature:_____ Pulse rate: _____ Respiratory rate: _____ Pain (0-10):____

MENTAL STATUS EXAMINATION:

DIAGNOSIS:

    Axis I:
    Axis II:
    Axis III:
    Axis IV:
    Axis V: GAF Current: Past year:

CURRENT POTENTIAL FOR HARM:

INTERPRETIVE SUMMARY:

                                  STAFF PSYCHIATRIST

County of San Diego	Patient Name:
Health and Human Services Agency	
Mental Health Services	MR#: Unit:
SAN DIEGO COUNTY PSYCHIATRIC HOSPITAL	
	D.O.B.: Date
PSYCHIATRIC ASSESSMENT	

HHSA:MHS-204 (01/02)

Major piece of documentation

Figure 12.9. **Initial mental health assessment.**

Assessment Date:_____

PRESENTING PROBLEM: (Identifying Data/Chief Complaint and History of Present Illness. Summarize client's request for services **including client's subjective description of the problem.**   Include precipitating factors, objective impairing behaviors, including experiences and stigma, if any, and prejudice and client's requests/needs.)

_____

_____

_____

_____

_____

_____

_____

_____

_____

_____

_____

_____

_____

_____

PAST PSYCHIATRIC HISTORY: (Previous mental health treatment; where, when, for how long. Include dates/providers related to any prior psychiatric treatment, history, traumatic and/or significant events, include immigration history, and impact if any).

_____

_____

_____

_____

_____

_____

_____

_____

_____

_____

_____

_____

_____

_____

_____

_____

_____

FAMILY HISTORY: _____

_____

_____

_____

Any family members with a history of any of the following? (Please, check all that apply)

	Depression	Schizophrenia	Bipolar	Substance Abuse	Suicide	Other	Effective Treatments
Parent							
Sibling							
Children							
Aunt/Uncle							
Grandparent							

County of San Diego Health and Human Services Agency Mental Health Services **INITIAL MENTAL HEALTH ASSESSMENT** HHSA:MHS-912 (6/2003)	**Client:**_____ **MR/Client ID #:**_____ **Program:**_____ Page 1 of 5

Figure 12.9. (*continued*)

<u>CULTURE/FAMILY and RECOVERY POTENTIAL:</u>

Birth place: ( ) San Diego ( ) USA ( ) **Other (fill in birth place and year moved to USA):**_____

Language of choice for therapy: ☐English ☐Spanish ☐Vietnamese ☐Other (fill in language) _____

Ethnicity: ☐ Latino/Hispanic ☐ African American ☐ Asian/Pacific Islander (fill in): _____

☐ White ☐ American Indian ☐ Other (fill in): _____

Culture specific symptomatology/explanations for behavior (may reference Appendix I of DSM-IV-TR): _____
_____
_____

Family/Community Support System: (Live alone? Describe it, including alternative relationship support, if any. Who is supportive? Community groups, e.g. AA/NA)
_____
_____

Socioeconomic Factors: (educational achievement, occupation, income source, and level)
_____
_____

Religious/Spiritual Issues: (Is R/S important in your life? If yes, is it a source of strength in your recovery process? Describe how/who: persons, practices.)
_____
_____
_____

ASSETS/STRENGTHS: (What abilities or skills do you have that you would choose to develop during your recovery? What new ones might you choose to develop?)
_____
_____
_____

[handwritten note in margin: what can we build on? use strengths to develop weaknesses]

MEDICAL HISTORY: (Indicate any significant medical history related to client's current mental health condition, including dates/providers related to prior treatment, as well as client's adjustment to co-occurring disabilities.)
_____
_____
_____
_____

Current Medication(s)	*Dose*	Frequency	Taken as Prescribed?
			☐YES ☐NO
			☐YES ☐NO
			☐YES ☐NO
			☐YES ☐NO

ALLERGIES AND ADVERSE MEDICATION REACTIONS:
☐ NKA(s)
☐ Other (s)_____

HEALING AND HEALTH: (Alternative healing practices/beliefs. Apart from mental health professionals, who-- or what-- helps you deal with disability/illness? Describe.)
_____
_____
_____

County of San Diego
Health and Human Services Agency
Mental Health Services

INITIAL MENTAL HEALTH ASSESSMENT

HHSA:MHS-912 (6/2003)

Client:_____

MR/Client ID #:_____

Program:_____

Page 2 of 5

Figure 12.9. (*continued*)

NAME OF CURRENT PRIMARY CARE PHYSICIAN:
May we consult? ☐Yes ☐No   Date Last Seen: _____   Release of Information Form: ☐Yes ☐No

_____

Name   Address   Phone number (including area code)

CLIENT'S HOSPITAL OF CHOICE:

_____

Name   Address   Phone number (including area code)

SUBSTANCE USE INFORMATION: Indicate if no history of use ☐   History unknown ☐

Type:	Date of Last Use	Amount of Last Use	Frequency and Amount of Use	Length of Time Using	Age of First Use
_____	_____	_____	_____	_____	_____
_____	_____	_____	_____	_____	_____
_____	_____	_____	_____	_____	_____
_____	_____	_____	_____	_____	_____
_____	_____	_____	_____	_____	_____
_____	_____	_____	_____	_____	_____

MENTAL STATUS EXAM:

Level of Consciousness:	☐ Alert	☐ Lethargic	☐ Stuporous		
Orientation:	☐ Person	☐ Place	Time ☐ Day ☐ Month ☐ Year	☐ Current Situation	☐ None
Appearance:	☐ Clean	☐ Well-Nourished	☐ Malodorous	☐ Disheveled	☐ Malnourished	☐ Reddened Eyes
Speech:	☐ Normal	☐ Slurred	☐ Loud	☐ Pressured	☐ Slow	☐ Mute
Thought Process:	☐ Coherent	☐ Tangential	☐ Circumstantial	☐ Incoherent	☐ Loose Association	
Behavior:	☐ Cooperative	☐ Evasive	☐ Uncooperative	☐ Threatening	☐ Agitated	☐ Combative
Affect:	☐ Appropriate	☐ Blunted	☐ Flat	☐ Restricted	☐ Labile	☐ Other
Intellect:	☐ Normal	☐ Below Normal	☐ Paucity of Knowledge	☐ Vocabulary Poor	☐ Poor Abstraction	☐ Uncooperative
Mood:	☐ Euthymic	☐ Elevated	☐ Euphoric	☐ Depressed	☐ Anxious	☐ Irritable
Memory:	☐ Normal	☐ Poor Recent	☐ Poor Remote	☐ Inability to Concentrate	☐ Confabulation	☐ Amnesia
Judgment:	☐ Normal	☐ Poor	☐ Unrealistic	☐ Unmotivated	☐ Uncertain	
Motor:	☐ Normal	☐ Decreased	☐ Agitated	☐ Tremors	☐ Tics	☐ Repetitive Motions
Insight:	☐ Normal	☐ Adequate	☐ Marginal	☐ Poor		

Note: A narrative mental status exam may be done on a progress note, in lieu of above.

County of San Diego Health and Human Services Agency Mental Health Services **INITIAL MENTAL HEALTH ASSESSMENT** HHSA:MHS-912 (6/2003)	**Client:**_____ **MR/Client ID #:**_____ **Program:**_____ Page 3 of 5

Figure 12.9. (*continued*)

Visual Hallucinations: ☐No ☐Yes Specify:_____

Auditory Hallucinations:☐No ☐Yes Specify:_____

Delusions: ☐No ☐Yes Specify:_____

Other Information (optional):_____

POTENTIAL FOR HARM: (Include risk factors, e.g. chronic illness, recent loss of job, age)

Current SI: ☐ No ☐ Yes Specify plan (method, vague, passive, imminent):_____

_____

_____

Access to means: ☐ No ☐ Yes Specify:_____

Previous Attempts: ☐ No ☐ Yes Specify:_____

_____

Client Contract for Safety: ☐ No ☐ Yes Specify in Progress Notes:_____

Current III: ☐ No ☐ Yes Specify Plan (vague, intent, with/without means):_____

_____

_____

Identified Victim: ☐ No ☐ Yes Name and Contact Information:_____

_____

☐ No ☐ Yes Tarasoff warning: _____

Client No Harm Contract: ☐ No ☐ Yes Specify in Progress Notes:_____

History of Violence: ☐ No ☐ Yes Specify Type (past, current):_____

_____

History of Domestic Violence:_____

History of Abuse: ☐ No ☐ Yes Specify Type (past, current):_____

_____

_____

Abuse Reported: ☐ No ☐ Yes

Probation Officer Contact Info:

_____

Name   Address   Phone (including Area Code)

CONVICTION OF FELONY AND JAIL TIME: ☐ No ☐ Yes

What was the conviction for? Length of jail time?

_____

_____

DSM IV DIAGNOSIS: Impairment/Disability Use DSM-IV-TR Codes. Indicate (P) – Primary and (S) – Secondary	Enter P in front of primary	DIAGNOSTIC CODE
AXIS I		
AXIS I		
AXIS I		
AXIS II		
AXIS III Relevant Medical Conditions:		
AXIS IV Psychosocial and Environmental Problems:		
AXIS V Current GAF: Highest in Past Year:		

County of San Diego
Health and Human Services Agency
Mental Health Services

INITIAL MENTAL HEALTH ASSESSMENT

HHSA:MHS-912 (6/2003)

Client:_____

MR/Client ID #:_____

Program:_____

Page 4 of 5

Figure 12.9. (*continued*)

INTERPRETIVE SUMMARY: (Justification for diagnosis. Summarize and integrate all information gathered from other sources to render clinical judgments regarding intensity, length of treatment, and recommendations for services. Clearly state those emotional or behavioral symptoms that interfere with normal functioning. Include evaluation of client's ability and willingness to solve the client's presenting problem.)

_____

_____

_____

_____

_____

_____

_____

_____

_____

_____

_____

_____

_____

_____

Medical Necessity Met: ☐ Yes ☐ No   NOA Issued: ☐ Yes ☐ No (Medi-Cal Clients only)

REHABILITATION/RECOVERY/RECOMMENDATIONS: (List in-house clinical services as well as names of agencies/clinicians currently being received or recommended.)

1. ☐ Assisted Living Services	7. ☐ Employment Services	13. ☐ RAP Plan
2. ☐ Community Services	8. ☐ Group Therapy	14. ☐ Recovery Programs/Socialization Services
3. ☐ Case Management Services	9. ☐ Housing Services	15. ☐ Substance Abuse
4. ☐ Crisis Residential/Hospitalization	10. ☐ Individual Therapy	16. ☐ Support Group
5. ☐ Day Rehabilitation	11. ☐ Medical Treatment	17. ☐ Other
6. ☐ Education/Support	12. ☐ Medication Management	

Number and explain below:

_____ ☐ Current: _____

_____ ☐ Proposed Referral: _____

_____ ☐ Current: _____

_____ ☐ Proposed Referral: _____

_____ ☐ Current: _____

_____ ☐ Proposed Referral: _____

_____ ☐ Current: _____

_____ ☐ Proposed Referral: _____

_____ ☐ Current: _____

_____ ☐ Proposed Referral: _____

Completed by: _____

        Signature   Title   Date   Time Spent

Cosignature: _____

(if required)   Signature   Title   Date

County of San Diego Health and Human Services Agency Mental Health Services	Client: _____
	MR/Client ID #: _____
INITIAL MENTAL HEALTH ASSESSMENT	Program: _____
HHSA:MHS-912 (6/2003)	Page 5 of 5

checking for outcomes and goals

receiving first priority, and are maintained in such a manner as to protect confidentiality. See chapter 5 for additional discussion of documentation policies and procedures. In the behavioral healthcare setting, policies and procedures will mirror those used in acute care, except for those situations as noted in this chapter.

American Osteopathic Association

deemed authority

The American Osteopathic Association (AOA) accredits mental health, substance abuse, and several other types of organizations under the Healthcare Facilities Accreditation Program (HFAP). It was developed in 1943 and implemented in 1945 for annual hospital surveys.

Eligibility requirements specify that the behavioral healthcare organization do as follows:

- Meets state licensing requirements

- Has bylaws that specify acceptance of the HFAP certification process

- Has operated for at least three months prior to application

- Meets basic service requirements as well as requirements based on the type of organization seeking accreditation

National Committee for Quality Assurance

The National Committee for Quality Assurance (NCQA) was established in 1990 and began its accreditation program for **managed behavioral healthcare organizations (MBHOs)** in 1997.

Its accreditation model is based on the specific organization type or services provided. For example, if providing medical care under a **managed care organization (MCO)** and behavioral health services, standards for both the MCO and MBHO are used in the accreditation survey. Eligibility requirements are specific to the type of accreditation or certification being sought.

Accreditation is based on quality documentation. For managed behavioral healthcare organizations, this includes the following:

- Implementing a quality-improvement process for members

- Providing comprehensive services for members across the continuum of care

- Operating for at least 18 months

- Having appropriate licensure and meeting state, local, and federal regulations, as applicable

- Operating without discriminatory practices on the basis of gender, race, creed, or national origin (NCQA 2003)

The NCQA's accreditation of MBHOs rewards organizations that focus on quality, which, in turn, may help improve the nation's healthcare. The NCQA has developed a report card for MBHOs in which they meet quality of care standards.

The NCQA MBHO Accreditation Program is designed to:

- Foster accountability among MBHOs for the quality of care and services that members receive

- Provide employers, public purchasers, plans, and consumers with meaningful information regarding MBHOs

- Strengthen MBHO systems for population-based continuous quality improvement (CQI) programs

- Encourage effectiveness in the provision of behavioral healthcare by addressing the need for prevention, early intervention, and coordination of behavioral healthcare with medical care

The NCQA approaches accreditation through the complementary strategies of accreditation and performance improvement. The focus is to provide information that enables consumers to make informed healthcare decisions and choices.

Council on Accreditation

The Council on Accreditation (COA) was founded in 1977 by Child Welfare League of America and Family Service America. There are currently 98 programs or services that can be accredited under COA. Those related to behavioral health include the following:

- Mental health services

- Psychosocial and psychiatric rehabilitation services

- Case management services

- Counseling services

- Treatment/therapeutic foster care

- Day treatment services

COA accredits human service and behavioral healthcare organizations using a community-based social services model. The healthcare organization, in general, is accredited as well as specific individual programs. Organizations seeking COA accreditation can be public or private, not-for-profit or for-profit, and must provide at least one service for which COA has developed standards. All required licensures or certifications must be obtained, and the organization must be able to demonstrate the ability to have independence for review as a legal entity.

An organization is evaluated against best-practice standards, which are developed using a consensus model with input from a wide range of service providers, funders, experts, policymakers, and consumers.

Accreditation is based on quality documentation. Required behavioral healthcare documentation elements include the following (COA n.d.):

Screening assessments:

- Identifying information, including name, date of birth, and Social Security number (if available)

- Current residence

- Emergency health needs

- Emergency contacts (if any)

- Safety, imminent danger or risk of future harm, as applicable

- Legal status

Comprehensive basic assessments

- Information gathered for a screening/intake assessment
- A preliminary evaluation of the request or need for service
- The person's and/or family's strengths and resources
- Family relationships and formal and informal support systems
- The person's past or current use of services from this organization or other organizations
- Independent living skills, activities of daily living assessment, as applicable
- A screening for family violence, abuse or neglect, or exploitation
- Mental health status and developmental screening, as applicable
- Trauma screening
- Alcohol and other drug use screening
- Educational and vocational information
- Financial status, including financial assistance and insurance coverage
- Housing status, history, and a description of living conditions
- Other information necessary to provide services

Comprehensive psychosocial assessments:

- Information gathered for the screening/intake assessment and basic assessment
- Psychiatric issues
- A mental status exam
- Alcohol and other drug use assessment
- Assessment of nonsubstance addictive behaviors

Government Regulation

Some of the more influential government agencies affecting delivery of behavioral healthcare are Centers for Medicare and Medicaid Services, Health Insurance Portability and Accountability Act Privacy Rule, and Substance Abuse and Mental Health Services Administration.

Centers for Medicare and Medicaid Services

The Centers for Medicare and Medicaid Services (CMS) is a division of the U.S. Department of Health and Human Services (HHS). CMS plays an integral role in the quality of care provided to those individuals utilizing the behavioral healthcare system. It monitors expenses related to behavioral healthcare and provides mental health benefits through its Medicare program to eligible recipients (CMS 2003). Additionally, CMS oversees the quality improvement organizations (QIOs), which monitor medical necessity, quality of care, and the appropriateness of reimbursed services in behavioral healthcare settings.

Behavioral healthcare organizations that participate in the Medicare program must comply with federal standards issued by the CMS called the *Conditions of Participation* (COP) (2006). Standard 482.61 addresses special medical record requirements for inpatient psychiatric hospitals and states, "the medical records maintained by a psychiatric hospital must permit determination of the degree and intensity of the treatment provided to individuals who are furnished services in the institution." In other words, the documentation must support the amount and level of services provided. A facility's documentation policies must be developed in alignment with these in order to be in compliance.

Documentation standards specified in the COP for psychiatric hospitals include the following:

- **Development of assessment/diagnostic data:** Medical records must stress the psychiatric components of the record, including history of findings and treatment provided for the psychiatric condition for which the patient is hospitalized.

- **Psychiatric evaluation:** Each patient must receive a psychiatric evaluation within 60 hours of admission. It must include a medical history noting the mental status of the patient, onset of illness and circumstances leading to admission, attitudes and behavior, and intellectual and memory functioning.

- **Treatment plan:** Each patient must have an individual comprehensive treatment plan based on an inventory of the patient's strengths and disabilities. The treatment must be documented in such a way to ensure that all active therapeutic efforts are included.

- **Recording progress:** Progress notes must be recorded by the doctor responsible for the care of the patient, nurse, social worker, and, when appropriate, others significantly involved in active treatment. The frequency of progress notes is determined by the condition of the patient but must be recorded at least weekly for the first 2 months and at least once a month thereafter. Progress notes must contain recommendations for revisions in the treatment plan as indicated as well as precise assessment of the patient's progress in accordance with the original or revised treatment plan.

- **Discharge planning and discharge summary:** The medical record must have a discharge summary that includes a summary of the patient's hospitalization and recommendations from appropriate services concerning follow-up or aftercare as well as a brief summary of the patient's condition on discharge.

Quality Improvement Organizations (QIOs)

Formerly known as peer review organizations (PROs), QIOs are entities operating under the funding of CMS. Their primary function is to assess and improve the quality of healthcare provided to consumers. Oftentimes functioning as advocates for healthcare consumers, QIOs perform retrospective record reviews, conduct national and local quality improvement studies, and investigate consumer complaints regarding the quality of care provided in a number of settings. The record reviews influence healthcare organizations to comply with governmental documentation standards.

Although QIOs do not specifically review mental health facilities, care provided to individuals with mental illness is monitored in other settings in which behavioral healthcare is sought, such as rehabilitation facilities and emergency departments. QIOs also protect the integrity of the Medicare funds by ensuring that services are provided only when medically appropriate or necessary. QIOs are dedicated to protecting the rights of individuals receiving behavioral healthcare services (CMS 2003).

Health Insurance Portability and Accountability Act Privacy Rule

Behavioral healthcare organizations are considered covered entities (CEs) under HIPAA. However, there may be additional privacy considerations in other federal laws. Substance-abuse programs must meet the HIPAA guidelines and the more stringent *Code of Federal Regulations*, 42 CFR 2. Some behavioral health organizations also provide **Early Childhood Intervention (ECI)** services. ECI services are currently exempt from HIPAA; the privacy of these records is covered by FERPA, (20 USC §1232g, 34 CFR 99), a federal law that protects the privacy of student education records.

Although HIPAA and FERPA do not necessarily influence the format of mental healthcare documentation, both of these laws restrict the release of mental health information about a person who may be a threat to self or others.

The federal law governing the confidentiality of alcohol and drug abuse clients requires that client authorization be obtained before disclosing PHI to any other entity that is not specifically permitted by these regulations. It is noteworthy that 42 CFR 2 does not permit authorized disclosures that would be self-incriminating, except when clients have been referred for services by the courts (42 CFR 2, §2.33 and §2.35). Figure 12.10 describes the circumstances in which information may be disclosed without authorization as long as the Privacy Rule and state law permit the disclosure. The HIM manager would do well to read the full text in 42 CFR 2.

Federal regulations covering the confidentiality of PHI on alcohol and drug abuse patients apply to recipients of the information. Recipients are prohibited from redisclosing information they have received under authorization (42 CFR 2, §2.12[d]). This is in contrast to the Privacy Rule (HIPAA 2003), which requires the CE to inform patients that their information is no longer protected after it has been disclosed. Because it is more protective, 42 CFR 2 supersedes the Privacy Rule.

One of the most difficult situations to deal with that illustrates the extent of the privacy afforded clients in a substance-abuse program occurs when state law generally permits—or even requires—disclosure in response to a subpoena or court order. A patient would need to enlist an attorney to respond to a court order. With the exception of a court order following a

Figure 12.10.   Disclosure and alcohol and drug abuse treatment programs.

Alcohol and drug treatment programs that are regulated under 42 CFR, Part 2, may only disclose protected health information *without* authorization in the following circumstances:

- Communication within and between a program and with an entity having direct administrative control over the program and its personnel who need the information in connection with their duties that arise out of the provision of services provided (Subpart B, §2.12[c][3])

- Communication between a program and a business associate/qualified service organization (§2.12[c][4])

- Limited information to law enforcement and the courts when a client has committed a crime on program property or against program staff (§2.12[c][5]

- Limited information to report suspected child abuse and neglect (§2.12[c][6]

- For medical emergency to medical personnel (Subpart D, §2.51)

- For research activities (Subpart D, §2.52)

- For program audit and evaluation activities (§2.53)

- Upon a court order following the special 42 CFR, Part 2, "good cause" hearing (Subpart E, §2.61 and §2.63) (Note: Other than for purposes of criminal investigation or prosecution, anyone having a legally recognized interest in a disclosure may apply for a hearing [§2.64].)

- Situations in which certain entities apply for the "good cause" hearing to criminally investigate or prosecute a client (§2.65) or the program (§2.66)

"good cause" hearing to which all parties have been notified to appear, including the provider, 42 CFR 2, §2.31, requires an authorization for the provider to respond to the subpoena, warrant, or court order that meets the requirements of the regulations. (HHS 2003)

Substance Abuse and Mental Health Services Administration

The **Substance Abuse and Mental Health Services Administration (SAMHSA)** is a federal agency of the HHS established to focus on assessing and improving the lives of individuals with or at risk for mental illness and/or substance abuse disorders. SAMHSA also offers public programs and funding to provide treatment, prevention efforts, and rehabilitation services for substance abuse and mental illness (SAMHSA 2003).

In 2004, SAMHSA issued a document titled "The Confidentiality of Alcohol and Drug Abuse Patient Records Regulation and the HIPAA Privacy Rule: Implications for Alcohol and Substance Abuse Programs" (HHS 2004). The document outlines the principle preemptive aspects of 42 CFR 2 over the HIPAA (2003) Privacy Rule. It provides helpful information to substance abuse healthcare providers and recipients of substance abuse patient information from substance abuse providers. The document is available online from www.samhsa.gov.

Additionally, SAMHSA provides grants for various programs. These grants are highly dependent on providing quality documentation. Information is available online from www.samhsa.gov/grants/.

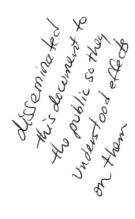
disseminated this document to the public so they understood effects on them

Healthcare Industry Forces

Healthcare industry forces focus on patient care and cost controls. These include managed care, integrated delivery systems, **healthcare reengineering**, performance improvement, outcomes assessment and management, and growth of outpatient and partial treatment settings. All of these focus areas influence a facility's documentation requirements and will vary from organization to organization.

Managed Care

As with other service types in the healthcare delivery system, behavioral healthcare must take measures to control the cost of services. Managed care entities have added behavioral health benefits to their plans and routinely monitor compliance with contractual agreements. In many circumstances, however, benefits provided for behavioral health services are less than those provided for traditional medical treatment. For this reason, many employers have opted to establish employee assistance programs (EAPs) to provide employees with access to brief and limited counseling or therapy services during times of need. This service is often fully paid for by the employer.

Integrated Delivery Systems

In today's healthcare environment, it is not uncommon for a provider or organization to offer a variety of healthcare services. For example, one organization may provide acute-care services, home healthcare services, and behavioral healthcare services under the same organizational name. As with any other healthcare provider, access to health information is critical to the successful delivery of care in such an **integrated delivery system (IDS)**. Reliable and timely access to information is essential for the delivery of high-quality client care and yet is one of the most significant challenges in this type of healthcare system.

It is not uncommon for the individual component disciplines to establish and maintain separate and distinct records of care (commonly referred to as clinical records) in the IDS. Thus, it is essential that the provider have a well-maintained information management system or other reliable client indexing system that allows for the identification of shared clients. This permits optimal communication among healthcare providers in each component discipline within the network or IDS arrangement and ensures continuity of care for the client.

Performance Improvement

Performance improvement (PI) activities are an important aspect of any industry in the healthcare delivery system. Behavioral healthcare facilities accredited by the Joint Commission or CARF demonstrate an excellence in high-quality service provision by maintaining compliance with hundreds of quality standards developed by the accreditation bodies. Accrediting bodies such as the Joint Commission and CARF closely monitor organizational policies and procedures related to PI activities.

Outcomes Assessment and Management

Outcomes assessment is an effective tool used to monitor the success of a plan from beginning to end. In behavioral health, it is a way to determine if care and services were prescribed appropriately and provided to assist the client in achieving the expected or desired outcome (Rudman 1997, 81–85).

Although behavioral healthcare experts report that individuals suffering from behavioral health conditions may never be "cured" in the traditional sense of the word, it is highly accepted that many of them can achieve a fairly independent lifestyle when diagnosed and treated properly.

Growth of Outpatient and Partial Treatment Settings

With the rising cost of inpatient services, many individuals are seeking behavioral health services through outpatient or partial-treatment settings. These options provide the client with a stable healthcare provider at a significantly lower expense. Unfortunately, the decision to move to the outpatient setting is not always made by the individual or provider but, rather, by the payer.

Organizations and Advocacy Groups

Several other organizations support, fund, and influence some behavioral healthcare services. These organizations may not have specific documentation requirements, but are included here because of their influence in the behavioral healthcare industry.

National Alliance on Mental Illness

The National Alliance on Mental Illness (NAMI) is a nonprofit organization dedicated to providing advocacy and support to individuals affected by mental illness (such as schizophrenia, bipolar disorder, major depressive disorders). NAMI not only assists individuals with the mental illness but also works with their families. NAMI's primary mission is to "eradicate mental illnesses and improve the quality of life for people of all ages affected by mental illnesses" (NAMI 2003).

Mental Health America

Mental Health America (MHA) (formerly National Mental Health Association) is a non-profit organization created to assist the more than 54 million Americans with mental disorders. Through its public advocacy, education, and research programs, MHA hopes to elevate public knowledge of mental health issues, encourage reform, and promote the effective use of qualified prevention and recovery programs (MHA 2007).

The Health Information Management Professional's Role in Behavioral Healthcare

The HIM professional is a vital part of any behavioral healthcare organization. From the onset of care, he or she is able to provide best-practice guidance and expertise on documentation issues, compliance issues, and general record maintenance issues.

Figure 12.11 lists several questions to assist in improving behavioral healthcare documentation.

Successful HIM practices throughout the continuum of care provided in the behavioral healthcare setting assist in the safety and quality of care provided to clients, effective outcomes monitoring, and positive customer satisfaction. As the keepers of information and data, HIM professionals play an integral, indispensable, and powerful role in meeting these challenges.

To provide accurate and timely assistance, it is critical that the HIM professional understands the complexity of the behavioral healthcare system, its rules and regulations, and its unique position in the healthcare delivery system.

Protecting the confidentiality, privacy, and security of mental health and substance abuse records, as well as all related PHI, has become a very complicated endeavor in the behavioral healthcare setting. Health information managers, who also may be privacy officers, have significant responsibilities within their healthcare organizations regarding implementation of the various laws regulating use and disclosure of PHI. For this reason, it is imperative that they be familiar with federal and state laws and keep abreast of new legislation in order to carry out the responsibilities entrusted to them.

Figure 12.11.   Questions for improving behavioral healthcare documentation.

• Is there documentation of medical necessity, in other words, does documentation indicate why services are necessary?
• Does the diagnosis warrant the particular treatment being offered?
• Are correct diagnostic codes being used?
• Does the patient have the cognitive or communication skills necessary to benefit from treatment?
• Could services be provided by someone other than a mental health professional?
• Is there documentation of symptoms, goals, and client's capacity to participate in treatment?
• Do progress notes relate to the interventions prescribed on the treatment plan?
• Do progress notes document all services being prescribed on the treatment plan?
• Does documentation justify the duration or frequency of services?
• Does documentation justify any extension of services?
• Are services being provided by a qualified professional?
• Is documentation timely, legible, and signed?
• Is billing timely and accurate?
• Are services provided within the standard payer definitions and do these align with correct CPT codes?

Source: Martins and Nicholson 2008, 242.

Because of their daily oversight of PHI use and disclosure in behavioral healthcare organizations, HIM professionals also are well qualified—and should therefore come forward—to take part in the revision and/or development of laws and standards of practice related to the privacy, confidentiality, and security of behavioral healthcare PHI. Their contribution is valuable and necessary (and perhaps sometimes overlooked) within the overall healthcare industry and beyond.

HIM managers working in substance-abuse programs must ensure that the organization's work force understands that with the exception of a court order following a "good cause" hearing, communication of PHI without an authorization is prohibited, and even when a judge finds reason for PHI disclosure, information is restricted to that which is essential to fulfill the purpose of the order. Without authorization, as stated in 42 CFR 2, §2.13, 2.31, 2.61ff, disclosure in response to a subpoena, court order, or warrant is prohibited. State laws that are less protective also are preempted.

Summary

Documentation is a critical component of the HIM profession. The need for HIM professionals working in the behavioral healthcare setting to have a thorough knowledge and understanding of documentation law, rules, regulations, standards, and best practices is crucial to the operation of the behavioral healthcare organization.

Traditionally, outpatient mental health and substance abuse organizations have little or no funding available for extensive compliance activities. The design of an organization's compliance program should be developed in accordance with available resources and compliance needs. Most organizations have an idea where they are most vulnerable and often start with a few audits per month, which can validate concerns and identify other problems if they exist.

References

Abdelhak, M., S. Grostick, M. A. Hanken, E. Jacobs. 2007. Health Information: *Management of a Strategic Resource*, 3rd ed. St. Louis, MO: Saunders.

American Osteopathic Association (AOA). 2007. *Accreditation of Colleges of Osteopathic Medicine: COM Accreditation Standards and Procedures*. Chicago, IL: American Osteopathic Association. Available online from www.osteopathic.org/pdf/acc_predocomstds07.pdf.

American Psychiatric Association. 2000. *Diagnostic and Statistical Manual of Mental Disorders DSM-IV-TR,* fourth edition (Text Revision) Arlington, VA: American Psychiatric Association.

American Psychiatric Association. 2003. *Practice Guideline for the Assessment and Treatment of Patients With Suicidal Behaviors*. Available online from www.psych.org/psych_pract/treatg/pg/SuicidalBehavior_05-15-06.pdf.

California Department of Justice. 2004. Assembly Bill (AB) 157 - Revised mental health reporting requirements. CCR AB 1587 (Chapter 578, Statutes of 1999) Chaptered September 29, 1999. Available online from www.dmh.ca.gov/DMHDocs/docs/notices99/99-17.pdf.

Center for Mental Health Services. 1992. Mental health information and statistics. Available online from www.mhsource.com.

Centers for Disease Control and Prevention, National Center on Birth Defects and Developmental Disabilities. 2003. *Developmental disabilities*. Available online from www.cdc.gov/ncbddd.

Centers for Medicare and Medicaid Services. 2003. Medicare and your mental health benefits. Available online from www.nimh.nih.gov.

Centers for Medicare and Medicaid Services. 2006 (Nov. 27). Conditions of participation for hospitals; Final rule. 42 CFR Part 482. *Federal Register* 71(227): 68672–68695. Available online from http://a257.g.akamaitech. net/7/257/2422/01jan20061800/edocket.access.gpo.gov/2006/pdf/E6-19957.pdf.

Commission on Accreditation of Rehabilitation Facilities. 2004. *What does CARF Accredit?* Available online from www.carf.org.

Council on Accreditation (COA). *COA Accreditation and Standards*. Available online from www.coanet.org/front3/index.cfm.

Department of Education, Department of Human Services, Department of Justice. 2007. Report to the President on issues raised by the Virginia Tech tragedy. Available online from www.hhs.gov/vtreport.pdf.

Department of Health and Human Services. 2002. Confidentiality of alcohol and drug abuse patient records; Final rule. 42 CFR Part 2.63 *Federal Register*. Available online from www.access.gpo.gov/nara/cfr/waisidx_02/42cfr2_02.html.

Department of Health and Human Services. 2004. The confidentiality of alcohol and drug abuse patient records regulation and the HIPAA privacy rule: Implications for alcohol and substance abuse programs. Available online from www.hipaa.samhsa.gov/download2/SAMHSAHIPAAComparisonClearedPDFVersion.pdf.

Family Educational Rights and Privacy Act (FERPA). 20 U.S.C. § 1232g; 34 CFR Part 99. 1974.

Grant, Jon E. 2007. Failing the 15-minute suicide watch: Guidelines to monitor patients. *Current Psychiatry Online* 6(6). Available online from www.currentpsychiatry.com/article_pages.asp?AID=5061#bib1.

Health Insurance Portability and Accountability Act (HIPAA) of 1996. Public Law 104-191. Available online from www.gpoaccess.gov/cfr/index.html.

Joint Commission on Accreditation of Healthcare Organizations. 2003. Facts about the Joint Commission on Accreditation of Healthcare Organizations. Available online from www.jointcommission.com.

Martins, L., and R. Nicholson, 2008. Compliance considerations in behavioral health facilities. Chapter 13 in *Health Information Management Compliance: Guidelines for Preventing Fraud and Abuse*. Edited by Sue Bowman. Chicago: AHIMA.

Mental Health America. 2007. In-patient care: Considering hospital care. Available online from www.nmha.org/.

National Alliance on Mental Illness. 2003. About NAMI. Available online from www.nami.org.

National Committee for Quality Assurance (NCQA). 2007. MBHO Standards and Guidelines. Available online from www.ncqa.org/tabid/378/Default.aspx.

National Council for Community Behavioral Healthcare. 2007. Principles for behavioral healthcare delivery. Available online from www.nccbh.org/SERVICE/Bookstore/Principles.pdf.

National Institute of Mental Health. 2001. The numbers count. Available online from www.nimh.nih.gov.

National Mental Health Association. 2004. About NMHA. Available online from www.nmha.org.

Rudman, William J. 1997. *Performance Improvement in Health Information Management Services*. Philadelphia: W. B. Saunders.

Shorter, Edward. 1997. *A History of Psychiatry*. New York: John Wiley & Sons.

Substance Abuse and Mental Health Services Administration. 2003. Overview of findings from the 2002 national survey on drug use and health. Office of Applied Studies, NHSDA Series H-21, HHS Publication No. SMA 03-3774. Rockville, MD: Substance Abuse and Mental Health Services Administration.

Substance Abuse and Mental Health Services Administration. 2004. The confidentiality of alcohol and drug abuse patient records regulation and the HIPAA privacy rule: Implications for alcohol and substance abuse programs. Available online from http://ncadistore.samhsa.gov/catalog/productDetails.aspx?ProductID=16873.

Tarasoff v. Regents of the University of California, 17 Cal. 3d 425, 551 P.2d 334, 131 Cal. Rptr. 14 (1976). Available online from http://www.publichealthlaw.net/Reader/docs/Tarasoff.pdf.

U.S. Public Health Service. 1999. Mental health: A report of the surgeon general. Available online from www.surgeongeneral.gov/library/mentalhealth.

Youngberg, Barbara J. 1998. *The Risk Manager's Desk Reference*, 2nd ed. Gaithersburg, MD: Aspen Publishers.

Glossary

Accreditation: A voluntary process whereby a healthcare organization seeks formal approval from an accrediting body (such as the **Joint Commission** or the **American Osteopathic Association [AOA]**). Approval is based on whether the organization meets a set of voluntary **standards** developed by the accrediting body. The purpose of **accreditation** is to confirm the quality of the services provided by healthcare organizations. Accreditation has a number of benefits for hospitals and other healthcare organizations. After a hospital receives accreditation by the Joint Commission, **Medicare** automatically allows the hospital to participate in the Medicare and **Medicaid** programs for **reimbursement** purposes. Accreditation, **certification,** and **licensure** processes are linked to how healthcare organizations operate, and these processes require **health record information**.

Accreditation Association for Ambulatory Health Care (AAAHC): A nonprofit organization incorporated in 1979, the association is dedicated to educating providers in quality assurance and **accreditation standards** and **procedures**. It has conducted thousands of accreditation surveys of all types of ambulatory-care organizations, including ambulatory surgical facilities, college and university health centers, single and **multispecialty group practices**, and health networks. The association currently accredits more than 3,700 organizations nationwide.

Accreditation organizations: Professional organizations that set the **standards** against which healthcare organizations are measured to ensure the quality and safety of their services. Accrediting organizations expect hospitals and other healthcare organizations to strive for the highest possible quality in customer care. The **Joint Commission** and the **American Osteopathic Association (AOA)** are two examples of accreditation organizations.

Activities of daily living (ADL): Basic activities such as self-care, including the ability to communicate with others, feed oneself, bathe and dress oneself, use the toilet, and move within one's environment.

Acute care: The short-term medical and nursing care provided in an **inpatient** hospital setting to treat the acute phase of a patient's injury or illness.

Administrative information: Patient-identifiable documentation used for administrative, regulatory, healthcare operations, and payment (financial) purposes. Administrative **information** should have the same level of **confidentiality** as the **legal health record**. Two types of administrative **information** are created and maintained by healthcare organizations. The first type consists of documentation that is typically part of the health record such as consents for treatment, surgery, and **research** forms that would be produced in response to a **subpoena**. The second type of administrative information should not be considered part of the legal health record and would not be produced in response to a subpoena for the health record.

Advance directive: A written document that describes the patient's healthcare preferences in the event that he or she is unable to communicate directly at some point in the future. The types of advance directives vary by state but include living wills and statements of the patient's wishes in case of a critical illness, such as life support, ventilator support, food and hydration, healthcare surrogate designation or durable power of attorney for healthcare (also called a healthcare power of attorney), and anatomical donation. Ideally, advance directives and organ donation forms should also be placed in the patient's chart before surgery. Advance directives are required in the long-term acute-care (LTCH) setting. Two examples of advance directives are the advance beneficiary notice (ABN) and **do-not-resuscitate (DNR) order**.

Advanced decision support: Resources that provide the latest clinical guidelines and **research** findings available to physicians. In an electronic health record system, these resources are integrated electronically and available at a click to the healthcare provider.

Agency for Healthcare Research and Quality (AHRQ): An agency within U.S. **Department of Health and Human Services (HHS)** that aims to improve the quality, safety, efficiency, and effectiveness of healthcare for all Americans. One of its functions is to support **health services research**. The AHRQ provides funding and **information** for health information technology projects, including grants to state and regional **health information exchange (HIE) initiatives**. In 2007, AHRQ and the **Centers for Medicare and Medicaid Services (CMS)** published a handbook to help providers set up **registries**, including recommendations for design and **data** source access and suggestions on ways to encourage participation in registries.

Aggregate data: Data are categorized as either primary or secondary data. Aggregate data are **secondary data.** Secondary data are taken from **health records** (without identifying any particular patients individually) and entered into **databases**, such as disease-oriented databases, for use by researchers. Aggregate data are used to determine the effectiveness of alternate treatment methods and demonstrate survival rates at different stages of diseases.

Allied health professional: Professionals who provide direct patient care. Examples of allied health professionals include nurse-anesthetists; respiratory therapists; and physical, occupational, and speech therapists. Allied health professionals document their services and author **health record** entries. They are allowed to accept physicians' orders for services within their area of practice.

Ambulatory care: The preventive, diagnostic, and therapeutic medical services provided on a nonresidential basis in healthcare practitioners' offices, group practices, private clinics, community-based clinics, and hospital-based **outpatient** departments.

Ambulatory surgical center (ASC): Elective surgical **procedures** are performed on patients in ambulatory surgical centers (ASC). Patients using these facilities are classified as **outpatients** and typically are released from the surgery center on the same day that the procedure is performed. Surgical procedures are scheduled in advance and usually take from 5 to 90 minutes. Generally, recovery following the procedure requires less than four hours; so patients can leave the same day. There are no emergency services available at ambulatory surgical centers, and patients in whom surgical **complications** develop are transported to an emergency department at an **inpatient facility**.

American Association for Accreditation of Ambulatory Surgery Facilities (AAAASF): Organization established in 1980 to develop an **accreditation** program to standardize and improve the quality of medical and surgical care in ambulatory-surgery facilities while assuring the public of high **standards** for patient care and safety in an accredited facility. Accreditation consists of a three-step review that includes a site visit, committee assessment of site visit findings, and successful participation in a peer review/quality assurance program, including mandatory semiannual online reporting to AAAASF.

American Health Information Community (AHIC): A federal advisory body established in 2005 by the U.S. **Department of Health and Human Services (HHS)**. The AHIC comprises nine public and eight federal representatives plus the HHS secretary. AHIC provides input and recommendations to HHS, digitizing **health records** for interoperability while ensuring **privacy** and security of those records.

American Osteopathic Association (AOA): A professional membership association that represents more than 56,000 osteopathic physicians (DOs) in practice in the United States. The AOA is also the primary **certification** agency for osteopathic physicians and the **accreditation** agency for all osteopathic medical colleges and many osteopathic healthcare facilities. The AOA first initiated its hospital accreditation program in 1945 to ensure the quality of residency training programs for doctors of osteopathy. Today, the association's **Healthcare Facilities Accreditation Program (HFAP)** accredits a number of healthcare facilities and services, including laboratories, ambulatory-care clinics, ambulatory-surgery centers, behavioral health and substance abuse treatment facilities, physical rehabilitation facilities, acute-care hospitals, and critical-access hospitals. Entities that have been accredited by the AOA are automatically granted **deemed status** by the **Medicare** program.

American Society for Testing and Materials (ASTM): Society that develops the standard for the content and structure of electronic **health records** (EHRs). In 1999, ASTM released the Standard Practice for Content and Structure of the **Electronic Health Record (EHR)**. It describes the basic **information** categories in EHRs and segments the categories into specific **data** elements. This standard has been revised several times. The current standard, E1384-07, was revised in October 2007. In addition to covering the content and structure of electronic health records, it provides guidelines for healthcare organizations planning and implementing new systems.

Analysis: The process of translating **data** into **information** utilized for an application. Analysis in the healthcare industry involves **qualitative analysis**, **quantitative analysis**, and **case-mix analysis**. According to AHIMA's Data Quality Management Model, analysis is one of the four key processes for data. The other key processes are **collection**, **application**, and **warehousing**.

Ancillary services: Procedures such as laboratory and imaging that are performed in separate departments in a healthcare facility.

Application: The purpose for which **data** are collected. According to AHIMA's Data Quality Management Model, application is one of the four key processes for data. The other key processes are **collection**, **analysis**, and **warehousing**.

Authentication: The process of providing proof of the authorship of documentation in the **health record**. Federal and state laws govern **standards** for authentication of health records. Some states have no requirements, while others outline specific **procedures** for authentication, including acceptable methods and time frames. Many state laws apply exclusively to physicians' orders for drugs and services. Additionally, hospitals address authentication requirements for health records in medical staff rules and **regulations**, which provide minimum authentication requirements for documentation including how it is authenticated. State and federal regulations require that physicians sign, date, and note the time of their orders for diagnostic and therapeutic services. The authentication requirements for physicians' orders are the same in paper-based and electronic health record systems.

Autopsy report: A description of the examination of a patient's body after he or she has died. Autopsies are usually conducted when there is some question about the cause of death or when **information** is needed for educational or legal purposes. The purpose of the autopsy is to determine or confirm the cause of death or to provide more information about the course of the patient's illness.

Behavioral healthcare: The psychiatric and/or psychological care provided to address mental disorders, developmental disorders, and substance-abuse disorders; provided in a variety of settings, including dedicated units in acute-care hospitals, psychiatric hospitals, community-based clinics, and physicians' offices. Behavioral healthcare poses unique challenges to patient rights and requires specific documentation that is unique to behavioral healthcare settings.

Biomedical research: The process of systematically investigating subjects related to the functioning of the human body. Biomedical **research** often leads to a greater understanding of disease processes and the development of new or improved treatments and medical technologies.

Biometric identifier: A **unique personal identifier** such as a fingerprint or retinal scan that is used by some **electronic health records systems** to validate a healthcare professional's authorization and access to documentation.

Birthing center: Center that provides delivery services for women who are expected to have normal deliveries. A patient must be screened for medical acceptability before she can be scheduled to deliver her child at a birthing center. Some hospitals also offer ambulatory obstetric services for women who are expected to have normal deliveries.

Board certification: Professional practice guidelines developed by a certification organization and generally accepted as the established standard of care for that specialty. A specific procedure performed by a board-certified physician or surgeon according to the practice guidelines established for that procedure is considered to have met the established standard of care. Physicians and other clinical professionals who earn board certification through a professional certification organization are generally assumed to be fully qualified to practice in their area of specialty.

Cancer treatment center: A facility that specializes in providing comprehensive cancer treatment, including radiation and chemotherapy. Many cancer treatment facilities also offer patient education and family counseling services.

Cardiology reports: Results of diagnostic tests performed by a cardiologist in the hospital on both **inpatients** and **outpatients**. Many patients treated primarily for noncardiac diagnoses may also have preexisting cardiac conditions that need monitoring through routine electrocardiography. Specialized tests performed and/or interpreted by cardiologists include exercise and pharmacological stress tests, tilt-table tests, Holter monitoring, pacemaker checks, electrocardiography, echocardiography, cardioradionucleide imaging, myocardial imaging, and cardiac catheterization.

Care plan: A multidisciplinary tool for organizing the diagnostic and therapeutic services to be provided to a patient. Care plans are required in the **long-term care** setting and other **inpatient** environments. The purpose of the care plan is to ensure the efficacy and efficiency of patient services and the quality of patient **outcomes**. Care plans usually include the following elements: initial assessment (medical and nursing) of the patient's immediate and long-term needs, statement of treatment goals based on the patient's needs and diagnosis, description of the activities planned to meet the treatment goals, patient education goals, discharge planning goals, timing of periodic assessments to determine progress toward meeting the treatment goals, and indicators of the need for reassessing the plan to address the patient's response to treatment and/or the development of **complications**.

Case management: A process of ongoing and concurrent review performed to ensure the **medical necessity** and effectiveness of the clinical services being provided to the patient.

Case-mix analysis: A method of grouping patients according to a predefined set of characteristics.

Census: A methodical accounting of current population, usually including **demographic data**, that is performed at regular intervals.

Centers for Disease Control and Prevention (CDC): A group of federal agencies that collect statistics about births, deaths, illnesses, and diseases and oversee health promotion and disease control and prevention activities in the United States. The CDC manages the WONDER **database**, an integrated information and communication system for public health. WONDER speeds and simplifies access to public health information for state and local health departments, the U.S. Public Health Service, and the academic public health community. It is a valuable tool for public health **research**, decision making, priority setting, program evaluation, and resource allocation.

Centers for Medicare and Medicaid Services (CMS): A federal agency of the U.S. Department of Health and Human Services. CMS is charged with developing and implementing Medicare and Medicaid **regulations**, such as the *Medicare Conditions of Participation*. CMS plays an integral role in the quality of care provided to individuals by monitoring expenses related to healthcare and providing health benefits to eligible recipients through its Medicare program. Additionally, CMS oversees the **quality improvement organizations (QIOs)** that monitor **medical necessity** and the appropriateness of reimbursed services in healthcare settings.

Certificate of destruction: Appropriate documentation of **health record** destruction must be maintained permanently no matter how the process is carried out. This documentation usually takes the form of a certificate of destruction, which should include the following details: date of destruction, method of destruction, description of the record(s) destroyed, including health record number(s), statement that the record(s) was destroyed during the normal course of business, signatures of the individuals who authorized and witnessed the destruction.

Certification: The process of granting an organization the right to provide healthcare services to a specific group of individuals. For example, healthcare organizations must meet certain federal **regulations** to receive funding through the **Medicare** program. These regulations are published in the *Medicare Conditions of Participation*.

Certification Commission for Healthcare Information Technology (CCHIT): Organization that certifies **electronic health records (EHRs)** and EHR network developments of EHR system **standards**.

Charting by exception: A system of documentation in which only abnormal or unusual findings are documented in the **progress notes**. Charting by exception focuses on abnormal events and describes interventions ordered and the patient's response. The purpose of charting by exception is to reduce the amount of routine record keeping required. Charting by exception is also called *focus charting*.

Civilian Health and Medical Program of the Uniformed Services (CHAMPUS): A public funding source for **home care** services.

Clinical data repository: A centralized **database** that captures, sorts, and processes patient **data** and then returns them to the user. These functions demand specialized database management capabilities. The most common type of **database management system** in use today is the relational database, which uses data tables to organize data.

Clinical decision support (CDS) systems: A system that automatically analyzes **health record data** and searches for unusual patterns. When a potential problem is identified (for example, a drug interaction), the system issues an alert or a reminder that includes a recommendation for specific corrective action.

Clinical information: The documentation of a patient's condition and course of treatment. The following types of clinical **information** are documented in the healthcare record: the patient's physical condition upon initial examination and the reason the patient's condition required treatment, the patient's medical **history**, the diagnostic and therapeutic orders given by the patient's physician(s), the observations made by clinicians over the course of the patient's treatment (**progress notes**), the **outcomes** of diagnostic and therapeutic services (including surgical interventions), and the patient's final diagnosis and condition at discharge.

Clinical pathways: Structured **plans of care** that help organizations implement clinical guidelines and **protocols**. Sometimes known as *critical paths*, *care paths*, and/or *care maps*, they are widely used by institutions hoping to reduce costs and improve quality through decreased variation in practices.

Clinical practice guidelines: Health record information that is used to develop **clinical pathways**.

Clinical privileges: Privileges granted to a practitioner by a hospital board, which authorize the practitioner to provide patient services in the hospital, but only those specific services that fall within his or her area of medical expertise. For example, a cardiovascular surgeon's clinical privileges would allow him or her to perform cardiac bypass surgery but not cataract surgery. Medical staff members typically must submit applications for reappointment to the medical staff every two years.

Clinical protocols: Treatment recommendations that are often based on **clinical practice guidelines**.

Clinical trial: A **research** project in which new treatments and tests are investigated to determine whether they are safe and effective. The trial proceeds according to a **protocol**, which is the list of rules and **procedures** to be followed. A clinical trials **database** provides the **data** that enable patients and practitioners to determine which clinical trials are available and applicable to the patients. The **Food and Drug Administration (FDA)** Modernization Act of 1997 mandated that a clinical trials database be developed. The National Library of Medicine has developed this database for use by both consumers and practitioners. The Clinical Trials database is available online at http://clinicaltrials.gov.

Closing practice policy: Policy that directs an organization to send out letters to patients of physicians who are closing their practice at a facility. Information should include options for the patients either continue receiving care from another physician at the facility or receive a copy of their medical record if they decide to transfer to another practice.

Code of Federal Regulations (**CFR**)*:* A daily publication of the U.S. Government Printing Office. Whenever federal **statutes** or **regulations** are added or changed in the U.S. *Code of Federal Regulations*, the rules are published in the *Federal Register.*

Collection: The processes by which **data** elements are accumulated. According to AHIMA's Data Quality Management Model, collection is one of the four key processes for data. The other key processes are **analysi**s, **application**, and **warehousing**.

Commission on Accreditation of Rehabilitation Facilities (CARF): A nonprofit organization that accredits organizations for quality excellence in rehabilitative and human services. Like the **Joint Commission**, CARF develops performance **standards** that must be met in order for a healthcare organization to pass the survey process. The organization surveys a variety of behavioral health settings, including mental healthcare, substance-abuse care, and other addiction programs.

Commission on Cancer (CoC): Entity that sets **standards** for quality multidisciplinary cancer care. The CoC Approvals Program encourages hospitals, treatment centers, and other facilities to improve their quality of patient care through various cancer-related programs. These programs are concerned with prevention, early diagnosis, pretreatment evaluation, staging, and optimal treatment, as well as rehabilitation, surveillance for recurrent disease, support services, and end-of-life care. The CoC was established by the American College of Surgeons (ACoS) in 1922.

Community Health Accreditation Program (CHAP): An organization that accredits **home care** and hospice organizations. CHAP's core **standards** concern information management, clinical records, and management information systems.

Community health center: Facilities usually located in low-income areas. They offer comprehensive, primary healthcare services (both therapeutic and preventive) to patients who otherwise would have limited access to healthcare. Community health centers frequently are operated by local and state **public health** departments, and most of the services are provided by public health nurses. Patients pay for services either on a sliding scale based on income or according to a flat-rate, discounted fee schedule supplemented by public funding. Community health centers are sometimes called *neighborhood health centers.*

Comorbidities: Preexisting conditions that affect a patient's care.

Complication: A condition that begins after a patient is admitted for inpatient care.

Comprehensive assessment: A patient-specific, comprehensive assessment that accurately reflects the patient's current health status and includes **information** that may be used to demonstrate the patient's progress toward achievement of desired **outcomes**. The comprehensive assessment must identify the patient's continuing need for **home care** and meet the patient's medical, nursing, rehabilitative, social, and discharge planning needs. For **Medicare** beneficiaries, the **home health agency (HHA)** must verify the patient's eligibility for the Medicare home health benefit, including homebound status, both at the time of the initial assessment visit and at the time of the comprehensive assessment. The comprehensive assessment must also incorporate the use of the current version of **OASIS** items, using the language and groupings as specified. The comprehensive assessment includes the collection of OASIS **data** items by a qualified clinician, such as a registered nurse, physical therapist, occupational therapist, or speech language pathologist.

Computer-based record (CPR): A term that was in use during the 1990s to refer to an **electronic health record (EHR)**.

Computerized physician order entry (CPOE): An electronic order-entry system that includes safeguards to ensure the authenticity, accuracy, and completeness of physicians' orders. Such computer-based order-entry systems are an integral part of electronic **health record** systems. **Computerized physician order entry (CPOE)** systems are gaining acceptance in the medical community.

Conditions of Participation for Hospitals: Medicare *Conditions of Participation for Hospitals* are published under title 42, part 482, of the ***Code of Federal Regulations (CFR)***. CMS works directly with **accreditation organizations** to coordinate the Medicare *Conditions of Participation* with national accreditation **standards**. As a result, the Medicare **acute-care** standards are similar to the acute-care standards published by the **Joint Commission** and the American Osteopathic Association. Medicare *Conditions of Participation for Hospitals* are available online at www.gpoaccess.gov/fr/index.html.

Confidentiality: Consumers have a right to control how information in their **health records** is used. Patients can review, copy, and amend their records when necessary. Outside healthcare providers, **third-party payers**, clinical researchers, and others who have a legitimate interest in the contents of health records need access. To meet the growing demand for healthcare information, hospitals and other healthcare providers must develop processes for fulfilling legitimate requests for health information while protecting the confidentiality of health records and the **privacy** of patients. Hospitals and providers in other healthcare settings must ensure records remain accessible for legitimate purposes for a reasonable period after the original healthcare episode is complete. The implementation of the **Health Insurance Portability and Accountability Act (HIPAA)** in 2003 established a consistent set of privacy and security rules for the first time. The rules are designed to protect the privacy of patients and to simplify the sharing of health information for legitimate purposes. However, only the minimum necessary **information** needed to satisfy the specified purpose can be used or disclosed. The release of information for purposes unrelated to treatment, payment, or healthcare operations still requires the patient's written authorization.

Consent to treatment: A signed, general consent form. Most healthcare providers ask patients or their legal representatives to sign a general consent to treatment. By signing a general consent to treatment, the patient agrees to submit to routine clinical **procedures** and medical and nursing care while he or she is a patient. Except in emergency situations, patients are usually asked to sign a general consent form during the admissions process. More specific consents are required for procedures that involve significant risk, such as invasive diagnostic tests, transfusions, and surgery. These specific consents are completed in addition to the general consent forms.

Conservatorship: When a person is unable to provide for personal needs such as food, shelter, or clothing as the result of a mental disorder, and thereby is gravely disabled and unwilling or incapable of accepting voluntary treatment, he or she may be recommended for conservatorship placement—that is, placed under the care of an appointed guardian. Mental health conservatorship requirements may vary from state to state. Acceptable conservatorship documents are created by attorneys and the courts in each state and may differ in format. Conservatorship documents become part of the medical record.

Consolidated Health Informatics (CHI) Initiatives: A federal initiative that addresses the development of **standards** and exchange of **information** for the healthcare information industry.

Consultation reports: A report provided by a consulting physician at the request of a patient's principal physician when seeking advice about diagnostic and therapeutic decisions for the patient. Consultation reports usually contain the following types of **information**: name of the physician who requested the consultation and the reason for the consultation; date and time the consultant examined the patient; pertinent findings of the examination; consultant's opinion, diagnosis, or impression; recommendations for diagnostic tests and/or treatment; and signature, credentials, and specialty of the consultant. The consultant's report becomes part of the patient's record.

Continuous quality improvement (CQI): Concept that emphasizes the critical importance of three factors: knowing and meeting customer expectations, reducing variation within processes, and relying on **data** to build knowledge for process improvement. Most healthcare organizations utilize some form of CQI.

Continuum of care: The sum of all the healthcare services provided in all settings, from the least intensive and specialized (the least expensive) to the most intensive and specialized (the most expensive). The services that make up the continuum can be further categorized into three levels of care: primary, secondary, and tertiary. The levels of care reflect the cost of the services as well as the intensity of the services provided.

Coordinated school health program: A school health program that works with students, their families, and their community to provide strategies, activities, and services in a coordinated, planned way. Ideally, a coordinated school health program includes a healthful environment; nursing and other health services that students need to stay in school; nutritious and appealing school meals; opportunities for physical activity that include physical education; health education that covers a range of developmentally appropriate topics taught by knowledgeable teachers; programs that promote the health of school faculty and staff; and counseling, psychological, and social services that promote healthy social and emotional development and remove barriers to students' learning.

Core measures: Measures used to assess the quality management efforts of healthcare organizations. For **accreditation** purposes, core measures are grouped into measure sets, which may include clinical performance, client perception of care, health status, and administrative or financial measures. The initial core measures focus primarily on clinical performance. The identification and use of core measures allow comparisons of processes and **outcomes** of patient care among healthcare organizations across the country, regardless of which **performance measurement** system the organization is using.

Corporate negligence: A legal doctrine that was established by a judicial decision handed down in a 1965 court case, *Darling v. Charleston Community Hospital*. The court's ruling established the hospital's obligation to appoint only highly qualified practitioners to the medical staff. Owing to that obligation, hospitals may be held liable when a member of the medical staff fails to meet established **standards** of patient care.

Correctional facility health clinic: An ambulatory-care clinic in which healthcare is provided to prisoners confined to a correctional facility. Neither **informed consent** nor payment is required to carry out treatment at a correctional facility health clinic. This exception is made for treating inmates so a facility will not be held hostage to a manipulative inmate seeking to obstruct healthcare operations.

Court order: A legal document issued in place of a **subpoena** that requires an individual or a representative of an organization to appear in court and/or to present an object to the court. With the advice of legal counsel, an HIM director may decide that it is inappropriate for a hospital to release a subpoenaed record. When the disclosure of such material would otherwise be prohibited by state or federal **statutes** or **regulations**, a court order must be issued.

Credentialing: The process of verifying the educational qualifications, **licensure** status, and experience levels of healthcare professionals who have applied for the **privilege** of practicing within a healthcare facility.

Data: Objective descriptions of processes, **procedures**, people, and other observable things and activities. Data are collected in the form of dates, numbers, symbols, images, illustrations, texts, lists, charts, and equations. The **analysis** of data for a specific purpose results in **information**. Data represent facts; information conveys meaning. In other words, data themselves have no meaning until they are considered in the context of a specific purpose or function.

Data dictionary: A descriptive list of names, definitions, and attributes of **data** elements to be collected in an information system or **database**. Guidelines must be established by the HIM professionals with input from the various departments in the organization so that data dictionaries provide standardize definitions and ensure consistency of use. Lack of a sound data dictionary can cause problems within and across organizations. Variances among the **data sets** that are not recognized across the system can affect the information flow as well as the workflow. These guidelines aid in the development of new and existing data content **standards** and support national standards harmonization efforts as they relate to data dictionaries.

Data Elements for Emergency Department Systems (DEEDS): A **data** set commonly used in hospitals. Other **data sets** used today include the **Uniform Hospital Discharge Data Set (UHDDS)**, the **Essential Medical Data Set (EMEDS)**, the **Health Plan Employer Data and Information Set (HEDIS)**, and the **Uniform Ambulatory Care Data Set (UACDS)**.

Data exchange standards: Established **messaging standards**, also called interoperability standards, which ensure that all of the organization's data are structured and formatted in the same way.

Data quality management: A process that ensures the integrity of **data** during **data collection**, **application**, **warehousing**, and **analysis**. In 2006, the AHIMA issued a revised position statement on "Quality Healthcare Data and Information" that calls for the improvement of data quality by developing and implementing **standards** for data content, data mapping, and documentation within the healthcare industry.

Data sets: The collection of uniform data and the development of **databases** made up of **aggregate data**. Healthcare data sets have two purposes: to identify data elements that should be collected for each patient and to provide uniform definitions for common terms. Characteristics of several healthcare data sets are detailed in table 4.7.

Database: An organized collection of **data** that has been stored electronically for easy access. **Databases** can reveal trends and contribute to improving healthcare for everyone. They can be used for statistical reports that guide decisions in a local facility, for reports to **public health** agencies, and can influence the health of a state and even a nation. Databases can be facility-specific, state wide, or national in scope. Sometimes they are called **indexes** or **registries**.

Database management system: An electronic system that makes it possible to create, modify, delete, and view the **data** in a **database**.

Day treatment: A program that provides individuals with mental health treatment that is more intense than the services provided on an **outpatient** basis. Day treatment is sometimes referred to as **partial stay** treatment. Most payers (including **Medicare**) cover this service when it is determined medically appropriate by the physician.

Deemed status: Status granted by the **Centers for Medicare and Medicaid Services (CMS)**. Hospitals accredited through the **Joint Commission** Hospital Accreditation Program or the **American Osteopathic Association (AOA) Healthcare Facilities Accreditation Program (HFAP)** may participate in the Medicare program because the accrediting agency has been granted deemed status by the Medicare program.

Deficiency system: System designed to track and report elements of documentation missing from **health records**, a deficiency system can be paper-based, computer-based, or electronic. Paper-based deficiency systems use a checklist to indicate missing reports, signatures, consents, and other documentation. Computer-based deficiency systems provide logs for reporting and tracking health record deficiencies. Deficiencies created in an electronic system are automatically placed in the physician in-box or work queue.

Demographic data: Basic factual details about the individual patient. The demographic **data** collected from the patient include last, first, and middle name; address; telephone number; gender; date of birth; place of birth; race or ethnic origin; marital status; name and address of next of kin; and Social Security number. The main purpose of collecting demographic data is to confirm the identity of the patient. Hospitals and other healthcare-related organizations use the demographic data collected from patients as the basis of statistical records, **research**, and resource planning.

Department of Health and Human Services (HHS): Department of the federal government that established a Data Council to coordinate and integrate **data** collection and **analysis** activities. HHS has taken a number of steps to address key data needs, promote a coordinated HHS-wide strategy on data issues, and strengthen collaboration with private sector entities, state and local governments, and other partners. The Data Council also supports HHS-wide implementation of the Health Insurance Portability and Accountability Act Administrative Simplification, an initiative to adopt national **standards** for electronic healthcare transactions.

Derived data: Factual details aggregated or summarized from a group of **health records** that provide no means to identify specific patients. These **data** should have the same level of **confidentiality** as the **legal health record**. However, derived data should not be considered part of the legal health record and would not be produced in response to a **subpoena** for the health record.

Descriptive outcome: Rates that are not adjusted. Observed (actual) **outcomes** are aggregated across all eligible patients served by **home health agencies** in each state and further aggregated to obtain national observed rates. These observed rates are what appear in the report. Descriptive outcomes are one of two kinds of outcomes defined by **Medicare**. The second type of outcome is **risk-adjusted outcome**.

Diagnosis-related groups (DRG): A prospective payment system, implemented in the 1980s, that started the movement to **outpatient** services.

Diagnostic codes: Specific diagnoses and clinical **procedures** identified on claims and encounter forms. The International Classification of Diseases, Ninth Revision, Clinical Modification (ICD-9-CM), Current Procedural Terminology, Fourth Edition (CPT®-4), and Healthcare Common Procedure Coding System (HCPCS) are examples of code sets for procedures and diagnoses. Diagnostic codes must comply with HIPAA format and content. Standardized transactions include items such as claims information, encounter information, payment, remittance advice, claim status inquiry and response, and eligibility inquiry and response.

Diagnostic imaging center: A freestanding facility that provides diagnostic imaging services including MRI (magnetic resonance imaging), CT (computed tomography), and PET (positron emission tomography), as well as ultrasound (ultrasonography), nuclear medicine, picture archival communication systems, digital mammography, and molecular imaging. These technologies enable physicians to diagnose diseases at earlier stages while avoiding more invasive and costly diagnostic **procedures**.

Digital signature: A digitized version of a handwritten signature. The author of the documentation signs his or her name on a pen pad, and the signature is automatically converted to a digital signature that is affixed to the electronic document. Digital signatures, also known as **electronic signatures**, use the same technology as automated credit card authentication systems.

Disaster recovery planning: The technological aspect of business continuity planning. HIM professionals assist in designing disaster recovery plans that address how **information** can be documented in the **health record** during down time or a disaster. A well-designed disaster-recovery plan should consider daily backups and removal of electronic **data/information** to offsite locations for protection; access to information needed to treat patients; backup plans to collect and document health information; protection of computer systems, data, and paper-based records from destruction; protection against unauthorized use and disclosure; safeguards to ensure integrity and **confidentiality** of information; provision for orderly recovery of information; and periodic testing of disaster recovery plans before a disaster strikes.

Discharge summary: A concise account of the patient's illness, course of treatment, response to treatment, and condition at discharge. (Other terms for this type of documentation include *discharge abstract* and *clinical resume*.) The physician principally responsible for the patient's hospital care writes and signs the discharge summary. The discharge summary must be completed within thirty days after discharge for most patients but within twenty-four hours for patients transferred to other facilities. Discharge summaries are not always required for patients who were hospitalized for less than forty-eight hours.

Disease index: Retrieval of patient **information** by diagnosis. A disease index is arranged by diagnostic or procedure codes that facilitate the study of patients with the same or similar conditions or treatment. This sorting guides the locating of **health records** to conduct quality improvement and **research** studies, as well as for monitoring quality of care. The index is also useful for retrieving records for research studies. To be useful for use in a disease index, the health record should provide the following information: **principal diagnosis** and relevant secondary diagnoses with codes; associated **procedures** and codes; patient's health record number; patient's gender, age, and race; attending physician's code or name; service rendered to the patient; the disposition following service; and dates of encounter.

Do-not-resuscitate (DNR) order: A physician's order documenting a patient's (or surrogate's) desire for no resuscitation attempts. A DNR order results from a desire expressed in an **advance directive**. A DNR is issued when it has been decided that the patient is near death and that no resuscitation attempts should be made when the patient stops breathing. In addition to the order, **health record** documentation must indicate that the decision to withhold resuscitation efforts was discussed with the patient or the patient's legal representative, when the decision was made, and who took part in making the decision.

Dumping: The once-common practice of private hospitals to transfer indigent patients to the emergency departments of nearby public hospitals with the sole purpose of avoiding the cost of providing emergency treatment to patients who were uninsured or underinsured and could not pay for the services themselves. Federal legislation (Emergency Medical Treatment and Active Labor Act [EMTALA]) passed in 1986 and implemented in 1990 contains provisions intended to curtail this practice. State and federal **regulations** require emergency facilities to thoroughly document the reasons for patient transfers to confirm that the transfers were not related to the patients' ability to pay for treatment or the source of payment.

Early Childhood Intervention (ECI): Services provided by some behavioral health organizations. Currently, ECI services are exempt from HIPAA; the **privacy** of these records is covered by the **Family Educational Rights and Privacy Act of 1974 (FERPA)**.

e-Discovery: The process by which electronic information is produced in response to threatened or impending litigation. Amendments to the **Federal Rules of Civil Procedure** and the Uniform Rules Relating to the Discovery of Electronically Stored Information are creating new responsibilities for legal counsel and HIM professionals. Organizations must begin thinking about how they will respond to e-discovery requests for information.

EHR Collaborative: Collaboration of organizations representing key stakeholders in healthcare that worked together with **Health Level Seven (HL7)** to publicize and refine a draft version of a new **electronic health record (EHR)** functional model in late 2003.

Electronic data interchange (EDI): The transaction and messaging activity that occurs among independent computer information systems.

Electronic document management system (EDMS): An electronic storage system. Source documents such as medical reports are scanned to create digital images of the original documents. The digital documents can then be stored electronically on optical disks. Some digital scanners can process hundreds or even thousands of documents per day. Access to images stored on optical disks is fast and easy, and scanned information can be made available simultaneously to any number of users. Document scanning is also used to convert stored **health record information** into images that can be loaded onto new electronic health record systems.

Electronic health record (EHR): An electronic documentation that replaces the paper-based **health record**. An electronic health record (EHR) contains all of the **information** found in a paper-based record, but it can be in multiple versions, have different views of displaying the same information, and contain features (such as alerts and reminders) that provide clinical decision support. These functions and features are not available in a paper-based health record. The biggest factors delaying the universal implementation of electronic health records (EHRs) have likely been the lack of shared vision and an absence of functional **standards**. The standard for EHRs has been revised several times since its initial release in 1999. The current standard, E1384-07, was revised in October 2007.

Electronic signature: A digitized version of a handwritten signature. The author of the documentation signs his or her name on a pen pad, and the signature is automatically converted to a **digital signature** that is affixed to the electronic document. Electronic signatures, also known as digital signatures, use the same technology as automated credit card authentication systems.

Elements of Performance (EP): The **Joint Commission's** specific performance expectations and/or structures or processes that must be in place for an organization to pervade safe, high-quality care, treatment, and services. The Joint Commission bases its **accreditation** outcome on the ability of the healthcare organization to demonstrate compliance with specific performance **standards**. Knowledge of EPs pertaining directly to the **health record** and documentation in the record are critical for the health information management (HIM) professional working in an accredited facility.

Emergency and trauma care: The medical–surgical care provided to individuals whose injuries or illnesses require urgent care to address conditions that could be life threatening or disabling if not treated immediately; provided through a network of designated hospitals and emergency transportation systems.

Emergency Medical Treatment and Active Labor Act (EMTALA): Requirement for emergency departments to complete a medical screening examination prior to collecting any information regarding the patient's ability to pay for the services. EMTALA was enacted as part of the Consolidated Omnibus Budget Reconciliation Act (COBRA) of 1986.

Employee Assistance Programs (EAPs): Outpatient programs designed to provide employees immediate access to psychological counseling on a limited basis. These services are often provided on-site or through local providers.

Encounter note: Documentation in the **health record**, which is often authored by more than one healthcare provider. For example, a nurse or alternate user can begin a patient's encounter note, and later, the examining physician can add comments. Encounter notes are also called **visit notes**.

Enterprise master person/patient index (EMPI): An electronic system that consolidates information from various software systems in a healthcare organization, such as registration, scheduling, financial, and clinical systems. EMPIs may also assist organizations in maintaining HIPAA patient identification and tracking requirements.

Essential Medical Data Set (EMEDS): A data set commonly used in hospitals. Other **data sets** used today include the **Uniform Hospital Discharge Data Set (UHDDS)**, the **Data Elements for Emergency Department Systems (DEEDS)**, the **Health Plan Employer Data and Information Set (HEDIS)**, and the **Uniform Ambulatory Care Data Set (UACDS)**.

Expressed consent: Consent for treatment that is either spoken or written by the patient. Although courts recognize both verbal and written consent, verbal consent is more difficult to prove.

Face sheet: Information about the patient as well as information about the patient's health insurance coverage is collected at the time of admission. The patient's **administrative information** is then recorded on an identification sheet, which is often called a **face sheet**. In paper-based record systems, a printout of the face sheet is used as the front page in the patient's record. In an electronic format, **data** collected from the face sheet may be captured on several screens but displayed in a logical manner to those who need it. For instance, clinical staff caring for the patient should be able to quickly identify the patient by name, **health record** number, and account number, as well as locate emergency contacts for the patient; whereas the billing office needs the patient's name, account number, and insurance information.

Facility-specific index: Databases established by healthcare facilities to meet their individual, specific needs for customer care or other reporting requirements. These **indexes** make it possible to retrieve **health records** in a variety of ways including by disease, physician, operation, or other **data** element. Prior to computerization in healthcare, these indexes were kept on cards. Today, most are compiled from databases routinely developed by the facility.

Facility-specific registry: Chronological listing of patients with a common characteristic. **Registries** are different from **indexes** because they contain information that is more extensive. These reports are typically generated from a facility's existing **database**. Registries are also used for patient follow-up as well as aggregate studies. Registry maintenance consists of the following activities: case definition (describing the patients that are to be included), case finding (identifying patients that are to be included), and case abstracting (extracting the **information** to be included from **health records**). Registries usually maintained by healthcare facilities are listed in chapter 4, figure 4.1. Creation and maintenance of these registries is often a responsibility of the HIM department.

Failed/missed appointment policy: Policy that tracks appointments that are canceled or missed. A failed/missed appointment policy should state the required documentation of information concerning the missed appointment.

Family Educational Rights and Privacy Act of 1974 (FERPA): A federal **statute** enacted in 1974 that clarifies how **information** can be shared legally.

Federal Register: Daily publication of the U.S. Government Printing Office that publishes final changes, updates, and proposed changes and updates to the *Code of Federal Regulations.* HIM professionals are advised to check the *Federal Register* for the most current version of the **Medicare *Conditions of Participation for Hospitals***, available online at www.gpoaccess. gov/fr/index.html.

Federal Rules of Civil Procedure (FRCP): A federal rule, enacted in 1938 with significant revisions in 2007, that governs civil proceedings in the U.S. federal court system.

Financial data: Details about the patient's occupation, employer, and insurance coverage are collected at the time of treatment. Healthcare providers use this **data** to complete claims forms submitted to **third-party payers**. Financial data includes the patient's name, name of the insured party and his or her relationship to the patient if the patient is a dependent of the insured party, insured party's member identification number, name of the insurance company and the group policy number, and the employer's name and address.

Flow charts: Graphic illustrations of **data** and observations that make it easy to visualize patterns and identify abnormal results. Flow charts are often used in addition to narrative **progress notes** for recording the patient's fluid consumption (input) and elimination (output) patterns. Input and output records are especially important in pediatric patients because medications are often based on the patient's weight and may affect input and output. Blood glucose records for diabetic patients are also maintained as flow charts. Pain assessments can be charted as well.

Food and Drug Administration (FDA): A federal agency of the U.S. Department of Health and Human Services. The FDA is charged with protecting and promoting health. The FDA **regulations** govern biologics, drugs, medical devices, and radiation-emitting devices used in the healthcare industry. The FDA Modernization Act of 1997 mandated that a **clinical trials database** be developed. The National Library of Medicine has developed this database for use by both consumers and practitioners. The Clinical Trials database is available online at http:// clinicaltrials.gov.

Functional independent measures (FIM): Measures used to evaluate the level of independence of patients in long-term acute-care (LTCH) settings where the focus of care is on extensive rehabilitation of the patient. FIM includes 18 items that are scored on a scale of 1 to 7, with 1 being the most dependent and 7 being the most independent. Total scores range between 18 and 126. FIM scores can be used as outcome measures by LTCHs.

Functionality standards: Standards that define the components that an **electronic health record (EHR)** needs to support the functions for which it is designed. **Health Level Seven (HL7)** draft **standards** for an EHR were developed in 2004.

Hand-off communication: Communication of patient **information** between caregivers. The **Joint Commission** developed a standard for hand-off communication as one of its Patient Safety Goals. Standard 2E recommends that each healthcare organization implement a standardized approach to "hand off" communications, including an opportunity to ask and respond to questions.

Health data repository: A **database** that will provide immediate nationwide access to local data in the event of primary system failure or system unavailability. In the aftermath of Hurricane Katrina in 2005, the Veterans Administration initiated the development of the Health Data Repository. It will contain real-time copies of local clinical data. The repository is an effort to improve data accessibility and increase disaster preparedness.

Health informatics standards: **Standards** that describe uniform methods for collecting, maintaining, and/or transferring healthcare **data** among computer information systems. Health informatics standards can be classified into five categories: **vocabulary standards**, **structure and content standards**, **transaction and messaging standards**, **security standards**, and i**dentifier standards**. Work completed to develop and establish health informatics standards ensures the successful implementation of electronic **health record** systems. Many organizations are currently working on the development of health informatics standards. Compliance with such industry standards continues to be voluntary.

Health information exchange (HIE): Public and private sector stakeholders are focusing efforts on health information exchange (HIE) because there is increasing evidence that health information technology can improve healthcare quality and customer safety by reducing errors and unnecessary expenditures.

Health Information Technology Standards Panel (HITSP): Federal organization established by the **Office of the National Coordinator of Health Information Technology (ONC)** that is charged with determining which sets of national **standards**, developed by **standards development organizations (SDOs)**, will be used in the United States and for what purpose. The results of this initiative are reviewed by the American Health Information Community (AHIC) and the **Department of Health and Human Services (HHS)** to further refine those standards for the healthcare industry.

Health Insurance Portability and Accountability Act (HIPAA): A federal **statute**, enacted in 1996 and amended in 2003, that establishes a consistent set of **privacy** and security rules that are designed to protect the privacy of patients, while at the same time simplifying the sharing of health **information** for legitimate purposes. For example, before implementation of HIPAA, a healthcare provider who needed access to a **health record** maintained by another provider usually could not directly request the information. The former provider required the patient's written authorization to release information to the current provider. In many cases, the patient or the patient's legal representative had to facilitate the transfer of medical information to a current healthcare provider. Under HIPAA privacy regulations, the healthcare provider can directly request protected medical information, and a written authorization from the patient is not required when the information is used for treatment purposes.

Health Level Seven (HL7): An organization that develops **standards** related to healthcare delivery. In late 2003, it released the draft version of a new EHR functional model.

Health maintenance organization (HMO): Organization that offers a wide range of healthcare services, including **acute care** and **ambulatory care**. HMOs provide health coverage to voluntarily enrolled individuals in return for prepayment of a fixed fee, regardless of the services the individual enrollees actually use.

Health Plan Employer Data and Information Set (HEDIS): A **data** set commonly used in hospitals. Other **data sets** used today include the **Uniform Hospital Discharge Data Set (UHDDS)**, the **Data Elements for Emergency Department Systems (DEEDS)**, **Essential Medical Data Set (EMEDS)**, and the **Uniform Ambulatory Care Data Set (UACDS)**.

Health record: The means that healthcare providers use to collect and store the clinical documentation they create for individual patients. Health records are sometimes called *medical records*. They serve many purposes such as providing documentation of healthcare services for **reimbursement**, **outcomes** management, and quality care; protecting legal interests; and supplying clinical **data** for **research**. It supports the operational management of the healthcare organization as it is used for training and education as well as planning of services that support community health needs.

Health record analysis: Review that ensures the quality and completeness of clinical documentation. The purpose of health record analysis is not an evaluation of the clinical care provided to the patient, but rather to review for completeness and accuracy of the health record and to ensure that **protocols** are met. Health record analysis comprises two separate but related processes: **quantitative analysis** and **qualitative analysis**.

Health record review process: An auditing procedure that examines clinical pertinence and **health record** completion. An examination of discharged records ensures compliance with documentation **standards**. Health records are typically examined at the point of care by various clinical and HIM staff; however, it is important to include discharge documentation monitoring in the health record review process to ensure that requirements and standards for discharge documentation are met.

Health services research: Research to improve the quality, safety, efficiency, and effectiveness of healthcare for all Americans. Health services **research** is one of the functions of the **Agency for Healthcare Research and Quality (AHRQ)**. In 2007, the AHRQ and the **Centers for Medicare and Medicaid Services (CMS)** published a handbook to help providers set up **registries**, including recommendations for design and **data** source access and suggestions on ways to encourage participation in registries.

Healthcare Facilities Accreditation Program (HFAP): The **American Osteopathic Association (AOA)** accreditation program. The AOA first initiated its hospital **accreditation** program in 1945 to ensure the quality of residency training programs for doctors of osteopathy. Today, the association's Healthcare Facilities Accreditation Program (HFAP) accredits a number of healthcare facilities and services, including laboratories, ambulatory-care clinics, ambulatory-surgery centers, behavioral health and substance abuse treatment facilities, physical rehabilitation facilities, acute-care hospitals, and critical-access hospitals. Healthcare facilities that have been accredited by the AOA earn **deemed status** from the **Centers for Medicare and Medicaid Services (CMS)**. CMS extended the AOA HFAP deemed status effective through September 25, 2009. Like hospitals accredited by the **Joint Commission**, AOA-accredited hospitals are not required to undergo yearly Medicare certification surveys.

Healthcare Integrity and Protection Data Bank (HIPDB): One of two federal **databases**. The HIPDB collects information on legal actions taken against licensed healthcare providers, including both civil judgments and criminal convictions. As part of every medical staff appointment process, hospitals and other healthcare organizations are required by federal law to send inquiries to the **National Practitioner Data Bank (NPDB)** and the Healthcare Integrity and Protection Data Bank (HIPDB).

Healthcare reengineering: A focus of the healthcare industry whose forces have turned their attention to patient care and cost controls, managed care, integrated delivery systems, performance improvement, **outcomes assessment** and management, and growth of **outpatient** and partial treatment settings. All of these focus areas influence a facility's documentation requirements and will vary from organization to organization.

History: A summary of the patient's illness from his or her point of view. The purpose of documenting the patient's medical history is to gather background **information** about the patient's condition before he or she is admitted to the facility. In most cases, the history is documented in the patient's record by the admitting physician. In teaching hospitals, the history may be collected and documented by a resident in the hospital. In other facilities, assigned personnel are responsible for collecting this initial information. Increasingly, patients have the responsibility of responding to questionnaires (on paper or electronically) to create this history.

Home Assessment Validation and Entry (HAVEN): A software application used by **home care** or hospice organizations to accurately compute and encode **OASIS data**. Encoding of all OASIS data items must be complete, or locked, in order to accurately compute the information (Health Insurance Prospective Payment System [HIPPS] code set) necessary for billing **Medicare** patients under the prospective payment system.

Home care: A diverse and dynamic service industry comprised of **home health agencies**, home care, personal-care providers, and hospices that have come to be known collectively as home care organizations. It should be noted that the term *home care* is often interchanged with **home health** and should be regarded as one and the same.

Home health: A diverse and dynamic service industry comprised of home health agencies, **home care**, personal-care providers, and hospices that have come to be known collectively as home care organizations. It should be noted that the term *home care* is often interchanged with home health and should be regarded as one and the same.

Home health agency (HHA): An organization that provides **home care**. More than 20,000 providers deliver home care services to some eight million individuals who require services because of acute illness, long-term health conditions, permanent disability, or terminal illness. **Medicare-certified home health agencies** are governed by the Home Health Initiative, a quality-monitoring system that makes highly specific **data** collection and **information** management demands on home care providers. The **prospective payment system (PPS)**, which became effective on October 1, 2000, changed **Medicare** and **Medicaid** home care **reimbursement** from a cost-based system to a system of fixed-fee reimbursement based on a patient-need classification system. Home care agencies can seek **accreditation** from the **Joint Commission** or the **Community Health Accreditation Program (CHAP)**.

Home health resource group (HHRG): A classification determined by **Medicare**, based on the input **data** from **home health** claims submitted by **home health agencies (HHAs)** that are paid under the Medicare HHA **prospective payment system (PPS)**. According to the CMS Medicare Claims Processing Manual, ROVER uses **health records** to verify that the **information** contained on an HHA-completed **OASIS** reflects the condition of the patient and the services actually delivered during a particular episode in time. The program guides medical review staff through a review of information in the clinical record. The reviewer can document whether the case-mix OASIS items have been validated by the information contained in the record. The end results are twofold: a recommended **home health resource group (HHRG)** classification based on the input data and a reporting **database** containing information from the reviews. Therefore, the information gained by the use of ROVER applies not only to data verification but also to intermediary data **analysis** and provider education.

Home healthcare: The medical and/or personal care provided to individuals and families in their place of residence with the goal of promoting, maintaining, or restoring health or minimizing the effects of disabilities and illnesses, including terminal illnesses.

Hospice care: The medical and/or personal care provided to individuals with life expectancies of six months or less who elect to receive palliative care in place of standard medical treatment for their illnesses; provided in patients' homes and in residential treatment facilities.

Hospitalist: A fully qualified physician hired by a hospital to coordinate patient care. In the past, resident physicians worked long hours and were responsible for providing much of the patient care in teaching hospitals. Starting in the 1980s, however, several highly publicized cases of patients dying while under the care of overworked and underqualified residents created significant concern about the way teaching hospitals operate. Recent changes in federal **regulations** now limit the number of hours residents may work. This has resulted in the need for a new category of physicians called hospitalists.

Hybrid: As hospitals transition to an electronic **health records** system, they find their records in a hybrid state. HIM professionals play an essential role in implementing systems and processes that permit timely access to clinical **data**, regardless of how records are documented or stored. Another key role is advocating for quality documentation and data in health records to improve customer care and safety.

Hybrid health record: A system with functional components that include both paper and electronic documents, and use both manual and electronic processes. Some types of documentation that compose the **health record** may physically exist in separate and multiple paper-based, electronic, or computer-based **databases**.

ICD-10-CM© and ICD-10-PCS: New diagnostic and procedural coding systems that are used to identify diagnoses and **procedures** and recorded electronically during the billing process. The ICD-10-CM codes replace the ICD-9-CM codes. The Official Guidelines for Coding and Reporting discuss the importance of determining the appropriate diagnoses to be reported in any setting. The official guidelines are updated regularly.

Identifier standards: Uniform methods for collecting, maintaining, and/or transferring healthcare **data** among computer information systems. Identifier standards are one of five categories of **health informatics standards**. The other categories include **vocabulary standards, structure and content standards, transaction and messaging standards**, and **security standards**. Work completed to develop and establish health informatics standards ensures the successful implementation of electronic **health record** systems. Many organizations are currently working on the development of health informatics standards. Compliance with such industry standards continues to be voluntary.

Imaging reports: Scans and x-ray images of various parts of the body and organs are frequently performed by **inpatient** and **outpatient** imaging departments. Most hospital imaging departments are equipped to perform x-ray examinations and computed tomography (CT) scans. Many large, urban hospitals also provide more advanced imaging services including magnetic resonance imaging (MRI) and positron-emission tomography (PET). Some imaging **procedures** require the administration of radiopharmaceuticals, radioactive contrast media administered to the patient before or during the procedure to make it possible to visualize physiological processes and tissues more clearly.

Implied consent: Consent that is assumed when a patient voluntarily submits to medical treatment. The rationale behind this conclusion is that it is reasonable to assume that patients must understand the nature of the medical care or they would not submit to it.

Incidence: Health record documentation is required for developing the **databases** used by **public health** departments to provide **data** on the incidence and **prevalence** of diseases, possible high-risk populations, survival statistics, and trends over time. Data elements for the databases may be collected using a variety of methods, including interviews, physical examinations of individuals, and review of health records. The HIM manager may have input in these databases through information provided from health records.

Incident: An event that is considered to be inconsistent with accepted **standards** of care. **Policies** should address the steps to be taken in response to an incident. Most hospitals institute policies that require the preparation of **incident reports**. Some facilities use the terms *occurrence* and *occurrence report* in this context.

Incident report: Report that describes the occurrence (time, date, and location); identifies the individual(s) involved (patients, visitors, and/or staff); and the current condition of the individual(s) who were affected. The report should include statements from witnesses and be completed as soon as possible after the **incident** to ensure accuracy and completeness. Incident reports are prepared for **risk management**, performance improvement, and staff education purposes but not for direct patient care. The report contains subjective information from witnesses and individuals involved in the incident. For these reasons, incident reports must never be included or mentioned in a patient's **legal health record**. Instead, incident reports should be stored in separate, secure **databases** or files in the facility's risk management or performance improvement department. In anticipation of future court action, incident reports should be marked as confidential and addressed to the hospital's attorney. Incident reports should not be disseminated internally or externally to anyone other than the individuals designated by the hospital's risk management **policies**. Incident reports are not disseminated because of the risk of copies being filed in another file, which would cause them to become discoverable. When kept as discussed, incident reports are generally not discoverable.

Index: Databases used to sort **data** in a variety of ways to assist study of certain data elements.

Individual tracer activity: One of two **tracer methods** used by **Joint Commission** surveyors in the **accreditation** process. Individual tracer activity permits the evaluation of the care experience of a specific patient while in the hospital. This method analyzes a hospital's system of providing care, treatment, and services used as the framework for assessing **standards** of compliance.

Individual-based system tracer activity: One of two **tracer methods** used by **Joint Commission** surveyors in the **accreditation** process. The individual-based system tracer activity explores a specific system or process across the organization. The surveyor evaluates the integration of related processes, coordination, and communication among disciplines and departments during the individual-based system tracer. **Data** use, infection control, and medical management are key components evaluated during the individual-based system tracer activity.

Industrial health clinic: Clinic that offers treatment to workers who are affected by work-related injuries and illnesses. Usually, industrial health clinics are financed through the employer's workers' compensation insurance plans. Sometimes they also provide preemployment physicals and testing, which are paid for directly by the potential employers. Finally, many industrial health centers collect **data** on patterns of work-related illness and injury and provide the information to employers on a contract basis.

Information: The **analysis** of data for a specific purpose results in **information**. Data are collected in the form of dates, numbers, symbols, images, illustrations, texts, lists, charts, and equations. The analysis of data for a specific purpose results in information. Data represent facts; information conveys meaning. In other words, data themselves have no meaning until they are considered in the context of a specific purpose or function.

Information exchange: Public and private sector stakeholders focusing efforts on health information exchange (HIE) because there is increasing evidence that health information technology can improve healthcare quality and customer safety by reducing errors and unnecessary expenditures. Health information exchange projects have brought a diverse group of stakeholders together to plan, finance, and implement systems to share electronic health information. Stakeholders include hospitals, clinicians, laboratories, pharmacies, payers, employers, **public health** departments, quality-improvement organizations, and consumers.

Informed consent: Documentation of a patient's consents for treatment and use of healthcare **information**. Hospitals and other healthcare organizations are required to obtain written consents and authorizations before they provide treatment or release confidential patient information. Acknowledgments usually apply to the patient's confirmation that he or she has received specific information. All consents, authorizations, and acknowledgments that have been signed by patients or their legal representatives in connection with services to be provided in a hospital should be stored in the patients' **health records**. The need to obtain the patient's consent before performing medical and surgical **procedures** is based on the legal concept of battery. Battery is the unlawful touching of a person without his or her implied or **expressed consent**. **Implied consent** is assumed when a patient voluntarily submits to medical treatment. The rationale behind this conclusion is that it is reasonable to assume that patients must understand the nature of the medical care or they would not submit to it. Expressed consent is permission that is either spoken or written. Although the courts recognize both spoken and written forms of consent, spoken consent is more difficult to prove in a legal proceeding. Most healthcare providers ask patients or their legal representatives to sign a general **consent to treatment**. By signing a general consent to treatment, the patient agrees to submit to routine clinical procedures and medical and nursing care while he or she is a patient. Except in emergency situations, patients are usually asked to sign a general consent form during the admissions process. More specific consents are required for procedures that involve significant risk, such as invasive diagnostic tests, transfusions, and surgery. These specific consents are completed in addition to the general consent forms.

The HIPAA (2003) **privacy** standard does not require healthcare organizations to obtain the patient's formal consent to use health information for treatment, **reimbursement**, operational, and reporting purposes. However, some state laws may still require hospitals and other healthcare providers to obtain a written consent from the patient or the patient's legal representative before sharing the patient's confidential health information with external healthcare providers and **third-party payers**. Even in the absence of state and federal requirements, many hospitals choose to document the patient's consent for routine uses and disclosures of confidential information. Patients are usually asked to sign general consents during the admissions process. (See chapter 3, figure 3.9 for an example of a general consent form.) Consents relevant to information are treated as separate documents rather than as elements of the general consent to treatment, which is obtained at admission.

Informed consent policy: A challenge to large multispecialty physicians' practices due to patients' multiple points of entry. One clinic may assume that another clinic has already had a patient sign the **informed consent**. Options for managing this challenge include having each patient sign a new consent upon each visit, or establishing a monitoring system that alerts clinics when consent is needed. Patients often respond negatively to the first option due to not wanting to sign a new release each time they visit the facility. The perception is that the organization should know when the consent has been signed. The second choice presents an economic challenge due to the high cost associated with the staff time required for monitoring and auditing for compliance.

Inpatient: An individual who receives healthcare services as well as room, board, and continuous nursing care in a hospital unit dedicated to providing around-the-clock patient care.

Inpatient facilities: Facilities that provide patients with around-the-clock care. Inpatient facilities may be a dedicated portion of a hospital or may stand alone. For individuals seeking mental health treatment, in some circumstances, they are in need of partial-stay services or partial hospitalization. Such services are provided to individuals who fall between the need for **inpatient** and **outpatient** services and would benefit from a short stay at an inpatient mental health facility or hospital.

Integrated delivery system (IDS): An organization that offers a variety of healthcare services. For example, one organization may provide acute-care services, **home healthcare** services, and **behavioral healthcare** services under the same organizational name. As with any other healthcare provider, access to health information is critical to the successful delivery of care in such an integrated delivery system (IDS). Reliable and timely access to information is essential for the delivery of high-quality client care and yet is one of the most significant challenges in this type of healthcare system.

Integrated health record: A format used for paper-based **health records** in which information is arranged so that the documentation from various sources is intermingled and follows a strict chronological or reverse chronological order. The advantage of the integrated format is that it is easy for caregivers to follow the course of the patient's diagnosis and treatment. The disadvantage is that the format makes it difficult to compare related information. The other formats for paper-based records are **source-oriented records** and **problem-oriented records**.

Integrated healthcare network: A network made up of hospitals, postacute-care facilities, and ambulatory-care facilities operated by the same corporate entity.

Interval note: Note that includes **information** about the patient's current complaint, any relevant changes in his or her condition, and the physical findings since the last hospital admission. Patients are sometimes readmitted to the same hospital for treatment of the same condition. When the readmission occurs within thirty days after the previous discharge, the admitting physician may add an interval note to the patient's record in place of a complete **history** and physical. However, when the patient is admitted for treatment of a different condition, a complete history and physical must be performed and documented. If a patient is admitted more than thirty days after the previous discharge for the same condition, a complete history and physical must be obtained.

Intraoperative anesthesia record: A record that is created while a surgical procedure is being performed. The record describes the entire surgical process and includes the following information: patient identification, including name and record number; name of the anesthesiologist or nurse-anesthetist; type and amount of anesthesia administered; induction mechanisms; medication log, including medical gases and fluid administration; usage of blood products; placement of lines and monitoring devices; patient's reaction to anesthesia; and results of continuous patient monitoring, including vital signs and oxygen saturation levels. The professional administering anesthesia during the procedure must also maintain the intraoperative anesthesia record.

Joint Commission: A not-for-profit, **standards**-setting organization whose primary mission is "to continuously improve the safety and quality of care provided to the public through the provision of health care **accreditation** and related services that support performance improvement in health care organizations." Currently, it accredits more than 15,000 healthcare organizations and programs in the United States. Joint Commission International expands that commitment worldwide by providing consultation, accreditation, publications, and education services to public and private healthcare organizations in more than 60 countries. The Joint Commission provides evaluation and accreditation services for the following types of healthcare organizations: acute-care hospitals, ambulatory-care organizations, **behavioral healthcare**, critical-access hospitals, children's hospitals, group practices, **home care** organizations, hospice services, independent or freestanding laboratories and medical equipment services, office-based surgery, **long-term care** (or skilled-nursing) facilities, psychiatric hospitals, and rehabilitation hospitals. Entities that have been accredited by the Joint Commission are automatically granted **deemed status** by the **Medicare** program.

Labor and delivery record: The hospital records for pregnant women admitted for labor and delivery contain elements similar to general **health records**. The obstetrician's records of prenatal care constitute documentation of the patient's preadmission **history** and physical. At admission, the physician also prepares a note describing the patient's progress since he or she last saw her for prenatal care. For normal deliveries, a labor and delivery record takes the place of an **operative report**.

Laboratory reports: The documented results of samples examined in the clinical laboratory. Samples include blood, urine, spinal fluid, and other fluids and substances collected from patients. Laboratory tests require a physician's order. The samples for testing are usually collected from patients by nurses or phlebotomists (technicians specially trained to draw blood samples) and then delivered to the laboratory. When the samples are received in the laboratory, a medical technologist or another laboratory **specialist** performs the standardized testing **procedures** ordered. Medical technologists receive training in four-year college programs, where they learn a combination of manual and automated biochemical **analysis** techniques. Large clinical laboratories may also employ bacteriologists, biologists, and other scientists to conduct more complex analyses, such as genetic testing. In hospitals, the results of most routine laboratory procedures are generated automatically by electronic testing equipment. Laboratory computer systems generate reports on the test results, which are returned to the physician who ordered the tests. Paper or electronic copies of the results are also placed in the patient's **health record**. Reports of laboratory results include the following information: patient identification, including name and record number, name of the test performed, date the test was performed and time in/time out of the laboratory, signature of the laboratory technologist or scientist who performed the test, name of the laboratory where the test was performed, and results of the test.

Legal health record: The contents of the **health record** that is the healthcare provider's legal business record of the services administered to the patient. As organizations transition to electronic health records, defining the "legal record" becomes complex. It is necessary for a healthcare organization to determine which parts of the EHR are included in the legal record and which parts are not.

Liability: The legal responsibility to compensate individuals for injuries and losses sustained as the result of negligence.

Licensure: The process of granting an organization the right to provide healthcare services. State governments establish licensure requirements. Unlike **accreditation**, which is a voluntary process, licensure is mandatory. Some individual healthcare practitioners are subject to state licensure requirements. For example, physicians, dentists, and nurses must obtain a license in an individual state in order to practice in that state. Specific licensure requirements are determined by state **regulations** and vary from state to state. However, it is illegal in all fifty states to operate healthcare facilities and practice medicine without a license.

Longitudinal health record: A **health record** that includes all of the health-related **information** generated for an individual during his or her lifetime. A longitudinal health record has many benefits for customers. However, the maintenance of such records for every American will be impossible until every healthcare provider in the country has implemented an EHR system.

Long-term acute care: The medical care provided to individuals who are clinically complex with multiple acute and chronic conditions requiring an average length of stay greater than 25 days in long-term care hospitals certified as acute-care hospitals.

Long-term acute-care hospital (LTCH): Hospitals that have an average **inpatient** length of stay greater than 25 days and typically provide extended medical and rehabilitative care for patients who are clinically complex and suffer from multiple acute or chronic conditions. The clinical documentation for **long-term care** encompasses a broad range of **information**, assessments, and medical services. Much of the information captured is similar to that for the short-term acute-care hospitals. The LTCH **Medicare Prospective Payment System** uses short-term acute-care hospital diagnosis-related groups (DRGs), but mandates the use of LTCH DRGs. While these DRGs are the same as those used in short-term acute-care, the LTCH DRGs have different weights and lengths of stay attached to them. The importance of the **principal diagnosis** is detailed.

Long-term care: The medical- and/or personal-care services provided to chronically ill, aged, disabled, or mentally handicapped individuals who reside in dedicated nursing facilities on a permanent basis.

Managed behavioral healthcare organizations (MBHOs): Organizations that provide **behavioral healthcare** services. The **National Committee for Quality Assurance (NCQA)** was established in 1990 and began its **accreditation** program for managed behavioral healthcare organizations (MBHOs) in 1997. Its accreditation model is based on the specific organization type or services provided. For example, if medical care is provided under a managed-care organization (MCO) and behavioral health services, **standards** for both managed-care organizations—MCO and MBHO—are used in the accreditation survey. Eligibility requirements are specific to the type of accreditation or **certification** being sought. Accreditation is based on quality documentation. The NCQA's accreditation of MBHOs rewards organizations that focus on quality, which, in turn, may help improve the nation's healthcare.

Managed-care facility: Facility that provides healthcare services. Many managed-care contractors require **accreditation** for **reimbursement, certification, licensure,** and participation agreement. Managed-care programs that provide acute-care services may be accredited through the National Committee for Quality Assurance. Ambulatory-surgery centers and **outpatient** diagnostic imaging and radiation oncology treatment facilities may be accredited through the Accreditation Association for Ambulatory Health Care (AAAHC). In April 1997, AAAHC adopted special **standards** for managed-care professional services delivery organizations. These standards focus on system-wide mechanisms for evaluating care providers that function within managed-care systems and for ensuring standards compliance. The standards address such critical issues as communication to patients, grievance resolution, consumer information, appeals procedures, and **utilization management.** In addition, the AAAHC has undertaken specialized reviews for state agencies in conjunction with state regulatory requirements, which has resulted in extensive involvement in external reviews of managed-care organizations. This environment challenges providers to develop information management systems that encourage documentation of standardized, high-quality, and accessible **data** and information to support patient and family care, quality improvement efforts, strategic planning, and other essential activities.

Managed care organization (MCO): Third-party payers who review information on services provided to their beneficiaries. The appropriateness and quality of care provided to customers is the focus.

Master patient (person) index (MPI): A computer-based registration system linked to a **database.** When a patient is readmitted to a healthcare facility, registration personnel check the patient's personal **information** against the **data** in the database to ensure that it is current and correct.

Master patient index (MPI): A **database** of patients within a facility or associated group of facilities (enterprise). The MPI, whether in paper or electronic format, may be considered the most important resource in a healthcare facility because it tracks patient activity across customer-care settings. The MPI identifies all patients who have been treated in a facility or enterprise and lists the **health records** or identification numbers associated with the names. An **index** can be maintained manually or as part of a computerized system. Retention of entries depends on the MPI's use. Typically, entries for healthcare facilities are retained permanently, while those for insurers, registries, or others may have different retention periods.

Medicaid: An amendment in 1965 to the Social Security Act established two federal programs, **Medicare** and Medicaid, to provide health insurance coverage to the aged and poor populations. With the implementation of Medicare and Medicaid, these federal programs played a pivotal role in the U.S. government becoming the largest payer for healthcare services.

Medical necessity: Determinations of medical necessity are based on whether the services can be expected to have a reasonably beneficial effect on the patient's physical needs and quality of life. Accurate clinical **data** collection is important because it becomes the basis of **care plans** and helps determine medical necessity. In all cases, **health record** documentation must support the medical necessity of the services and materials ordered.

Medical record delinquency rate: Accreditation standards require that hospitals track the number of delinquent medical records. The **Joint Commission** requires hospitals to monitor the medical record delinquency rate at least quarterly. During the Joint Commission accreditation process, delinquency statistics **data** are used during accreditation surveys to show past evidence of compliance with record completion standards. The delinquency rate is calculated by dividing the monthly average number of discharges by the monthly average number of delinquent records.

Medical specialties: Areas of medicine that include the following: Internal medicine, Pediatrics, Cardiology, Endocrinology, Psychiatry, Oncology, Nephrology, Neurology, Pulmonology, Gastroenterology, Dermatology, Radiology and nuclear medicine.

Medical staff bylaws: The rights and responsibilities of individual members and the means by which medical staff leaders govern the conduct of members.

Medical staff bylaws, rules, and regulations: Methods that govern the conduct of the independent healthcare professionals who provide patient-care services in acute-care facilities. Bylaws are similar to **policies** in that they describe general guidelines. Rules and **regulations**, like **procedures**, describe the specific activities to be performed to carry out the bylaws. The bylaws describe the structure of the medical staff and its membership qualifications, rights, and responsibilities. Rules and regulations are generally easier to amend and therefore should be used to communicate elements that are likely to change frequently. Medical staff rules and regulations establish the medical staff's specific responsibilities for patient care and **health record** documentation.

Medicare: An amendment in 1965 to the Social Security Act established two federal programs, Medicare and **Medicaid**, to provide health insurance coverage to the aged and poor populations. With the implementation of Medicare and Medicaid, these federal programs played a pivotal role in the U.S. government becoming the largest payer for healthcare services.

Medicare Prospective Payment System (PPS): Designed to promote efficiency and help prevent waste and abuse within the home health payment system. The Balanced Budget Act of 1997 (BBA) and the Omnibus Budget Reconciliation Act of 1986 (OBRA) mandated the implementation of a new prospective payment system for skilled-nursing facilities, **home healthcare** agencies, **outpatient** rehabilitation services, and other outpatient services provided to Medicare beneficiaries. The PPS became effective on October 1, 2000. It changed **Medicare** and **Medicaid home care reimbursement** from a cost-based system to a system of fixed-fee reimbursement based on a patient-need classification system. The BBA bundled all services covered and paid for on a reasonable cost basis under the Medicare home health benefit, including medical supplies, into the prospective payment. Medicare home care benefit drives documentation requirements for patient care, home health **certification**, CMS form 485, Medicare home care surveys, and the prospective payment system. The prospective payment system did not change the plan of care. It remains the beneficiary's physician's responsibility to develop a plan of care based on his or her intimate knowledge of the medical condition of the **home health** patient. The plan of care developed in consultation with the agency staff covers all pertinent diagnoses, mental status, types of services and equipment required, frequency of visits, prognosis, rehabilitation potential, functional limitations, activities permitted, nutritional requirements, medications and treatments, safety measures to protect against injury, instructions for timely discharge or referral, and any other appropriate items.

Medicare-certified: Medicare/Medicaid certification programs are conducted by state **licensure** agencies working under contract with the **Centers for Medicare and Medicaid Services**

(CMS). Organizations that have been accredited by the **Joint Commission** or the **American Osteopathic Association (AOA)** are automatically granted **deemed status** by the Medicare program. Hospitals must undergo a Medicare certification survey annually if they do not qualify for deemed status. Such facilities may have chosen not to participate in one of the **accreditation** programs, or they may have lost their accreditation temporarily because of compliance deficiencies. The Joint Commission and other **accreditation organizations** work with the CMS in an attempt to coordinate their accreditation **standards** with the **Medicare *Conditions of Participation***. However, some inconsistencies still exist. Regardless of an organization's Medicare certification status, a **care plan** conforms to the physician's plan-of-care orders. The care plan is based on the nursing initial assessment, as well as the initial assessments of other disciplines involved in the care of the patient. An interdisciplinary care plan is recommended, but separate discipline care plans may be documented when they are filed together in the **health record**.

Medication administration records (MARs): Tools used to capture the delivery of each drug to the resident of a long-term care facility. The MAR identifies medications a resident is scheduled to take, how often they should be administered, and at what dose they are to be administered. Due to the extended length of stay in an LTCH setting and multiple medications that the patient is prescribed, medication administration records may be voluminous.

Medication list: An ongoing record of the medications a patient has received in the past and is taking currently. This list is required by the **Joint Commission**, the Accreditation Association for Ambulatory Health care (AAAHC), and the **National Committee for Quality Assurance (NCQA)**. Key **data** elements include names of medications, dosages and amounts dispensed, dispensing instructions (with signature), prescription dates and discontinued dates, and problem numbers for which each medication was prescribed.

Medication record: Record that indicates the date and time a drug is administered, the name of the medication, the form of administration, and the medication's dosage and strength. The entry for each medication in the record is signed or initialed and dated by the person who administered the drug. The medication record includes all of the medications administered to a patient while the patient is in the nursing unit. The surgery department and ancillary departments that perform diagnostic and therapeutic **procedures** also maintain records of the medications administered to patients under their care. Surgical patients and others who experience severe levels of pain are sometimes treated with patient-controlled analgesics such as morphine. The medications are administered through a pump that delivers continuous doses controlled manually by the patient. Monitoring equipment automatically records the patient's respiration rate, level of sedation, and pain level as well as pump volume, dose received, and cumulative dosage since the beginning of the monitoring period. New requirements from the **Joint Commission** focus on medication reconciliation within the medical record. Medications must be reconciled on admission to include name of medication, route, and dosage. Medication reconciliation must include any over-the-counter medications the patient may be taking in addition to those medications prescribed by a physician. In addition, medications must be reconciled upon moving from one level of care to another, such as from ICU to a step down unit and on discharge.

Mental Health America (MHA): A nonprofit organization created to assist the more than 54 million Americans with mental disorders. Through its public advocacy, education, and **research** programs, MHA hopes to elevate public knowledge of mental health issues, encourage reform, and promote the effective use of qualified prevention and recovery programs. The Mental Health America (MHA) was formerly called the National Mental Health Association.

Messaging standards: Established messaging **standards**, also called interoperability standards or **data exchange standards**, which ensure that all of the organization's data are structured and formatted in the same way.

Minimum Data Set (MDS 3.0): A resident assessment instrument required by **long-term care** facilities that are certified to participate in the **Medicare** and **Medicaid** programs. The MDS is the first component of the **Resident Assessment Instrument (RAI)**. It is used to gather **information** about specific health status factors and include information about specific risk factors in the resident's care. This comprehensive MDS is used to plan the ongoing care and treatment of the resident in the long-term care facility. It must be printed and placed in the resident's paper record and also sent electronically to the state for reporting. The three components of the RAI are the MDS, the **Resident Assessment Protocols (RAPs)**, and the utilization guidelines, which provide a comprehensive tool for the assessment of each resident.

Multispecialty group practice: Practice that includes providers who represent a variety of **medical specialties**. Physician offices are the most common site for the delivery of **ambulatory care**. Physicians of many specialties deliver ambulatory care. These physicians include **specialists** in family medicine, internal medicine, obstetrics, gynecology, cardiology, gastroenterology, ophthalmology, and dermatology.

National Alliance for Health Information Technology (NAHIT): Organization that has compiled a comprehensive list of current health-related **standards** in its Alliance Standards Directory. Available online from www.hitsdir.org, the directory overviews the extent of the many standards used in the healthcare industry.

National Association for Home Care & Hospice (NAHC): Organization that represents the interests of **home health** care, hospice, and **home care** aid organizations.

National Center for Health Statistics (NCHS): Center that compiles statistical information to guide actions and **policies** to improve health. NCHS uses health statistics to document the population's and subgroups' health status, identify differences in health status and use of healthcare by demographics (such as race/ethnicity, socioeconomic status, or region), describe NCHS's experiences with the healthcare system, monitor health status and delivery trends, identify health problems, support medical and HIM **research**, suggest changes in public policies and programs, and evaluate the impact of health policies and programs.

National Committee for Quality Assurance (NCQA): An organization that provides **behavioral healthcare** services. The National Council for Community Behavioral Healthcare lists the following principles for recording information regarding their consumers. Documentation from mental health and mental retardation (MHMR) centers should reflect the consumer's strengths, competencies, problems and needs; reflect the recognition of family strengths and individuality of family caregivers and others in the consumer's support network; use respectful and nonjudgmental language regarding consumers and their support network; and be treated as a mechanism for enhancing communication.

National Committee on Vital and Health Statistics (NCVHS): Group that provides help in connecting the interests of the U.S. government, the health industry, and **research** and **public health** entities as well as connecting to those working on health information policy in other countries. The mission of the NCVHS, which was formed in 1949, is to advise the federal government on the information needs underlying health policy. It designs and coordinates improvements in national and international vital and health statistics.

National Council for Community Behavioral Healthcare (NCCBH): An organization of **behavioral healthcare** providers.

National Council for Prescription Drug Programs (NCPDP) Script: Program that specifies SCRIPT **standards** for the electronic transmission of prescription drug information between providers and pharmacies. **Medicare** has mandated e-prescribing for Medicare plans to reduce prescription errors due to illegible handwriting. The NCPDP is the official standard for HIPAA pharmacy claims.

National Guideline Clearinghouse (NGC): A comprehensive **database** of evidence-based **clinical practice guidelines** and related documents. The NGC is an initiative of the **Agency for Healthcare Research and Quality (AHRQ)**. Its purpose is to provide physicians, nurses, and other healthcare professionals; healthcare facilities and networks; health insurance plans; and healthcare consumers with an accessible source for objective, authoritative, and detailed information on effective clinical practices. The NGC's mission also includes facilitating the dissemination, implementation, and use of clinical guidelines in the United States.

National health information infrastructure (NHII): A concept advanced when the **National Committee on Vital and Health Statistics (NCVHS)** began exploring a national health information infrastructure (NHII) in 1997. The framework of an NHII would support the appropriate and secure exchange of health information.

National Health Information Network (NHIN): The primary objectives of the NHIN are to interconnect networks of clinicians, make information portable, and move consumers from one healthcare provider to another. This requires an interoperable infrastructure that allows clinicians access to critical healthcare information to make clinical or treatment decisions. The NHIN has developed and released prototype architecture that contains functional requirements, security, and business models for information exchange. State and regional health information networks will compose the NHIN.

An executive order in spring 2004 created the **Office of the National Coordinator for Health Information Technology (ONC)** within the **Department of Health and Human Services (HHS)**. One of the coordinator's initial duties was to oversee development of an NHII. Within 90 days of its creation, ONC released "The Decade of Health Information Technology," which became better known as the "Strategic Framework." Soon after this, NHII disappeared as ONC referenced the National Health Information Network (NHIN). The following year, the title was tweaked, switching from *national* to *nationwide,* reflecting an integration of locally managed networks rather than a single, national **database**. Today, much of the activity in health information technology concerning the private sector comes from within the HHS.

National Practitioner Data Bank (NPDB): One of two federal **databases**. The NPDB collects information on medical malpractice settlements, clinical privilege actions, and medical society actions taken against licensed healthcare providers in the United States. As part of every medical staff appointment process, hospitals and other healthcare organizations are required by federal law to send inquiries to the National Practitioner Data Bank (NPDB) and the **Healthcare Integrity and Protection Data Bank (HIPDB)**.

National Resource Center for Health Information Technology: A resource of the **Agency for Healthcare Research and Quality (AHRQ)** within the **Department of Health and Human Services (HHS)**, it provides technical assistance on health information projects to information technology stakeholders.

National Vital Statistics System (NVSS): A federal agency that operates within the **Centers for Disease Control and Prevention (CDC)**. In the United States, official **vital statistics** are maintained under the National Vital Statistics System (NVSS).

Nationwide network for health data exchange: A vision that began more than a decade ago with the Institute of Medicine's report, *The Computer-Based Patient Record*. In that study, the institute recommended a major, coordinated national effort, with federal funding and strong private-sector advisory support, to accelerate the adoption of computerized medical records. In the years that have followed, consensus has emerged that the nation's medical system must replace its outdated and frequently error-plagued, paper-based approach to information management. Because moving patient **data** from paper to electronic methods dramatically increases its potential mobility, discussion has turned to ways that data can be organized and shared to improve care and decrease cost. The current surge in activity began with President Bush's January 2004 State of the Union Address, which contained a mention of the benefits of computerized **health records**. In spring 2004, the **Office of the National Coordinator for Health Information Technology (ONC)** was created within the **Department of Health and Human Services (HHS)**. One of the coordinator's initial duties was to oversee development of nationwide network for health data exchange. Today, much of the activity in health information technology concerning the private sector comes from within the HHS. The **Agency for Healthcare Research and Quality (AHRQ)** provides funding and information for health information technology projects, including grants to state and regional **health information exchange (HIE)** initiatives. The **National Resource Center for Health Information Technology** provides technical assistance. The HHS plays an active role promoting industry discussion, **research**, and demonstrations. The universal adoption of an electronic health records system may still be years off, but the change is inevitable.

Neurology reports: Evaluation of neurological status of patients being treated for different types of illnesses to help distinguish neurological impairment from other illnesses.

Notice of privacy practices: Notice that describes how the patient's health **information** will be used and provides examples of those uses in hospital treatment and operations as well as **reimbursement**. Since the implementation of the **Health Insurance Portability and Accountability Act (HIPAA)**, hospitals and other healthcare organizations have been required to provide information to patients about the facilities' use of confidential health information. The explanation must be provided in the form of a notice of privacy practices.

Notifiable diseases: Communicable illnesses that must be reported to the **Centers for Disease Control and Prevention (CDC)**. National **data** on these diseases are reported weekly. Case-specific **information** is included in the CDC's reports. The CDC investigates cases where the cause of an illness or the source of an epidemic cannot be determined at the local level.

Nursing assessment: Documentation of the level of nursing assistance and personal care needed by the patient. An initial nursing assessment is always performed to obtain clinical and personal **information** about the patient shortly after he or she has been admitted to the nursing unit. State, **Joint Commission**, and federal guidelines now require nursing assessments within 24 hours. At a minimum, the initial nursing assessment summarizes the date, time, and method of admission as well as the patient's current condition, symptoms (including level of pain), and vital signs. Most hospitals develop and use a nursing assessment instrument to collect additional information about the patient's physical condition and psychosocial status at admission. Information in the nursing assessment can include patient's reason for being in the hospital; patient's current and past illnesses; patient's current medical condition, including the condition of his or her skin and the level of pain; patient's current cognitive status, including his or her ability to communicate and to understand and follow instructions; patient's current functional status, including his or her level of physical activity and ability to walk, move, and perform personal care; patient's current psychosocial status, including his or her marital status, living arrangements, personal habits (such as smoking, alcohol consumption, and use of illegal drugs), and occupation; patient's family history, including information about his or her parents, children, and siblings and their current health status or cause of death; patient's current nutritional status, including his or her ability to feed himself or herself and any special dietary requirements or food allergies; patient's known drug allergies, including any sensitivity to latex products; patient's current medications; and patient's need for special discharge planning.

Nursing facility: A comprehensive term for long-term care facilities that provide nursing care and related services on a 24-hour basis for residents requiring medical, nursing, or rehabilitative care.

Nutritional assessment: Assessment of the patient's diet history, weight and height, appetite and food preferences, and **information** on food sensitivities and allergies. A nutritional assessment is performed by a registered dietitian.

Office of the National Coordinator for Health Information Technology (ONC): Entity created within the **Department of Health and Human Services (HHS)** in spring 2004. One of the coordinator's initial duties was to oversee development of **nationwide network for health data exchange**. Today, much of the activity in health information technology concerning the private sector comes from within the HHS. The **Agency for Healthcare Research and Quality (AHRQ)** provides funding and information for health information technology projects, including grants to state and regional **health information exchange (HIE)** initiatives. The **National Resource Center for Health Information Technology** provides technical assistance. The HHS plays an active role promoting industry discussion, **research**, and demonstrations. The universal adoption of an electronic **health records** system may still be years off, but the change is inevitable.

Omnibus Budget Reconciliation Act of 1987 (OBRA): Federal **statute** that mandated the implementation of a **prospective payment system (PPS)** for skilled-nursing facilities, **home health** agencies, **outpatient** rehabilitation services, and other outpatient services provided to **Medicare** beneficiaries. OBRA focuses on the health and safety of patients and emphasizes **patient's rights** and the competency of home health aides. It requires organizations receiving Medicare and **Medicaid** funds to inform patients of their rights under state law to make advance decisions concerning medical care by activating **advance directives**. Additionally, in mental illness/mental retardation (MI/MR) care settings, OBRA requires that the Preadmission Screening Assessment and Annual Resident Review (PASARR) be completed preadmission and annually.

Ongoing record review: Process that assists organizations in meeting **accreditation** and regulatory requirements so that identified documentation issues are timely addressed. Utilizing clinical staff for ongoing record review at the point of care may be used as a means to educate staff on regulatory documentation requirements and improves the overall quality of **health record** documentation. Oftentimes, organizations develop health record review **policies** to define the scope of reviews and to analyze the collection and reporting of **data** for use within the organization.

Operation index: The retrieval of patient **information** by surgical procedure. An operative index is arranged by diagnostic or procedure codes that facilitate the study of patients with the same or similar conditions or treatment. This sorting guides the locating of **health records** to conduct quality improvement and **research** studies, as well as for monitoring quality of care. The **index** is also useful for retrieving records for research studies. To be useful for use in an operative index, the health record should provide the following information: **principal diagnosis** and relevant secondary diagnoses with codes; associated **procedures** and codes; patient's health record number; patient's gender, age, and race; attending physician's code or name; service rendered to the patient; the disposition following service; and dates of encounter.

Operative report: A formal document prepared by the principal surgeon to describe the surgical procedure(s) performed for the patient. Each report includes the following **information**: patient identification, including name and record number; patient's preoperative and postoperative diagnoses and indications for surgery; descriptions of the **procedures** performed; descriptions of all normal and abnormal findings; descriptions of any specimens removed; descriptions of the patient's medical condition before, during, and after the operation; estimated blood loss; descriptions of any unique or unusual events that occurred during the course of the surgery; names of the surgeons and their assistants; date and duration of the surgery; and signature of principal physician, credentials, and date the report was written.

ORYX®: Data sets provided by the **Joint Commission** that function as benchmarks of **performance improvement (PI)** within and among organizations. The initial phase of the ORYX initiative offers accredited healthcare organizations significant flexibility by allowing them to select the **performance measurement** system and individual measures that best serve their strategic measurement goals. ORYX initiatives are designed so that expectations should increase over time. The next phase of the ORYX initiative includes the identification of specific core performance measures and the opportunity for listed systems to embed some, or all, of these measures in their own systems. **Core measures** are grouped into measure sets. In time, measure sets may include clinical performance, client perception of care, health status, and administrative or financial measures. The initial core measures focus primarily on clinical performance. The identification and use of core measures allow comparisons of processes and **outcomes** of patient care among healthcare organizations across the country, regardless of which performance measurement system the organization is using. The Joint Commission is gradually transitioning core measure sets into ORYX requirements. In the future, the Joint Commission intends to create a balanced set of measures applicable to all types of healthcare organizations.

Outcome and Assessment Information Set (OASIS): A group of **data** elements that represents core items in a **comprehensive assessment** for an adult **home care** patient. The data elements form the basis of patient outcome measurements used for outcome-based quality improvement. In 1993, the National Association for Home Care's board of directors charged the information resources and quality assurance committee with the task of developing standardized definitions for home care and hospice data elements through a consensus conference process. The board recognized that a uniform minimum data set was a necessary first step toward achieving standardized, comparable home care and hospice data. The consensus conference was held in December 1993. In 1997, the information resources and quality assurance committee added the Outcome and Assessment Information Set (OASIS) to the uniform minimum **data sets** (UDS). For patients to whom OASIS applies, **Medicare** CoP 484.55 requires that the comprehensive assessment must be completed in a timely manner, consistent with the patient's immediate needs, but no later than five calendar days after the start of care. Every month, agencies must electronically report all OASIS data collected on all applicable patients in a format that meets CMS electronic data and editing specifications. OASIS data on non-Medicare and non-Medicaid patients receiving skilled services must be reported once the masking requirement is effective. Medicare CoP 484.20 requires OASIS data collection by a qualified clinician as part of the comprehensive assessment at start of care, resumption of care, follow-up, transfer to **inpatient facility** with or without discharge, significant change in clinical condition, discharge to community, and death at home. Encoding of OASIS data items must be complete and locked in order to accurately compute the information (health insurance prospective payment system [HIPPS] code) necessary for billing Medicare patients under the **prospective payment system**.

Outcomes: A change (lack of change) in a patient's condition during an episode of care. **Medicare** divides outcomes into the two groups: **risk-adjusted outcomes** and **descriptive outcomes.**

Outcomes assessment: An effective tool used to monitor the success of a plan from beginning to end. In behavioral health, it is a way to determine if care and services were prescribed appropriately and provided to assist the client in achieving the expected or desired outcome.

Outpatient: An individual who receives healthcare services in a hospital-based clinic or department but who is not admitted to a dedicated acute-care unit. For example, a patient treated exclusively in the emergency department of a hospital is considered an outpatient rather than an **inpatient**. However, if that same patient is admitted to an acute-care unit of the hospital after receiving emergency services, the patient is then considered an inpatient for the rest of his or her hospital stay.

Outpatient facilities: Services to provide clients with access to a stable treatment provider on an **outpatient** basis. Such care may occur in a formal office setting or in the comfort of the individual's home or residence. In some circumstances, outpatient services are provided in homeless shelters in an effort to reach the estimated hundreds of thousands of homeless individuals in America who suffer from mental illness.

Outstanding record policy: Policy that details the time frame in which a medical record can be kept in the clinic or physician's office. The recommended time is no longer than 48 hours.

Partial stay: A program that provides individuals with mental health treatment that is more intense than the services provided on an **outpatient** basis. Partial stay treatment is sometimes referred to as **day treatment**. Most payers (including **Medicare**) cover this service when it is determined medically appropriate by the physician.

Pathology report: A microscopic and macroscopic (or gross) evaluation of a specimen, which is fully described in a report. Pathology examinations must be performed on every specimen or foreign object removed or expelled from a patient during a surgical procedure. Some hospitals have established medical staff rules that exempt some types of specimens from microscopic examination. Examples of such specimens include normal placentas, tonsils, and foreign bodies such as bullets.

Patient assessment instrument (PAI): Standardized assessment tool used by **inpatient** rehabilitation hospitals and rehabilitation units within acute-care hospitals that are subject to a **Medicare prospective payment system** based on documentation. The PAI must be completed shortly after the patient's admission and upon discharge. Payment level is based on the patient's medical condition and diagnostic profile as well as the services provided.

Patient outcome measures: Calculation based on a completed "episode of care," which begins with admission to a **home health agency** (or a resumption of care following an **inpatient**

facility stay) and ends with discharge or transfer to an inpatient facility. This is different than a Home Health Prospective Payment episode of 60 days.

Patient Self-Determination Act (1990): A federal **statute** that requires **home care** and hospice organizations receiving **Medicare** and **Medicaid** funds to inform patients of their rights under state law to make advance decisions concerning medical care by activating **advance directives**.

Patient's rights: The patient's healthcare rights include the right to know who is providing treatment, the right to **confidentiality**, the right to receive information about treatment, the right to refuse treatment, the right to participate in care planning, and the right to be safe from abusive treatment. Some hospitals ask patients to sign an acknowledgment that they have received patient's rights information. The signed acknowledgment then becomes a permanent part of the patient's record. State **regulations** often require similar explanations and stipulate additional patient's rights, such as the right to **privacy** in treatment. The **Medicare** *Conditions of Participation* documents requirements for patient's rights for all environments of care.

Patient-specific/identifiable data: Data categorized as primary data. Data are categorized as either **primary** or **aggregate data**. The **health record** consists entirely of primary or patient-specific/identifiable data. Aggregate data (also referred to as **secondary data**) includes compiled information on groups of people or patients without identifying any particular patient individually.

Performance improvement (PI): Quality assurance efforts. Present-day performance improvement (PI) efforts emphasize the importance of identifying the shortcomings of processes and systems rather than individuals. Healthcare organizations use a number of different PI models, and the models tend to go in and out of fashion rather quickly. Regardless of the chosen model, PI processes driven by patient-care information are the most effective. Currently, most healthcare organizations utilize some form of **continuous quality improvement (CQI)**. The CQI philosophy emphasizes the critical importance of three factors: knowing and meeting customer expectations, reducing variation within processes, and relying on **data** to build knowledge for process improvement. CQI entails a continuous cycle of planning, measuring, and monitoring performance and making periodic knowledge-based improvements. Quality managers use a number of tools to monitor performance and identify areas for improvement. Many hospitals use a model known as FOCUS-PDCA®: **F**ind a clinical process to improve; **O**rganize a team made up of people who understand the process; **C**larify the team's current knowledge of the process; **U**nderstand the causes of the undesired variation; **S**elect the improvement to be made in the process.

Performance measurement: Considered to be at the heart of all **performance improvement (PI)** activities. Through evaluation of measurement **data**, healthcare organizations address the need for improved processes. **Joint Commission** requires certain measurements to be conducted systematically for the following factors: processes and **outcomes**, performance of processes pertaining to the functions addressed in the **accreditation** manual, and quality control activities in at least the following areas, where applicable: clinical laboratory services, equipment provided to patients, equipment used in providing care, and pharmacy equipment and preparations.

Periodic Performance Review (PPR): A key component in the continuous **accreditation** process. The PPR helps hospitals incorporate **Joint Commission standards** as part of routine operations and ongoing quality-improvement efforts. Hospitals have access to the PPR tool continuously throughout the accreditation cycle. Hospitals evaluate compliance with applicable standards, elements of performance, National Patient Safety Goals and Accreditation Participation Requirements. Organizations are required to submit an update to its PPR annually to the Joint Commission. However, hospitals may select different options for compliance. The annual due dates for the PPR update is at one-year intervals after the hospital's last full survey.

Personal health information (PHI): Disclosure of personal health information is governed by federal and state laws. Some states permit minors to admit themselves into mental health treatment facilities without parental consent; they also permit minors to authorize disclosure of personal health information (PHI). Likewise, according to 42 CFR 2, Subpart B, 2.14, if state law permits minors to seek admission for services in a substance-abuse program without parental consent, unless the minor lacks the capacity to make rational choice, only the minor can authorize disclosure of his or her PHI, including the disclosure of information to parents. The federal law governing the **confidentiality** of alcohol and drug abuse clients requires that client authorization be obtained before disclosing PHI to any other entity that is not specifically permitted by these **regulations**. Federal regulations covering the confidentiality of PHI on alcohol and drug abuse patients apply to recipients of the information. Recipients are prohibited from redisclosing information they have received under authorization (42 CFR 2, §2.12[d]). This is in contrast to the Privacy Rule, which requires the CE to inform patients that their information is no longer protected after it has been disclosed. Because it is more protective, 42 CFR 2 supersedes the Privacy Rule.

Personal health record (PHR): An electronic, universally available, lifelong resource of health **information** needed by individuals to make health decisions. Individuals own and manage the information in the PHR, which comes from healthcare providers and the individual. The PHR is maintained in a secure and private environment, with the individual determining rights of access. The PHR is separate from and does not replace the legal record of any provider.

Physician acknowledgment statement: Notification to physicians that **Medicare** payment to the facility is partly based on the patient's principal and secondary diagnoses, as well as the major **procedures** performed, and that falsification of records can lead to fines, imprisonment, or civil penalty under federal laws.

Physician certification: Certification required by **Medicare** upon patient's admission to **skilled-nursing facility (SNF)**, or as soon as possible thereafter. Staff and attending physicians must periodically certify the need for **long-term care** services within an SNF. The first recertification is required no later than the fourteenth day of the patient's stay, and additional recertifications are required every 30 days.

Physician index: Index that categorizes patients by physician. It guides the retrieval of cases treated by a particular physician. Creating the **index** simply involves sorting patients by physician. Facilities can designate which physician(s) are recorded as the **data** element. Information required in a physician index include physician's name or code, **health record** number, diagnosis, operations, and disposition of the patients the physician treated, the dates of admission and discharge, patient's gender and age, and other demographic information deemed useful by the facility. For example, with a physician's index in place, a facility can retrieve all of Dr. Anderson's patients with melanoma and compare their treatment with Dr. Bradford's patients with the same diagnosis.

Physician query form: Form used to help clarify principal and secondary diagnoses. A physician query form clarifies conflicting, ambiguous, or incomplete information about significant conditions or **procedures** in the **health record**. Use should be kept to a minimum in any healthcare setting. It should be guided by AHIMA's **Standards** of Ethical Coding and official guidelines. Medical staff in conjunction with coding professionals should develop the specific clinical criteria for a valid query.

Physician query process: Response to problems that were revealed as prospective payment systems (PPS) have become the rule (rather than the exception) for **reimbursement**. Lack of a uniform language or guidelines for **health record** documentation have made it necessary to create the **physician query form** to satisfy health record documentation requirements. The physician query form provides a means of addressing requests for additional information from physicians as part of the coding and reimbursement process. It is a communication tool and an educational mechanism that provides a clearer picture of specific diagnoses when in question. Coders can use notes and one-on-one training to teach the clinical team to use terms that are acceptable and recognizable to payers, thus leading to codes that enhance reimbursement.

Physician's orders: The instructions that the physician gives to the other healthcare professionals who perform diagnostic and therapeutic **procedures**, provide nursing care, formulate and administer medications, and provide nutritional services to the patient.

Picture archiving and communications systems (PACS): System used to store portions of the **electronic health record (EHR)** such as x-rays, fetal trace archives and digitally produce scanned images. Picture archiving and communications systems (PACs) provide pointers from the clinical portal (EHR) to the various repositories (such as labs, cardiology information systems, results reporting systems, computerized provider order entry systems, nurse care-planning systems, word-processing systems) for quick access to patient information that cannot be electronically stored in the EHR.

Plans of care: May also be referred to as **physician's orders**. The plan of care or *impression* should discuss what specific treatments and services will be provided for the patient's care. **Clinical pathways** are an example of structured plans of care that help organizations implement clinical guidelines and **protocols**. Sometimes known as critical paths, care paths, and/ or care maps, they are widely used by institutions hoping to reduce costs and improve quality through decreased variation in practices. In **home health** services, the term plans of care refers to the **Medicare** requirements that are documented on CMS form 485. Although the form is no longer required, the information contained within the form is required. Agencies may choose to use form 485 to meet the required documentation.

Policies: General written guidelines that dictate behavior or direct and constrain decision making within the organization.

Population-based registry: Chronological listing of patients with a common characteristic. **Registries** are different from **indexes** because they contain information that is more extensive. These reports are typically generated from existing **databases**. Registries are also used for patient follow-up as well as aggregate studies. Registry maintenance consists of the following activities: case definition (describing the patients that are to be included), case finding (identifying patients that are to be included), and case abstracting (extracting the information to be included from **health records**). Databases reveal patterns that may be used for **research** and improvement in customer care. Examples of population-based registries include The International Implant Registry and the cancer registry.

Population-based statistics: Estimates of the **incidence** of a disease as a percentage of the total population that could have been affected. For example, the crude birth rate for a community can be calculated by dividing the number of live births in the community during a specified time period by the estimated population of that community during the same time.

Postoperative anesthesia record: Information on any unusual events or **complications** that occurred during surgery. The postoperative anesthesia record also documents the patient's condition at the conclusion of surgery and after recovery from anesthesia.

Preoperative anesthesia evaluation: An evaluation that addresses the patient's risk factors, allergies, and drug usage; considers the patient's general medical condition; stipulates the type of anesthesia to be used; and becomes the basis for an anesthesia plan. Preoperative anesthesia evaluations are performed by anesthesiologists (who are physicians) and certified nurse-anesthetists.

Prevalence: Health record documentation is required for developing the **databases** used by **public health** departments to provide information on the **incidence** and **prevalence** of diseases, possible high-risk populations, survival statistics, and trends over time. Data elements for the databases may be collected using a variety of methods, including interviews, physical examinations of individuals, and review of health records. The HIM manager may have input in these databases through information provided from health records.

Primary care: The most appropriate setting for routine healthcare services falls at the **primary-care** level. Physicians working in private offices, group practices, private clinics, or community-based clinics generally provide primary-care services.

Primary data source: The **health record** is considered a primary **data** source because it contains patient-specific data and information about a patient that has been documented by the professionals who provided care or services to that patient. Data taken from the health record and entered into registries and **databases** are considered a **secondary data source**.

Principal diagnosis: The actual reason for a patient's admission to the healthcare facility. The principal diagnosis is established after study and evaluation of the medical **data**.

Principal procedure: The procedure that is performed for the definitive treatment (rather than the diagnosis) of the main condition or a **complication** of a patient's condition.

Priority focus areas (PFAs): Processes, systems, and structures that have the most substantial effect on patient-care services. The **Joint Commission** designates priority focus areas in its **accreditation** process. Information management is one of fourteen PFAs vital to successful operation in hospitals.

Priority focus process (PFP): The **Joint Commission** focuses survey activities on the organization-specific issues that are most relevant to safety and quality of care. Internal and external **data** about the organization are integrated to identify clinical service groups and priority focus areas for each hospital. The Joint Commission provides the hospital information about its top clinical service groups and priority focus areas on its secure extranet site.

Privacy: Information that is protected by federal and state laws and **regulations**. The HIPAA privacy standard is widely applicable. It has established a consistent set of rules that apply to virtually every healthcare facility, healthcare professional, healthcare information clearinghouse, and health plan in the United States. The standard supersedes state regulations that permitted less stringent privacy practices. Although the federal privacy standard has preempted some state **health record** regulations, many state regulations are still relevant. The federal regulations constitute a minimum standard for protecting confidential records. When state regulations require stricter privacy practices, hospitals and other healthcare organizations must continue to follow state regulations in addition to the federal privacy standard. Healthcare organizations must continue to comply with **public health** reporting regulations and **licensure/certification** requirements in their geopolitical area.

Privileged communication: A legal concept. Many states base the **confidentiality** rights of patients on the concept of privileged communication. According to this concept, medical practitioners, like lawyers and other professionals, are not allowed to disclose the confidential information that they learn in their capacity as professional service providers. There are very few exceptions to this basic rule for medical practitioners.

Problem list: List that captures relevant past and current problems of the patient. It provides a mechanism to organize each of the patient's medical or physical issues. The problems are listed numerically, with the date each problem was identified and the date the problem was resolved. In some healthcare facilities, it may be nursing driven or physician driven. The list is patient specific and includes the patient and problems. It may also contain the attending physician, **principal diagnosis**, allergies and adverse drug reactions, and symptoms of allergic/drug reactions. Not all facilities utilize problem lists.

Problem-oriented health record: The key characteristic of this format is that it is arranged according to a **problem list.** A problem list is an itemized description of the patient's past and present social, psychological, and medical problems. Each problem is **indexed** with a unique number, and reports and clinical documentation are keyed to the numbers representing the problems they address. The documentation is arranged in chronological or reverse chronological order. In addition to the problem list, the problem-oriented **health record** contains a prescribed set of patient **data**, an initial **care plan**, and **progress notes**. The content of the problem-oriented health record is basically the same as the content of the **source-oriented health record**. Content includes chief complaint, present illness(es), social history, medical **history**, physical examination, and diagnostic test results.

Problem/Summary list: A valuable tool in patient care management. It should always be visible and easy to read. A single page summarizes all of the major medical and surgical problems that have long-term clinical significance for the patient, including social and psychiatric problems. The dates of onset and resolution are recorded for each problem. The healthcare provider can use the **problem list** to determine at a glance which problems are active or resolved and can adjust treatment plans accordingly. As a communication tool, the problem list helps specialty physicians make evaluation and treatment decisions about the patients referred to them for care; having this information often eliminates the need to duplicate costly tests. Each provider documents his or her care of the patient on the same list, thereby creating a comprehensive overview of the patient's medical status. For consistency and clarity, facilities should develop guidelines for recording several key elements in the problem list, including problems, dates of onset, active versus inactive status, and resolution dates.

Procedural codes: Specific diagnoses and clinical **procedures** identified on claims and encounter forms. The International Classification of Diseases, Ninth Revision, Clinical Modification (ICD-9-CM), Current Procedural Terminology, Fourth Edition (CPT®-4), and Healthcare Common Procedure Coding System (HCPCS) are examples of code sets for **procedures** and diagnoses. **Diagnostic codes** must comply with HIPAA format and content. Standardized transactions include items such as claims information, encounter information, payment, remittance advice, claim status inquiry and response, and eligibility inquiry and response.

Procedures: Detailed written instructions on how functions and processes are implemented. Procedures should explicitly fulfill the stipulations of general **policies**.

Professional certification organizations: Private societies and membership organizations that establish professional qualification requirements and clinical practice **standards** for specific areas of medicine, nursing, and allied health professions.

Progress notes: Records of clinical observations. Progress notes must contain recommendations for revisions in the treatment plan as indicated as well as precise assessment of the patient's progress in accordance with the original or revised treatment plan.

Prohibited abbreviations: Abbreviations that have more than one meaning or can easily be misinterpreted in handwritten form, with potentially dangerous results for patients. The **Joint Commission** now requires hospitals to prohibit the use of the following abbreviations in all handwritten, patient-specific documentation: **U** (for unit), **IU** or **iu**, **-QD** or **qd**, **QOD** or **qod**,**.0** (zero after a decimal point), **0.** (zero before a decimal point), and **MS, MSO4, MgSO4**.

Prospective payment system (PPS): System of payment for **Medicare**-reimbursed healthcare providers. Providers must meet all of the requirements set by Medicare for **reimbursement** of services, and they must encode and transmit **OASIS data** items to accurately compute the information (Health Insurance Prospective Payment System [HIPPS] code set) necessary for billing under the prospective payment system.

Protected health information: As defined by the HIPAA **Privacy** Act of 1996, Title 45 of the *Code of Federal Regulations*, Part 160 and Subparts A and E of Part 164, protected health information is "individually identifiable health information, held or maintained by a covered entity or its business associates acting for the covered entity, that is transmitted or maintained in any form or medium (including the individually identifiable health information of non-U.S. citizens). This includes identifiable demographic and other information relating to the past, present, or future physical or mental health or condition of an individual, or the provision or payment of health care to an individual that is created or received by a health care provider, health plan, employer, or health care clearinghouse. For purposes of the Privacy Rule, genetic information is considered to be health information." The full text of the Privacy Rule is available from http://privacyruleandresearch.nih.gov/pr_02.asp.

Protocol: A list of rules and **procedures** to be followed.

Public health: Health of populations in geopolitical locations is the domain of public health. One of the duties of public health agencies is surveillance of the health status of the population within their jurisdictions.

Qualitative analysis: A review of the **health record** to ensure that **clinical protocols** are met and to determine the adequacy of entries documenting the quality of care. Qualitative **analysis** and **quantitative analysis** are the two activities that complete **health record analysis**. Many hospitals are applying a new quality review technique that combines quantitative and qualitative review.

Quality improvement organization (QIO): Groups that work under contract with the **Centers for Medicare and Medicaid Services (CMS)**. Their mission is to improve the effectiveness, efficiency, economy, and quality of services delivered to beneficiaries. QIO contracts set related targets at the state level based on a focused set of publicly reported quality measures. Healthcare organizations submit patient information collected from **health records** to the QIOs, which then review the appropriateness of delivered care. The QIO launched its 8th Statement of Work (SOW) in August 2005. The 8th SOW is a comprehensive document that describes the requirements for QIOs over a three-year cycle. Based on these requirements, the document describes the national quality improvement projects led by CMS. These deliverables and **data** submission requirements assist providers in developing the capacity for achieving excellence in healthcare. The statement of work has specific tasks for providers in settings such as nursing homes, **home health**, hospitals, critical-access hospital/rural PPS hospitals, and physicians' practices. In the physician practice setting, tasks are further defined to include underserved populations and pharmacies.

Quantitative analysis: A review of the **health record** to determine its completeness and accuracy. Quantitative **analysis** and **qualitative analysis** are the two activities that complete **health record analysis**. Many hospitals are applying a new quality review technique that combines quantitative and qualitative review.

Recovery room record: Documents the patient's reaction to anesthesia and condition after surgery. Information on the patient's level of consciousness, overall medical condition, vital signs, and medications and intravenous fluids is documented by nurses when the patient enters the recovery room. The same information is documented when the patient is ready to be transferred or discharged. The status of any surgical dressings, catheters, tubes, and drains is also recorded. The patient's surgical record should also include documentation that demonstrates that the patient met the facility's discharge criteria before being discharged or transferred. The name of the physician or surgeon who was responsible for the discharge must be included on the discharge order.

Redisclosure: The process of disclosing **health record** documentation originally created by a different provider. Federal and state **regulations** provide specific redisclosure guidelines; however, when in doubt, follow the same principles as the **release and disclosure** guidelines for other types of health record information.

Regional health information organizations (RHIOs): Health information exchange collaborations are known by many names, but the most common is regional health information organizations (RHIOs). Although the term, *RHIO,* has become standard language in healthcare, there is no legal definition in federal or state law. Roles that RHIOs play in the region or community vary broadly, and collaborations range from relatively simple to complex structures.

Regional Home Health Intermediary (RHHI): Auditors for the **Centers of Medicare and Medicaid Services (CMS)**. RHHI auditors assess Medicare claims and monitor services in Medicare-reimbursed healthcare facilities.

Registry: A chronological listing of patients with a common characteristic. Registries usually maintained by healthcare facilities are listed in chapter 4, figure 4.1. Creation and maintenance of these registries is often a responsibility of the HIM department. Registries are different from **indexes** because they contain information that is more extensive. These reports are typically generated from a facility's existing **database**. Registries are also used for patient follow-up as well as aggregate studies.

Regulation: A rule established by an administrative agency of government. The difference between a **statute** and a regulation is regulations must be followed by any healthcare organization participating in the related program. Administrative agencies are responsible for implementing and managing the programs instituted by state and federal statutes.

Rehabilitation care: The therapeutic medical services (speech, physical, and occupational therapy) provided to patients who have been disabled by injuries or illnesses; provided in dedicated rehabilitation hospitals, community-based facilities, patients' homes, and hospital-based **outpatient** departments with the goal of helping patients recover as much function as possible.

Reimbursement: Payment based on the documentation contained in the **health record**. By referring to the records of individual patients, coding specialists identify the patients' diagnoses as well as the therapeutic **procedures** they underwent and the services they received. Using this information, coding specialists assign appropriate **diagnostic** and **procedural codes**. The coded information is then used to generate a patient bill and/or a claim for reimbursement to a third-party payer, such as a commercial health insurance company or government-sponsored health program such as **Medicare**. Some **third-party payers** require billers to submit copies of portions of the health record along with the claims. The health record documentation substantiates the need for services and the fact that such services were provided.

Release and disclosure: A process that makes **health record** information available to legitimate users. **Release of information (ROI)** is another term used when disclosing patient information. These processes are subject to specific regulations in many states. Federal **regulations** and **accreditation standards** also include specific guidelines on the release and disclosure of patient-identified health information.

Release of information (ROI): A process that makes **health record** information available to legitimate users. **Release and disclosure** is another term used when disclosing patient information. These processes are subject to specific **regulations** in many states. Federal regulations and **accreditation standards** also include specific guidelines on the release of patient-identified health information.

Request for anticipated payment (RAP): Initial percentage payment requested by a **home health agency (HHA)**. Rather than submitting a **Medicare** claim for home health **prospective payment (PPS)** purposes, the first percentage payment under home health PPS does not require a physician-signed plan of care before submission. The RAP for the episode may be submitted based on verbal orders. To request anticipated payment for the initial percentage based on a physician's verbal orders, a copy of the plan of care with all the physician's verbal orders—in writing with the date of receipt by the registered nurse or qualified therapist responsible for furnishing or supervising the ordered services—must be completed and immediately sent to the physician for signature. The RAP may be submitted when the HHA has a signed referral prescribing the physician's detailed orders for services and the patient's condition. Signed orders must be obtained as soon as possible and before the claim for services is submitted for the final percentage payment of each episode. The claim for the final percentage payment requires a signed plan of care prior to billing. The RAP will be canceled and recovered unless the claim for the episode is submitted within 60 days from the end of the episode or the issuance of the anticipated payment. This split-percentage payment approach helps alleviate cash flow concerns but increases the need for timely signed orders.

Research: Scientific investigation of disease. **Data** contained in the **health record** are required for **research**, statistical reporting, cancer registries, and trauma registries to name a few **public**

health uses. Documentation needed for research ranges from identification of candidate health records for projects to actual review of selected records and abstract preparation or collection of data from them for the physician or clinical researcher.

Resident Assessment Instrument (RAI): A federally mandated resident assessment that must be done for every resident in a nursing home. During the RAI process, several assessments should be considered to support the **Minimum Data Set (MDS)** documentation and may include the following: physician **history** and physical exam, **nursing assessment**, wound and skin assessment, fall assessment, bowel and bladder assessment, pain assessment, basic mental/cognitive examination, restraint assessment (only if applicable), **nutritional assessment**, therapy assessments (as required), therapeutic recreation assessment, and pastoral care assessment.

Resident Assessment Protocols (RAPs): A federally mandated resident assessment that must be done for every resident in a nursing home. RAPs are administered in an effort to capture supporting documentation of the **Resident Assessment Instrument (RAI)**. RAPs include the principal components of a **long-term care** resident's **care plan**. They are used to further define the resident's care-planning needs and treatment. Moreover, they are used in conjunction with the MDS to ensure that the resident's assessment is comprehensive and the care-planning process is complete.

Residential facility: Often referred to as *group homes* or *foster homes*, these **facilities** are staffed by behavioral health professionals who provide supervision and training to the residents in an alternative to the **inpatient** setting. Clients of such facilities are often encouraged to achieve independence in daily functions with little assistance from the provider. The residence provides a somewhat stable environment that helps many individuals with mental illness to assimilate into the "real world."

Retention and destruction: Processes entailed in storing health information and destroying it when it is no longer needed. These processes are subject to specific **regulations** in many states. Federal regulations and **accreditation standards** also include specific guidelines on the retention and destruction of patient-identified health information.

RHHI Outcomes and Assessment Information Set Verification (ROVER) protocol: An automated accuracy software application used to assist in the medical review of **home health** claims submitted by home health agencies (HHAs) that are paid under the HHA **prospective payment system (PPS)**.

Risk management (RM): Prevention of situations that might put hospital patients, caregivers, or visitors in danger. Risk management includes investigating reported **incidents**, reviewing **liability** claims, and working with the hospital's legal counsel. Hospitals employ professional risk managers, who may manage the hospital's safety programs and disaster planning depending on size and complexity of the organization.

Risk-adjusted outcome: Rates that are adjusted to compensate for differences in the patient population served by different **home health** agencies, including differences between states. Risk-adjusted **outcomes** are one of two kinds of outcomes defined by **Medicare**. The second type of outcome is **descriptive outcome**.

RxNorm: Provision for standard names for clinical drugs and administered dose forms.

Secondary care: Encompasses the diagnostic and therapeutic services provided by medical **specialists** working in private offices, specialty group practices, private clinics, community-based clinics, and general and community hospitals. Patients may arrange to consult specialists directly. However, it is more common for primary-care physicians to refer patients to specialists for the diagnosis and treatment of complex conditions that require more intensive services than the primary-care physician can provide.

Secondary data: Data taken from **health records** and entered into registries and **databases**.

Secondary data source: Information that is not easily available by looking at individual **health records**. **Data** taken from health records and entered into disease-oriented **databases** can help researchers determine the effectiveness of alternate treatment methods. They can also quickly demonstrate survival rates at different stages of diseases. Types of **secondary data** sources are listed in chapter 4, table 4.6.

Security standards: Uniform methods for collecting, maintaining, and/or transferring healthcare **data** among computer information systems. Security standards are one of five categories of **health informatics standards**. The other categories include **vocabulary standards**, **structure and content standards**, **transaction and messaging standards**, and **identifier standards**. Work completed to develop and establish health informatics standards ensures the successful implementation of electronic **health record** systems. Many organizations are currently working on the development of health informatics standards. Compliance with such industry standards continues to be voluntary.

Sentinel event: An undesired variation in performance. This variation may be represented by a important single event, such as a blood transfusion reaction, or by a significant variation from either the **standards** or comparative performances of other organizations. Several terms are used to describe unforeseen events that lead to injuries and other losses, including *incidents, adverse events, potentially compensable events*, and *adverse occurrences*. The **Joint Commission** uses the term sentinel event to describe such events and requests that the most serious events be reported to the Joint Commission as well as to government agencies as required by federal or state law. The Joint Commission requires intensive assessment when any of the following sentinel events occur: confirmed transfusion reactions, significant adverse drug reactions, or significant errors related to medication use. When systematic **data** assessment reveals that an individual's performance presents an opportunity for improvement, the person responsible for patient services ensures that steps for assessing and improving competence are followed.

Shadow chart policy: Policy that requires that all original information and medical reports be kept in the medical record located in the health information management department. Physicians should be discouraged from keeping copies of records or reports in a shadow chart in their offices. Incorporating and reconciling shadow charts from a physician's practice places an economic burden on the healthcare facility and the HIM department.

Skilled-nursing care: The professional nursing care and related medical, therapeutic, psychosocial, and personal services provided in a residential setting to individuals recovering from injuries or illnesses or the residual effects of injuries or illnesses after the acute phase of the condition has resolved; sometimes called **subacute care.**

Skilled nursing facility (SNF): A long-term care facility with an organized professional staff and permanent facilities (including inpatient beds) that provides continuous nursing and other health-related, psychosocial, and personal services to patients who are not in an acute phase of illness but who primarily require continued care on an inpatient basis.

Source system data: Data from which interpretations, summaries, and notes are derived. Examples of source system data are radiological film or scans, laboratory values, pathology slides, video and/or audio recordings, and EKG tracings. They may be designated part of the **legal health record**, whether or not they are integrated into a single system or maintained as part of the source system.

Source-oriented health record: Documents that are grouped together according to their point of origin. That is, laboratory records are grouped together, radiology records are grouped together, clinical notes are grouped together, and so on. Thus, physicians' **progress notes** for a single episode of patient care are arranged, usually in reverse chronological order, and filed together in the patient's **health record**. Similarly, notes prepared by nursing services, social services, and other clinical services are grouped according to service and arranged sequentially. Under this format, the individuals charged with filing reports in paper-based records can do so simply by looking at the source and date of the report. However, the users of information filed in this type of record have more trouble. To follow or document information on the patient's course of treatment, they must search by date of occurrence in each of the sections (that is, laboratory, radiology, and every group of clinical notes). The more departments a hospital has, the more sections the source-oriented health record can have. It is left to the end user to tie together information from the various sections of the record to get a full picture of the patient's course of treatment.

Specialist: A physician who offers specialized treatment in **ambulatory care**. **Specialists** include physicians offering services in family medicine, internal medicine, obstetrics, gynecology, cardiology, gastroenterology, ophthalmology, and dermatology.

Standards: Preestablished, written criteria. Standards describe minimum performance levels and include specific guidelines to ensure the safety of patients and achieve quality of medical care.

Standards development organizations (SDOs): Groups that design scientifically based models against which structures, processes, and **outcomes** can be measured. The American National Standards Institute (ANSI) coordinates the development of **standards** in the United States. The United Nations International Standards Organization (ISO) coordinates international standards development efforts.

State Operations Manual: Interpretive guidelines published by the **Centers for Medicare and Medicaid Services (CMS)**.

Statute: A piece of legislation written and approved by a state or federal legislature and then signed into law by the state's governor or the president.

Statute of limitations: A law that dictates the maximum period of time that may elapse between an event (for example, an injury or a crime) and any consequent legal action. In most states, the statute of limitations requires legal action in less than ten years. Therefore, in the absence of other state retention guidelines, hospitals and other healthcare providers may decide to maintain **health records** for a minimum of ten years.

Structure and content standards: Uniform methods for collecting, maintaining, and/or transferring healthcare **data** among computer information systems. Structure and content standards are one of five categories of **health informatics standards**. The other categories include **vocabulary standards**, **transaction and messaging standards**, **security standards**, and **identifier standards**. Work completed to develop and establish health informatics standards ensures the successful implementation of electronic **health record** systems. Many organizations are currently working on the development of health informatics standards. Compliance with such industry standards continues to be voluntary.

Subacute care: The professional nursing care and related medical, therapeutic, psychosocial, and personal services provided in a residential setting to individuals recovering from injuries or illnesses or the residual effects of injuries or illnesses after the acute phase of the condition has resolved; sometimes called **skilled-nursing care**.

Subpoena: A direct command that requires an individual or a representative of an organization to appear in court and/or to present an object to the court.

Subpoena duces tecum: A direct command that requires an individual or a representative of an organization to appear in court and/or to present an object to the court. In the healthcare context, subpoena duces tecum directs a hospital's representative (usually the director of health information management) to submit a specific **health record** or other business record to the court that holds jurisdiction over the pending proceedings.

Substance Abuse and Mental Health Services Administration (SAMHSA): A federal agency of the Department of Health and Human Services, established to focus on assessing and improving the lives of individuals with or at risk for mental illness and/or substance abuse disorders. SAMHSA offers public programs and funding to provide treatment, prevention efforts, and rehabilitation services for substance abuse and mental illness. In 2004, SAMHSA issued a document titled "The Confidentiality of Alcohol and Drug Abuse Patient Records Regulation and the HIPAA Privacy Rule: Implications for Alcohol and Substance Abuse Programs." The document outlines the principle preemptive aspects of 42 CFR 2 over the HIPAA **Privacy** Rule. It provides helpful information to substance abuse healthcare providers and recipients of substance abuse patient information from substance abuse providers. Additionally, SAMHSA provides grants for various programs. These grants are highly dependent upon providing quality documentation. Information is available online from www.samhsa.gov.

Surgical specialties: Medical specialties that include the following: Obstetrics/gynecology, Ophthalmology, Orthopedics, Cardiovascular surgery, Otorhinolaryngology, Trauma surgery, Neurosurgery, Thoracic surgery, Urology, Plastic and reconstructive surgery, Anesthesiology, and Pathology.

Systematized Nomenclature of Medicine–Clinical Terms® (SNOMED CT®): A standardized, controlled medical vocabulary that provides a common language for indexing, storing, retrieving, and aggregating clinical **data** across specialties and healthcare providers. The National Library of Medicine purchased a license for SNOMED CT that allows its free use in the United States. This purchase is intended to accelerate the adoption and interoperability of EHR systems. The **National Committee on Vital and Health Statistics (NCVHS)** supports the adoption of SNOMED CT as the standard for nonlaboratory interventions and **procedures**, laboratory test results, anatomical locations, diagnoses, **problem list**s, and nursing care. The adoption of SNOMED CT supports the inevitable transition from paper and mixed media to electronic **health record** systems.

Tax Equity and Fiscal Responsibility Act of 1982 (TEFRA): **Medicare** coverage for **hospice care** began with enactment of section 122 of public law 97–248, the **Tax Equity and Fiscal Responsibility Act of 1982 (TEFRA)**. The *Code of Federal Regulations* defines the Medicare hospice benefit and documentation requirements. Interpretive guidelines provide additional guidance on required documentation.

Technical standards: Standards that provide the rules, often called **protocols**, for how **data** are actually transmitted from one computer system to another. Technical standards are the next step in making interoperability possible. For **health record** systems to function beyond one healthcare facility, several types of health information system (HIS) standards must be established and followed. Technical standards complement **structure and content, functionality,** and **vocabulary standards.**

Telephone encounter: Telephone conversations between patient and healthcare providers. From a **risk management** perspective as well as a patient-care perspective, it is critical to document any advice (instructions, prescriptions, orders, medication changes, and such) or patient follow-up that is communicated by telephone. Documentation should include the date and time of the call, the caller's name and telephone number, the patient's name and identifying information, reason for the call, the date and time of the response (or attempts to return the call), the response given, and the signature of the person returning the call. Because messages may be relayed among several people, a standard **telephone encounter** form should be used to document all information regarding phone calls with every patient.

Tertiary care: Care centered on the provision of highly specialized and technologically advanced diagnostic and therapeutic services in **inpatient** and **outpatient** hospital settings. Medical **specialists** working in large, urban hospitals and specialty clinics affiliated with nearby medical schools and universities provide most tertiary care. Tertiary-care services include medical–surgical services such as trauma care; burn care; organ transplantation; and medical–surgical intensive care for neonatal, pediatric, and adult patients. In addition, tertiary-care hospitals perform medical **research** and conduct resident-training programs for physicians and other healthcare practitioners.

Tethered record: Sometimes called a **personal health record (PHR)**, it is a subset of information compiled by the healthcare provider and offered to the customer, often through the healthcare provider's Web site. A tethered record functions as a customer's view into the provider's electronic record. Some providers offer consumers the opportunity to build and maintain their PHRs through the providers' Web sites. Like untethered PHRs, tethered records offer customers the benefit of two-way sharing of health information between themselves and their healthcare provider. Unlike an **untethered record**, the content of the PHR is controlled, to a certain extent, by the provider.

Third-party payers: Entities that reimburse healthcare organizations for care provided to their beneficiaries. Third-party payers require that professional services be provided under a plan of care that a physician has established. The appropriateness and quality of care provided to customers is the focus. Many third-party payers will only reimburse for conditions of an acute nature. Third-party payers review the quality of care their members receive, have a legitimate interest in the contents of **health records**, and like **Medicare**, often review copies of health record documentation for information on services provided to their beneficiaries. Diagnostic and **procedural codes** are used for determining **reimbursement** to healthcare facilities. Some third-party payers require billers to submit copies of portions of the health record along with the claims. Additionally, some third-party payers cannot be billed unless signed orders are present. The health record documentation substantiates the need for services and the fact that such services were provided. Therefore, complete documentation of the **medical necessity** and length of services is particularly important.

Tracer methodology: A procedure used by **Joint Commission** surveyors in the **accreditation** process. The tracer method incorporates the priority focus procedure, follows the experience of care through the organization's entire healthcare process, and allows the surveyor to identify performance issues. Surveyors may perform two different types of tracers: **individual tracer activity** or **individual-based system tracer activity**. Individual tracer activity permits the evaluation of the care experience of a specific patient while in the hospital. This method analyzes a hospital's system of providing care, treatment, and services used as the framework for assessing **standards** of compliance. The individual-based system tracer activity explores a specific system or process across the organization. The surveyor evaluates the integration of related processes, coordination, and communication among disciplines and departments during the individual-based system tracer. **Data** use, infection control, and medical management are key components evaluated during the individual-based system tracer activity.

Transaction and messaging standards: Uniform methods for collecting, maintaining, and/or transferring healthcare **data** among computer information systems. Transaction and messaging standards are one of five categories of **health informatics standards**. The other categories include **vocabulary standards**, **structure and content standards**, **security standards**, and **identifier standard**s. Work completed to develop and establish health informatics standards ensures the successful implementation of electronic **health record** systems. Many organizations are currently working on the development of health informatics standards. Compliance with such industry standards continues to be voluntary.

Transcriptionist: Specially trained typists who understand medical terminology. Before the widespread use of computer technology in healthcare, all of the information in healthcare records was collected and stored in paper format. Each record was a compilation of handwritten **progress notes**, paper forms, photographs, graphic tracings, and typewritten reports. Many of the typewritten reports of medical findings and operative **procedures** were originally dictated by physicians and surgeons and subsequently converted into written format by medical **transcriptionists**.

Transfusion record: Information on the type and amount of blood products a patient receives, the source of the blood products, and the patient's reaction to the transfusion. The record also documents the blood group and Rh status of the patient and the donor, the results of cross-matching tests, and a description of the transfusion process. Every adverse reaction to a transfusion must be fully documented in the patient's **health record**.

Unannounced survey: The **Joint Commission** defines an unannounced survey as one in which an accredited organization will receive *no notice*. The Joint Commission transitioned to an unannounced survey process for hospitals in 2006. This was a significant change from the triennial **accreditation** and survey process. The change to unannounced surveys has caused hospitals to move toward a continuous ongoing performance improvement process that supports reversing (internet-only manuals) IOM findings of medical error and death. This redesign of the accreditation process more accurately measures efforts toward quality care delivery and patient safety.

Uniform Ambulatory Care Data Set (UACDS): A **data** set commonly used in hospitals. Other **data sets** used today include the **Uniform Hospital Discharge Data Set (UHDDS)**, **Data Elements for Emergency Department Systems (DEEDS)**, the **Essential Medical Data Set (EMEDS)**, and the **Health Plan Employer Data and Information Set (HEDIS)**.

Uniform Hospital Discharge Data Set (UHDDS): A **data** set commonly used in hospitals. Other **data sets** used today include the **Data Elements for Emergency Department Systems (DEEDS)**, the **Essential Medical Data Set (EMEDS)**, the **Health Plan Employer Data and Information Set (HEDIS)**, and the **Uniform Ambulatory Care Data Set (UACDS)**.

Unique identifier: A method of identifying a patient in the healthcare setting. Social Security numbers are often used to help positively identify patients because they are one type of unique identifier that represents one and only one individual. Hospitals assign unique identifiers to individual **health records** to make sure information in the records is easily retrievable and not misplaced or lost. Due to the growing issue of identity theft, the collection and use of Social Security numbers as a unique identifier is controversial. Healthcare providers are finding alternative solutions to uniquely identify their customers.

Unique personal identifier: A means of securely logging on to an electronic records system. The logon procedure is accomplished through an **authentication** process. Some systems require a code or password. Other systems may require another form of unique personal identifier such as an **electronic signature** or a **biometric identifier**, for example, a fingerprint or retinal scan. Authentication identifies the user and protects the security of the system. Each personal identifier must be assigned exclusively to a specific clinician, and a master list of the electronic identifiers must be maintained in a secure environment. This is the responsibility of the HIM professional.

Untethered record: A **personal health record (PHR)** that is maintained by the customer. It is the customer's compilation of his or her health information from one or more healthcare providers, past and present. Untethered PHRs offer customers the benefit of two-way sharing of health information between themselves and their healthcare providers. The content of an untethered PHR is completely controlled by the customer.

Urgent Care Association of America (UCAOA): Association that works to promote urgent care in the United States through bylaws and **standards**.

Urgent-care centers: A facility that is designed to evaluate and treat conditions that are not severe enough to require treatment in a hospital emergency department but still require treatment beyond normal physician office hours or before a physician's appointment is available. The **Urgent Care Association of America (UCAOA)** estimates that more than 15,000 urgent-care centers deliver urgent care in the United States.

Utilization management (UM): A process that focuses on how healthcare organizations use their resources. Hospital utilization management programs ensure that customers receive appropriate levels of services and that the services are performed in an efficient and cost-effective way. State and federal government **regulations** require hospitals to conduct utilization management reviews. Most commercial health insurance plans conduct their own UM reviews for both **inpatient** and **outpatient** services. **Health record** information is used as the basis for utilization management review of a healthcare organization's resources.

Utilization review (UR): A formal process conducted to determine the **medical necessity** of the services provided to, or planned for, an individual patient.

Visit note: Documentation in the **health record**, which is often authored by more than one healthcare provider. For example, a nurse or alternate user can begin a patient's encounter note, and later, the examining physician can add comments. Visit notes are also called **encounter notes**.

Vital statistics: Data on births, deaths, fetal deaths, marriages, and divorce. Responsibility for the collection of vital statistics rests with the states. The states share information with the **National Center for Health Statistics (NCHS)**. The state serves as the official repository for birth and death certificates and provides vital statistics information to the NCHS. From the vital statistics collected, states and the national government develop a variety of **databases**.

Vocabulary standards: Uniform methods for collecting, maintaining, and/or transferring healthcare **data** among computer information systems. Vocabulary standards are one of five categories of **health informatics standards**. The other categories include **structure and con-**

tent standards, transaction and messaging standards, security standards, and **identifier standards**. Work completed to develop and establish health informatics standards ensures the successful implementation of electronic **health record** systems. Many organizations are currently working on the development of health informatics standards. Compliance with such industry standards continues to be voluntary.

Warehousing: The processes and systems used to store and maintain **data** and data journals. According to AHIMA's Data Quality Management Model, warehousing is one of the four key processes for data. The other key processes are **collection, analysis,** and **application.**

Working documents: Administrative information not considered part of the **health record,** such as abbreviation and prohibitive abbreviation lists, audit trails related to the **electronic health record (EHR)**, authorization forms for release of information, birth and death certificate worksheets, correspondence concerning requests for records, **databases** containing patient **data**, event history and audit trails, financial and insurance forms, **incident** or patient safety reports, **indexes** (disease, operation, death), institutional review board lists, logs, **notice of privacy practices** acknowledgments (unless the organization chooses to classify them as part of the health record), patient-identifiable claims, patient-identifiable data reviewed for quality assurance or **utilization management, protocols** and **clinical pathways**, practice guidelines and other knowledge sources that do not imbed patient data, psychotherapy notes, registries, staff roles and access rights, and work lists and works in progress.

World Health Organization (WHO): The United Nations' agency that oversees global health initiatives. International health **regulations** require **incidence** reporting from participating nations so that WHO can track potential worldwide epidemics. The SARS epidemic that spread from China to Europe, Canada, and the United States in 2003 is an example of how quickly communicable diseases can be carried from continent to continent via international transportation systems.

Index

517